Biochemistry and Oral Biology
Second edition

We shall not cease from exploration
And the end of all our exploring
Will be to arrive where we started
And know the place for the first time
> from *Little Gidding*, in *Four Quartets* by T. S. Eliot

This we know. All things are connected like the blood which
unites one family. All things are connected.
Whatever befalls the earth befalls the sons of the earth. Man
did not weave the web of life; he is merely a strand in it.
Whatever he does to the web, he does to himself.
> From Chief Seattle's letter to
> the Great White Chief in Washington
> in 1854 in reply to an offer for
> a large area of Indian land.

Biochemistry and Oral Biology

Second edition

A. S. Cole, B.Sc., Ph.D.,
Senior Lecturer in Biochemistry (retired), University of Bristol

J. E. Eastoe, D.Sc., Ph.D., F.D.S.R.C.S., D.I.C.A.R.C.S.,
Professor of Oral Biology, University of Newcastle upon Tyne

with contributions by
John McGivan, M.A., Ph.D.
M. L. Hayes, B.D.S., M.Sc., Ph.D.,
A. C. Smillie, M.D.S., Ph.D.

WRIGHT

London   Boston   Singapore   Sydney   Toronto   Wellington

Wright

is an imprint of Butterworth Scientific.

First edition published by John Wright, Bristol, 1977
Reprinted, 1978, 1979, 1980, 1983
Second edition, 1988

Butterworth International Edition, 1988
ISBN 0 7236 1751 1

British Library Cataloguing in Publication Data

Cole, A. S.
  Biochemistry and oral biology—2nd ed.
  1. Biochemistry—For dentistry
  I. Title   II. Eastoe, J. E. (John Eric)
  574.19′2′0246176

  ISNB 0-7236-0834-2

Library of Congress Cataloging in Publication Data

Cole, Anne S.
  Biochemistry and oral biology/A. S. Cole and J. E. Eastoe;
  with contributions by M. L. Hayes and A. C. Smillie—2nd ed.
  p.   cm.
  Bibliography: p.
  Includes index.
  ISBN 0-7236-0834-2
  1. Biochemistry.   2. Mouth.   3. Dental chemistry.
  I. Eastoe, John E.   II. Hayes, M. L.   III. Smillie, A. C.
  IV. Title.
  QP514.2.C64   1988
  612′.015′0246176—dc 19

Typeset by EJS Chemical Composition, Midsomer Norton, Bath
Printed and bound in Great Britain by Anchor Brendon Ltd, Tiptree, Essex

Foreword

Professor G. N. Jenkins

Department of Oral Physiology, Dental School, Newcastle upon Tyne

Textbooks in pre-clinical subjects for dental students have always presented a problem. Very few books in physiology and biochemistry have been written specifically for dental students. This has meant that they have had to use texts designed for medical or science students containing more detail on many topics while omitting altogether or discussing superficially subjects of outstanding dental importance. Although a number of books are now available covering these dentally orientated topics the present book by Anne Cole and John Eastoe, and other contributors, is, I believe, the first work covering both the general and the dental aspects of a pre-clinical subject and will be warmly welcomed on that account. I am particularly pleased to note that prominence has been given to nutrition, a subject clearly of outstanding importance to all humanity yet frequently neglected in medical and dental courses. This subject, bristling with challenging intellectual and practical problems, has inexplicably become the Cinderella of biochemistry. The unique combination of a modern exposition of biochemistry at a level eminently suitable for dental students, linked with nutrition and with the fascinating but highly controversial questions of dental biochemistry will, I am sure, be a very valuable addition to the dental literature. I congratulate the authors on their book and wish it every success.

November 1976

Preface to the second edition

It is eleven years since the appearance of the first edition of *Biochemistry and Oral Biology* during which time there have been many notable advances not only in biochemistry and molecular biology but also in dental science. This has meant that large parts of the book have had to be rewritten or extensively revised. The text follows the same general pattern as the first edition but some of the material has been rearranged and a completely new chapter 'The prevention of plaque-induced diseases' has been added. The team of authors has been strengthened by the inclusion of John McGivan who is responsible for Chapter 16 (Bioenergetics) and for rewriting the chapters on the control of metabolism. He also revised the chapters on enzymes and amino acid metabolism. The updating of other parts of the book would have been impossible without the help of various friends and former colleagues mostly in the Department of Biochemistry at Bristol. The chapters on nucleic acids and protein synthesis have been rewritten and that on mutations, evolution and inherited disease revised by Dr L. Hall. Invaluable help with other sections of the book was given as follows: Chapter 1 – Dr W. Walder, Chapter 15 – Dr M. J. A. Tanner, Chapters 17 and 18 – Dr T. Hopkirk, Chapter 25 – Dr M. Luscombe. Dr H. C. Watson provided the computerized diagrams from which Figures 5.5 and 5.6 were drawn and Dr Hilary Muirhead those for Figures 5.7c and d. Dr E. H. Batten provided Figure 26.1. Others whose help is gratefully acknowledged are Professor O. T. G. Jones and Dr J. Williams. Finally we would like to thank Mrs Brenda Fowler, Mrs Rosemary Musgrave and Miss Karen Short for help with the typing.

A.S.C. and J.E.E.
May, 1988

Note I would like to record the fact that owing to increased pressure of administrative work, the editing of the greater part of this second edition (other than the chapters for which I was originally responsible) was undertaken by Anne Cole during her retirement.

J.E.E.

Preface to the first edition

While many books cater for the biochemical needs of science and medical students, no modern introductory biochemistry text appears to be available that meets the specific requirements of those whose main interest is dentistry. We feel that there is a need for a book which, while explaining the basic principles of biochemistry, also includes topics that are of specifically dental interest. Also relevant are subjects, such as nutrition, that were once considered as areas of 'physiological chemistry' but which now, despite their importance, tend to be neglected as far as basic science courses for dentists and doctors are concerned.

The plan of our book proceeds from the structural basis of biochemistry, via metabolism and its control towards an increasing degree of specialization on dental topics – soft tissues, hard tissues and the biology of the mouth. Thus, after a preliminary look at the aims of biochemistry, some basic chemical facts and the role of water, comes Section 2 on Molecular Architecture. Section 3, concerning Nutrition, includes a discussion of fluoride, giving the main facts on which arguments for or against a policy of water fluoridation are based. Section 4, Molecular Organization and Interactions, starts with Chapters on general principles of metabolism and the biochemical organization of the cell and ends with an outline of biochemical individuality and the molecular basis of inherited disease. The last subject is rarely dealt with in textbooks of biochemistry, though it is of obvious importance to clinicians.

Once the basic metabolic pathways have been considered, the book continues with Section 5, Control Processes, which covers regulatory mechanisms operating within the cell and also the hormones responsible for integrating the body's various component systems. Section 6 on Soft Tissues contains chapters on body fluids, epithelium and connective tissue and deals with areas rarely covered in detail in textbooks of biochemistry.

The two final sections are specifically concerned with aspects of Oral Biology. Section 7 on the Calcified Tissues, which includes chapters on calcium and phosphorus metabolism, biological apatite, mineralized tissues and the mineralization process, helps to bridge the gap between chemistry and dental histology. Finally in Section 8, Biology of the Mouth, consideration is given to biochemical aspects of saliva, the oral flora and the formation and properties of dental plaque. A chapter on plaque diseases completes this survey of dental biochemistry.

Throughout the book we have tried to avoid undue detail and excessive numbers of formulae and equations, and also to show how biochemistry is relevant not only to dentistry but also to many wider aspects of life today.

In most instances SI units are used, although, when dealing with energy, at this time of transition it was thought helpful to give values in both joules and calories. For very small measurements of length, nanometres are nearly always used despite the fact that X-ray crystallographers understandably continue to prefer Ångströms. The one instance where we have intentionally used units other than SI is for pressure. It seems to us that millimetres of mercury are, for most people, a more meaningful method of expression than pascals. For concentrations of material we have sometimes preferred mg or g per 100 ml to molar concentrations. This is either a matter of common usage, as with blood glucose concentrations, or because the exact composition of such mixtures as plasma proteins is unknown. A table of units is given on page ix.

January, 1977   A.S.C. AND J.E.E.

Contents

Units

Table of units used

Physical quantity	Unit	Symbol
Volume	litre	l
Length	metre	m
	ångström	Å* ($1\,Å = 0{\cdot}1\,nm$)
Mass	gram	g
Time	second	s
Energy	joule	J
	calorie	cal*
Pressure	millimetres of mercury	mmHg*

* Not SI units.

Prefixes for multiples and submultiples of units

Multiple	Prefix	Symbol
10^6	mega	M
10^3	kilo	k
10^{-3}	milli	m
10^{-6}	micro	μ
10^{-9}	nano	n
10^{-12}	pico	p

Amounts and concentrations

Amounts of material are usually expressed as *moles* which are equivalent to the molecular (or atomic) weight of the substance in grams.

Concentrations are expressed in terms of molarity, i.e. the number of moles present in 1 litre of the solution or $g\,(mg)\,l^{-1}$ (decilitres).

Section 1

Some preliminary considerations

Chapter 1
Introduction

The scope of biochemistry

The aims of biochemistry are to describe the nature of living forms and living processes in terms of chemistry and physics. Biochemists believe that the existence and activities of living organisms can be explained on the basis of the interaction of their component molecules. These may be divided very broadly into two groups, namely *small molecules* and *macromolecules*.

The main types of macromolecule are proteins, nucleic acids and polysaccharides, all of which are long, chain-like molecules built up from a large number of linked subunits. These *bio-polymers* tend to associate into still larger complexes with other molecules which may or may not be of the same type. The small molecules act not only as the building units from which macro-molecules are synthesized but also as sources of energy, messengers and regulators. Macro-molecules are the essential basis of the elaborate structures in and around which the life processes occur; they also control and regulate these processes. Thus macromolecules are responsible for the energy exchanges and chemical reactions that comprise *metabolism*, for the *irritability* which enables the organism to respond to changes in its environment, for *mobility* and for *reproduction*.

Since molecules do not function alone but by interaction with other molecules, living processes require specific arrangements of molecules and 'life' resolves itself into a question of molecular organization.

This organization is based on certain general principles, e.g.:

1. That biological molecules have been 'selected' for specific functions.
2. That biological events always tend to happen in a manner that will lead to an overall decrease in free energy.
3. That biological systems are open, dynamic and self-ordering.

In the higher forms of life biological organization falls into a series of levels arranged in a discontinuous order. At each level there appear to be units of a fairly definite size which become associated to form a unit at the next level, and as each successive level of organization is achieved new properties emerge. The levels may be listed as follows:

(*a*) Small molecules
(*b*) Macromolecules

(*c*) Subcellular structures
(*d*) Cells
(*e*) Tissues
(*f*) Organs
(*g*) Organisms
(*h*) Societies.

For the most part, biochemical studies are concentrated at the levels of molecules, subcellular structures and cells, but, in order to explain 'life' in chemical and physicochemical terms every level of organization must be studied and it is where discontinuities exist that the most challenging problems occur. For example, how do cells differentiate? What makes cells of the same and different types associate to form tissues? Why do cells, organs and organisms grow to a certain size and then stop growing? Why are partially constructed subcellular components, e.g. mitochondria, membranes, cilia etc., never seen within cells? Such structures are either present in their completed form or not present at all. This suggests that assembly of the components into the single appropriate configuration depends on the existence of a precise set of conditions under which they fall into their proper place in the right numbers and orientation for the assembly of the complete structure.

Biological organization therefore seems to require the provision of a suitable environment where the individual molecules can interact in such a way that they become specifically orientated. The mitotic spindle is formed in just this way since it appears spontaneously in response to a set of critically determined environmental conditions. Another example is seen in the formation of collagen fibres, where a self-ordered fabric is produced by the mutual interaction of collagen molecules (Chapter 27). Furthermore molecular organization depends on appropriate *molecular architecture* since, for molecules to interact, they must be suitably designed. In fact, natural selection has ensured that biological macromolecules are uniquely fitted for their functional role. The simplest function of a macromolecule is perhaps the storage of energy. A substance which fulfils this role in the animal world is glycogen, a biopolymer of glucose. To serve its purpose the structure of glycogen does not need to be very precisely defined provided that it can be degraded rapidly when extra energy is required. It is significant, therefore, that the molecular weight of glycogen is variable and that it possesses a highly branched structure, which means that the molecule is vulnerable to enzymic attack at many points simultaneously (Figure 7.2).

Proteins, the most ubiquitous of the biological macromolecules, perform an enormous variety of functions, and have structures which are not only complicated but also highly specific. They are composed of a large but definite number of *amino acid* units selected from twenty or so different types joined together in a specific sequence. Although the protein molecules are linear and unbranched the properties of their amino acid side chains are such that highly specific interactions occur. These take place between different protein molecules so that they are able to associate to form sheets and bundles and also between different parts of the same molecule so that it may assume an elaborately folded configuration. As a consequence, protein molecules have well-defined geometrical shapes, and as a result of ionization effects they also have characteristic patterns of electric charge. Such patterns are believed to play an important part in their interaction with other molecules.

Proteins fulfil both structural and metabolic functions within the organism. The requirements for *structural proteins* are that they should be insoluble, chemically stable and possess a rigid structure capable of orientation. The long chain-like molecules of structural proteins are usually only slightly folded and have specific bonding sites so that the molecules can join together both in series and in parallel to form molecular aggregations with great tensile strength and varying elasticity. Muscle proteins are able to slide over one another so that the fibres can shorten or lengthen in response to appropriate stimuli.

Even more complex and varied in their structure and functions are the enzymic proteins which are designed for the accomplishment of molecular changes. To achieve these they must have structures that are closely related to those of the molecules with which they interact. Here, where very delicate mechanisms are involved, large stable aggregations of protein molecules are not appropriate, but the association of a small number of subunits may give the molecule flexibility and enable it to react to its environment.

Molecular biology defines the area where structure and function meet since it includes the enzymic, aggregational or genetic information which macromolecules contain by virtue of their structure. It is in the preservation of genetic information that the *nucleic acids* come into the picture since it is they that carry the coded information which ensures the supply of specifically designed macromolecules needed for the organization of subcellular structures, cells, tissues, organs and organisms which enable cells to replicate.

Biochemistry in relation to dentistry

The aims, attitudes and techniques of biochemistry are as relevant to dentistry as to medicine or any other aspect of biology. Only when the normal structures of the mouth and their development and reactions are understood is it possible to appreciate the true nature of dental disease. All disease has a biochemical basis regardless of whether its origin is nutritional or genetic or it is caused by an infectious or toxic agent.

Normal tooth development and dental health require that the body shall be well nourished, so that dentists need a knowledge of nutrition in order that they may give their patients appropriate dietary advice. Exposure of the teeth to bacteria is inevitable and the degree of colonization of the tooth surface, the types of bacteria present and their effects on the teeth all depend on their biochemical environment. Whether or not the bacterial colonization of the surfaces of the teeth is damaging to them and to their supporting tissues is largely determined by the environmental changes brought about by bacterial metabolism and the effect of the diet, including the 585 000 tons of sweets consumed each year. The products of bacterial metabolism act by changing the physicochemical factors which influence the solubility of various calcium phosphates at the tooth surface. Increased solubility of the calcium phosphate component of the teeth results in the demineralization characteristic of *dental caries*. Decreased solubility of various calcium phosphates deposited from saliva causes calculus formation, which in turn may lead to *periodontal disease*, the main cause of tooth loss in older subjects. For this reason dentists must be aware of the physicochemical factors that operate in the mouth and how these affect the solubility of calcium phosphates. Not only this, but the fact that tooth extraction leaves an empty bony socket which needs to be filled, while orthodontic procedures involve the movement of one calcium phosphate structure (the tooth) through another calcified structure (the bone) show that an understanding of the physiological processes underlying the resorption and deposition of bone mineral and its matrix is essential. Other areas of biochemistry which are of special relevance to dentists are blood clotting and the effects of drugs and other injected materials on cells.

As for the future, methods to prevent or cure tooth decay are likely to involve a biochemical approach. The role of fluoride is now well established, and means of remineralizing a carious lesion or chemically modifying the tooth, the enamel surface and its bacterial population offer scope for further investigation.

Biological principles and current concerns

Many of the technological problems that have confronted, and still confront, mankind have as regards their basic principles been solved by Nature in the course of evolution. The scales may be different but the problems are essentially the same and many instances can be cited where men have arrived at solutions based on principles that have subsequently been found to have been operating in Nature for thousands of years. Examples range from principles of molecular design, e.g. ropes, sheets, extensible springs, templates, ion-exchange materials, to ball and socket joints, assembly lines, feedback controls, amplification devices and computers.* Biological principles might, with advantage, be used to find solutions to some of our present ecological and other problems. What better example could there be of the efficient use of resources than the human body? Economists and politicians should accept the need for steady state conditions for prolonged survival and realize that nothing can grow indefinitely. Natural systems make it clear that, in the long run 'nothing fails like excess'. Recycling, a process known since biology first became a serious study, is at last being considered as an answer to some of our resource and waste disposal problems. On the other hand a biological principle that few people have yet grasped is that for any organization there is an optimal size which, although it may not be, in the short term, the most cost-effective, is in the long term most likely to achieve its purpose. Such considerations provide an excellent reason for studying the principles of biology and biochemistry and might even enable us to become as successful at the level of societies and populations as at the lower levels of organization.

* A further amusing example is the 'tin opener' device used by the crow-blackbird or purple grackle, *Quiscalus purpureus*, to cut the shells of acorns in half in order to free the kernel. The device takes the form of a sharp downward-pointing projection from the horny roof of its mouth.

Chapter 2
From atoms to molecules

Before proceeding to the study of the macromolecules which characterize living organisms it may be helpful to give a brief review of the types of compound found in living systems.

Life is based on carbon compounds and is only possible on account of their variety and complexity. Since carbon atoms can form stable covalent bonds with other carbon atoms, chains and ring structures can be built up; also because carbon is tetravalent, branched as well as straight chain compounds are possible.

The parent substances for all other organic compounds are the *hydrocarbons* which contain hydrogen as the only other element besides carbon. Their molecules contain a number of carbon atoms linked to give either an open chain structure or a closed form containing one or more rings.

Open chain hydrocarbons

These may or may not be branched and may or may not contain double bonds.

Straight chain saturated hydrocarbons

Ethane   Propane   Butane

Long hydrophobic chains of this type containing from two to more than 20 carbon atoms are attached to a –COOH group to form the *saturated fatty acids* (page 100).

Branched chain saturated hydrocarbons

$$CH_3$$
$$\overset{|}{C}H-CH_3$$
$$\overset{/}{C}H_3$$

$$CH_3-CH_2$$
$$\overset{|}{C}H-CH_3$$
$$\overset{|}{C}H_3$$

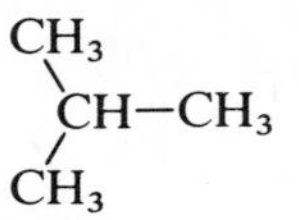

2-Methylpropane 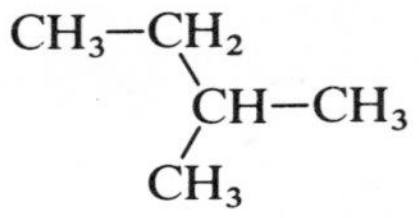   2-Methylbutane

The amino acids, *valine, leucine and isoleucine* (page 35) contain a branched hydrocarbon side chain.

Unsaturated hydrocarbons

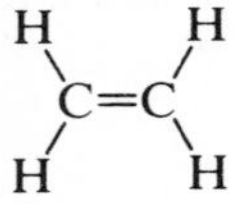

$$\underset{H}{\overset{H}{C}}=\underset{H}{\overset{H}{C}}$$

$$CH_3-CH=CH-CH_3$$

$$CH_3$$
$$\overset{|}{C}=CH-CH_3$$
$$\overset{|}{C}H_3$$

Ethene   But-2-ene   2-Methylbut-2-ene

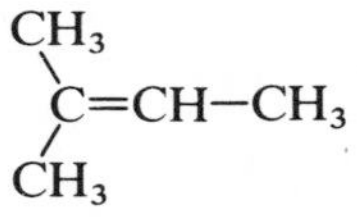

The unsaturated hydrocarbons are more reactive than the saturated and may add 2H to become saturated or water to give a hydroxy derivative. They may also be cleaved by oxidation at the double bond. The essential fatty acids are unsaturated (page 102).

Ring Compounds

Hydrocarbon ring compounds

Certain derivatives of ring hydrocarbons containing five or six carbon atoms and their unsaturated counterparts are biologically important.

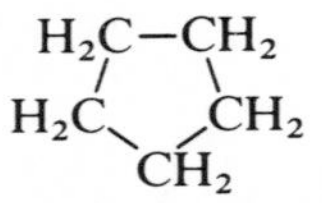

$$H_2C-CH_2$$
$$H_2C \qquad CH_2$$
$$CH_2$$

$$CH_2$$
$$H_2C \qquad CH_2$$
$$H_2C \qquad CH_2$$
$$CH_2$$

$$CH$$
$$HC \qquad CH$$
$$HC \qquad CH$$
$$CH$$

Cyclopentane 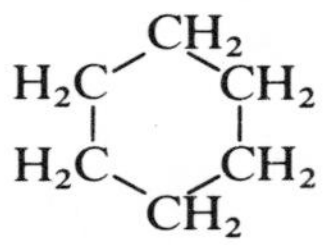   Cyclohexane 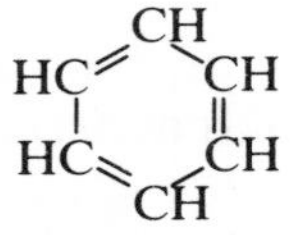   Benzene

Benzene, which contains alternate resonating double bonds, so that all the –C–C– bonds are equivalent, is the parent substance of the *aromatic series of compounds.*

As distinct from benzene and other ring systems which contain carbon as the only ring constituent are a number of *heterocyclic ring compounds* in which one or more of the carbons is replaced by an oxygen, nitrogen or sulphur atom. These too may be either saturated or unsaturated.

Oxygen-containing ring compounds

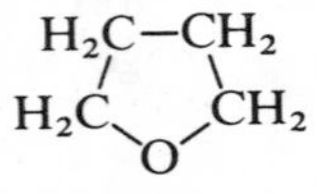

$$H_2C-CH_2$$
$$H_2C \qquad CH_2$$
$$O$$

$$HC-CH$$
$$HC \qquad CH$$
$$O$$

Tetrahydrofuran 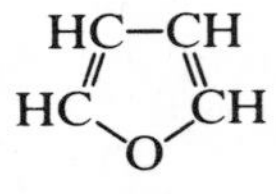   Furan

and also

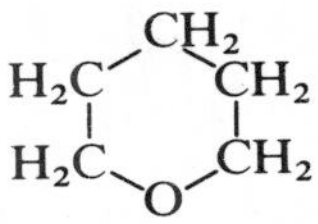

Tetrahydropyran 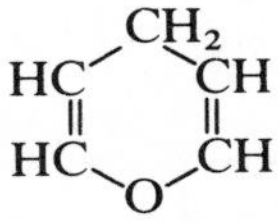   Pyran

Oxygen-containing ring structures of this type occur in the *carbohydrates*.

Nitrogen-containing ring compounds

These are found in the proteins and nucleic acids. The rings may be five- or six-membered and may contain one or two nitrogen atoms.

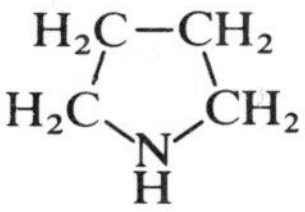

Pyrrolidine 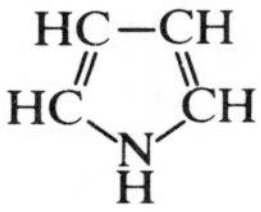   Pyrrole 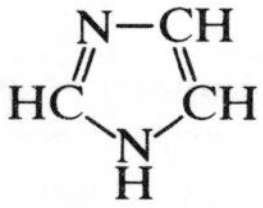   Imidazole

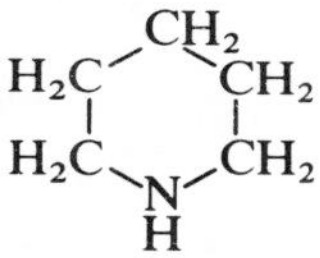

Piperidine 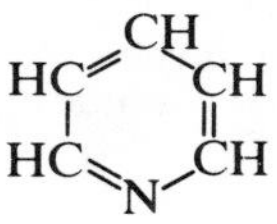   Pyridine 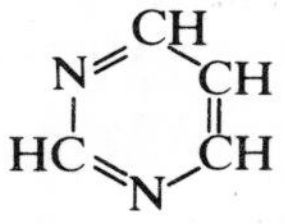   Pyrimidine

The imidazole ring occurs in the amino acid *histidine* (page 36) and the pyrrole ring in *haem* (page 371). Pyrimidine derivatives are found in the *nucleotides* and *nucleic acids*.

Fused ring systems

In addition to the simple ring systems described above, certain more complex systems consisting of two or more rings fused together are found in Nature. The steroids, which include the membrane constituent *cholesterol* as well as the *adrenocortical* and *sex hormones*, are derived from the sterane ring composed of three six-membered and one five-membered hydrocarbon rings containing 17 carbon atoms altogether.

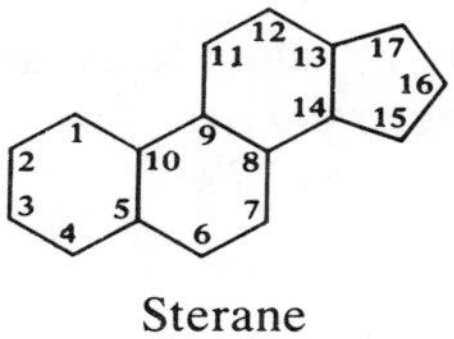

Sterane

Heterocyclic fused ring systems are found in a variety of biological compounds. The amino acid *tryptophan* (page 38) contains the indole nucleus, *adenine* and *guanine* (page 110) are purine derivatives and *riboflavin* (page 163) contains the alloxazine ring.

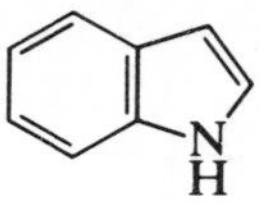

Indole
(1 benzene
+ 1 pyrrole)

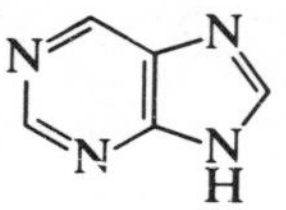

Purine
(1 pyrimidine
+ 1 imidazole)

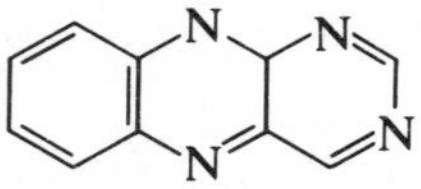

Alloxazine
(1 benzene + 1 pyrazine
+ 1 pyrimidine)

Functional groups

The hydrocarbons and heterocyclic ring compounds described above are rather inert and unreactive but they become more reactive if one or more of their hydrogens is substituted by other groupings, notably those containing oxygen or nitrogen. Biochemically speaking the most important of these functional groups are shown in Table 2.1.

Table 2.1 Some important functional groups

N containing	O containing	Carbonyl containing	S containing	P containing
$-NH_2$ (amino) $=NH$ (imino)	$-OH$ (hydroxyl) $=CO$ (carbonyl)	$-COOH$ (carboxylic) $-CONH_2$ (amide)	$-SH$ (sulphydryl) $-S-S-$ (disulphide) $-SO_3H$ (sulphonic acid)	$-PO_4H_2$ (singly esterified phosphate) $-PO_4H-$ (doubly esterified phosphate)

Hydroxyl groups

Compounds containing a hydroxyl group are known as *alcohols*. They are customarily referred to as primary, secondary and tertiary alcohols according to the number of hydrocarbon groups

$$R-CH_2OH$$

Primary

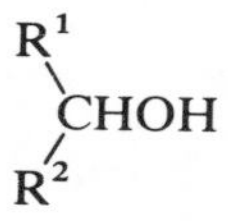

$$\overset{R^1}{\underset{R^2}{|}}CHOH$$

Secondary

$$R^2-\overset{R^1}{\underset{R^3}{|}}COH$$

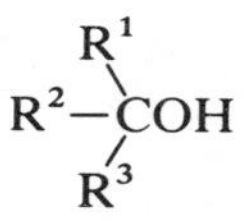

Tertiary

on the C atom which bears the hydroxyl group. Alcohols react with acids to form *esters* and two important classes of biological substance are compounds of this type, namely the triglycerides and the phosphoric acid esters.

Hydroxyl groups which are directly attached to an aromatic nucleus have rather different properties from aliphatic hydroxyl groups since they can act as proton donors and are therefore weakly acidic as in the case of *tyrosine* (page 37).

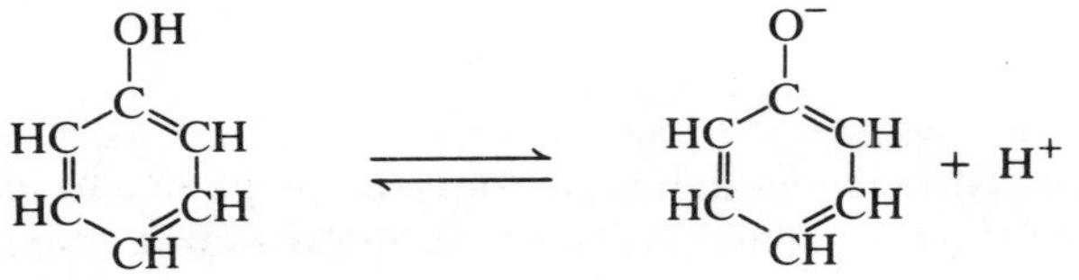

$+ H^+$

Phenolic substances also resemble the alcohols in their ability to react with acids to form esters.

Aldehydes and ketones

If alcohols are dehydrogenated they yield two types of compound, both of which contain the reactive carbonyl $-C=O$ group. Thus removal of 2H from a primary alcohol will yield an aldehyde:

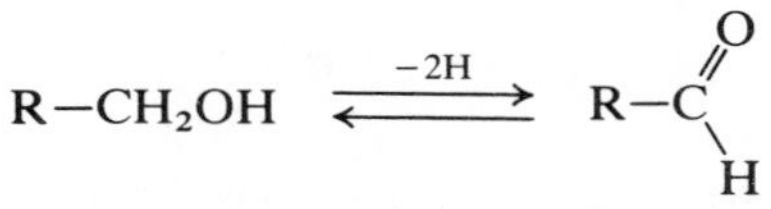

$$R-CH_2OH \xrightleftharpoons{-2H} R-C\overset{O}{\underset{H}{\diagdown}}$$

while removal of 2H from a secondary alcohol yields a ketone:

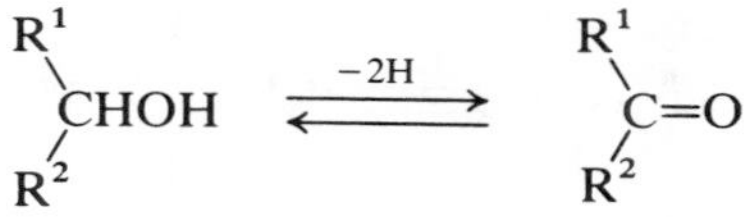

$$\underset{R^2}{\overset{R^1}{\diagup}}CHOH \xrightleftharpoons{-2H} \underset{R^2}{\overset{R^1}{\diagup}}C=O$$

Dehydrogenation reactions of this type frequently occur in metabolic processes and are readily reversible.

Aldehydes and ketones are tautomeric compounds and, as a result of a shift in the position of the double bond and of a hydrogen atom, may exist in either *keto* or *enol* forms.

Propionaldehyde
(propanal)

$$CH_3-CH_2-C\overset{O}{\underset{H}{\diagdown}} \rightleftharpoons CH_3-CH=C\overset{OH}{\underset{H}{\diagdown}}$$

Acetone
(propanone)

$$CH_3-CO-CH_3 \rightleftharpoons CH_3-C\underset{OH}{\overset{H}{=}}C\overset{H}{\underset{H}{\diagdown}}$$

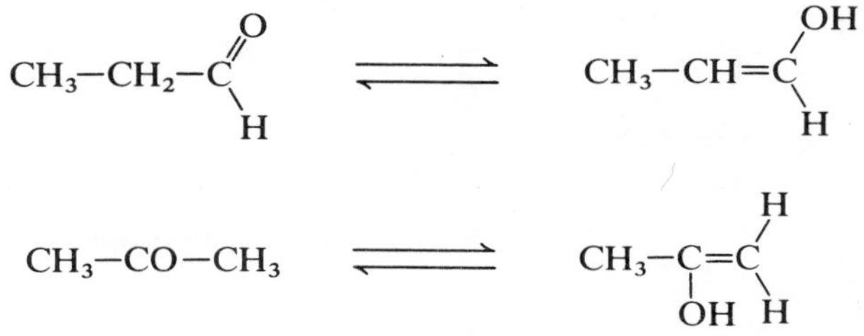

Keto form   Enol form

Acetone is formed in the body by the decarboxylation of acetoacetate when this is present in relatively large amounts in the condition of *ketosis* (page 262).

Instead of the addition of 2H to the carbonyl group of aldehydes and ketones, water may be introduced into the molecule to form hydrates that are unstable but that may be important intermediates in the formation of *carboxylic acids* by subsequent dehydrogenation.

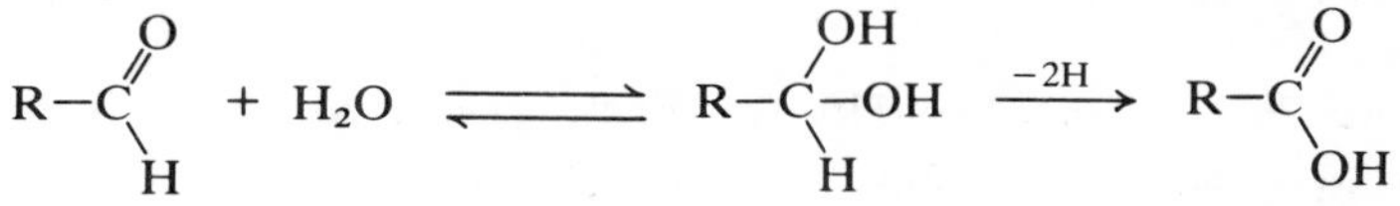

$$R-C\overset{O}{\underset{H}{\diagdown}} + H_2O \rightleftharpoons R-\underset{H}{\overset{OH}{C}}-OH \xrightarrow{-2H} R-C\overset{O}{\underset{OH}{\diagdown}}$$

Aldehyde   Aldehyde   Carboxylic
                         hydrate   acid

Oxidation reactions in the body are commonly performed in this manner, i.e. by the addition of water at a double bond followed by removal of 2H atoms.

Carboxylic acids

The carboxylic acid grouping ($-COOH$), as its name suggests, has acidic properties and dissociates in water to form H^+ and $-COO^-$ ions. Compounds containing a $-COOH$ group can therefore form salts and, in the physiological pH range, most of the organic acids exist in their salt forms, e.g. citrate, oxaloacetate, acetoacetate.

In the body the carboxylic acids can react with NH_3 and amines to form *acid amides*.

$$R^1COOH + R^2NH_2 \rightarrow R^1CONH_2 + R^2OH$$
Acid amide

Unlike the carboxylic acids, amides do not readily dissociate.

Asparagine and glutamine (page 37) are the acid amides of aspartic acid and glutamic acid.

Acetals and hemiacetals

In a reaction analogous to that with water, aldehydes will react with alcohols to form *hemiacetals* and *acetals*, which may be represented as follows:

| Aldehyde hydrate | Aldehyde | Hemiacetal | Acetal |

The sugars exist in ring structures in which the carbon atom of the potential aldehyde group bears the four substituents $-H$, $-OH$, $-R^1$ and $-OR^2$ so that their structure is essentially that of hemiacetals.

Furanose   Pyranose

Typical ring structures of sugars

Nitrogen-containing groups

These include amino and imino groups and quaternary ammonium bases, all of which may be regarded as derivatives of ammonia. There are several different types of amine according to the number of H atoms of the ammonia which have been replaced.

| Ammonia | Primary amine | Secondary amine | Tertiary amine |

The amines have basic properties and can bind protons, so becoming positively charged.

$$RNH_2 + H^+ \rightleftharpoons RNH_3^+$$

this reaction may be compared with the formation of ammonium ions

$$NH_3 + H^+ \rightleftharpoons NH_4^+$$

and amines can form salts of the type $RNH_3^+Cl^-$. Such reactions are used for buffering in the body.

Replacement of all four of the H atoms of an ammonium salt such as NH_4Cl with organic radicals yields a *quaternary ammonium salt*, which acts as a strong electrolyte and is completely ionized over a wide range of hydrogen ion concentrations. An example is choline (page 107).

$$\begin{array}{c} CH_3 \\ | \\ H_3C-\overset{+}{N}-CH_3 \quad Cl^- \\ | \\ CH_3 \end{array} \qquad \text{Tetramethyl ammonium chloride}$$

The free bases or hydroxides, e.g. $(CH_3)_4N \cdot OH$, of the quaternary ammonium ion also exist.

Dehydrogenation of a primary amine group converts it into an *imino* group which is unstable and hydrolyses spontaneously to yield an aldehyde (or ketone) and ammonia.

$$R-CH_2-NH_2 \xrightarrow{-2H} RCH=NH \xrightarrow{+H_2O} R-CHO + NH_3$$

Enzyme-catalysed dehydrogenations of this type occur frequently in metabolism.

Phosphate groups

Phosphoric acid and its derivatives have a special place in biochemistry, not only because inorganic phosphates are constituents of calcified tissues and the buffering systems of the body, but also because phosphoric acid is incorporated in many types of biologically important organic compound. Phosphate derivatives of sugars are essential metabolic intermediates, phosphate-containing lipids are components of membranes and phosphate-containing nucleotides are constituents of many coenzymes and building blocks for the construction of nucleic acids. Furthermore, changes in the activity of certain enzymes may be brought about by the reversible phosphorylation of specific amino acid residues.

Apart from calcium phosphates only two of the three possible types of inorganic orthophosphate occur under physiological conditions, e.g. NaH_2PO_4 and Na_2HPO_4. Similarly although three series of phosphoric esters are known, only mono- and di-esters occur in the body.

$$\begin{array}{cc} \begin{array}{c} OH \\ | \\ R^1O-P-OH \\ \| \\ O \end{array} & \begin{array}{c} OH \\ | \\ R^1O-P-OR^2 \\ \| \\ O \end{array} \\ \text{Monoester} & \text{Diester} \end{array}$$

Since phosphate esters are very reactive, relatively inert materials may be activated by esterification with phosphate.

Of even greater significance than the monophosphoric esters are the di- and tri-phosphates which contain two or three phosphate groupings linked together.

$$\begin{array}{ccc} \begin{array}{c} OH \\ | \\ R-O-P-OH \\ \| \\ O \end{array} & \begin{array}{c} OH \quad OH \\ | \quad\quad | \\ R-O-P-O-P-OH \\ \| \quad\quad \| \\ O \quad\quad O \end{array} & \begin{array}{c} OH \quad OH \quad OH \\ | \quad\quad | \quad\quad | \\ R-O-P-O-P-O-P-OH \\ \| \quad\quad \| \quad\quad \| \\ O \quad\quad O \quad\quad O \end{array} \\ \text{Monophosphate} & \begin{array}{c}\text{Diphosphate}\\ \text{(or pyrophosphate)}\end{array} & \text{Triphosphate} \end{array}$$

The di- and tri-phosphates are even more reactive than the monophosphates and act as sources of energy in the body (Chapter 16).

Sulphur-containing groups

Small quantities of inorganic sulphate are found in the body, and sulphuric acid esters of polysaccharides are present notably in the connective tissues. Sulphur also occurs in sulphydryl and disulphide groupings. The sulphydryl group is weakly acidic and can ionize

$$R \cdot SH \rightarrow R \cdot S^- + H^+$$

Mild oxidation of sulphydryl compounds converts them into disulphides.

$$2R \cdot SH \rightarrow R \cdot S - S \cdot R$$

The disulphide linkage is covalent and compounds containing it are stable.

Chemical bonds

In order to understand the nature of living processes it is first necessary to consider the forces responsible for the atomic and strong molecular interactions involved. These occur at two levels, namely interactions that hold atoms together to form molecules and weak interactions that bind molecules together to form larger systems. Although all bonding between atoms and molecules is a result of attractive forces between electric charges there are several types of chemical bond. Broadly these may be divided into strong and weak bonds. Biochemically speaking the strong interatomic bonds are *covalent* while weak interatomic and intermolecular bonds are of several different types, notably *ionic bonds* and *hydrogen bonds*. Intermolecular bonds between covalent compounds are weak *Van der Waals' forces*. Bond formation is accompanied by the release of energy and conversely energy must be supplied in order to break bonds. The stronger the bond the greater the energy involved.

Covalent bonds

Strong covalent bonds, which are responsible for welding atoms together to form stable molecules, do not rupture spontaneously under physiological conditions, although they may be broken by the action of specific enzymes. Covalent bonding between two atoms results from the sharing of a pair of electrons so that their electron shells overlap. The electrons may be envisaged as a sort of 'negatively charged cement holding two positively charged nuclei together'. Thus a covalent bond is a strong short-range attraction between atoms and is of definite length dependent on the nature of the atoms involved.

In a normal covalent bond each atom provides one electron thus making up a shared pair:

$$A \cdot + \cdot B \rightarrow A : B$$

The dative bond

In some instances one atom donates both the electrons:

$$D : + E \rightarrow D : E$$

This is still a covalent bond but it is referred to as a *dative covalence* or *coordinate bond* and is indicated by an arrow pointing in the direction in which the electrons are donated, e.g.

$$D \rightarrow E$$

This type of bond is found in *metal complexes* and *chelates*. A metal chelate (Greek *chela*, a crab's pincer) is a special kind of metal complex in which donor groups coordinated to the metal are also covalently bound to each other.

$$M{\kern-0.4em\raise0.3ex\hbox{$\swarrow$}\atop\kern-0.4em\raise-0.3ex\hbox{$\nwarrow$}}{A \atop B}\qquad\qquad M{\kern-0.4em\raise0.3ex\hbox{$\swarrow$}\atop\kern-0.4em\raise-0.3ex\hbox{$\nwarrow$}}{\overset{|}{A} \atop B}$$

Metal complex   Metal chelate

In this way a closed ring compound is formed. In some cases one of the groups may be attached to the metal by a normal covalent bond and to the other by a dative bond, thus

$$M{\kern-0.4em\raise0.3ex\hbox{$\diagup$}\atop\kern-0.4em\raise-0.3ex\hbox{$\nwarrow$}}{\overset{|}{A} \atop B}$$

Chelates do not necessarily have properties which distinguish them from ordinary metal compounds, but in many cases the stability of the coordination compound is extremely high. Important examples of chelates are found in biological systems, e.g. the haem group of haemoglobin and the cytochromes. Ethylenediaminetetra-acetic acid (EDTA) forms chelates with calcium ions that are both soluble and very stable. This substance can therefore dissolve highly insoluble calcium phosphates in neutral solution and EDTA is sometimes used to demineralize bone and the hard tissues of teeth because it avoids damage to the organic matrices which may occur when acids are used.

If an atom is covalently bound to more than one other atom the angle between the covalent bonds is always the same for any particular pair of bonds, e.g.

$$-\overset{|}{\underset{|}{C}}-\overset{|}{\underset{|}{C}}-, \quad -\overset{|}{\underset{|}{C}}-O- \quad \text{or} \quad -\overset{|}{\underset{|}{C}}-H$$

The number of covalent bonds which an atom can form is small and definite and is known as its *valency*, but in addition atoms can form a variable number of weak bonds which break easily and spontaneously. Only when weak bonds are present in ordered groups and large numbers do they collectively have any long-term existence.

Carbon with its valency of four can only form covalent interatomic bonds. However, one carbon atom can join to another and each can form covalent bonds with further carbon atoms or with atoms of other elements, mainly hydrogen. In this way chains and ring structures may arise and large molecules be produced. However, the overall shape and often the function of large molecules, notably of protein molecules, are determined by weak interatomic linkages that occur both within individual molecules and/or with adjacent molecules.

Weak bonds and interactions

The ionic bonds, hydrogen bonds and Van der Waals' forces which constitute the main types of secondary bond differ from covalent bonds in a number of respects.

1. They are much weaker having only 1–10% of the strength of covalent bonds.

Energy released in the formation of bonds of different types

Covalent bonds	210–460 kJ (50–110 kcal) mol^{-1}
Ionic and hydrogen bonds	12·6–29·4 kJ (3–7 kcal) mol^{-1}
Van der Waals' forces	4·2–8·4 kJ (1–2 kcal) mol^{-1}

2. They break spontaneously under physiological conditions so that enzymes are not required to disrupt them. (In a stable system the number of weak bonds broken is exactly equalled by the number of new bonds formed.)
3. They are longer and their length is not fixed and definite since they can be stretched, but when this happens the attractive force, i.e. the strength of the bond, is decreased as the distance between the participating atoms is increased.
4. The angle between weak bonds is much more variable than that between covalent bonds.
5. They are responsible for determining the specific conformation of macromolecules and also the associations which occur between different molecules and different parts of the same molecule.
6. Ionic and hydrogen bonds are pH sensitive.

Salt linkages (ionic bonds)

Organic molecules which contain ionized groups bearing opposite charges, e.g. amino (NH_3^+) and carboxyl (COO^-) or phosphate ($H_2PO_4^-$ and HPO_4^{2-}) groups, can react like inorganic ions to form salt linkages.

$$Na^+ : Cl^-$$

$$\boxed{}-NH_3^+ : {}^-OOC-\boxed{}$$

When such ions are formed one of the groupings acts as an electron donor and becomes positively charged and the other accepts the electron and becomes negatively charged. The ions are then held together by electrostatic forces. The direction of ionic bonds is in a straight line between charged centres. They are very sensitive to the pH of the surrounding medium since the charged state of the contributing ions is pH dependent.

Hydrogen bonds

This type of bond occurs between hydrogen atoms and oxygen or nitrogen atoms both of which are electronegative. All molecules which are not composed of identical atoms, e.g. H_2, N_2, Cl_2, have dipoles due to the uneven distribution of electrons which results from the differing electron-attracting forces of the component atoms.

Thus, covalently bound atoms may carry a residual charge and a covalently bound hydrogen atom with some positive charge will be weakly attracted to a covalently bound oxygen or nitrogen atom bearing some negative charge.

$$>N-\boxed{\overset{\delta+}{H}----\overset{\delta-}{O}}=C<$$

In the instance shown the H which is covalently bound to the N atom of the imino group is attracted to the covalently bound O of the carbonyl group and the two are said to be united by a hydrogen bond. Such bonds are individually weak but when molecules of particular kinds come together they arrange themselves so as to form the maximum number of hydrogen bonds. Hydrogen bonds are much weaker than covalent bonds, but stronger than Van der Waals' forces. They are also more specific than the latter and virtually only the three most electronegative elements – oxygen, nitrogen and fluorine – take part in hydrogen bonding. Hydrogen bonds play an integral part in the structure of both proteins and nucleic acids.

Van der Waals' forces

These are unspecific and operate regardless of whether molecules are polar or non-polar. They result from the attractive force (through the formation of mutually induced dipoles) that atoms exert on one another when they come close together. The number of such bonds that an atom can form is limited only by the number of other atoms with which it can be in contact at any given moment. The bond energy is only slightly greater than the average thermal energy of the molecules which keeps them in constant motion. As a result Van der Waals' forces are only effective when a large number of the atoms belonging to one molecule interact with a large number of atoms belonging to another molecule. Van der Waals' forces may also operate between different parts of the same molecule, if it is sufficiently large and is folded back on itself. Formation of the bond requires that the molecules or their parts should have complementary shapes and fit precisely into one another, so that where one projects its partner must be recessed and vice versa. Some molecules are designed so that 'like bonds with like', e.g. proteins made up of identical subunits. In other instances molecules interact with others of a different kind, e.g. the lipid–protein complexes of which membranes are composed.

Hydrophobic bonds

Hydrophobic bonds between two hydrophobic portions of organic molecules involve local changes in the structure of water and are discussed on page 55. Unlike other types of bond, hydrophobic bonds decrease in strength as the temperature is lowered.

Chemical nomenclature

Biochemists often use shorter common names for compounds rather than their standard chemical ones. This may be confusing for students in the initial stages of their studies and for this reason the alternative names for some important biochemical compounds are given in Table 2.2.

Table 2.2 Alphabetical list of common current biochemical names and their recommended names in modern chemical terminology

Common current name	Recommended name
Acetaldehyde	Ethanal
Acetic acid	Ethanoic acid
Acetoacetic acid	3-Oxobutanoic acid
Acetone	Propanone
Alanine	2-Aminopropanoic acid
γ-Aminobutyric acid	3-Aminobutanoic acid
Aspartic acid	Aminobutanedioic acid
Benzoic acid	Benzenecarboxylic acid
Butyric acid	Butanoic acid
Carbon tetrachloride	Tetrachloromethane
Citric acid	2-Hydroxypropane-1,2,3-tricarboxylic acid
Diglyceride	Diacylglycerol
Dihydroxyacetone	1,3-Dihydroxypropanone
Diphosphoglyceric acid	1,3-Diphosphoglyceric acid
Elaidic acid	*trans*-Octadec-9-enoic acid
Ethyl acetic acid	Ethyl ethanoic acid
Ethyl alcohol	Ethanol
Ethylene glycol	Ethane-1,2-diol

Table 2.2 (*cont.*)

Common current name	Recommended name
Formaldehyde	Methanal
Formic acid	Methanoic acid
Fumaric acid	*trans*-Butenedioic acid
Glutamic acid	2-Aminopentanedioic acid
Glyceraldehyde	1,2-Dihydroxypropanal
Glycine	Aminoethanoic acid
Glycerol	Propane-1,2,3-triol
β-Hydroxybutyric acid	2-Hydroxybutanoic acid
Lactic acid	2-Hydroxypropanoic acid
Malic acid	2-Hydroxybutanedioic acid
Malonic acid	Propanedioic acid
Methyl alcohol	Methanol
Oxalic acid	Ethanedioic acid
Oxaloacetic acid	2-Oxobutanedioic acid
α-Oxoglutaric acid	2-Oxopentanedioic acid
Propionic acid	Propanoic acid
Pyruvic acid	2-Oxopropanoic acid
Salicylic acid	2-Hydroxybenzoic acid
Stearic acid	Octadecanoic acid
Succinic acid	Butanedioic acid
Sulphanilamide	4-Aminobenzenesulphonamide
Triglyceride	Triacylglycerol
Urea	Carbamide

Chapter 3
The molecular environment

The biological ubiquity of water

Life is essentially a watery affair. Its aquatic origins are reflected in the high water contents of the cells and tissues even of terrestrial plants and animals. Mammalian cells contain some 70–75% of water, while soft tissues range from 65 to 80% in water content. Considering extremes, whole blood contains about 80% of water while heavily mineralized compact bone may have only 15%. The lowest content is reached in dental enamel which, when mature, contains only 4% by weight (approximately 10% by volume) of water. A man weighing 65 kg contains about 40 kg (or litres) of water (i.e. 62%) of which 25 kg are within cells and 15 kg are extracellular. Water in the plasma accounts for only 3 kg the remaining 12 kg of extracellular water being interstitial and bathing the cells within the tissues. The approximate composition of the body is given in Table 3.1.

Water thus provides an all-pervading environment which surrounds and interacts with the whole gamut of biological molecules, small and large. Most biochemical reactions take place within or near this aqueous continuum, indeed their very occurrence often depends upon the

Table 3.1 Approximate values for the chemical composition of the adult human body

Tissue or organ	Percentage of body weight	Water	Protein	Lipid	Ash
Whole body	100	61·5	18	15	4·0
Muscle	36	75	18	6	1·0
Skeleton	16	30	19	21	28·1
Adipose tissue	12	36	7	57	0·3
Blood	8	79	20	1	0·2
Skin	7	61	25	13	0·6
Nervous tissue	3	74	12	12	0·7
Liver	3	75	18	3	1·1
Heart	0·6	68	17	13	0·7
Kidneys	0·5	79	15	4	1·0

In these organs 0–5% of carbohydrate may also be present

presence and special nature of water. Although water is commonplace and familiar, its apparent simplicity is deceptive.

The structure and properties of water

The structural form of complex molecules such as those of proteins depends upon water, which also acts as a directing and orientating influence on cell and tissue development. For its own part, water is not simple and homogeneous, its properties being greatly influenced by temperature and the molecular environment. The structure of pure water depends upon the ease with which its molecules form hydrogen bonds with each other. Water molecules may be considered as bent rods which by means of their two hydrogen atoms and the two lone pairs of electrons on the oxygen atom may participate in the formation of up to 4 hydrogen bonds with neighbouring water molecules. The maximum number is achieved in ice, which, as can be seen in snowflakes, is highly crystalline. Thus, in ice, water has a coordination number of 4 and the tetrahedral lattice has a highly regular pattern and an open structure of low density.

When ice melts, its continuous crystalline structure is partially broken down and becomes more complex. Water consists partly of free molecules and partly of 'clusters' or 'icebergs' in which a number of molecules are joined together by hydrogen bonds (Figure 3.1).

These clusters are short-lived, however, and soon break down to individual molecules while new clusters are continually being formed. Thus there is a dynamic equilibrium between molecules and clusters. The molecules inside the clusters are in the tetrabonded form while those on the surface of the clusters may have one, two or three hydrogen bonds with neighbouring molecules. Since the second hydrogen bond is formed more easily than the first, the formation of new clusters is a cooperative phenomenon between many molecules. Consequently there are no small units (dimers, trimers, etc.) but only rather large and uniform clusters of approximately spherical shape in equilibrium with individual molecules. The size of the clusters, and the proportion of the water within them, both decrease as the temperature rises; at 37°C, about two-thirds of the molecules are in clusters with approximately 40 molecules per cluster.

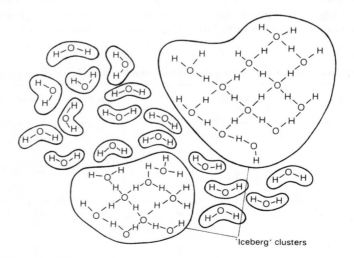

'Iceberg' clusters

Figure 3.1 The structure of liquid water showing 'icebergs'

Interaction between water and biological molecules

As a result of interaction between water and organic substances including proteins, the structure of the water at the interface is modified (page 55) so that it differs from the structure of bulk water. This interaction may also modify the structure of the organic molecules. Consequently not only do biological molecules themselves take on a preferred configuration but they become surrounded by layers of water which behave in a different manner from the bulk of free water. Almost all of the large amount of water present in living cells is in the form of orientated multi-layers on the surfaces of cell proteins and the special properties of orientated water are intimately concerned with the chemical changes that are the basis of life.

The general action of anaesthetic agents is believed to result from their stabilizing effect on the pre-existing layers of orientated water molecules near protein molecules, including those of various cell membranes. Molecules of the anaesthetic penetrate into these layers where their hydrates have an ordering effect on the water structure and oppose the changes it normally undergoes as a result of the biochemical functioning of associated protein structures.

The mechanism whereby the carious process penetrates healthy dental enamel is intimately related to the structure and properties of the water within the 'spaces' of the enamel. This water is presumably partially orientated with respect to both hydroxyapatite crystals and the small amount of protein present. An appreciation of the significance of water in this rather special situation, however, still awaits further advances in our knowledge of both the physicochemical and biological behaviour of water.

Water as an ionizing solvent

Water is a good solvent for a variety of inorganic substances and also for many organic substances except for those that are predominantly hydrocarbon in nature. The specific solvent properties of water arise from its highly polar character and unequal charge distribution, which result from an excess of electrons near the oxygen atom and a deficiency near the hydrogen atoms. The molecule thus acts like a small dipole with its negative charge near the oxygen and its positive charge midway between the two hydrogen–oxygen bonds (page 14).

Like all dipoles, water molecules become orientated in an electric field such as exists in the neighbourhood of molecules of other polar substances. When these are dissolved in water each of their molecules is surrounded by a little cloud of orientated water molecules, which stabilizes the solution by the so-called 'solvation' effect. For this reason water is a good solvent for most polar substances.

When salts dissolve in water they are almost completely dissociated into ions, e.g.

$$NaCl \rightarrow Na^+ + Cl^-$$

Because of their high local concentration of charge, ions would be very unstable were it not for the solvation effect whereby they become effectively hydrated. Thus, in the presence of water, the sodium ion exists in the form $Na^+ \leftarrow O \begin{smallmatrix} ..H \\ .. \\ ..H \end{smallmatrix}$ and the chloride ion as $Cl^- \begin{smallmatrix} H.. \\ \nearrow \\ H. \end{smallmatrix} O$, the arrow denoting donation of a free electron pair from the complete outer shell.

Ions that have more than one charge produce a larger local concentration of charge than the monovalent ions, e.g.

$$MgSO_4 \rightleftharpoons Mg^{2+} + SO_4^{2-}$$
$$Na_3PO_4 \rightleftharpoons 3Na^+ + PO_4^{3-}$$

This effect of the local charge concentration of a solution is expressed as its *ionic strength I* defined as

$$I = \tfrac{1}{2} \sum_i c_i z_i^2$$

Thus ionic strength is equal to one-half of the sum of the products of the concentration of each ion and the square of its valency. Thus a 0·1 M solution of NaCl has $I = 0·1$, but 0·1 M $MgSO_4$ has $I = 0·4$ and 0·1 M Na_3PO_4 has $I = 0·6$. It is the ionic strength of its environment that determines the solubility of a protein.

When any electrically neutral molecule dissociates, equal numbers of positive and negative charges are produced on the ions. Similarly, the solution containing the ions, considered as a whole, is electrically neutral. Thus, in any system that is sufficiently large the sum of the positive charges equals the sum of the negative charges.

Hydrogen ions and the idea of acidity

There is something special about hydrogen ions which distinguishes them from all other ions and which has long been recognized in the chemical idea of 'acidity'. Essentially, the hydrogen ion is a proton, i.e. a hydrogen nucleus that has lost its orbital electron, and exists in aqueous solution in the hydrated form, H_3O^+ formed by the water oxygen donating a lone pair of electrons to the proton

$$\begin{matrix} H \\ \end{matrix} \!\!\!\diagdown\!\!\! O \rightarrow H^+ \diagup\!\!\! H$$

This hydrated form is sometimes referred to as a 'hydronium' or 'oxonium' ion but, provided it is understood that aqueous solutions are under consideration, the term 'hydrogen ion' (H^+) is less confusing. In one respect hydrogen ions in solution seem to retain the characteristics of subatomic smallness and mobility associated with the proton; they are subject to two distinct transfer processes: (1) by diffusion like all other ions and (2) by transfer between adjacent molecules, often water molecules, by a mechanism which, though not completely understood, probably accounts for their high mobility.

An *acid* was defined by Bronsted in 1923 as a molecule or ion with a tendency to give up protons in solution and a *base* as a molecule or ion which has a tendency to acquire protons and thereby form an acid. There is a complementary relationship between *conjugate pairs* of acid and base. Thus considering the equilibrium

$$HX \rightleftharpoons H^+ + X^- \tag{3·1}$$

HX is an acid, since on ionization it loses a proton, whereas the ion X^- is a base since it has a tendency to acquire a proton and form HX. HX is the conjugate acid to base X^- and conversely X^- is the conjugate base to acid HX.

Different acids vary considerably in their strength. A strong acid is one that gives up protons readily whereas a weak acid gives them up reluctantly. A strong base acquires protons avidly and a weak base less readily. Strong acids have relatively weak conjugate bases (i.e. when the equilibrium of Equation (3·1) lies to the right), whereas weak acids have strong conjugate bases (equilibrium lying to the left).

The strength of an acid can be expressed as its *dissociation constant, K_a*, by applying the *law of mass action** to the equilibrium of Equation (3·1). Thus the velocity of the reaction from left to

---

* The law of mass action states that the velocity of a chemical reaction is proportional to the product of the 'active masses' (or concentrations) of the reacting substances. Equations (3·2) and (3·3) are mathematical expressions of this law.

right (V_1) is given by the equation

$$V_1 = k_1[HX] \tag{3.2}$$

where k_1 is the velocity coefficient for the forward reaction and $[HX]$ is the 'activity' of the acid HX which for dilute solutions, such as occur in living organisms, can to all intents and purposes be considered as equal to the concentration of the acid. Considering the reverse reaction, its velocity (V_2) is given by

$$V_2 = k_2[H^+][X^-] \tag{3.3}$$

where k_2 is the velocity coefficient of the reaction from right to left and $[H^+]$ and $[X^-]$ are the concentrations of hydrogen ions and the conjugate base respectively.

When equilibrium is reached the velocities $(V_1$ and $V_2)$ of the forward and reverse reactions are equal, so from Equations (3.2) and (3.3)

$$k_1[HX] = k_2[H^+][X^-]$$

by cross multiplying we obtain the definition of the acid dissociation constant K_a:

$$K_a = \frac{k_1}{k_2} = \frac{[H^+][X^-]}{[HX]} \tag{3.4}$$

k_1 and k_2 are both constants so that k_1/k_2 will also be a constant which is denoted by K_a. For strong acids the concentrations of products $[H^+]$ and $[X^-]$ will be large and the concentration of acid $[HX]$ small so the dissociation constant K_a will be large. Conversely, the dissociation constant of a weak acid will be small.

In Table 3.2 a number of acids of biochemical interest are listed, together with their dissociation constants and conjugate bases. There is a considerable range of acid strengths, represented by the dissociation constants. These range from values greater than unity for the very strong mineral acids to very small values indeed, where K_a involves large negative powers of ten, e.g. for the third ionization of phosphoric acid and for water itself. Examination of the formulae in the first column of the table shows that acids may be either electrically neutral molecules, anions with one or more negative charges (e.g. the ion HPO_4^{2-}), zwitterions (such as

Table 3.2 Dissociation constants and pK_a values at 25°C of some common acids of biochemical importance

Formula of acid		K_a	pK_a	Formula of conjugate base
HCl	Hydrochloric acid	>2.9	<-0.46	Cl^-
$CH_3 \cdot COOH$	Acetic acid	1.75×10^{-5}	4.76	$CH_3 \cdot COO^-$
$CH_3CH(OH)COOH$	Lactic acid	8.32×10^{-4}	3.08	$CH_3 \cdot CH(OH)COO^-$
$C_3H_5O(COOH)_3$	Citric acid	9.20×10^{-4}	3.04	$C_3H_5O(COOH)_2COO^-$
$C_3H_5O(COOH)_2COO^-$	Citric acid	2.69×10^{-5}	4.57	$C_3H_5O(COOH)(COO^-)_2$
$C_3H_5O(COOH)(COO^-)_2$	Citric acid	1.34×10^{-6}	5.87	$C_3H_5O(COO^-)_3$
H_2CO_3	Carbonic acid	4.31×10^{-7}	6.37	HCO_3^-
HCO_3^-	Carbonic acid	5.61×10^{-11}	10.25	CO_3^{2-}
H_3PO_4	Phosphoric acid	7.52×10^{-3}	2.12	$H_2PO_4^-$
$H_2PO_4^-$	Phosphoric acid	6.23×10^{-8}	7.21	HPO_4^{2-}
HPO_4^{2-}	Phosphoric acid	5.0×10^{-13}	12.30	PO_4^{3-}
NH_4^+	Ammonium ion	5.5×10^{-10}	9.26	NH_3
$NH_3^+ \cdot CH_2 \cdot COOH$	Glycine	4.5×10^{-3}	2.35	$NH_3^+CH_2COO^-$
$NH_3^+ \cdot CH_2 \cdot COO^-$	Glycine	1.6×10^{-10}	9.78	$NH_2 \cdot CH_2COO^-$
H_2O	Water	1.8×10^{-16}	15.74	OH^-

the zwitterionic form of glycine, $NH_3^+ \cdot CH_2 \cdot COO^-$) (page 41) and even cations (such as the ammonium ion NH_4^+ which is an acid because it has a tendency to lose a proton to form an electrically neutral ammonia molecule). Polybasic acids such as carbonic, citric and orthophosphoric acids have distinct values of K_a for each of their dissociable protons. These dissociation constants may lie close together as in citric acid, where they differ only by a power of ten, or spread far apart as in phosphoric acid, where the K_a values differ by factors of 10^5. The intermediate ions formed from polybasic acids can behave either as acids or bases according to their environment. Thus the dihydrogen phosphate ion $H_2PO_4^-$ acts as an acid when it loses a proton to form the monohydrogen phosphate ion HPO_4^{2-} but as a base when it gains one to form orthophosphoric acid.

The concept of pH

The wide range of concentrations of hydrogen ions which may be encountered in different solutions, together with the very low numerical values for many of them, means that hydrogen ion concentration is a cumbersome unit. This is also apparent when comparing dissociation constants of different acids and may be further illustrated by considering the hydrogen ion concentrations of two solutions towards the extreme values for biological situations. Gastric juice is an acidic secretion with a concentration of hydrogen ions which may be expressed as either $0 \cdot 08$ or 8×10^{-2} g-ions per litre. Blood, by contrast, is a more nearly neutral fluid with a hydrogen ion concentration of $0 \cdot 0000000398$ or 3.98×10^{-8} g-ions per litre. For comparative purposes, the first mode of expression is clumsy as it involves several noughts following the decimal point. The second method is also mathematically clumsy since it involves the combination of a numerical value with a negative exponent of ten. The disadvantages of these modes of expression were overcome by Sorensen when, in 1908, he introduced the concept of pH. The pH of a solution is a convenient measure of its hydrogen ion concentration on a condensed scale which readily permits the comparison of different solutions. The *pH (or hydrogen ion exponent)* is defined by the equation:

$$pH = -\log_{10}[H^+] = \log_{10}\left(\frac{1}{[H^+]}\right) \qquad (3 \cdot 5)$$

Thus pH is the negative value of the logarithm to base 10 of the hydrogen ion activity (or for dilute solutions the hydrogen ion concentration). Hydrogen ion concentration and pH are readily interconvertible by means of Equation (3·5) as in the following calculation for the pH of blood:

$$
\begin{aligned}
[H^+] &= 3 \cdot 98 \times 10^{-8} \\
&= 10^{0 \cdot 60} \times 10^{-8} \quad \text{(since } \log_{10} 3 \cdot 98 = 0 \cdot 6\text{)} \\
&= 10^{0 \cdot 60 - 8} \\
&= 10^{-7 \cdot 40} \\
pH &= -\log_{10}[H^+] \\
&= -\log_{10}[10^{-7 \cdot 40}] \\
&= 7 \cdot 40
\end{aligned}
$$

The ionization of water

To appreciate the reasons behind the length of the pH scale and the positions of various fixed points on it, it is necessary to consider the ionization of water in more detail. So far we have seen that water is a good ionizing solvent but no mention has yet been made of the fact that water itself is capable of ionization to a very slight extent and is in fact an extremely weak acid, as is shown in Table 3.2. To study this it is necessary to prepare water free from all dissolved impurities. Pure water can be prepared by passage through a bed of mixed cation- and anion-exchange resins, which remove all ionic impurities. As water is progressively purified its electrical conductivity falls to a minimum value which results from the ions produced by the ionization of water itself.

$$H_2O \rightleftharpoons H^+ + OH^-$$

By applying Equation (3·4) the dissociation constant for water can be calculated

$$K_a = \frac{[H^+][OH^-]}{[H_2O]}$$

the value given in Table 3.2 having been calculated in this way. Further simplifications are possible, however. Since $[H^+]$ and $[OH^-]$ are very small, the comparatively large concentration of undissociated water $[H_2O]$ will be effectively constant therefore

$$[H^+][OH^-] = K_w \tag{3·6}$$

where K_w is a constant at a given temperature known as the *ionic product for water*. Equation (3.6) applies not only to pure water but to all dilute aqueous solutions, and, since if the concentration of hydrogen ions is known, that of the hydroxyl ions can be calculated or vice versa. Values of K_w have been calculated from the conductivity of pure water; it varies with temperature being $1·00 \times 10^{-14}$ at 25°C and $2·51 \times 10^{-14}$ at 37°C. In pure water the concentrations of hydrogen and hydroxyl ions must be equal since equal numbers of these two kinds of ion are produced by dissociation.

Therefore at 25°C, $K_w = 10^{-14}$ and $[H^+] = [OH^-]$ and inserting these values in Equation (3·6).

$$[H^+]^2 = 10^{-14}$$

and therefore, taking square roots

$$[H^+] = 10^{-7}$$

Thus the hydrogen ion concentration of pure water at 25°C is 10^{-7} g-ions per litre. By inserting this value in Equation (3·5) we obtain the pH value of water at 25°C:

$$\begin{aligned} pH &= -\log_{10}[H^+] \\ &= -\log_{10}[10^{-7}] \\ &= 7 \end{aligned}$$

The pH scale

This value of 7·0 at 25°C represents an important reference point on the pH scale, the point of neutrality where equal concentrations of hydrogen and hydroxyl ions are present. There are no definite ends to the pH scale but we can visualize approximately where these lie by calculating the pH of a strongly acid and a strongly alkaline solution respectively.

A molar solution of hydrochloric acid is 78·4% ionized, its $[H^+]$ is thus 0·784 M and its pH, $-\log_{10} 0·784$, i.e. $-(0·894-1) = 0·106$. If it were completely ionized and its hydrogen ion activity were exactly equal to its concentration it would have a pH of zero. Similarly a normal solution of sodium hydroxide is 73% ionized; its $[OH^-]$ is thus 0·73 M and its $[H^+]$ can be calculated from Equation (3·6):

$$[H^+] = \frac{K_w}{[OH^-]} = \frac{10^{-14}}{0·73} = 1·37 \times 10^{-14}$$

Therefore

$$pH = -\log_{10}(1{\cdot}37 \times 10^{-14})$$
$$= 13{\cdot}863$$

Again if the solution were ideal and completely ionized it would have a pH of 14 at 25°C.

The pH scale thus stretches from somewhere below 0 on the strongly acid side through a neutral point at pH 7 to somewhere above 14 on the alkaline side. Some useful pH values for various biological fluids and buffer solutions are given in Figure 3.2. The pH scale is easy to use,

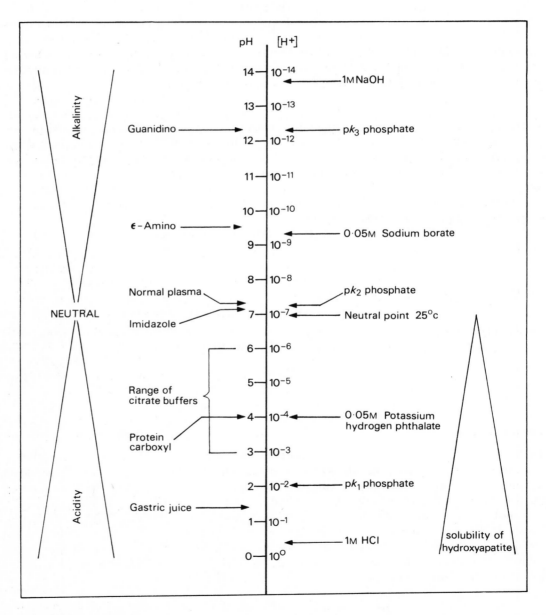

Figure 3.2 The pH scale

but it has a few peculiarities that can cause confusion if they are not recognized. Firstly as a result of the negative sign in Equation (3·5), an *increase* in hydrogen ion concentration means that a solution has a *lower* pH whereas a *higher* pH corresponds to *fewer* hydrogen ions. Secondly, it is a logarithmic scale so that a decrease in the pH value of one unit corresponds to a 10-fold increase in $[H^+]$, a decrease of two pH units to a 100-fold increase in $[H^+]$ and so forth. The pH scale is thus very much compressed and fairly small changes in pH correspond to substantial changes in hydrogen ion concentration. When the pH rises or falls by only 0·3 of a pH unit the hydrogen ion concentration is halved or doubled respectively.

For practical purposes pH is measured by comparing the properties of the unknown solution with those of a reference buffer solution of known composition. The pH values of such reference solutions have been accurately determined and are recorded in the literature. Comparisons may be carried out by means of a potentiometric pH meter which measures the d.c. potential produced when a porous glass electrode, permeable only to hydrogen ions, is placed in contact with the solution. The difference in the potentials produced by two solutions (e.g. the standard and the unknown) is a direct measure of their difference in pH. For less accurate work a colorimetric method may be used, based on colour changes undergone by an added indicator, the colour of which changes according to the concentration of hydrogen ions in equilibrium with it. For potentiometric measurements, two solutions only, e.g. 0·05 M-potassium hydrogen phthalate and 0·05 M-sodium borate having pH values of 4·00 and 9·175 at 25°C (Figure 3.2) are sufficient to standardize the pH meter.

Buffering effects and buffer solutions

Addition of even minute quantities of impurities may bring about large changes in the pH of pure water. Thus by adding one drop (say 0·05 ml) of 0·1 M HCl to 1 litre of pure water its pH is reduced from 7·0 to 5·3 while addition of one drop of 0·1 M NaOH would raise the pH to 8·7.

A *buffer solution* is one that resists changes in pH when moderate amounts of foreign substances, especially hydrogen or hydroxyl ions, are added to it or when it is diluted. Buffer solutions are used in biochemistry to maintain a constant pH by minimizing changes that would otherwise be brought about by substances produced or removed in the experiment or by accidental contamination. Certain buffer solutions are also used as exact pH reference standards, as already mentioned. Natural buffer systems operate in living organisms and play an important part in homeostasis by maintaining the pH constant within narrow limits. This applies especially to blood and also to cell contents and saliva.

Considering the design of an artificial buffer solution, a moderately concentrated solution of a fairly weak organic acid such as 1 M acetic acid will be partially ionized according to the equation

$$CH_3COOH \rightleftharpoons H^+ + CH_3COO^- \tag{3.7}$$

but, since the acid is weak, the equilibrium will lie mainly to the left and there will be a relatively high concentration of undissociated acetic acid. If the dissociation constant of acetic acid is known ($1·75 \times 10^{-5}$ from Table 3.2) the concentrations of ions can be calculated. From Equation (3·4)

$$K_a = 1·75 \times 10^{-5} = \frac{[H^+][CH_3COO^-]}{[CH_3COOH]} \tag{3.8}$$

If two approximations are made and (a) the concentration of acetic acid before dissociation is taken as 1 and (b) the very small association of hydrogen ions with hydroxyl to form water is ignored, $[CH_3COO^-] = [H^+]$, and it follows that

$$\frac{[H^+]^2}{1 - [H^+]} = 1.75 \times 10^{-5}$$

or since $[H^+] \ll 1$

$$
\begin{aligned}
H^+ &= \sqrt{(1.75 \times 10^{-5})} \\
&= \sqrt{(10^{0.243} \times 10^{-5})} \\
&= 10^{-2.38} \\
&= 4.27 \times 10^{-3}
\end{aligned}
$$

Thus the concentration of hydrogen and of acetate ions will each be only 4.27×10^{-3} g-ions per litre and that of undissociated acetic acid molecules will be 0.996 g-ions per litre, approximately 250 times greater. The pH of the solution will be 2.37.

When hydroxyl ions are added to 1 M acetic acid the first effect is that they combine with hydrogen ions already present to form water:

$$OH^- + H^+ \rightleftharpoons H_2O$$

This markedly reduces the concentration of hydrogen ions which is already low and disturbs the equilibrium represented by Equation (3·7). The equilibrium therefore moves to the right; more acetic acid dissociates, although since its concentration is high its value remains almost constant. The concentration of acetate ions will increase substantially. The hydrogen ion concentration will be partially but not completely restored because of the increased acetate concentration. If, on the other hand, hydrogen ions are added to the system, equilibrium (3·7) is disturbed in the opposite direction and moves from right to left. Acetic acid is formed with little effect on its total concentration but the small acetate concentration rapidly falls to a small fraction of its original value, the hydrogen ion concentration being increased reciprocally. Thus while 1 M acetic acid offers a slight buffering power towards addition of hydroxyl ions, it has very little indeed towards added hydrogen ions.

The main reason for the failure of buffering is seen to be the rapid change in acetate ion concentration. This may be overcome by adding a large excess of acetate, e.g. by making the solution 1 M with respect to sodium acetate, as well as to the acetic acid already present. The effects of making this change are that the salt, sodium acetate, will dissociate almost completely in solution so that $[Na^+]$ and $[CH_3COO^-]$ will each be approximately unity. This large increase in the value of $[CH_3COO^-]$ will disturb the equilibrium of Equation (3·7) driving the reaction to the left with a very slight increase in the concentration of undissociated acetic acid towards the original value of unity and a marked fall in the value of $[H^+]$.

Referring once more to Equation (3·8)

$$K_a = 1.75 \times 10^{-5} = \frac{[H^+][CH_3COO^-]}{[CH_3COOH]} \tag{3·8}$$

but

$$[CH_3COO^-] = 1 = [CH_3COOH]$$

therefore

$$[H^+] = K_a = 1.75 \times 10^{-5} \tag{3·9}$$

Equations of this type apply generally to any concentrated solution containing a weak acid with an equal concentration of its soluble salt (giving rise to an equal concentration of the anion, which is the conjugate base). In such a solution the hydrogen ion concentration will be equal to the acid dissociation constant. The pH of the solution assumes a unique value for each particular weak acid, which is known as the pK_a of that acid.

$$pH = -\log_{10}[H^+] \tag{3.5}$$

from Equation (3.9)

$$pH = -\log_{10}K_a = pK_a \tag{3.10}$$

The pK_a of a weak acid is the pH of a solution containing equal concentrations of that acid and its conjugate base. The pK_a may be evaluated from Equation (3.10) if the dissociation constant is known or vice versa. Thus for acetic acid

$$\begin{aligned}
pK_a &= -\log_{10} K_a \\
&= -\log_{10}(1.75 \times 10^{-5}) \\
&= -\log_{10}(10^{0.243} \times 10^{-5}) \\
&= 4.757
\end{aligned}$$

The pK_a values for a number of acids are included in Table 3.2.

It thus appears that the addition of sufficient sodium acetate to make the solution 1 M with respect to this salt increases the pH of acetic acid from 2.37 to 4.76. The modified solution is a very good buffer at this pH. The concentrations of both undissociated acid and acetate ions are high and equal to 1 and the hydrogen ion concentration is much lower at 1.75×10^{-5}. Addition of a small number of hydroxyl ions removes an equal number of hydrogen ions as water. The original concentration of hydrogen ions is then restored by the dissociation of more acetic acid, the equilibrium of Equation (3.7) moving to the right. There is a slight increase in acetate concentration and a slight decrease in acetic acid concentration but since both concentrations are high, their ratio remains nearly constant and the hydrogen ion concentration (given by Equation (3.8)) is also practically constant. Conversely, addition of hydrogen ions moves the equilibrium of Equation (3.7) to the left with a slight decrease in acetate concentration and a slight increase in that of acetic acid. The ratio of these high concentrations again remains almost constant as does the hydrogen ion concentration and pH of the buffer solution.

The effect on the pH of buffer solutions of more substantial additions of hydroxyl and hydrogen ions than those just considered is given by the *Henderson–Hasselbalch equation*, which, in the case of acetic acid–acetate buffer, may be derived as follows:

$$K_a = \frac{[H^+][CH_3COO^-]}{[CH_3COOH]} \tag{3.8}$$

Therefore

$$\log_{10}K_a = \log_{10}[H^+] + \log_{10}\frac{[CH_3COO^-]}{[CH_3COOH]}$$

Therefore

$$-\log_{10}[H^+] = -\log_{10}K_a + \log_{10}\frac{[CH_3COO^-]}{[CH_3COOH]}$$

and therefore

$$pH = pK_a + \log_{10}\frac{[CH_3COO^-]}{[CH_3COOH]}$$

In the general case

$$pH = pK_a + \log_{10}\frac{\text{concentration of anion (conjugate base)}}{\text{concentration of undissociated acid}} \tag{3.11}$$

or more approximately

$$\text{pH} = pK_a + \log_{10} \frac{[\text{salt}]}{[\text{acid}]} \text{ (the Henderson–Hasselbalch equation)}$$

Adjustment of the ratio of anion to undissociated acid permits the adjustment of the pH of a buffer system over a definite range. When anion and acid concentrations are equal, the pH of the solution will be equal to the pK_a of the acid. This represents the centre point of the range of the buffer system at which buffering is maximum (Figure 3.3). Concentration ratios for anion to acid of 10 and 0·1 correspond to pH values of one unit above and below the pK_a respectively. The system will have reasonable buffering power between these extremes. Similarly concentration ratios of 100 and 0·01 correspond to pH values two units above and below the pK_a but under these conditions the buffering power is greatly reduced.

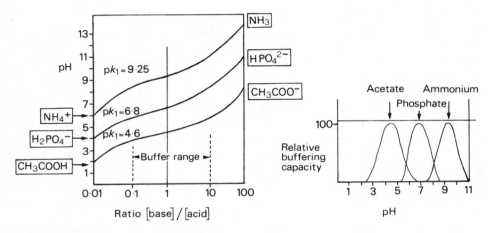

Figure 3.3 Titration curves and buffering capacity of acetate, phosphate and ammonium ions

There is a wide range of dissociation constants and hence pK values among the acids and to obtain a buffer solution of a given pH it is necessary to select an acid having a pK value close to that pH (preferably within half a unit) and then adjust the ratio of salt to acid to obtain the exact pH required. Use of polybasic acids considerably extends the range of buffer solutions that can be prepared with a limited number of acids. Each dissociable hydrogen of a polybasic acid has its own pK value corresponding to the centre point of its buffering range. Where these are spaced some way apart, as are the pKs of the tribasic phosphoric acid, the acid will have discrete buffering ranges (centred around pH 2·1, 7·2 and 12·3 respectively) and intermediate ranges with very little buffering power (Figure 3.4). Tris buffer is used in biochemical experiments when phosphate addition would upset the conditions. When the pK values are more closely spaced as for the tribasic citric acid, the buffering ranges overlap and reinforce each other. Thus, citric acid has a long almost linear buffer range from pH 3·0 to 6·0 and is useful for preparing buffers throughout this region. Since ammonium ions and substituted ammonium ions are also acids, a very wide range of buffer solutions can be prepared based on solutions containing weak acids and conjugate bases. Tables showing the composition and corresponding pH values of a variety of buffers throughout the entire pH range are available.

The Henderson–Hasselbalch equation can be used to work out the pH of dilute solutions of acid. Since there is no added salt

$$[\text{H}^+] = \text{concentration of anion}$$

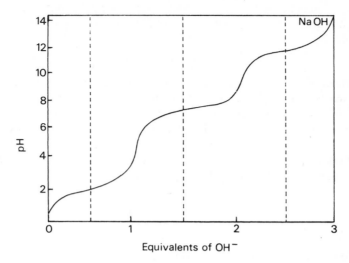

Figure 3.4 Titration curve of phosphoric acid

From Equation (3·11)

$$pH = pK_a - pH - \log_{10} \text{(concentration of undissociated acid)}$$

Therefore

$$pH = \tfrac{1}{2}[pK_a - \log_{10} \text{(concentration of undissociated acid)}]$$

Thus in the example for 1 M acetic acid ($pK = 4·76$)

$$pH = \tfrac{1}{2}(4·76 - 0) = 2·38$$

Biological buffer systems

Normal human arterial blood plasma at pH 7·40 ± 0·04 is on the alkaline side of neutrality by over half a pH unit since at 37°C the ionic product for water corresponds to a neutral point at pH 6·80. The pH range for plasma which is compatible with survival extends from pH 7·0 to 7·8. Expressed on an arithmetic scale this is quite a considerable range, from 40 to 250% of the normal hydrogen ion concentration. However, persons whose blood pH is at either of these extremes suffer severe physical and mental effects. The maintenance of blood pH within closer limits is therefore essential for health.

This close control of hydrogen ion concentration in blood is maintained by three distinct buffer systems. The first system is made up of the mixed proteins of the plasma and blood cells, the molecules of which have both negatively and positively charged groups:

$$\text{Prot}_{m+}^{n-} \rightleftharpoons \text{Prot}_{(m-1)+}^{n-} + H^+$$

In the physiological pH range, changes in the dissociation of proteins are due mainly to the imidazole group of histidine (page 36) which has a pK_a value of 7·3. Haemoglobin, which is present at high concentration in the red blood cells, is a particularly effective buffer on account of its special properties (page 375). The second buffer system is the equilibrium between dihydrogen phosphate and monohydrogen phosphate ions which has a pK_a of 6·8 and so is near its point of maximum buffering under physiological conditions:

$$H_2PO_4^- \rightleftharpoons HPO_4^{2-} + H^+$$

The third buffer system is the equilibrium between carbonic acid and bicarbonate ions (i.e. the first dissociation of carbonic acid). Carbonic acid is itself in equilibrium with carbon dioxide dissolved in the plasma.

$$H_2O + CO_2 \rightleftharpoons H_2CO_3 \rightleftharpoons HCO_3^- + H^+$$

This bicarbonate buffer system is quantitatively the most important of the three because of the high bicarbonate concentration in blood which results from the large amounts of CO_2 produced by the metabolic activity of cells. Loss of CO_2 in the lungs displaces the equation to the left once more and prevents build up of hydrogen ions. The pK value of this system is considerably below pH 7·4, the normal physiological value for blood, and can be evaluated by applying the Henderson–Hasselbalch equation. The normal plasma bicarbonate value is 27 m-equiv per litre, approximately twenty times the total solubility of carbon dioxide of 1·35 mmol per litre (at a partial pressure of 40 mmHg) From Equation (3·11)

$$pH = pK_a + \log_{10} \frac{[HCO_3^-]}{[H_2CO_3]} \tag{3·12}$$

Therefore inserting pH = 7·4 and $[HCO_3^-]/[H_2CO_3] = 20$ and rearranging

$$pK_a = 7\cdot4 - \log_{10} 20 = 7\cdot4 - 1\cdot3 = 6\cdot1$$

This value of pK_a assumes that all the carbon dioxide in solution is present as carbonic acid.

The solubility of carbon dioxide in water is directly proportional to its partial pressure in the gas phase. The solubility in mmol per litre at 37°C is $0\cdot0334P$ where P is the partial pressure of carbon dioxide in mmHg. Substituting this value for the carbonic acid concentration in Equation (3·12) we obtain

$$pH = 6\cdot1 + \log_{10} \frac{[HCO_3^-]}{0\cdot0334P} \tag{3·13}$$

Equation (3·13) shows that the equilibrium pH of the bicarbonate buffer system of plasma can be to some extent controlled by varying the partial pressure of carbon dioxide in the air to which the blood is exposed (i.e. in the lungs). Reduction in partial pressure results in carbon dioxide leaving the blood with a rise in the last term of Equation (3·13) provided that the bicarbonate concentration remains constant. The equilibrium pH of the buffer system and hence the pH of the blood consequently rise. Conversely an increase in partial pressure of carbon dioxide in the alveolar air will result in a fall in the pH of blood plasma. In practice the partial pressure of carbon dioxide in the alveolar air is controlled by the rate of pulmonary ventilation in relation to the rate of production of carbon dioxide by metabolic oxidation within the body. Increased ventilation (i.e. hyperventilation) will lower the partial pressure of carbon dioxide and raise the blood pH, while decreased ventilation raises the partial pressure, making the blood more acid (metabolic acidosis). Normally the respiratory centre controls the rate of ventilation to keep the partial pressure of carbon dioxide close to the normal value of 40 mmHg.

Experiments in which a 0·027 M solution of sodium bicarbonate (to simulate the isolated bicarbonate buffer system of plasma) was brought to equilibrium with air having various partial pressures of carbon dioxide showed that doubling the partial pressure reduced the pH by 0·3 unit, whereas halving it increased the pH by the same amount. When the experiment was repeated with blood, smaller changes in the same directions were observed, a reduction of 0·2 pH unit on doubling the partial pressure and the same increase on halving it. The smaller effect was due to the additional presence of the protein and the phosphate buffer systems in blood. These experiments, however, show the importance of pulmonary ventilation in controlling the pH of blood.

Equation (3·13) shows that the concentration of bicarbonate ions is also an important factor in the control of blood pH. The pH is increased by 0·3 to pH 7·7 by doubling the bicarbonate concentration from 27 to 54 m-equiv per litre and reduced by 0·3 to pH 7·1 by halving the bicarbonate concentration to 13·5 m-equiv per litre. Again with blood itself, the pH changes are rather smaller as a result of the effect of the other buffer systems. The bicarbonate concentration of plasma is in effect controlled by the kidneys (page 395).

Thus both renal and pulmonary activity are involved in maintaining the pH of blood at its normal level and their cooperative effects are typical of the many biochemically balanced systems which are dynamically integrated within organisms.

Bicarbonate is the most important buffer system in saliva and is especially so in stimulated saliva, since much CO_2 is produced by the increased metabolic activity of the cells (see page 480).

Section 2

Molecular architecture – The building materials

Chapter 4
The amino acids

The amino acids are the building materials for the proteins which are the most characteristic constituents of living matter and among the most complex substances known. Proteins are irregular polymeric compounds made up from a selection of twenty different amino acids joined together by peptide linkages. They may contain anything from one hundred to several thousand amino acid units joined in a specific genetically determined order and each protein has unique chemical and biological properties.

The amino acids are amphoteric compounds and, as the name suggests, contain both a potentially basic amino ($-NH_2$) group and a potentially acidic carboxyl ($-COOH$) group. All the amino acids found in proteins are α-amino acids, the $-NH_2$ and $-COOH$ groups both being attached to the α-carbon atom. They conform to the general formula:

$$H_2N-\underset{\underset{R}{|}}{\overset{\overset{COOH}{|}}{C}}-H \qquad \alpha\text{-amino acid}$$

All the amino acids except glycine (in which $R = H$) contain at least one asymmetric carbon atom, i.e. one that has four different groups attached to it and exist in stereoisomeric forms. The amino acids in proteins belong to the L-series, since they are related in their three-dimensional configuration to the reference compound L-glyceraldehyde (page 91). The D and L forms, which are mirror images of each other and cannot be superimposed, may be represented on a flat sheet of paper as shown in Figure 4.1. The hatched circle represents the asymmetric C atom which is in the plane of the paper, and the –COOH and R– groups of the amino acid project behind the plane of the paper and the –H and $-NH_2$ in front of it.

Once these structures are understood a simpler convention known as *projection formulae*, because the atoms are projected on to the plane of the paper, may be adopted.

$$H_2N-\underset{\underset{R}{|}}{\overset{\overset{COOH}{|}}{C}}-H \qquad\qquad H-\underset{\underset{R}{|}}{\overset{\overset{COOH}{|}}{C}}-NH_2$$

L-Amino acid   D-Amino acid

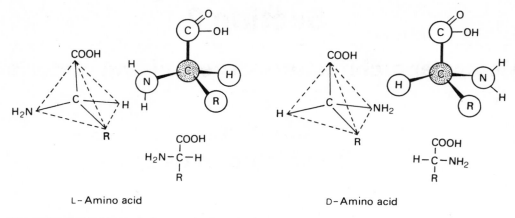

Figure 4.1 Optical isomers (or D and L forms) of an amino acid

The D- forms of the amino acids do not occur in proteins although they are constituents of certain bacterial products, e.g. the antibiotic gramicidin.

The side chains of the amino acids, which are designated in the above formula as R, are of many different types. Several contain reactive groupings such as a second acidic or basic grouping, or a hydroxyl, amide or thiol group or a heterocyclic ring. Others have aliphatic and aromatic side chains that are strongly hydrophobic. The common ancestry of living organisms is indicated by the finding that the same twenty amino acids occur in the proteins of all living forms. Although rather more amino acids are known to occur in the entire range of proteins there are only twenty whose occurrence and arrangement in peptide chains are determined by the genetic coding mechanism.

The amino acids may be divided into:

1. Those with a non-polar hydrocarbon side chain: glycine, alanine, valine, leucine, isoleucine, phenylalanine and proline.
2. Acidic amino acids which have two acidic groups and only one basic group: aspartic acid and glutamic acid.
3. Basic amino acids which possess two basic and only one acidic group: lysine, arginine and histidine.
4. Amino acids with un-ionized but polar substituents in their side chains, e.g.:

hydroxyl ($-OH$)	serine, threonine and tyrosine
sulphydryl ($-SH$)	cysteine
acid amide ($-CONH_2$)	asparagine and glutamine
others	tryptophan and methionine (contains S)

Characteristics of the individual acids

Certain features of the individual amino acids have an important bearing on the structure, and hence on the function, of proteins.

Amino acids with non-polar side chains

In the simplest of the amino acids, *glycine*, the radical R is a hydrogen atom. For various reasons glycine is not a very typical amino acid. More typical is *α-alanine* (where R = CH_3) from which all the other amino acids found in proteins may be regarded as being derived by substitution on the CH_3- group.

$$
\begin{array}{cc}
\text{COOH} & \text{COOH} \\
| & | \\
H_2N-C-H & H_2N-C-H \\
| & | \\
H & CH_3 \\
\end{array}
$$

Glycine (Gly)   α-Alanine (Ala)

Valine, *leucine* and *isoleucine* have branched hydrocarbon side chains which are unreactive and hydrophobic. *Phenylalanine* has a bulky aromatic side chain and this too is hydrophobic. As a result of their water-repellant properties these amino acids tend to orientate towards the interior of folded polypeptide chains.

Valine (Val)   Leucine (Leu)   Isoleucine (Ile)   Phenylalanine (Phe)

Another of the amino acids with an essentially unreactive side chain is *proline*. Strictly speaking proline is not an amino acid but a cyclic secondary amino acid and it is commonly, but incorrectly, called an *imino acid*. It contains a pyrrolidine ring and may be visualized as being derived from norvaline, a straight chain amino acid containing five carbon atoms in which the amino group has become involved in ring formation with the δ-C atom.

$$
\overset{\delta}{CH_3} \cdot \overset{\gamma}{CH_2} \cdot \overset{\beta}{CH_2} \cdot \overset{\alpha}{CH}NH_2 \cdot COOH
$$

Norvaline   Proline (Pro)

Replacement of one of the H atoms on C-4 by a hydroxyl group gives *hydroxyproline*, which is found in the connective tissue proteins collagen and elastin but not in other proteins. As will be apparent later, the ring structure of proline and hydroxyproline imposes certain restrictions on the folding of the polypeptide chain in their vicinity.

Acidic amino acids

The acidic amino acids, *aspartic acid* and *glutamic acid*, represent the aminated forms of oxaloacetic and α-oxoglutaric acids respectively and have two carboxyl groups but only one amino group. Like other amino acids, when they are present in peptide chains the amino group

$$
\begin{array}{cc}
\text{COOH} & \text{COOH} \\
| & | \\
\beta CH_2 & \gamma CH_2 \\
| & | \\
\alpha CHNH_2 & \beta CH_2 \\
| & | \\
\text{COOH} & \alpha CHNH_2 \\
 & | \\
 & \text{COOH} \\
\end{array}
$$

Aspartic acid (Asp)   Glutamic acid (Glu)

and the α-COOH group are unreactive since they are combined in peptide linkage (page 39) with the adjacent amino acids. However, the second (β or γ) –COOH group remains free and reactive.

A carboxylated derivative of glutamic acid, γ-carboxyglutamic acid, has been found in a number of proteins, notably in prothrombin and other blood-clotting factors (page 391).

Basic amino acids

Three of the amino acids that occur in proteins, lysine, arginine and histidine, contain an amino or substituted amino group in their side chains which gives them basic properties, i.e. enables them to act as proton acceptors.

Lysine is a six-carbon diamino-monocarboxylic acid, having two amino groups and only one carboxyl group. It may be modified in various ways after its incorporation into polypeptide

$$
\begin{array}{cc}
\mathrm{CH_2NH_2} & \\
| & \mathrm{CH_2NH_2} \\
\mathrm{CH_2} & | \\
| & \mathrm{CH_2} \\
\mathrm{CH_2} & | \\
| & \mathrm{CH_2} \\
\mathrm{CH_2} & | \\
| & \mathrm{CHNH_2} \\
\mathrm{CHNH_2} & | \\
| & \mathrm{COOH} \\
\mathrm{COOH} & \\
\text{Lysine (Lys)} & \text{Ornithine (Orn)}
\end{array}
$$

chains. Its derivatives include hydroxylysine, desmosine and isodesmosine (Chapter 27). *Ornithine*, a lower homologue of lysine, which contains five instead of six carbon atoms is not found in proteins although small quantities occur free in the liver where it is involved in the synthesis of urea.

Arginine is even more strongly basic than lysine owing to the presence of the guanidino group. No protein has yet been discovered which does not contain arginine. The free amino acid, like ornithine, is involved in the urea cycle. *Histidine* owes its basic properties to the presence of

$$
\left.
\begin{array}{l}
\mathrm{NH_2} \\
\mathrm{C}{=}\mathrm{NH} \\
\mathrm{NH}
\end{array}
\right\} \text{Guanidino group}
$$
$$
\begin{array}{l}
\mathrm{CH_2} \\
| \\
\mathrm{CH_2} \\
| \\
\mathrm{CH_2} \quad \text{Arginine (Arg)} \\
| \\
\mathrm{CHNH_2} \\
| \\
\mathrm{COOH}
\end{array}
$$

the imidazole ring. This grouping is only weakly basic and within the physiological pH range (6·5–7·5) where dissociation occurs histidine may function either as a proton donor or proton acceptor. This is probably the reason for the crucial role of histidine residues in the activity of many enzymes, including trypsin and chymotrypsin (page 86).

$$
\underset{\text{Histidine (His)}}{\mathrm{HC}{=}\mathrm{C}{-}\mathrm{CH_2CHNH_3}^{+}{\cdot}\mathrm{COO}^{-}} \xrightleftharpoons[pK'\,6{\cdot}04]{} \mathrm{HC}{=}\mathrm{C}{-}\mathrm{CH_2CHNH_3}^{+}{\cdot}\mathrm{COO}^{-}
$$

Amino acids with other non-ionizable substituents

Those containing a hydroxyl group

The three amino acids in this group are serine, threonine and tyrosine. *Serine* contains an alcoholic hydroxyl group and is β-hydroxyalanine. *Threonine* is the next higher homologue to serine. It has two asymmetric carbon atoms and can therefore exist in four forms but only one of these, L-threonine, is found in proteins. The –OH group of some serine and threonine residues in certain proteins may be phosphorylated to give phosphoserine and phosphothreonine. *Tyrosine* is an aromatic amino acid and in this respect may be classified with phenylalanine and tryptophan. In addition, it contains a phenolic hydroxyl group which is weakly acidic and loses a proton above pH 9. Thyroxine and other iodinated derivatives of tyrosine are found in the thyroid gland (page 360).

Serine (Ser)   Threonine (Thr)   Tyrosine (Tyr)

The sulphur-containing amino acids

These are cysteine, cystine and methionine. *Cysteine* is the sulphur analogue of serine and is the only amino acid to contain a sulphydryl (–SH) group. The activity of a number of enzymes has been found to depend on the presence of the –SH group of cysteine. If this group is oxidized these enzymes lose their activity.

Cysteine (Cys)   Cystine   Methionine (Met)

When two cysteine residues are oxidized they become united by a disulphide (–S–S–) bond to form the diamino acid *cystine*. The disulphide bond is a covalent bond and is found in some proteins, e.g. insulin (page 53). It is very important since it serves to form stable cross-linkages between different polypeptide chains or different parts of the same chain.

Methionine, which possesses sulphur in thioether linkage, cannot be synthesized in the animal body. It plays an important part in metabolic processes as a donor of methyl groups.

Acid amides

Also belonging to the group of amino acids with non-ionizable side chains are *asparagine* and *glutamine*, the acid amides of aspartic acid and glutamic acid respectively. Owing to the amide substitution on the β or γ group their side chains are no longer ionizable and like all but the basic and acidic amino acids they therefore come in the category of *neutral amino acids*. The acid amides are also found in the free form. In animals glutamine provides a small reserve of readily available nitrogen while asparagine occurs abundantly in plants where it fulfils a similar role.

$$\begin{array}{l} CONH_2 \\ | \\ \beta\, CH_2 \\ | \\ \alpha\, CHNH_2 \\ | \\ COOH \end{array} \qquad\qquad \begin{array}{l} CONH_2 \\ | \\ \gamma\, CH_2 \\ | \\ \beta\, CH_2 \\ | \\ \alpha\, CHNH_2 \\ | \\ COOH \end{array}$$

Asparagine (Asn)   Glutamine (Gln)

Miscellaneous

Of the three *aromatic amino acids* phenylalanine, tyrosine and tryptophan, phenylalanine has been classified with the hydrophobic amino acids which have a non-polar side chain and tyrosine with those containing a hydroxyl group. This leaves *tryptophan*, the largest and rarest of the amino acids which contains the heterocyclic indole nucleus as its bulky R group. Trytophan is the parent compound for the neurotransmitter serotonin which is 5-hydroxytryptamine.

$$CH_2CH(NH_2)\cdot COOH$$

Tryptophan (β-indole alanine) (Trp)

Unusual amino acids

The following amino acids are not coded for genetically and are only found in proteins of rather special types:

Amino acid	*Where found*
Hydroxyproline	Collagen and elastin
Hydroxylysine	Collagen
Phosphoserine	Various enzymes, caseinogen
Desmosine	Elastin
Isodesmosine	Elastin
Thyroxine	Thyroglobulin
γ-Carboxyglutamic acid	Blood-clotting factors and some other calcium-binding proteins

They are formed by modification of one of the common amino acids after the peptide chain has been assembled.

A few more amino acids take part in metabolic reactions but are not present in proteins. They include ornithine, citrulline, γ-aminobutyric acid and dihydroxyphenylalanine.

Abbreviated notations for the common amino acids are given in Table 4.1.

Table 4.1 Abbreviated notations for amino acids

Amino acid	Three-letter abbreviation	One-letter abbreviation	Molecular weight of residue	pK value of R groups
Alanine	Ala	A	71	—
Arginine	Arg	R	157	12·5
Aspartate	Asp	D	114	3·9
Asparagine	Asn	N	114	—
Cysteine	Cys	C	103	—
Glutamate	Glu	E	128	4·3
Glutamine	Gln	Q	128	—
Glycine	Gly	G	57	—
Histidine	His	H	137	6·0
Isoleucine	Ile	I	113	—
Leucine	Leu	L	113	—
Lysine	Lys	K	128	10·5
Methionine	Met	M	131	—
Phenylalanine	Phe	F	147	—
Proline	Pro	P	97	—
Serine	Ser	S	87	—
Threonine	Thr	T	101	—
Tryptophan	Trp	W	186	—
Tyrosine	Tyr	Y	163	10·1
Valine	Val	V	99	—
		Weighted mean	108·7	

Some properties and reactions of amino acids

The properties and reactions of the amino acids may be broadly divided into three types: those due to the presence of (1) the acidic α–COOH group, (2) the basic α–NH_2 group, and (3) the side chain grouping. Reactions of types (1) and (2) are general reactions and may be expected to be given by all amino acids, whereas those of type (3) differ according to the particular amino acid.

Peptide bond formation

The most important reaction of the amino acids is their ability to condense together to form peptides. The presence of the two different types of functional group means that the amino group of one amino acid can join covalently with the carboxyl group of a second to give a *dipeptide* containing two amino acid residues.

$$\underset{\substack{| \\ H_2N-CH-COOH}}{R'} + \underset{\substack{| \\ H_2N-CH-COOH}}{R''} \longrightarrow \underset{\substack{| \\ H_2N-CH \vdots CO-NH \vdots CH-COOH}}{R' \qquad\qquad R''}$$

peptide bond

$+\ H_2O$

The resulting combination of a carbonyl group and an imino group is known as a *peptide bond*. The dipeptide is left with a free –NH_2 group at one end of the molecule and a free –COOH group at the other, so that further amino acids can be added at either end of the molecule. In this way molecules containing three, four or more amino acids may be built up to give *tri-*, *tetra-*, *oligo-* or *poly-peptides* according to the number of amino acid residues that they contain. In protein biosynthesis addition always occurs on the free –COOH group.

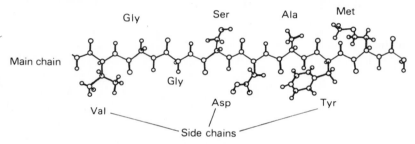

$$\underset{\substack{\text{N-terminal}\\\text{residue}}}{\text{H}_2\text{N}-\underset{\text{R}^1}{\text{CH}}-\text{CO}-}\text{HN}-\underset{\text{R}^{28}}{\text{CH}}-\text{CO}-\text{NH}-\underset{\text{R}^{29}}{\text{CH}}-\text{CO}-\text{NH}-\underset{\text{R}^{30}}{\text{CH}}-\text{CO}-\text{NH}-\underset{\substack{\text{R}^{127}\\\ \\\text{C-Terminal}\\\text{residue}}}{\text{CH}}-\text{COOH}$$

An essential feature of proteins and peptides is that they have a regular backbone structure with repeated triple groupings (–NH·CHR·CO–). The amino acid residue bearing the free –NH$_2$ group is known as the *N-terminal amino acid* and by convention is given on the left, while the amino acid at the other end of the chain with the free α-COOH group is known as the *C-terminal amino acid* and is shown on the right. The amino acid residues are arranged in a specific linear sequence so that the side chains of the constituent amino acids project on alternate sides of the backbone giving a different pattern for each protein (Figure 4.2).

Figure 4.2 Part of an extended polypeptide chain with projecting side chain groups

The ninhydrin reaction

Amino acids react with ninhydrin which is a strong oxidizing agent with the release of CO$_2$ and NH$_3$ and the production of an aldehyde with one less C atom than the original amino acid.

$$\text{R}\cdot\text{CHNH}_2\cdot\text{COOH} \xrightarrow{\text{O}} \text{R}\cdot\text{CHO} + \text{NH}_3 + \text{CO}_2$$

The reaction is the basis of various methods for the determination of amino acids since it is possible to measure (1) the CO$_2$ produced, (2) the NH$_3$ produced and (3) the colour intensity obtained when the liberated ammonia reacts with a further molecule of ninhydrin to produce a purple compound which can be assayed photometrically. This is the method by which amino acids are estimated using an amino acid analyser. The imino acids (proline and hydroxyproline) give yellow products instead of a purple one. Amino acids give a strong reaction with ninhydrin, but proteins and polypeptides, which contain far fewer free amino groups, give a much weaker reaction.

Ionization of amino acids

Amino acids have amphoteric properties and can function both as proton donors as a result of dissociation of the carboxyl group

$$\text{–COOH} \rightarrow \text{–COO}^- + \text{H}^+$$

and as proton acceptors, i.e. bases due to the presence of the amino group.

$$-NH_2 + H^+ \rightarrow -NH_3^+$$

In solutions at low pH the amino acid acts as a proton acceptor and becomes positively charged, while at high pH values it loses a proton and becomes negatively charged. The intermediate pH at which the amino acid carries no net charge varies with the amino acid in question and is known as its *isoelectric point*. Although at this pH the amino acid is electrically neutral this is not because it is uncharged but because it exists in a dipolar or *zwitterion* form and carries positive and negative charges in equal amounts.

$$
\begin{array}{ccc}
\text{R} & \text{R} & \text{R} \\
| & | & | \\
\text{CHNH}_3^+ & \text{CHNH}_3^+ & \text{CHNH}_2 \\
| & | & | \\
\text{COOH} & \text{COO}^- & \text{COO}^-
\end{array}
$$

Cationic form $(+1)$	*Dipolar form* (0)	*Anionic form* (-1)
at low pH	at isoelectric	at high pH
(fully protonated)	point	(all protons lost)

Earlier it was seen that at the half-equivalence point of the titration of a weak acid in dilute solution, i.e. when the acid and its salt are present in equal amounts $pH = pK_a$ and at this point the buffering action is most efficient. It follows therefore that amino acids, which each have at least two pK values, will have at least two buffer ranges, one in the range of pK_{a1} where $R \cdot CHNH_3^+ \cdot COOH$ and $R \cdot CHNH_3^+ COO^-$ are present in equal amounts and the other in the region of pK_{a2} where $R \cdot CHNH_3^+ COO^-$ and $R-CHNH_2 \cdot COO^-$ are present in equal amounts. This is illustrated by the titration curve for glycine shown in Figure 4.3, where it may be seen that $pK_{a1} = 2 \cdot 4$ and $pK_{a2} = 9 \cdot 8$. The isoelectric point of glycine, i.e. the pH at which all the molecules carry equal numbers of positive and negative charges, will be given by

$$pI = \frac{pK_{a1} + pK_{a2}}{2} = \frac{2 \cdot 4 + 9 \cdot 8}{2} = 6 \cdot 1$$

The situation is more complicated for amino acids that carry extra ionizable groupings, e.g. the basic and acidic amino acids. For example, glutamic acid which has a second –COOH group in

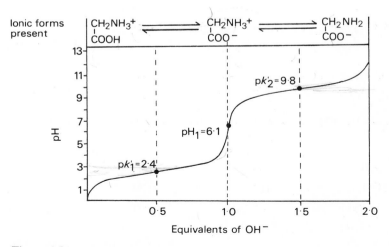

Figure 4.3 Titration curve of glycine

the γ-position may exist in four distinct forms according to the degree of ionization of its various polar groups.

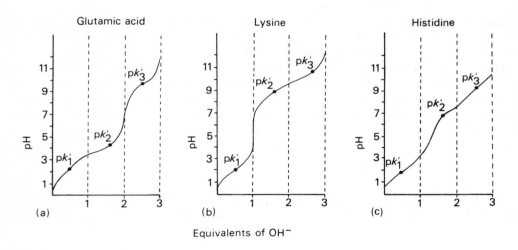

Thus glutamic acid has three dissociation constants $pK_{a1} = 2\cdot19$, $pK_{a2} = 4\cdot25$ and $pK_{a3} = 9\cdot67$ and its isoelectric point lies midway between pK_{a1} and pK_{a2} and is therefore $3\cdot22$ (Figure 4.4). At physiological pH values glutamic and aspartic acids are negatively charged and exist in the form of glutamate and aspartate.

Figure 4.4 Titration curves of glutamic acid, lysine and histidine

Other groupings which may dissociate to leave a negatively charged group are the β-carboxyl group of aspartate, the sulphydryl (–SH) group of cysteine, and the phenolic hydroxyl group of tyrosine.

The basic amino acid lysine also exists in four different ionic forms which may be represented as:

Starting with the dipolar form it can be seen that two equivalents of acid are required to convert it to the cationic (2+) form and one equivalent of alkali for its conversion to the anionic form. The isoelectric point of lysine falls between pK_{a2} and pK_{a3} (Figure 4.4b).

$$pI = \frac{8\cdot95 + 10\cdot53}{2} = 9\cdot74$$

Certain properties of amino acids (and consequently of proteins) depend on their ionization characteristics and so are affected by pH. These include solubility, optical rotation, their ability to chelate metals and to take part in biological reactions. Most amino acids are least soluble at their isoelectric point probably because of mutual attraction between the oppositely charged groups of neighbouring molecules, the number of charges being greatest in the dipolar form. From what has been said it will be clear that, within the physiological pH range, all the amino acids exist in a charged form and from now on this is how they will be written.

The separation of amino acids

Amino acids may be separated by various methods. Separation is achieved on the basis of such characteristics as adsorption, partition between partially miscible phases, ion-exchange and electrophoresis. Details of the techniques can be found in text books of practical biochemistry.

Chapter 5
Peptides and proteins

From the biological point of view the most important reaction which the amino acids undergo is condensation and the formation of peptide bonds (page 39). This reaction is responsible for a vast spectrum of compounds containing anything from two to many hundreds of amino acid residues. The smaller members of the group containing less than 10–20 residues are classed as *oligopeptides* while above this they are known as *polypeptides*. It is customary, however, to refer to polypeptides which have a molecular weight of more than 10 000 as *proteins* and those with lower values simply as *peptides*. This distinction is arbitrary but convenient. The average molecular weight of the amino acid residues present in polypeptides is rather less than 110 (Table 4.1), so that a molecular weight of 10 000 is roughly equivalent to 100 residues.

Although the mammalian peptides normally contain only those amino acids that are found in proteins linked by normal peptide bonds, some of the peptides produced by micro-organisms show unusual features such as the presence of ornithine and of D-amino acids.

Peptides

Peptides are widely distributed in nature and show a great range of biological activities. Most tissues contain them and more than 30 have been found in the mammalian nervous system. They are also present in plants, fungi and bacteria and include some of the most biologically active compounds known. Some of the antibiotics, e.g. penicillin, gramicidin and chloramphenicol, are essentially peptide in character as are some extremely toxic substances, e.g. the fungal poisons amanitin and phalloidin. The botulinus, tetanus and black widow spider toxins are all polypeptide neurotoxins. A list of some of the best characterized peptides is given in Table 5.1. They include hormones, released from the hypothalamus, posterior pituitary, gut and pancreas and neuropeptides such as the opioids and tissue growth factors.

The mammalian peptides often occur in families which may be products of a single gene or of closely related multiple genes. Peptides are currently arousing considerable interest because *neuropeptides* are now thought to play a part not only in pain perception, in feeding and temperature control but also in memory and learning ability! More is said about the neuropeptides and tissue growth factors in Chapter 24.

Table 5.1 Some biologically active peptides of animal origin

Substance	No. of amino acid residues	Source	Activity
Glutathione	3	Wide distribution	Maintenance of –SH groups
Oxytocin	9	Posterior pituitary	Contraction of uterus. Let-down of milk
Vasopressin	9	Posterior pituitary	Vasoconstrictor, Antidiuretic
Calcitonin	10	Thyroid	Lowering of blood Ca^{2+}. Inhibition of bone resorption
Gastrin	17	Pyloric region of stomach	Secretion of HCl by stomach
Glucagon	29	α-Cells of pancreatic islets	Raising of blood sugar. Increase of glycogen breakdown in liver
ACTH	39	Anterior pituitary	Release of adrenal cortical hormones
Parathormone	84	Parathyroid	Mobilization of Ca^{2+}. Increase of blood Ca^{2+}

Proteins

Proteins comprise more than half the solid matter of the body. They are responsible for virtually all the reactions which occur within the tissues as well as being of structural importance. Proteins are macromolecules and have colloidal properties but their molecules are not necessarily very large. Their molecular weights range from an arbitrary lower limit of 10 000 to several million and from its DNA content it has been estimated that the human body contains some 100 000 different types of protein. Proteins are, moreover, usually unique to the species from which they are derived so that human serum albumin is distinct from that of a duck, dog, hen or horse and, although similar in structure and function, they have slight differences in composition and are immunologically distinct. From this it can be seen that proteins must exist in almost infinite variety and some idea of the range of their functions may be obtained from Table 5.2. Nevertheless all proteins are derived from the same selection of 20 amino acids which are joined by peptide linkages into long unbranched polypeptide chains. Their main distinguishing characteristics lie in the precise selection of amino acids and the sequence or order in which they follow one another in the polypeptide chain which is genetically determined.

Although the polypeptide chains are linear and unbranched, their component amino acids interact with one another in a number of different ways causing the molecules to assume highly specific shapes and/or combinations of chains. Interactions may occur

1. between different parts of the same chain
2. between two or more chains which may be of the same or different types
3. between a polypeptide chain and a non-protein molecule or molecules. This latter type of interaction produces the so-called *conjugated proteins*, e.g. haemoglobin, the lipoproteins of cell membranes and the nucleoproteins of the chromosomes. The non-protein part of the molecule is known as the *prosthetic group*.

Proteins can be broadly divided into two categories – fibrous and globular.

Table 5.2 Functional classification of proteins

1. Enzyme and enzyme precursors
2. Structural proteins:
   a. Keratin: found in epidermal structures,
      e.g. hair, nails, surface layers of the skin
   b. Collagen: main protein of connective tissues present in bone and dentine
   c. Elastin: present in elastic fibres of connective tissue, especially in arterial walls
   d. Fibrin: protein of blood clots formed from soluble precursor, fibrinogen
   e. Silk fibroin: constituent of silk fibres
3. Transport proteins:
   a. Oxygen-carrying: haemoglobin
   b. Hydrogen-carrying: flavoproteins
   c. Electron-transporting: cytochromes
   d. Fatty acid-transporting: serum albumin
   e. Metal-carrying serum proteins: transferrins (iron), caeruloplasmin (copper)
4. Receptor proteins
5. Hormones:
   a. Protein hormones: insulin, growth hormone, follicle-stimulating hormone
   b. Polypeptide hormones: gastrin, vasopressin, oxytocin, calcitonin, glucagon, adrenocortico-
      tropic hormone
6. Contractile proteins: actomyosin of muscle
7. Lubricants: glycoproteins present in saliva and dental plaque and generally in secretions of the
   gastrointestinal, respiratory and urinary tracts
8. Storage proteins:
   a. Myoglobin: O_2 storage in red muscle
   b. Ferritin: iron reserves in liver and spleen
   c. Phosvitin: phosphate reserves in egg yolk
9. Chromosomal protein:
   a. Histones: basic proteins found in association with DNA and somehow involved in the control
      of gene activity
   b. Acidic proteins believed to be concerned in the more precise aspects of gene control
10. Immunity-conferring proteins: immunoglobulins of various types
11. Bactericidal proteins: lysozyme present in tears, nasal mucus and other secretions and also in
    egg-white
12. ? Memory proteins: long term memory in higher animals *may* be encoded in some brain proteins
13. Virus proteins: these form a protective coat round the viral nucleic acid
14. Controlling proteins: e.g. nerve growth factor
15. Miscellaneous: e.g. proton conductance protein of brown adipose tissue

Fibrous proteins

These include nearly all the structural proteins which have molecules with a high axial (length/width) ratio. Most of them are very insoluble and metabolically unreactive. They include the various *keratins* found in the skin and its appendages, the *fibrin* of blood clots, and *collagen* and *elastin* the protein constituents of connective tissues. *Myosin* the fibrous protein of muscle contains both fibrous and globular regions and is both metabolically reactive and relatively soluble.

In the fibrous proteins a large number of molecules of the same type associate to form sheets or bundles. Association of the molecules occurs in the first instance as the result of the formation of weak non-covalent bonds but, subsequently, strong covalent bonds develop which convert the structure into a rigid insoluble aggregate usually of considerable strength. The structure of keratin is dealt with on page 401, fibrin on page 386 and collagen and elastin in Chapter 27.

Globular proteins

There are an enormous number of soluble proteins each of which fulfils a specific function or functions. They are usually more or less globular in shape and have highly characteristic conformations which are designed to bring particular reactive chemical groups together or to force them apart. To do this the molecules must be folded in a complex manner in order to produce a specific shape and charge pattern. The larger proteins often consist of two or more separate chains which may or may not be identical. Such proteins are said to be *oligomeric* and their constituent chains are known as *subunits* or *monomers*. Oligomeric proteins usually have more complex functions than single chain proteins. They are often able to react appropriately to physiological changes and hence play an important part in the control of metabolism (Chapter 23). The folded shapes of the globular proteins are inherently flexible and are able to undergo subtle changes which relate to their biological function. The normal biologically active form of such proteins is known as the *native* form and when major changes in its three-dimensional characteristics are induced by some external agent and cause a marked reduction in its biological activity, the protein is said to be *denatured* (page 63).

The ionization of proteins

Proteins in aqueous solution behave as giant polyions, with positively and negatively charged groups projecting from the molecule at various points. These are associated with various small *counterions* which help to maintain local and general electrical neutrality. The charged groups on a protein markedly affect its behaviour and the configuration which it adopts, since like charges repel and unlike ones attract each other.

Nearly all the ionizable groups of proteins are contributed by the side chain groups of amino acid residues because all but the terminal α-amino and α-carboxyl groups are involved in peptide linkages which do not ionize. The properties of the main ionizable groups in proteins are summarized in Table 5.3.

Below pH 1·5 the protein is fully protonated and has maximum positive charge, since at this pH it possesses no negatively charged groups and a maximum number of cationic groups on the

Table 5.3 The ionizable groups of proteins

Ionizable group	Acid form	pK_a value at 25°C	Conjugate base
α-COOH (*C*-terminal)	–COOH	3·0–3·2	–COO$^-$
β-COOH (Asp)	–COOH	3·0–4·7	–COO$^-$
γ-COOH (Glu)	–COOH	4·4	–COO$^-$
Imidazole (His)	$-C=CH$ ^+HN NH C H	6·2–7·6	$-C=CH$ N NH C H
α-amino (*N*-terminal)	–NH$_3^+$	7·6–8·4	–NH$_2$
ε-amino (Lys)	–NH$_3^+$	9·4–10·6	–NH$_2$
Sulphydryl (Cys)	–SH	9·1–10·8	–S$^-$
Phenolic hydroxyl (Tyr)	–OH	9·8–10·4	–O$^-$
Guanidinium (Arg)	$-NH-C\!\!<^{NH_3^+}_{NH}$	11·6–12·6	$-NH-C\!\!<^{NH_2}_{NH}$

basic amino acid residues. As the pH is increased, hydrogen ions are lost so that its charge, originally highly positive, is progressively reduced to zero, after which the protein molecule gradually acquires an increasing net negative charge. Each type of ionizable group has its own characteristic pK value and a buffering effect centred at the pK value and extending about 1·5 units on either side of it.

Proteins thus act as buffers at many regions of pH and make a significant contribution to total buffering in cells and tissues. Most importantly, the imidazole side chains of the histidine residues lose their positive charge between pH 6·5 and 8·0 and, since this change in ionization occurs within the physiological range, it is highly significant both as a buffering factor and in causing changes in charge distribution and molecular configuration in living cells and tissue.

Proteins, like amino acids, have an isoelectric point at which they are 'self-neutralized' and have zero net charge. The isoelectric point is largely determined by the ratio of the free acidic (Asp and Glu) to basic (Lys and Arg) amino acid residues. The majority of proteins contain a preponderance of the acidic amino acids, that is Glu + Asp, so that their isoelectric point (pI) is less than 7·0, and they are negatively charged at neutral pH. On the other hand, basic proteins such as the histones, which have a marked preponderance of lysine and arginine, are positively charged at neutral pH. Proteins with different isoelectric points will interact, and a basic protein will tend to form a precipitate with an acidic one. Insulin protaminate formed by combination of insulin (pI 5) with protamine (pI 12) is relatively insoluble and is more slowly absorbed in the body; consequently it has a more prolonged action than ordinary insulin. In the cell nucleus, basic histones are bound to the nucleic acids and may function as regulators of gene activity (Chapter 21).

Protein purification and identification

Before the structure and properties of a protein can be studied it must be obtained in a pure condition. Protein purification is laborious and difficult for three reasons.

1. With a few exceptions, such as haemoglobin, myosin and collagen, individual proteins are present to an extent of less than 0.5% of the starting material.
2. Proteins rarely, if ever, occur singly and, since they differ essentially only in the proportions and sequence of their constituent amino acids, their reactions are very similar so that their separation requires highly selective methods.
3. Owing to the reactivity and instability of most proteins many of the chemical and physical agents which might otherwise be employed cause their denaturation (page 63). Proteins are, for example, sensitive not only to heat and extremes of pH but also to the presence of organic solvents, detergents, heavy metals and many other substances.

The first stage in the isolation of a protein which is not already in solution, e.g. in plasma or milk, is to release it from cell structures. Cells may be disrupted by homogenization, exposure to hypo-osmotic solutions or to ultrasonic vibrations, or by drying them to a powder with acetone at low temperatures. This latter process also serves to remove lipids and facilitates subsequent extraction of the protein.

Once the cells have been disintegrated, the proteins may be extracted with a dilute buffer solution of appropriate pH and ionic strength. From this crude extract means must be found of isolating the required protein from others present. Methods for separating proteins include differential precipitation, ion-exchange chromatography, electrophoresis, gel filtration and ultracentrifugation.

One of the difficulties encountered in protein purification is how to test for the desired protein among other protein contaminants. This is relatively simple if the protein is an enzyme or a hormone, since *the specific activity* of the preparation may be followed. Specific activity, defined as the activity per unit weight of total protein, increases as the protein becomes progressively purer until no further purification occurs. This may result either because purification has been completed or because the method is not effecting any further purification. The problem of determining whether or not a protein is pure is extremely difficult since ordinary criteria (such as melting point determination) cannot be applied, and, although crystalline preparations of proteins can sometimes be obtained, these may nevertheless still be mixtures. A further complication arises because polypeptide chains may interact specifically with other polypeptide chains. Criteria of purity for proteins are therefore necessarily negative, a protein being assumed to be pure or at least homogeneous if it cannot be shown to be impure. With the development of the highly sensitive technique SDS-PAGE (sodium dodecyl sulphate–polyacrylamide gel electrophoresis) if the protein shows as a single band, it is almost certainly homogeneous. This method which is the one which is now most commonly used depends mainly on molecular size.

Since the only criterion of protein purity is consistent failure to detect inhomogeneity, a protein should be tested by at least two methods that depend on different molecular characteristics as the basis of separation. Thus techniques such as ion-exchange chromatography or electrophoresis, which depend on charge differences, should be used in conjunction with others such as ultracentrifugation and gel filtration, which are based on differences in molecular size and shape.

Affinity chromatography

This valuable technique which may be used to purify certain proteins is very simple in principle. It depends on the highly specific binding affinity of pairs of compounds such as enzymes and inhibitors, hormones and their receptors or antigens and antibodies. It is first necessary to attach covalently one of the pair of high-affinity compounds (ligands) to an insoluble matrix without interfering with its specific binding properties. This may not be easy but, once it has been achieved, the high-affinity material to which, for example, a trypsin inhibitor has been attached, can be packed into a column; then, when an appropriately buffered solution containing trypsin is passed through the column the trypsin is strongly bound to the resin via the inhibitor while the impurities pass through it freely. The trypsin may subsequently be eluted from the solid phase, e.g. by changing the buffer in the column to one having a pH at which the inhibitor has no affinity for trypsin. This liberates the trypsin which is eluted in a pure state. The method can be used not only for the separation of proteins but also for peptides, nucleic acids and polysaccharides or any other substance which takes part in highly specific interactions with a substance which can be covalently linked to an appropriate stationary phase.

The size and shape of protein molecules

Methods which give absolute values for the molecular weight of a protein depend upon determination of their osmotic pressure, their rate of diffusion or their rate of sedimentation in the ultracentrifuge. Such methods, though simple in theory, require expensive equipment and meticulous technique for accurate results. However, under reducing conditions which break –S–S– bridges and with the use of marker proteins of known molecular weight the SDS-PAGE method mentioned earlier provides a means by which the approximate molecular weight of a protein may be simply and rapidly determined.

The molecular weight of a single molecular species is, of course, independent of the method used for its determination. However, owing to the tendency of protein molecules to associate and form aggregates, e.g. gels and fibres, or complexes with other cell constituents such as lipids and nucleic acids, one of the problems of the protein chemist is to decide whether the entities under any given conditions represent a single molecular species or a molecular aggregate. For example, it has been established that the molecule of haemoglobin is made up of four separate polypeptide chains that may only be separated under conditions which are outside the physiological range. The individual chains are consequently regarded as subunits of the haemoglobin molecule. It is now recognized that many large proteins are built up of smaller subunits (Table 5.4). The subunits are held together by non-covalent bonds which are weak enough to be broken by reagents, such as urea, that are unable to break covalent bonds. The construction of large units from a number of smaller ones is a sound building principle which increases the flexibility of the resulting structure and reduces the likelihood of errors. Thus if any single unit is defective either it has little effect on the structure as a whole or it may be rejected in favour of a normal one.

Table 5.4 Molecular weights and subunit constitution of various proteins

Protein	Molecular weight	Number of subunits
Ribonuclease	12 600	1
Lysozyme (egg white)	13 900	1
Myoglobin	16 900	1
Malate dehydrogenase	66 300	2
Glycerol-1-phosphate dehydrogenase	78 000	2
Creatine kinase	80 000	2
Enolase	82 000	2
α-Amylase	97 600	2
Haemoglobin	64 500	4
Hexokinase	102 000	4
Lactate dehydrogenase	150 000	4
Fumarase	194 000	4
Catalase	232 000	4
Pyruvate kinase	237 000	4
Glucose-6-phosphate dehydrogenase	240 000	6
Mitochondrial ATPase	284 000	10
Phosphorylase *a*	370 000	4
Glutamine synthetase	592 000	12

Information regarding the shape of protein molecules may be obtained from measurements of viscosity, light scattering or streaming birefringence, aided by electron microscopy and X-ray diffraction analysis. This last technique is specially valuable since it can be used to provide not merely the overall shape of a protein molecule but also a detailed picture of its molecular architecture.

The generation of individuality in protein molecules

There are a number of ways in which proteins, which as we have seen are basically very similar, are stamped with individual characteristics. Differences may be summarized as follows:

1. The sequence of the amino acids. It would in theory be possible to have two proteins of identical amino acid composition with completely different properties if the amino acids were strung together in a different order.

2. The presence (or not) of stable intrachain and/or interchain cross-linkages, e.g. disulphide bonds.
3. The loose non-covalent association of two or more polypeptide chains of the same or different types.
4. The presence of non-protein prosthetic groups as in glycoproteins, phosphoproteins, lipoproteins, chromoproteins and nucleoproteins.

The structural organization of globular proteins

Both the structural and functional properties of a protein depend ultimately on the nature and sequence of amino acids in the polypeptide chain or chains of which it is composed. This is referred to as its *primary structure* and the peptide bonds that join the various amino acids together are strong covalent bonds. The primary structure of a protein may be compared with the structural formula of a small molecular compound, but protein chains do not usually exist either in a simple extended linear form or as a random coil. Instead they have a specific three-dimensional structure which is predetermined by the primary structure and which, in turn, determines their biological characteristics.

Three further levels of organization may be superimposed on the primary structure of globular proteins; these are known as the *secondary*, *tertiary* and *quaternary* levels respectively.

The *secondary level of organization* results from the formation of a regular pattern of hydrogen bonds between the –CO and –NH groups which occur on either side of the peptide bonds of the backbone structure. The hydrogen bonds may join different parts of the same chain, or may serve to link different polypeptide chains. As a result of these *regular patterns of hydrogen bonding*, the chains become either helically coiled or united into sheet-like structures. Secondary structuring tends to occur in all proteins but, superimposed upon it are interactions between side chain R groups that may profoundly modify the secondary structure. These *R group interactions* are specific for the protein in question and are responsible for folding the chain into the compact globular shape which constitutes its *tertiary structure*. Thus short stretches of regular helical coiling or sheet-like structure are interspersed with irregularly folded segments.

The quaternary level of organization, which is not found in all proteins, refers to the association of a number of polypeptide chains or subunits to form a single complex molecule.

The primary structure

The primary structure of every protein is specified by a gene, i.e. it is a linear transcript, in terms of amino acids of a linear sequence of bases in DNA, and as already mentioned the primary structure is responsible both for the overall conformation of the protein and for its biological function. The first protein to have its complete amino sequence established was *insulin* the hormone produced by the pancreatic islets. The insulin of most mammals has been found to be a small zinc-containing protein. Its individual polypeptide chains have a molecular weight of just under 6000 but these associate to give a polymeric complex containing six separate chains. Each monomeric unit contains 51 amino acid residues. (It may be noted that the approximate number of residues in a protein may be calculated by dividing its molecular weight by 110. This figure, allowing for the loss of a molecule of water during the formation of the peptide bonds, represents the average molecular weight of the amino acid residues present in proteins.) As a result of ten years' work at Cambridge, Sanger, in 1955, was able to specify the precise sequence in which the amino acids are arranged within the bovine insulin molecule. Since the peptide bonds linking the amino acids together are covalent, sequence determination has to be tackled by chemical or enzymic methods and Sanger's first step was to identify the *N*-terminal amino acid. He did this by coupling its free amino group to dinitrofluorobenzene (DNFB) to give a dinitrophenol (DNP) derivative. The protein was then broken down by acid hydrolysis into its component amino acids which were separated by paper chromatography. The labelled DNP amino acid could readily be identified.

$$O_2N-\!\!\bigcirc\!\!-F \ + \ H_2N-\underset{\underset{R^2}{|}}{CH}-CO-NH-\underset{\underset{R^2}{|}}{CH}-CO\cdots\cdots COOH$$

DNFB   Protein

$$O_2N-\!\!\bigcirc\!\!-NH-\underset{\underset{R^2}{|}}{CH}-CO-NH-\underset{\underset{R^2}{|}}{CH}-CO\cdots\cdots COOH \ + \ HF$$

DNP-protein

Acid hydrolysis

$$O_2N-\!\!\bigcirc\!\!-NH\cdot\underset{\underset{|}{R^1}}{CH}\cdot COOH \ + \ _x(NH_2-\underset{\underset{|}{R}}{CH}-COOH)$$

DNP-amino acid   Unlabelled amino acids

The *C*-terminal amino acid could likewise be identified using the pancreatic enzyme carboxy-peptidase which is highly specific and attacks the peptide bond which joins the *C*-terminal amino acid to the rest of the chain. Once liberated the *C*-terminal amino acid could be separated and identified.

By the application of such methods of *end group analysis* Sanger discovered that the insulin monomer contained two *N*-terminal and two *C*-terminal amino acids and that it consists of two polypeptide chains joined securely together by covalent disulphide bridges. In order to study their amino acid sequence it was necessary to break the S–S bonds by oxidizing them to $-SO_3^-$ groups with performic acid. The two chains (A and B) could then be separated and independently analysed. For the sequence determinations Sanger used mild methods of hydrolysis in order to split the polypeptide chain into a number of relatively small fragments which could be isolated and their amino acid composition and sequence determined. By using more than one method of hydrolysis so that the chain was broken at a number of different points it was possible, by identifying overlapping sequences of amino acids, to deduce an unequivocal sequence for the original chain. For example from one stretch of the B chain the following peptides were derived:

Dipeptides   His-Leu   Glu-Ala   Leu-Val   Ala-Leu   Ser-His   Val-Glu
Tripeptides   Val-Glu-Ala   Ser-His-Leu   Leu-Val-Glu
Tetrapeptides   Leu-Val-Glu-Ala   Ser-His-Leu-Val

From this it is clear that the original sequence must have been

Ser-His-Leu-Val-Glu-Ala-Leu

Even when the complete amino acid sequence of both A and B chains, which were found to contain 21 and 30 residues respectively, had been worked out, the problem of determining the position of the –S–S– bridges, which link the chains together, remained. Although this proved to be difficult, it was eventually solved and the primary structure of bovine insulin was found to be as shown in Figure 5.1. Its interesting double chain structure results from the fact that, although synthesized as one continuous chain, a portion is subsequently excised from the middle of the chain (Figure 24·6).

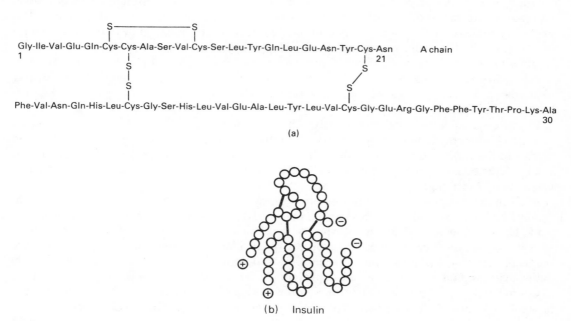

(a)

(b)   Insulin

Figure 5.1 The structure of insulin. (a) The amino acid sequence; (b) folding as determined by the disulphide bonds

Sanger had chosen insulin for his work for several reasons: (1) The smallness of its molecule; (2) supplies were available in a reasonably pure form; (3) on account of its hormonal effect it is a substance of great physiological interest and medical importance.

However, insulin is not a very typical protein because of the shortness of its polypeptide chains and the –S–S– bridge which links residues 6 and 11 of the A chain. Similar loops containing six residues are found in the posterior pituitary hormones oxytocin and vasopressin, while one containing seven residues is found in calcitonin. Their special significance, if any, is not known.

Since Sanger's original breakthrough, amino acid sequence studies have been carried out on a great variety of proteins. Polypeptide chains that are much longer than those of insulin must initially be split into several shorter reproducible fragments for sequence determination. The pancreatic enzyme trypsin is widely used for this as it is highly specific and acts only on peptide bonds which involve the carbonyl group of the basic amino acids, i.e. of either lysine or arginine (page 36). Thus, polypeptide chains are cleaved by trypsin into a number of fragments in all of which, excepting the one which contains the original C-terminal residue, either lysine or arginine is C-terminal. For example a polypeptide containing 121 residues with arginine at positions 7, 56 and 72 and lysine at positions 29 and 101 would give the following fragments when digested with trypsin.

1—7, 8—29, 30—56, 57—72, 73—101, 102—121
Arg   Lys   Arg   Arg   Lys

The peptides may be separated by electrophoresis on filter paper followed by chromatography at right angles to the direction of electrophoresis. When the paper is sprayed with ninhydrin the peptides show up as a characteristic pattern of spots which is known as the *fingerprint* of the protein in question (Figure 22·2).

Once their positions have been established the various peptides may be eluted from unstained chromatograms run under identical conditions and their amino acid sequences determined. It is necessary to cleave the original polypeptide chain into large specific peptide fragments by more than one method in order to produce the overlapping sequences that allow their order in the original molecule to be worked out. Other *endopeptidases* (page 274) such as chymotrypsin, which hydrolyses peptide bonds in which an aromatic amino acid supplies the –CO– group, may be used or cyanogen bromide which hydrolyses bonds in which the –CO– group of a methionine residue is involved.

Improved methods for end group analysis have become available, notably the use of *dansyl chloride* (5-dimethylaminonaphthalene-1-sulphonyl chloride) for labelling *N*-terminal amino acids and the *Edman technique*. Dansyl-amino acids fluoresce strongly in ultraviolet light and can be detected in very small amounts so that the method is much more sensitive than Sanger's original DNP technique.

In Edman's method, the *N*-terminal amino group is allowed to react with phenylisothiocyanate and the terminal amino acid is then removed by reaction with anhydrous trifluoroacetic acid (TFA) and identified, leaving the rest of the chain intact. Repetition of the process allows stepwise removal of the residues and progressive elucidation of their sequence. An automatic *sequenator* is now available which can be used to determine the sequence of as many as 100 amino acid residues in as little as 1 mg of protein. Such methods are, however, rapidly becoming 'fossil technology'! Methods of determining the base sequence of cloned DNA fragments are now so quick and simple that, instead of carrying out laborious amino acid sequencing, it may be easier to sequence the gene and use the genetic code (page 300) to work out the amino acid sequences. Using this technique it is possible to determine the primary structure of a protein even when no sample is available!

The primary structure of a large number of proteins is now known. They include ribonuclease, cytochrome *c*, myoglobin, haemoglobin, collagen, an amelogenin and lysozyme as well as various proteolytic enzymes, such as trypsin, chymotrypsin and pepsin and the single chain of human serum albumin which contains 582 residues.

With a selection of twenty different amino acids and chain lengths of up to several hundred residues it is possible to see how a bewildering variety of proteins may be formed. A rough analogy has sometimes been drawn between the alphabet of 26 letters, from which an infinite number of sentences and meanings can be derived, and the amino acid sequence of proteins. Just as the order of the letters defines the construction and meaning of a sentence, so the order of amino acid residues in a protein defines its molecular architecture and biological significance.

Bonds involved in the higher orders of protein structure

The super-structuring of polypeptides occurs mainly as the result of a large number of weak interactions, i.e. the formation of non-covalent bonds, although covalent –S–S– bonds may also be involved.

Hydrogen bonds can occur between the oxygen atom of a –CO group and the proton of an –NH or –OH group when they are in sufficiently close proximity. For example they may be formed between the –NH and –CO groups of the peptide bonds and also between –NH, –CO and –OH radicals present in the R groups.

Salt linkages (ionic or electrostatic bonds) result from the interaction of the positively charged side chains of lysine, arginine or to a lesser extent of histidine, and the negatively charged carboxyl groups of the side chains of glutamic and aspartic acids.

Hydrophobic bonding occurs as a result of the tendency of water to exclude non-polar groups which consequently arrange themselves in the interior of folded molecules. A hydrophobic bond is formed when two hydrocarbon side chains approach one another and there is a sudden reduction in the number of water molecules near the hydrocarbon groups. Bond formation thus causes a local rearrangement of water structure with corresponding changes in energy. Hydrophobic bonds help to stabilize the configurations of proteins in an analogous manner to hydrogen bonds, though by a different mechanism.

Disulphide bonds which are covalent may also play an important part. These bonds are formed between two cysteine residues, which may be constituents of either the same or different chains. Owing to their covalent nature, disulphide bonds resist cleavage and are an important means of conferring stability on protein molecules. In insulin, ribonuclease, lysozyme and the immunoglobulins they serve to link different portions of the same chain causing it to adopt a looped configuration. In other proteins, e.g. chymotrypsin and fibrinogen, they are responsible for holding separate chains firmly together.

Secondary structures

Certain characteristic structural patterns have been found to occur in proteins. This finding arose from the work of Pauling and Corey who examined amino acids and small peptides by physical techniques such as X-ray diffraction and infrared spectroscopy and made accurate determinations of the bond lengths and bond angles in the *polypeptide backbone structure*. As a result they discovered that, although the chain is flexible, it can bend only at certain points: namely round the α-C atoms of the constituent amino acids. The peptide bonds are partial double bonds and are therefore rigid and their constituent carbonyl and imino groups always lie in the same plane. Thus polypeptides can be envisaged as a series of rigid plates hinged at one corner.

Pauling and Corey also came to the conclusion that in stable arrangements of peptide chains, e.g. polyglycine, in which no side chain interactions are involved (i) as many hydrogen bonds as possible are formed; (ii) all the amino acids are arranged symmetrically with respect to one another, and all play an equivalent part in the structure.

On this basis, using information provided by X-ray diffraction patterns of polyglycine and other synthetic polypeptides containing only one type of amino acid so that R group interaction is reduced to a minimum, Pauling and Corey built models of various possible structures. Three main types of secondary structure result from regular patterns of hydrogen bonding, and these are major features in various types of fibrous protein. They are:

1. *The pleated sheet* which is found in silk fibroin where great suppleness and flexibility are required.

2. *The α-helix* which is found in proteins which need to be extensible as well as strong, such as the keratins present in hair and other epithelial structures, myosin in muscle and fibrin in clotted blood.

3. The *triple helix* or three-stranded cable which is found only in collagen, the main protein of connective tissue, where great strength is required but little or no extensibility.

The triple helical structure is associated with special features of amino acid composition but the α-helix can accommodate nearly all the amino acids and short stretches of α-helix and of pleated sheet occur in globular proteins which have a predominantly irregular arrangement.

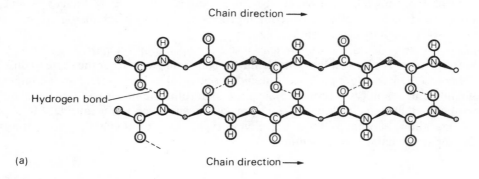

(a)

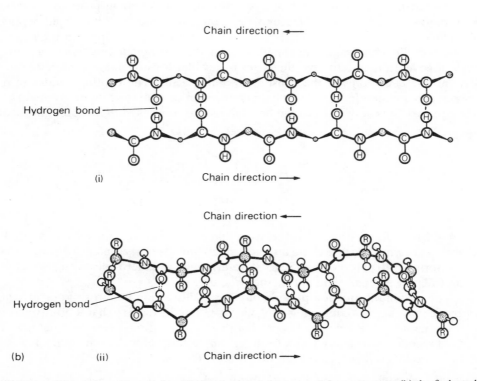

(b)   (ii)

Figure 5.2 Secondary structures in proteins. (a) The β-pleated sheet – parallel arrangement; (b) the β-pleated sheet – antiparallel arrangement: (i) schematic, (ii) actual configuration

The pleated sheet

Even when polypeptide chains are fully extended they take a zigzag course that gives a pleated effect. If a number of these chains are placed side by side their respective –CO and –NH groups come into alignment. Hydrogen bonding can occur between the chains and a sheet-like structure results. If the chains all run in the same direction they lie parallel and give rise to the type of structure shown in Figure 5.2a, while if they run alternately in opposite directions the arrangement is antiparallel as shown in Figure 5.2b. The latter arrangement is found in silk fibroin.

To produce a silk fibre a number of sheets are packed on top of one another with the side chain groupings projecting alternately above and below the sheet. This arrangement is possible because silk fibroin contains a marked preponderance of glycine, alanine and serine residues which have small side chains. In fact every alternate residue is glycine so that the R groups projecting from one side of the sheet are merely H atoms and this allows the sheets to pack together very closely. A thread of silk is thought to contain close-packed regions of this sort interspersed with less regular regions where the amino acid composition is more varied.

The α-helix

The α-helical configuration provides the structural basis for fibres of the α-keratin type with X-ray diffraction patterns which are quite different from those given by silk fibroin. Polypeptides composed of L-amino acids take up the right-handed α-helical configuration which is more stable than the left-handed form.

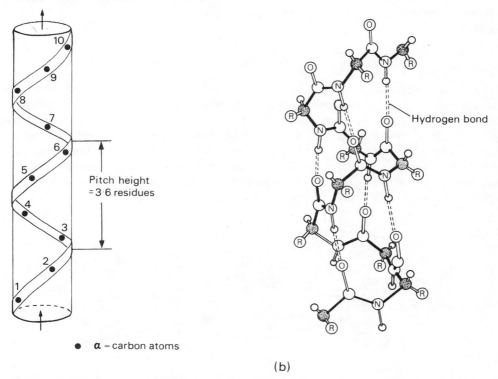

(a) (b)

Figure 5.3 Secondary structures in proteins. The right-handed α-helix: (a) simplified representation; (b) actual configuration

Whereas in sheet structures hydrogen bonding occurs between different chains or different sections of the same chain and is essentially perpendicular to the long axis of the chains, in the α-helix hydrogen bonding is intrachain and the bonds run more or less parallel with the fibre axis. The polypeptide chain in the α-helix can be visualized as having been wound round an imaginary cylinder in such a way that the –CO of each peptide bond is in a suitable position for hydrogen bonding with the –NH group of the third peptide bond beyond it along the chain. Since the chain is pleated and can only bend at the bonds involving the α-C atoms, the helix is angular and the side chains of the amino acids project outwards from the angles (Figure 5.3). It takes 3.7 residues to make one complete turn of the helix so that the side chains of amino acids that are three or four residues distant in linear sequence are brought quite close together while those which are two apart project outwards from opposite sides of the helix. Consequently residues with bulky side chains as well as those with small side chains can take part in the configuration. The imino acid proline (page 35) cannot, however, be readily accommodated in the α-helix, not only because when the imino (–NH) group is joined in the peptide linkage there is no H atom available for hydrogen bonding but also because the rigid ring structure in which its α-C atom is involved will not allow it to fit into such a regular coiled structure. Thus, if proline is present there will be no α-helical conformation in its immediate vicinity.

The elucidation of the α-helix by Pauling and Corey has turned out to be a landmark in protein chemistry. The release of energy when bonds are formed makes the helical configuration, which allows maximum hydrogen bonding, a very stable structure which polypeptide chains tend to adopt whenever possible. Most proteins have some part of their molecule coiled in this way although the helical regions, which are of varying length, are interspersed with regions of irregular folding. The proportion of a polypeptide chain which is held in this configuration varies from 0 to more than 90% and depends on the number, strength and importance of the side chain interactions.

The triple helix

This type of secondary structure is found in collagen which is very tough and has enormous tensile strength. It has an unusual and restricted amino acid composition, the imino acids, proline and hydroxyproline accounting for about one-quarter of the residues. Not surprisingly therefore the chains do not adopt an α-helical configuration. However, owing to the presence of the numerous proline and hydroxyproline residues, each chain itself takes the form of a loose extended coil in which no hydrogen bonds are involved. Three of these loosely coiled chains become wound round each other to give a molecule of *tropocollagen* in the form of a three-stranded cable (Figure 5.4). Close association of the chains is only possible because, in each

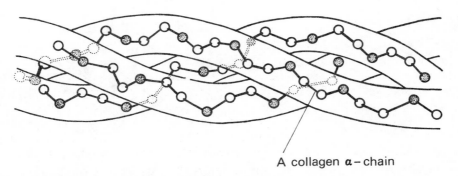

A collagen α – chain

Figure 5.4 Secondary structures in proteins: the triple helix of collagen

chain every third residue is Gly where R = H. The bulky R group of the amino acids on either side of the Gly residues can be accommodated because they project outwards from the cable. The strands are held together by hydrogen bonds in which the hydrogen donors are the peptide –NH groups in one chain and the acceptors are peptide –CO groups in one of the other chains. Further details of collagen structure are given in Chapter 27.

Tertiary structure

Regular linear polymers tend to adopt a helical conformation since this places each monomer in an identical orientation within the molecule and in a position to make the same non-covalent bonds. Helical conformations are adopted not only by proteins but also by nucleic acids and amylose. Proteins are *irregular polymers* since they have 20 different side chains attached to a regular backbone and the three-dimensional configuration which they assume is the result of two tendencies: (1) for the regular backbone to adopt a helical or sheet formation, and (2) for the irregularly placed side chains to twist the backbone into the most energetically favourable configuration which allows maximum side chain interaction within the molecule and with the aqueous environment. In fibrous proteins of the keratin group, the tendency of the backbone to assume a helical structure largely overrules the tendency of the side chains to cause irregular folding. In the globular proteins, on the other hand, side chain interactions usually predominate, many of the R groups are tucked into the interior of the molecule and stretches of helix or pleated sheet are short and may be few and far between. In fact since a large proportion of their constituent amino acids are non-polar, a significant amount of energy would be needed to force them into the strongly hydrogen-bonded water lattice. The repulsion between hydrophobic groupings and the aqueous environment is believed to be one of the principal forces causing a polypeptide chain to assume a particular conformation and globular proteins have been likened to oily droplets made water-soluble by a coat of polar residues.

Interactions between various parts of a protein molecule and its aqueous environment are as important in determining its tertiary structure as are the mutual interactions between these parts themselves. In its biological environment, the range of conformations which it exhibits results from the two types of interaction complementing each other. Hydrophilic (ionized and polar) side chains will spread out among the water molecules, while hydrophobic ones will seek one another within the protein molecule. The backbone structure also interacts with water; unbonded carbonyl and imino groups are hydrophilic, since they form hydrogen bonds with water, while pairs of such groups, already hydrogen-bonded together within the protein, are hydrophobic.

X-ray diffraction analysis

X-ray diffraction analysis is the only method available for discovering the specific configuration of protein molecules. All matter diffracts X-rays, which are scattered by electron clouds surrounding the atoms. When the atoms are arranged in regularly repeating groups as *unit cells* the rays are scattered in a regular manner giving a pattern of spots on a photographic plate. From the position and intensity of the spots the crystallographer can, by a series of very complicated calculations, construct maps of electron density from which the shape of the molecule can be deduced. The technique is complex even for simple compounds, but the problems involved in its application to large protein molecules are formidable. In the first place the compound is required in pure crystalline form and many proteins do not crystallize at all readily. In addition, for the complete elucidation of the structure of a protein, it is necessary to prepare and study several isomorphous derivatives containing heavy atoms. A heavy atom such as Hg must be introduced into the crystal structure in such a way that its exact position is known and so that it causes no appreciable distortion of the molecular shape. This is a chemical problem, but until it is solved for any particular protein it is not possible to work out its structure.

The significance of tertiary folding

The exact three-dimensional character of metabolic proteins is crucial since, as mentioned earlier, their function is to orientate reactive groupings in a very precise manner. By separating their reactive groupings by regions of non-reactivity highly specific spatial and charge patterns may be developed which give the protein its unique and individual character. Large proteins may be folded into a number of compact functional regions or *domains* which are connected by relatively flexible non-specific linking regions (Figure 5.5). It is noteworthy that proteins with similar functions occur in families and are probably derived from a common ancestral protein. For example all proteins that bind nucleotides have a common nucleotide-binding domain. Nevertheless it is possible that unrelated proteins with different amino acid constitutions might assume a similar overall structure and perform a similar function.

It should be noted that proteins have certain *critical positions* in their amino acid sequence. At such positions a change in the nature of the amino acid will almost always have an effect on its function, whereas at other non-critical positions amino acid substitutions seem to have little or no effect. A position may be critical either because its amino acid provides an essential reactive group on which the function of the protein depends, or because it is structurally important in that it helps to ensure the exact stereochemical position of a reactive group. It is usually found that positions within helical sections are non-critical.

The folding process

The unique tertiary structure of globular proteins usually results from the interspersion of regions of secondary structure with apparently non-ordered regions. It is now generally accepted that in a physiological environment all the information needed to specify the tertiary structure is contained in the amino acid sequence of the polypeptide chain and also that folding occurs sequentially as the chain is released from the ribosomes (page 302). In theory, therefore, once the amino acid sequence is known, it should be possible to predict the manner in which a protein will fold. The difficulty of making such predictions can, however, be imagined when it is realized that even a small polypeptide might adopt any of a large number of different conformations. One of the current challenges of protein chemistry is to determine the rules by which tertiary folding is specified. The following are thought to be among the most important:

(i) Energy considerations

Folding is believed to occur so as to result in the conformation having the minimum free energy although this might be a local minimum within a domain rather than an overall minimum.

(ii) Nucleation sites

It is thought that portions of the chain, such as small stretches of secondary structure, might serve as nucleation sites around which the rest of the protein will fold so that folding may be *cooperative*.

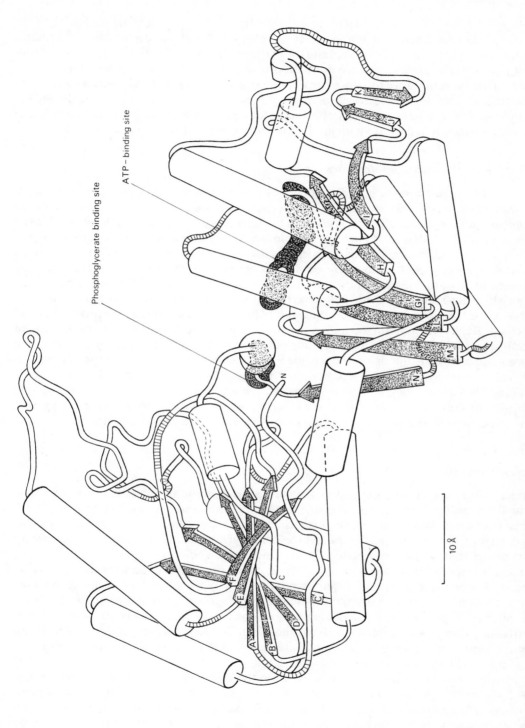

Phosphoglycerate binding site

ATP – binding site

10 Å

Figure 5.5 The structure of the enzyme phosphoglycerate kinase showing its two domains. The cylinders represent regions of α-helix and the stippled arrows regions of β-pleated sheet. The drawing, provided by Dr H. C. Watson, was produced with the help of a computer program written by Lesk and Hardman (1982) *Science*, **216**, 539–540

(iii) Hydrophobicity

It seems to be a general rule that, as far as possible, hydrophobic side chains are buried in the interior of protein molecules leaving the polar and charged side chains on the surface. Proteins are, in the main, close packed structures and the hydrophobic amino acids take up space without interacting with water so that they are useful in providing bulk and shape to the interior of the molecule. However, there are usually more non-polar side chains than can be accommodated in the interior and some are exposed on the surface. If these are concentrated in a particular area to give a hydrophobic patch they may be important in the development of quaternary structure and also in the association of proteins with lipids as in membrane structures.

(iv) Short range sequence considerations

Whereas tertiary structure is largely determined by interactions occurring between amino acids that are widely separated in the amino acid sequence, secondary structuring which as we have seen, might have a nucleating effect, is affected by short range sequence considerations. Not all sequences of amino acids can fold to form a stable α-helix or β conformation since, for example, blocks of amino acids of similar charge such as closely spaced glutamate residues carrying a negative charge will repel one another and clusters of amino acids with bulky side chains may either electrostatically or physically interfere with helix formation. Furthermore proline residues which have no substituent H atom on their peptide N and whose bulky pyrrolidine side chain has a fixed orientation (Figure 27.4) cannot fit into the α-helix and usually produce a bend in the chain. Bends and loops in the folded structure may thus be determined by the position of proline residues and also of certain other amino acids such as the hydroxy amino acids, serine and threonine, and also asparagine and leucine which, owing to the bulk and shape of their side chains, tend to prevent α-helix formation if they occur close together in the chain.

Modern DNA technology is now being used to study the folding rules. The amino acid composition of a protein may be altered at a specific point or points by *site-directed mutagenesis* and the effect of the alteration on the tertiary structure of the protein determined.

Quaternary structure

Quaternary structure may be defined as the specific association of subunits to form a single functional molecule. The arrangement of the subunits (monomers) and the way they pack together is of great importance since small changes in their relative orientations can cause marked changes in the properties of the protein. Such alterations occur in response to environmental changes and are usually of great functional significance.

The forces responsible for the formation of oligomeric proteins are the same as those which are responsible for secondary and tertiary structuring. Why a protein such as myoglobin (see following section) remains as a single unit whereas haemoglobin, whose polypeptide chains are very similar in shape and amino acid composition, consists of four associated subunits is not entirely clear. Complementariness of shapes and Van der Waals' forces are bound to be an important consideration while hydrophobic interactions and electrostatic attraction of surface charges are also likely to be implicated (Figure 5.6).

As mentioned earlier two advantages arise from the assembly of polypeptide subunits into complex molecules: (1) new characteristics are conferred upon them which make them more sensitive to their environment; (2) the chance of mistakes occurring in the synthesis of several copies of a relatively short chain are considerably less than those of making a copying error in the synthesis of a single chain several times as long.

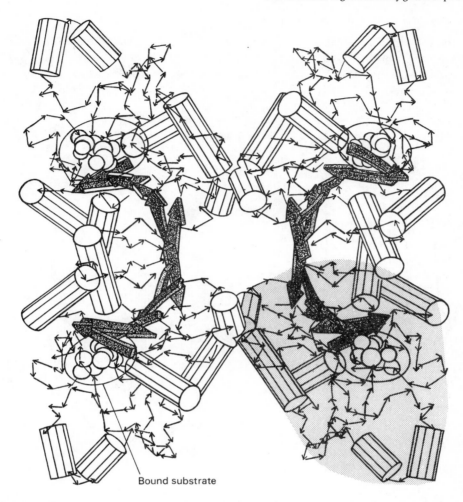

Bound substrate

Figure 5.6 The strtucture of the enzyme phosphoglycerate mutase showing the complementariness of the four subunits of which it is composed. The shaded area represents one subunit. The cylinders represent regions of α-helix and the shaded arrows regions of β-pleated sheet. (Computer drawing supplied by Dr H. C. Watson)

The various levels of structural organization in globular proteins are illustrated in Figure 5.7.

It has been suggested that a clear understanding of tertiary and quaternary structures and the principles of self assembly may enable the pharmaceutical industry to design better drugs, e.g. hormone agonists (activators) and antagonists and neuromuscular blocking agents. Furthermore knowledge of cell surface and viral coat structure might aid the design of antitumour and antiviral agents capable of attaching themselves specifically to malignant cells or virus particles.

Finally it should be noted that many proteins are subject to modification after the polypeptide chains have been assembled, e.g. by hydroxylation, phosphorylation or partial proteolysis (page 316).

Denaturation

Since both the tertiary and quaternary levels of protein structure depend on weak interactions within the molecule and between the molecule and its environment, it is easy to understand why

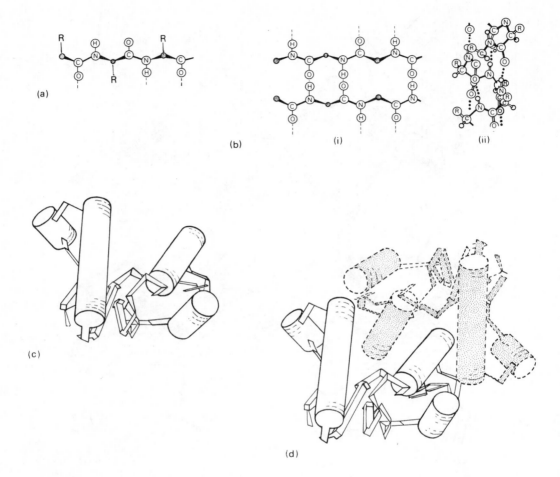

Figure 5.7 Levels of organization within globular protein (pyruvate kinase) molecules. (a) Primary level; (b) secondary level: (i) pleated sheet, (ii) α-helix; (c) tertiary level; (d) quarternary level

they should be so readily disturbed. During denaturation the specific architecture of some or all of the molecule is lost and replaced by *random coiling* and this may cause groupings that were previously buried in the interior of the molecule to become exposed. Denaturation therefore represents a transition from a highly ordered state to a less ordered one, as the result of the disorganization of non-covalent linkages. It may be brought about by a wide variety of physical agents, including heat, extremes of pH and radiation, as well as by many chemicals including organic solvents, detergents and heavy metals. The method of denaturation may affect different types of bond preferentially so that denaturation of a protein by different agents may result in different denatured forms. Whereas denaturation by urea results essentially from the rupture of hydrogen bonds and is often reversible, heat treatment, as witnessed by its effect on egg proteins, may cause much more extensive molecular alteration and is usually irreversible.

It should be stressed that it is only the higher levels of structural organization that are disrupted when a protein is denatured and no peptide bonds are broken. On this basis it might be thought that, if the natural configuration of a protein is the most stable one, it should revert to this form as soon as the denaturing reagent is removed. In certain cases this does occur and the enzyme ribonuclease is notable for the ease and completeness with which it can be renatured. Ribonuclease is a small protein containing only 124 residues and it has four disulphide bonds that link various parts of the chain and stabilize its looped structure.

When ribonuclease is dissolved in a strong urea solution the disulphide bridges are broken and the enzyme loses its activity, but, if the urea is removed and the reduced –SH groups are reoxidized, the original activity is almost completely regained. It is found that instead of the eight CySH groups joining up randomly, they reassociate with their original partners. The specific groups must have been brought into close contact by forces inherent in the primary structure, which cause the chain to fold so that the four disulphide bridges form in their original positions. The disulphide bridges are not a cause of specific folding but act as a means of stabilizing the folded molecule. However, ribonuclease is rather exceptional and renaturation, if it occurs at all, is, in most proteins, only partial. Native proteins are, in general, more resistant to proteolysis than denatured ones. Presumably their folded shape makes them less accessible to the proteolytic enzymes. This is, of course, one of the reasons why one cooks one's food!

The oxygen-binding proteins

Our first real knowledge of protein structure at the tertiary and quaternary levels resulted from work on myoglobin and haemoglobin. In the 1950s, at a time when computers were only just becoming available, Perutz, and later Kendrew, working at Cambridge, first had the courage to apply X-ray techniques to the study of globular proteins well knowing the enormous amount of work entailed. Both myoglobin and haemoglobin are O_2-carrying conjugated proteins with *globin* as the apoprotein and *haem* as the prosthetic group. Globin is a basic protein which contains relatively large amounts of lysine and arginine.

Myoglobin

Myoglobin, which is simpler both in structure and function (page 66) than haemoglobin, consists of a single polypeptide chain of 153 amino acid residues and has a molecular weight of 17 000. The chain is folded into eight helical sections which are joined by regions of apparently random coiling where the chain makes a major directional change (Figure 5.8). The four proline residues are all in the random coil regions but not all the corners contain a proline residue. This confirms the belief that, although the presence of a proline residue is a sufficient reason for a change of direction in the chain, it is not essential for loop formation. The interior of the myoglobin molecule consists entirely of non-polar residues except for two histidine residues which are critically concerned with the attachment and function of the haem group (page 371). The folding of the chain results in the formation of an oily pocket into which the haem group fits. The pocket is lined by hydrophobic side chains derived from amino acids present in several of the surrounding helical segments. Its function is to provide a special microenvironment for the haem group and to protect it from oxidation since it is essential that the iron atom should be kept in the ferrous state.

The intimate relationship between the haem and the globin parts of the molecule is illustrated by the fact that if the haem group is removed there is an appreciable change in the tertiary structure of the globin and its helical content is reduced from about 75% to 60%. The molecule can, however, be quite readily renatured. The importance of the relationship is further apparent from the fact that other haem-containing proteins such as cytochrome oxidase (page 217) and catalase (page 159) have different properties and serve different functions in the body.

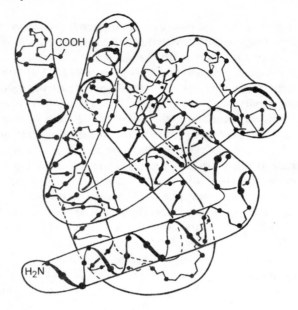

Figure 5.8 The structure of myoglobin

Haemoglobin

Unlike myoglobin haemoglobin has a quaternary structure and consists of two pairs of polypeptide chains (two α and two β) each of which is folded in a characteristic shape which bears a close resemblance to that of myoglobin. The four chains are fitted together to give a spheroidal molecule with approximate dimensions $64 \times 55 \times 50$ Å (Figure 5.9). The four haem groups lie on the surface of the molecule in individual pockets and are separated from one another by appreciable distances. The α chains each contain 141 amino acid residues and the β chains 146 residues. The molecular weight is 65 000. Each α subunit is in contact with both

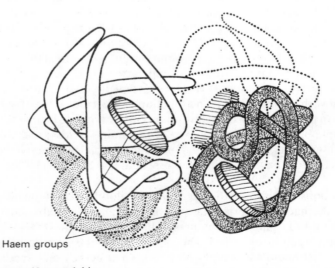

Haem groups

Figure 5.9 The structure of haemoglobin

β chains but there are few interactions between the two α or two β chains. Since the $\alpha_1\beta_1$ and $\alpha_2\beta_2$ half-molecules are irregularly shaped they leave a central open channel when fitted together.

The association of the haemoglobin subunits has an appreciable effect on the O_2-binding properties of the protein so that release of O_2 occurs much more readily than with myoglobin. A further consequence of the quaternary structure is that, as described elsewhere, the structure and properties of the molecule undergo modifications in response to environmental changes.

It is believed that myoglobin and haemoglobin are derived from a common ancestral gene and that the pattern of folding of the globin chain represents Nature's basic design for O_2-carrying proteins (see the next section).

Haemoglobin variants and protein evolution

Proteins responsible for similar functions in different forms of life are species specific and have different amino acid compositions. For example, 42 of the amino acids found in specific positions in horse haemoglobin are different from those in human haemoglobin while, in fish haemoglobin, nearly half of the residues are different from those in human haemoglobin. In spite of such differences, the tertiary structure of O_2-binding proteins, e.g. vertebrate myoglobins and haemoglobins, the haemoglobins of lower vertebrates and also of leguminous plants is similar, whatever their source. The reason is that it is vitally important to preserve the characteristics of the haem-containing pocket and consequently the quaternary structure of haemoglobins has remained almost invariant throughout their evolution. Most of the amino acid substitutions that have occurred are of no functional significance although a few have led to differing responses to chemical stimuli and appear to have evolved from a small number of amino acid replacements in key positions.

An interesting example of this is seen in the haemoglobins of two related species of geese. The greylag goose (*Anser anser*) lives on the plains and its blood has a normal O_2 affinity while the bar-headed goose (*Anser indicus*) migrates across the Himalayas at a height of 9000 m and is enabled to do so because its haemoglobin has a very high O_2 affinity. The haemoglobins of the two species differ by only four amino acids and only one of these substitutions has not been found in any other bird. Thus the difference may be due solely to the replacement of a single proline in the α chain of the haemoglobin of the greylag goose by alanine in that of the bar-headed goose.

Another functional adaptation is seen in teleost fish which use haemoglobin both for respiration and for the secretion of O_2 into the swim bladder and the eye. Such fish have two different types of haemoglobin. One of these functions in the normal way to provide a continuous supply of O_2 to the tissues in general. The other has an unusually low O_2 affinity at low pH values and discharges O_2 when and where there is an accumulation of lactic acid, thus ensuring an ample supply of O_2 at all times to the highly active swim bladder and eye. This 'Root Effect' may be regarded as an exaggerated Bohr effect (page 374) and Perutz believes that it results from a single amino acid substitution, namely of a CySH residue by a serine residue.

These examples of haemoglobin differences and adaptations may seem far removed from the interests of the dental profession as such but they illustrate important biochemical principles relating to protein structure and protein evolution.

In myoglobins and haemoglobins which are closely related in both form and function there are certain *conserved positions* at which the amino acid is always the same and is said to be *invariant*. Thus the haemoglobins of more than 20 species contain nine invariant amino acids which have special functional importance, several of them being directly involved in the O_2-binding site.

Invariant amino acids seem to be points at which molecular form and function are indissolubly linked.

The presence of closely related types of haemoglobin, not only in the fish mentioned above but also in humans (page 371), suggests that at certain stages in evolution the haemoglobin gene must have become duplicated and that there were subsequent mutations in one or both of the gene products. Instances are known where a number of proteins which have different functions show great similarities in their three-dimensional configuration and amino acid sequence. The *serine proteases* (page 86) are a good example. They include trypsin, chymotrypsin, elastase, thrombin and certain other blood-clotting factors. All of them possess the ability to cleave peptide bonds but they differ in their substrate specificities and the mode of activation of their precursors. Such *protein families*, like the haemoglobin variants, are believed to have arisen by *gene duplication* followed by *divergence*.

Other proteins which possess two or more distinct globular domains are believed to have arisen by the joining of two or more separate segments of DNA which are together responsible for the production of a single large polypeptide with new and important properties. The enzyme *phosphoglycerate kinase* illustrates this. It has two separate domains and binds both ATP and 3-phosphoglycerate. While the binding site for ATP is on one of the domains, that for the 3-phosphoglycerate is situated where the two domains are juxtaposed (Figure 5.5).

Some protein molecules have evolved a design which endows them with special aggregating properties so that they form large functional complexes or *supramolecular structures* in which the individual polypeptide chains are held together, as in the haemoglobin molecule, by noncovalent interactions. These complexes may be composed either of several different proteins as with *multienzyme complexes* such as pyruvate dehydrogenase and fatty acid synthetase or of numerous copies of the same protein as with the fibrous proteins fibrinogen, collagen and actin. The diversity of protein form and function is awe-inspiring and, in biology the proteins are preeminent. It is the proteins that are responsible for most of the attributes of living matter since heredity is essentially only an expression of the ability of an organism to make particular types of protein. Moreover, while most proteins can perform their functions in the absence of nucleic acids, the nucleic acids cannot operate in the absence of proteins.

Glycoproteins

These are a heterogeneous group of carbohydrate-containing proteins which are important components of cell membranes (page 194) and also of extracellular fluids and matrices. They occur not only in animals but also in viruses, bacteria, fungi and plants and, as shown in Table 5.5, they fulfil a great variety of functions. These range from unspecific effects such as acting as lubricants and antifreeze agents, which depend solely on their physicochemical properties, to the highly specific interactions involved in cellular recognition processes.

The glycoproteins are characterized by having one or more oligosaccharide chains, which may be linear or branched, attached covalently to their polypeptide chains. Their molecular weights range from 15 000 to more than one million and their carbohydrate contents from 1% in collagen to 50% in mucin and 85% in the blood group substances. The individual oligosaccharide chains do not usually contain more than 15 sugar units and altogether only nine of the many types of monosaccharide which occur in Nature are known to occur in glycoproteins. These are glucose, galactose, mannose, arabinose, xylose, fucose, *N*-acetylglucosamine, *N*-acetylgalactosamine and sialic acid. The sialic acid residues are usually situated at the ends of the oligosaccharide chains and are mainly responsible for the negative charge which exists on the surface of all eukaryotic cells (page 194). The method of attachment of the oligosaccharide units to the

Table 5.5 Some examples of glycoproteins classified according to function

Function	Examples
Structural	Collagen, elastin, bone matrix glycoprotein, fibrin
Lubricating	Mucins
Antifreeze	Present in certain polar fish
Hormones	Thyrotropin, thyroglobulin, chorionic gonadotropin
Enzymes	Ribonuclease, prothrombin, β-glucuronidase
Transport	Ceruloplasmin, transferrin
Cell surface glycoproteins	Glycophorin, fibronectin, hormone receptors
Immunological	Blood group substances, histocompatibility antigens, γ-globulins, complement
Lectins	Concanavalin A, ricin
Antiviral	Interferons

peptide chain is either by an *O*-glycosidic linkage (page 95) through the –OH group of serine or threonine (or, in the case of collagen, of hydroxyproline or hydroxylysine) or, more frequently, by an *N*-glycosidic linkage through the amide group of an asparagine residue.

The glycoproteins may be very simple or very complex. The antifreeze glycoprotein found in the blood of certain polar fish comes in the former category since it consists of the tripeptide sequence -Ala-Ala-Thr- repeated up to 50 times with each Thr residue bearing the disaccharide D-galactosyl-*N*-acetyl-D-galactosamine. Conversely the carbohydrate moieties of the glycoproteins which are responsible for recognition processes may be very complex. The reasons why glycoproteins can exist in such diversity are as follows.

1. The polypeptide chain may bear a variable number of oligosaccharide units.
2. The oligosaccharide units vary in the number and types of sugar they contain.
3. The units may be linear or branched.
4. Each sugar may have either the α or β configuration.
5. The sugars may be linked by any of their several –OH groups.

Interferons

In 1957 it was discovered that cells exposed to a virus release a protein that enables other cells to resist viral attack. This substance was called *interferon*. Since then it has been found that the interferons constitute a family of small glycoproteins which are produced in multiple forms varying both within a species and also from one species to another. Virtually all viruses, as well as some non-viral inducers, can stimulate the production of interferon which is non-toxic and has a broad spectrum of antiviral activity. In addition it has been found that interferons stimulate the activity of certain cells of the mammalian immune system and inhibit cell proliferation so that they are potentially valuable antitumour agents. Problems encountered in the production and purification of material which is active at very low concentrations, and the heavy cost of such work, has so far limited their study and therapeutic evaluation. However recombinant DNA technology (page 308) is now being used for their production, and monoclonal antibodies (page 384) for their purification and some clinical trials are in progress.

Interferons exert their antiviral effects on the cells that they protect rather than on the virus as such. The interferon binds to the surface of the host cells and initiates the synthesis of a number of proteins whose encoding genes are normally repressed. The proteins include several enzymes that block virus replication, assembly and release.

Blood group substances

More than 20 blood group systems are known having 160 distinct antigenic oligosaccharide groupings. They are present on other cells as well as red blood corpuscles and are found attached to mucous secretions including saliva.

Fibronectin

This is an extracellular glycoprotein containing about 5% carbohydrate which exists as large aggregates. It is present on the surface of normal fibroblasts but, when these cells are derived from tumours, the amount of fibronectin is greatly reduced. Fibronectin is believed to promote cell adhesion and hence to reduce cell migration (see also Chapter 27).

Lectins

Lectins are glycoproteins that were first discovered in plants and subsequently in invertebrates and other types of organism. They possess two or more binding sites that recognize specific sugar groupings and bind to cell surface glycoproteins and glycolipids. More than 1000 lectins have now been identified. Many of the plant seed lectins are toxic and may serve to deter animals from eating the seeds. The *haemagglutinins* present in leguminous plants bind to and agglutinate red blood cells, and beans containing them cause poisoning if eaten raw or insufficiently cooked. *Concanavalin A* from the jack bean and *ricin* from the castor oil bean, and one of the most toxic substances known, are both lectins.

Salivary glycoproteins

See page 479.

Chapter 6
Enzymes

Living organisms continuously tranform energy and materials and are able to do so only because of the innumerable enzymes that they contain. Enzymes act as catalysts whose function is to make or break covalent bonds which otherwise could only be created or destroyed under conditions of temperature and pH that are incompatible with life. For example, in order to oxidize glucose directly to carbon dioxide and water *in vitro* the temperature must be raised to several hundred degrees to provide enough energy to tear apart the atoms in the glucose molecule. Even the formation of water from hydrogen and oxygen, which releases so much energy that the reaction is explosive, will not occur unless it is sparked off. The energy provided by the spark breaks covalent bonds releasing oxygen and hydrogen atoms from their molecules, so enabling them to recombine as water, which has a lower energy content. The energy released during the reaction sets off the disintegration of other oxygen and hydrogen molecules and initiates a chain reaction.

Catalysts act by reducing the stability of bonds and consequently lowering the amount of energy required to break them. This energy is known as the *activation energy* and the greater it is the less reactive the compound or system. A catalyst lowers the activation energy by combining with the substrate and forming an unstable intermediate whose rapid decomposition provides an alternative pathway with a lower energy barrier. Whether the activation energy is high or low the overall change in *free energy* in the reaction will be the same (Figure 6.1).

Enzymes are proteins and, while they resemble inorganic catalysts in reducing the activation energy and in remaining unchanged at the end of the reaction, they are much more specific, more efficient and more readily inactivated. They achieve their effects by providing a surface on which their substrates are specifically adsorbed and orientated. As a result of the formation of this *enzyme–substrate complex*, a substrate which is to be broken down (lysed) becomes strained just at the point where fission is to take place. In condensation reactions instead of being dependent on random collisions the reactants are attracted and held by the enzyme in exactly the position needed for the reaction to occur.

While some enzymes are composed solely of protein, others require one or more non-protein substances of low molecular weight for their activity. If the non-protein moiety is firmly bound to the protein part it is known as a *prosthetic group* and the protein is a *conjugated protein*; but where the enzyme is only active in the presence of a discrete small organic molecule, separable by dialysis, the non-protein substance is known as a *coenzyme*.

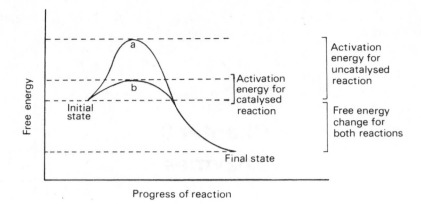

Figure 6.1 The effect of a catalyst on the activation energy of a reaction

Enzyme specificity

The property which especially distinguishes enzymes from other catalysts is their specificity. Whereas inorganic catalysts may speed up more than one reaction, enzymes usually accelerate a reaction involving particular molecules or closely related types of molecule. The specificity of enzymes ensures the close control and coordination of reactions that are necessary for the existence of living organisms. Of the numerous chemical reactions that a compound may undergo, an enzyme reduces the activation energy for only one of them, i.e. enzymes possess *reaction specificity*. Different enzymes are needed to initiate different reactions involving the same compound. For example, an amino acid will undergo quite different reactions according to whether it is acted upon by an oxidase, a transaminase or a decarboxylase.

Apart from being specific for a particular reaction, enzymes show varying degrees of *substrate specificity*. This ranges from the *absolute specificity* shown by urease, which has urea as its one and only substrate, to *group specificity* in which an enzyme will act upon a general type of substrate, e.g. alcohols, esters or peptide bonds. The lipases have a broad specificity and will act on the esters of most fatty acids, while hexokinase catalyses the phosphorylation of a variety of aldohexoses.

Since enzyme action depends on the closeness with which the structure of the enzyme and its substrate complement each other, most enzymes are stereochemically specific. They act on only one of a pair of optical isomers or, if both should be attacked, one reacts much more readily than the other. For example, maltase is a group-specific enzyme that attacks several other α-glucosides as well as maltose but has no effect on β-glucosides.

Classification of enzymes

Enzymes are classified into six main groups according to the type of reaction that they catalyse.

1. *Oxidoreductases* catalyse oxidoreduction reactions, and include dehydrogenases, oxidases, oxygenases, peroxidase and catalase.
2. *Transferases* catalyse the transfer of groups such as amino groups and phosphate.
3. *Hydrolases* hydrolyse glycosides and esters as well as peptide and other amide bonds, e.g. amylase, maltase, dextranase, lipase and trypsin.

4. *Lyases* either remove groups from their substrates leaving double bonds or alternatively add groups to existing double bonds, e.g. aldolase, fumarase.
5. *Isomerases* catalyse various intramolecular rearrangements such as the conversion of an aldose to a ketose sugar, or alteration of the position of a phosphate group, e.g. phosphohexoisomerase, phosphoglucomutase.
6. *Ligases or synthetases* catalyse the joining together of two molecules in a reaction that is coupled with the hydrolysis of a nucleoside triphosphate such as ATP (page 210), e.g. acetyl-CoA carboxylase, glycogen synthetase, succinic thiokinase.

According to the method of classification that has been adopted by the International Union of Biochemistry the systematic name of an enzyme consists of two parts, the first being the name of the substrate or substrates and the second indicating the type of reaction catalysed and ending in -ase. Thus the systematic name for hexokinase is ATP:hexose 6-phosphotransferase.

Coenzymes

A considerable number of enzymes require the presence of one or more small organic molecules which participate in the overall reaction. These molecules are usually termed *coenzymes*, but since they react in stoichiometric proportions with the substrate(s), they are more accurately regarded as *cosubstrates*. The function of such molecules is to link reactions. They do this by acting as carriers of particular groups such as phosphate or acyl groups, or of reducing equivalents, e.g. electrons or hydrogen atoms (Table 6.1).

The function of a coenzyme is well illustrated by the role of pyridoxal phosphate in the transfer of amino groups. The enzyme *alanine aminotransferase* (*glutamate–pyruvate transaminase*) catalyses the reaction of glutamate with pyruvate to form 2-oxoglutarate and alanine. In this reaction, the amino group of glutamate is transferred first to pyridoxal phosphate and then to pyruvate with the formation of alanine.

Table 6.1 Coenzymes

Full name	Abbreviation	Group transferred	Corresponding vitamin
I. Hydrogen-transferring coenzymes			
a. Nicotinamide–adenine dinucleotide	NAD	$H^+ + 2e$	Nicotinamide
b. Nicotinamide–adenine dinucleotide phosphate	NADP	$H^+ + 2e$	Nicotinamide
c. Flavin mononucleotide	FMN	2H	Riboflavin
d. Flavin adenine dinucleotide	FAD	2H	Riboflavin
e. Ubiquinone	CoQ	2H	?
f. Lipoic acid		2H + acyl	—
II. Group-transferring coenzymes			
a. Pyridoxal phosphate	PALP	Amino	Pyridoxine (B_6)
b. Tetrahydrofolate	CoF	Hydroxymethyl (formyl)	Folic acid
c. Biotin	—	Carboxyl (CO_2)	Biotin
d. Cobalamin	B_{12}	Carboxyl	Cobalamin (B_{12})
e. Coenzyme A	CoA	Acetyl and other acyl groups	Pantothenic acid
f. Thiamine pyrophosphate	TPP	Acetaldehyde	Thiamine

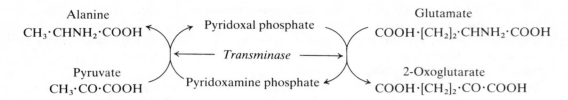

The pyridoxal phosphate returns to its original form at the end of the reaction. In the case of other coenzymes, a second enzyme reaction must occur before the coenzyme is reconverted to its original form. For example, with NAD (page 214), which is a coenzyme for many dehydrogenase enzymes, the oxidized form of the coenzyme is reduced in the first enzyme reaction to NADH which must then be reoxidized by a second enzyme-catalysed reaction before it is able to participate again in the first type of reaction.

Thus reduced NAD formed during glycolysis is usually reconverted to the oxidized form by passing its H atoms into the electron transport chain with the agency of a special NAD dehydrogenase. Alternatively if O_2 is in short supply the NAD is regenerated by the reduction of pyruvate to lactate.

$$CH_3 \cdot CO \cdot COOH + \text{reduced NAD (NADH)} \rightleftharpoons CH_3 \cdot CHOH \cdot COOH + \text{oxidized NAD (NAD}^+)$$
    Pyruvate   Lactate

Pyridoxine, the parent substance of pyridoxal phosphate, is also known as vitamin B_6 (page 165). Many coenzymes contain a derivative of one or other of the B vitamins as an essential part of their structure. Coenzymes may react with a number of different enzymes which are specific for different substrates but which catalyse the same general type of reaction.

The types of reaction which require a coenzyme include group transfers, isomerizations, oxidoreductions and reactions resulting in the formation of covalent bonds. Hydrolytic enzymes do not usually require a coenzyme.

Enzyme kinetics

A great deal of information about enzymes may be obtained by measuring the velocity of the reactions they catalyse under different conditions, i.e. by studying their kinetics. The velocity is measured in terms of the amount of substrate reacting or product formed in unit time under specified conditions, and it is usually expressed in micromoles of substrate transformed per minute. The quantity of enzyme which in 1 minute acts upon 1 micromole of substrate or produces 1 micromole of product under the prescribed conditions is said to possess 1 *unit of enzyme activity*.

Progress curves

If the progress of an enzyme reaction is plotted against time it is found that the velocity is initially high but soon begins to decrease so that a curve such as A in Figure 6.2 is obtained. If lower concentrations of enzyme are used similar curves (B) and (C) are obtained but the time taken to reach the same final concentration of product is increased.

This is a closed system and the falling off in the speed of the reaction can be accounted for by the disappearance of substrate S and the accumulation of products P so that eventually equilibrium conditions are established when

$$[S] \rightleftharpoons [P]$$

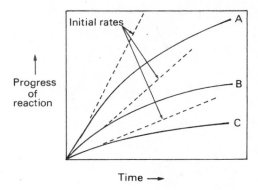

Figure 6.2 Typical progress curves for enzyme-catalysed reactions

and the forward and backward reactions are occurring at an equal rate. The slowing may also result from other changes in conditions occurring as a result of the reaction, such as an alteration in pH. Since enzyme studies are almost always comparative, it is possible to design the experiments so as to ensure that these factors apply equally in all cases. This is usually achieved by measuring the *initial velocity* (V_i) of the reaction, i.e. the slope of the curve in the earliest stages when the substrate concentration [S] is virtually unchanged, insignificant amounts of product have been formed, the original pH is maintained and the enzyme is not denatured, i.e. conditions approximate to those operating in an open system in a steady state.

The effect of enzyme concentration

If a series of progress curves are plotted over a whole range of enzyme concentrations it is found that, provided the substrate is in excess, the initial velocity of the reaction (V_i) is directly proportional to the enzyme concentration and a straight line relationship is obtained.

The effect of temperature

Most enzyme reactions only occur at temperatures between 0 and 60°C. At the lower end of the range, enzyme reactions behave like ordinary chemical reactions and the rate increases as the temperature rises, the velocity being approximately doubled for every 10°C rise as a result of the increased kinetic energy of the reacting molecules. A typical curve relating the activity of an enzyme measured over a constant time, e.g. 5 or 10 minutes, with the temperature is shown in Figure 6.3 from which it may be seen that there is a definite *optimum temperature* which is usually related to the temperature of the environment of the cell from which the enzyme was derived. In mammals the optimum is about 37°C while, curiously, for many plant and bacterial enzymes it is higher than this. The rapid decrease in activity seen at temperatures above the optimum is due to heat denaturation, which occurs progressively as the temperature rises.

The effect of pH on enzyme activity

In view of the importance of pH in determining the ionization of proteins, it is not surprising that enzymes are extremely sensitive to it. Changes in their charge distribution may affect activity by altering either the overall conformation of the protein or the reactivity of amino acid side chain groupings involved in the active site. Each enzyme has a characteristic optimum pH

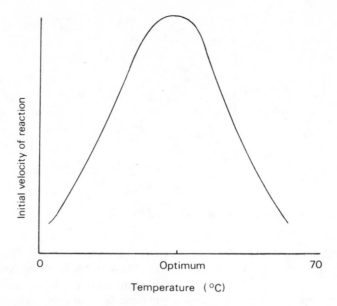

Figure 6.3 The effect of temperature on the rate of an enzyme-catalysed reaction measured over a constant time

although, if an enzyme acts on two different substrates, the optimum pH values may differ slightly. Pepsin is unusual in acting at very low pH values and has an optimum pH varying from 1.5 to 2.5 according to the protein being digested. Most enzymes have an optimum pH between 5 and 9 (Figure 6.4). The loss of activity at pH values at either end of the range may be reversible but most enzymes, if they are subjected to extremes of pH, will be denatured, when the loss of activity is usually permanent.

In addition to pH effects on the enzyme there may be pH effects on the substrate. In enzyme studies it is therefore essential to control the pH with a suitable buffer system.

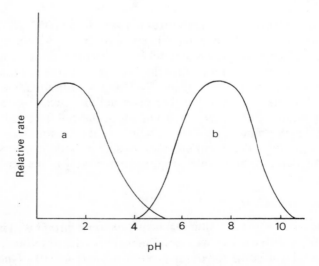

Figure 6.4 The effect of pH on the rate of enzyme-catalysed reactions. (a) Pepsin; (b) liver glucose-6-phosphatase

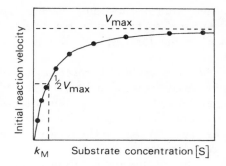

Figure 6.5 The effect of substrate concentration on the initial velocity of an enzyme-catalysed reaction

The effect of substrate concentration

The velocity of an enzyme-catalysed reaction is greatly influenced by the concentration of the substrate [S]. At low values of [S] the initial velocity V_i is usually proportional to [S] but, as the substrate concentration is increased, the rate of increase of reaction velocity slows down and finally a point is reached beyond which further increase in [S] has no effect on the rate. This is the *maximum velocity* or V_{max} of the reaction under the conditions specified.

A typical substrate concentration curve is shown in Figure 6.5 and can be described by the mathematical equation for a hyperbola.

$$V_i = \frac{V_{max}[S]}{K_m + [S]}$$

This is the *Michaelis–Menten equation* which contains two constants V_{max} and K_m. The latter is known as the *Michaelis constant* and is defined as the molar substrate concentration at which the velocity of the reaction is half-maximal. This can be shown by substituting the values $V_{max}/2$ for V_i in the equation as follows:

$$\frac{V_{max}}{2} = \frac{V_{max}[S]}{K_m + [S]}$$

therefore

$$K_m + [S] = 2[S]$$

and therefore

$$K_m = [S]$$

The relationship expressed in the Michaelis–Menten equation can be explained by the theory that the enzyme E combines reversibly with the substrate to form an enzyme–substrate complex (E–S) which can either dissociate to regenerate E and S or can react to form the product P and release the enzyme for further use.

$$E + S \rightleftharpoons E\text{–}S \rightarrow E + P$$

Michaelis and Menten postulated that the breakdown of E–S to E + P occurred more slowly than the formation of E–S, so that the overall speed of the reaction depended on the concentration of the enzyme–substrate complex. Considering the first stage of the reaction, when [S] is low, most of the enzyme molecules exist in the free state and the concentration of E–S is directly related to the concentration of substrate, which is therefore the limiting factor. However, at high substrate concentrations the enzyme becomes saturated with the substrate so that all the enzyme is present in the form of E–S and further increase in the substrate concentration can have no effect.

At point X on the graph at which the reaction is proceeding at half-maximal velocity half the molecules of enzyme will be in the free form E and half combined as E–S, and the substrate concentration (K_m) at this point is related to the dissociation constant of E–S while its reciprocal $1/K_m$ gives an indication of the affinity of the enzyme for its substrate. Enzymes with high K_m values have a low affinity for their substrate and will be relatively inactive within a cell unless the substrate is present at a high concentration.

It is not easy to obtain an accurate value for K_m from a direct plot of V_i against [S] and Lineweaver and Burk (1934) pointed out that both K_m and V_{max} could be more accurately determined by means of a double reciprocal plot, i.e. by plotting $1/V$ against $1/[S]$. This gives a straight line relationship in which $1/V_{max}$ is given by the intercept on the y-axis and $-1/K_m$ by the intercept on the x-axis, as shown in Figure 6.6.

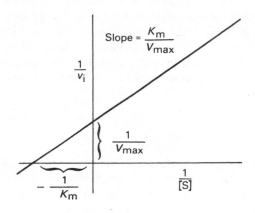

Figure 6.6 A typical Lineweaver–Burk (double-reciprocal) plot

The Michaelis constant is a fundamental value in enzyme chemistry; not only can it be used to estimate the [S] needed to give maximal reaction velocity but it can also be used in the identification of enzymes, to examine the conditions under which an enzyme will operate within the cell and to give information on the mode of action of the enzyme and of substances that affect its activity.

The idea that an intermediate enzyme–substrate complex is formed in the course of enzyme-catalysed reactions is supported by evidence other than that provided by data satisfying the Michaelis–Menten equation. Thus, certain enzymes are protected from denaturation in the presence of their substrates suggesting that the substrate increases the stability of a particular conformation. Furthermore, direct observations using special rapid mixing techniques showed that the absorption spectrum of the complex formed between peroxidase and its substrate hydrogen peroxide differs from those of the enzyme, substrate and products.

When the molecular weight of a pure enzyme is known it is possible to determine the *molecular activity* or *turnover number*, i.e. the number of molecules of substrate transformed per minute per molecule of enzyme. These are usually of the order of several thousand, although acetyl cholinesterase has a value of 950 000 and catalase 5 000 000.

The active site

The high degree of specificity of enzymes for their substrates and the formation of an enzyme–substrate complex strongly suggest that the substrate must become attached to the surface of the enzyme molecule. Furthermore, since the enzyme molecule is usually much larger than its substrate it is believed that the latter can only occupy a limited area on the enzyme surface, e.g.

Enzyme		*Substrate*	
Catalase mol. wt	250 000	Hydrogen peroxide mol. wt	34
Urease mol. wt	480 000	Urea mol. wt	60

This area to which the substrate becomes bound is known as the *active site* or *active centre* of the enzyme and must bear a specific complementary relationship to the structure of the substrate(s) which allows an almost precise fit between them.

The active site is made up of a *binding site* and a *catalytic site* since only a few of the amino acids in the peptide chain take part in the catalytic mechanism, while others, which presumably adjoin or overlap the catalytic site, must be responsible for binding the substrate and thus for determining the specificity of the enzyme. As might be expected, the active site usually includes amino acids, such as serine, histidine and cysteine, which have reactive side chain groupings.

In the formation of the enzyme–substrate complex it is believed that some deformation of the enzyme molecule takes place which, in the case of hydrolytic enzymes, places a strain on the geometry of the substrate molecule, rendering it susceptible to attack by H^+ or OH^- ions or by specific functional groupings belonging to the enzyme. As a result of this the susceptible bond in the substrate snaps and the products diffuse away allowing the enzyme to return to its original shape.

Enzyme molecules probably possess a measure of flexibility, and Koshland has proposed that when the enzyme–substrate complex is formed there is a fairly extensive change in the form of the enzyme, i.e. that the substrate causes a conformational change which results in an *induced fit* between the enzyme and its substrate. This would explain why certain groupings that were previously buried inside the molecule become exposed and active during enzyme activity.

The amino acids which constitute the active site of certain enzymes can be labelled and identified. For example, the enzyme may form a stable complex with labelled reagents, which are structurally related to the normal substrate, and the complex may then be degraded in such a way that one or more of the points of attachment can be identified.

In most cases, however, such complexes are not stable enough to allow identification of the reactive groupings and the labelled compound has to be sufficiently different from the normal substrate for the complex not to decompose. Di-isopropyl fluorophosphate (DFP) has been used for labelling the active sites of proteolytic enzymes but it is unspecific and might easily combine with residues other than those present at the active site. However, in the case of chymotrypsin, DFP reacts with a single specific serine residue which it does not do with either chymotrypsinogen or denatured chymotrypsin. α-Chymotrypsin contains 28 serine residues altogether and the DFP complex is enzymically inactive so that it is believed that the serine to which the DFP is attached must form part of the active site. There is considerable evidence that two histidine residues are also implicated in the catalytic activity of chymotrypsin. While these three amino acids are not sequentially adjacent to one another, they are brought close together by folding of the chain.

Factors that influence enzyme activity *in vitro*

The activity of enzymes may be affected by a great variety of substances. Apart from agents which act as general protein denaturants, many substances that affect enzymes are more or less specific for one enzyme or group of enzymes and such inhibitors may be broadly classified according to how they exert their effects.

Zymogen activation

A very specialized form of inhibition is seen in the case of certain enzymes which must remain inactive until they are specifically required. This applies to many proteolytic enzymes which would otherwise break down the cells that produce them and also to the enzymes required in blood clotting. Such enzymes are synthesized and secreted from the cells as an inactive proenzyme or *zymogen* which only becomes active when conditions are appropriate, such as after the ingestion of food or when a blood vessel has been damaged. Activation results from the splitting of a small number of peptide bonds, i.e. *limited proteolysis* which unmasks the active site and frees it from conformational restraints. The process is irreversible, extracellular and usually autocatalytic so that once initiated a chain reaction occurs forming progressively increasing amounts of active enzyme.

Metal ion effects

Metal ions may act as both activators and inhibitors of enzymes. For example, the kinases which mediate the ATP $\rightleftharpoons$ ADP conversion nearly always require Mg^{2+} and many peptidases are activated by divalent cations such as Mn^{2+}, Zn^{2+} or Co^{2+}. On the other hand, amylases require an activating anion, namely Cl^-, although Br^- and I^- will do nearly as well.

Heavy metals frequently act as enzyme inhibitors particularly when free –SH groups participate in the reaction. Papain, urease, myosin, triose phosphate dehydrogenase and many other enzymes fall into this category and are readily inactivated by Ca^{2+}, Hg^{2+} etc. The inhibition may sometimes be overcome by removing the metal ion, e.g. with H_2S or with a chelating agent such as EDTA.

Sulphydryl enzymes are also inactivated by oxidation to the –S–S– form but addition of a mild reducing agent may serve to reactivate the enzyme. Sulphydryl groups are irreversibly inactivated by iodoacetamide and *N*-ethylmaleimide.

Non-competitive inhibitors

The inhibitory effects of heavy metals, and of cyanide on cytochrome oxidase and of arsenate on glyceraldehyde phosphate dehydrogenase, are examples of non-competitive inhibition. This type of inhibitor acts by combining with the enzyme in such a way that for some reason the active site is rendered inoperative. The inhibition may or may not be reversible but it is not affected by the addition of extra substrate.

If a substrate concentration curve is constructed for the enzyme in the presence of sufficient non-competitive inhibitor to cause partial but not complete inhibition, as shown in Figure 6.7, it is found that the K_m of the reaction is unaffected although V_{max} is greatly reduced. The effect may be explained in terms of a reduction in the concentration of enzyme, i.e. that whereas some of the enzyme molecules are rendered completely inactive by combination with the inhibitor, others remain uncombined and normally reactive.

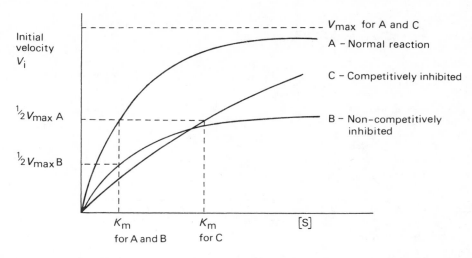

Figure 6.7 The relationship between substrate concentration and the initial velocity of an enzyme-catalysed reaction under normal conditions (A), and in the presence of a non-competitive inhibitor (B) and a competitive inhibitor (C)

Competitive inhibition

This type of inhibition is caused by substances (I) which bear a close structural relationship to the normal substrate for the enzyme and compete with it for the active site. Thus the enzyme may either form E–S or E–I, but, whereas the E–S complex reacts normally to give E + P, no products can be formed from E–I

$$E + S \rightleftharpoons E\text{–}S \rightarrow E + P$$

but

$$E + I \rightleftharpoons E\text{–}I$$

The presence of I reduces the amount of E–S formed but, if more substrate is added, I competes less effectively and the inhibition may be overcome. A notable example of this type of inhibition is the effect of malonate on succinate dehydrogenase which catalyses the reaction

$$
\begin{array}{ccccc}
\text{COOH} & & \text{COOH} & & \text{COOH}\\
| & & | & & |\\
\text{CH}_2 & \rightleftharpoons & \text{CH} & + 2\text{H} & \text{CH}_2\\
| & & \parallel & & |\\
\text{CH}_2 & & \text{HC} & & \text{COOH}\\
| & & | & & \\
\text{COOH} & & \text{COOH} & & \\
\text{Succinate} & & \text{Fumarate} & & \text{Malonate}
\end{array}
$$

In spite of its close structural similarity to succinate, malonate cannot be dehydrogenated by removal of 2H atoms. The rate of formation of fumarate will depend on the concentration of E–S so that if the concentration of succinate is increased sufficiently the effect of the malonate will become insignificant. Inhibitors of this type are known as *competitive inhibitors, structural analogues, metabolic antagonists* or *antimetabolites* and can be recognized by measuring the reaction velocity at varying substrate concentrations in the presence of a fixed concentration of inhibitor. In this instance the inhibitor has no effect on V_{max} but K_m is significantly increased (Figures 6.7 and 6.8). The actual rate of the reaction is strictly dependent on the relative amounts of S and I.

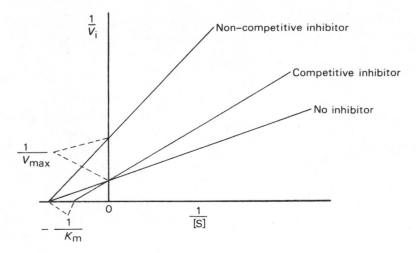

Figure 6.8 Lineweaver–Burk plots showing the effects of competitive and non-competitive inhibitors

There are two areas of experimental biochemistry in which competitive inhibitors are of practical significance.

1. They may be used as tools in the study of metabolic pathways, notably in microorganisms. If a pathway is blocked by the structural analogue of a postulated metabolite it may then be possible to identify precursors that will be likely to accumulate. Moreover, addition of substances involved in the pathway beyond the block should overcome the effect of the inhibitors so far as the final product is concerned.

$$A \rightarrow B \rightarrow C \longrightarrow\!\!\mid\!\!\longrightarrow D \rightarrow E \rightarrow F$$
Block

Thus, in the sequence represented above, B and C would tend to accumulate whereas addition of D or E would allow the normal production of F.

2. If competitive inhibitors can be found for reactions that are essential to pathogenic organisms or abnormal tumour cells, but are not required by the normal cells of the host, they might be developed as chemotherapeutic drugs. The antibacterial effect of the sulphonamide group of drugs results from the structural relationship of the parent substance, sulphanilamide, to *p*-aminobenzoic acid which is an essential growth factor for many microorganisms but not for Man.

p-aminobenzoic acid   Sulphanilamide

On the whole this 'antienzyme guided missile' approach to chemotherapy has been disappointing because the essential metabolic pathways are common to almost all forms of life, whereas effective chemotherapy is necessarily based on metabolic differences between microorganisms and Man and between normal and malignant cells. However, with increasing knowledge of the differences in structure and reactivity that occur between enzymes which fulfil the same function in different species greater success may be achieved in the future.

Allosteric effectors

While competitive inhibition depends on a close structural relationship between the inhibitor and the normal substrate, certain enzymes may have their activity modified by metabolites which bear no structural relationship to the substrate and which bind reversibly to a site on the enzyme surface which is quite distinct from the substrate-binding site. This is known as the *allosteric site*. It is believed that allosteric regulators act by modifying the conformation of the active site so that it binds the substrate either more (*positive effectors* or *activators*) or less (*negative effectors* or *inhibitors*) strongly. The allosteric site is not necessarily close to the active site and may even be situated on a different type of subunit from the active site.

Enzymes that are subject to allosteric regulation have been found to have certain features in common.

1. All those that have been investigated have a quaternary structure (i.e. are made up of a number of subunits) and possess more than one substrate-binding site.
2. The allosteric effectors produce an alteration in the spatial relationship of the subunits.
3. Allosteric enzymes show anomalous kinetics. Instead of the usual simple hyperbolic substrate concentration curve a sigmoid curve is obtained, which means that at low [S] values the reaction is slow but as [S] increases so the rate of reaction is greatly increased (Figure 6.9).

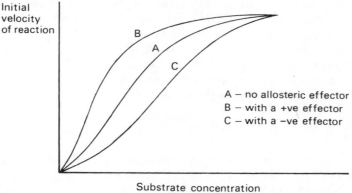

Figure 6.9 Substrate concentration curves for an allosteric enzyme (A) and for the same enzyme in the presence of positive (B) and negative (C) effectors

In other words the binding of the substrate S is *cooperative* in that its binding on the first subunit facilitates its binding on the other subunit(s) showing that there is some form of communication between them. This phenomenon is also seen in the binding of O_2 by haemoglobin (page 373).

Factors that affect enzyme activity *in vivo*

The factors mentioned in the previous section can all be shown to affect the activity of enzymes *in vitro* but it is, of course, even more important to understand the processes by which enzyme activity is altered *in vivo*. These may be listed as follows.

The concentrations of the reactants

Substrate availability

Obviously no reaction can occur unless substrate is available and the presence or absence of substrate must be the ultimate determinant of whether or not a particular reaction for which the necessary enzymes are available will take place. However, when substrate is available the extent to which its concentration controls the rate of a reaction depends on the nature of the reaction.

Many enzymes catalyse physiologically reversible reactions which proceed sometimes in one direction and sometimes in the other, depending on the relative concentrations of the reactants. Typically these reactants are involved in the central area of metabolism (page 189) and are present at all times, although their concentrations are subject to appreciable variation as a result of food ingestion or physical activity. Examples of this type of reaction are:

$$\text{Glucose 6-phosphate} \underset{}{\overset{\text{Phosphoglucomutase}}{\rightleftharpoons}} \text{Glucose 1-phosphate}$$

$$\text{Creatine + ATP} \underset{}{\overset{\text{Creatine kinase}}{\rightleftharpoons}} \text{Phosphocreatine + ADP}$$

Coenzyme availability

Many of the enzymes involved in metabolic pathways require coenzymes to act as carriers of electrons, atoms or groups of atoms. The coenzymes act alternately as acceptors and donors and exist in alternative states, e.g. $NAD^+/NADH$, $NADP^+/NADPH$, pyridoxal/pyridoxamine, CoA/acetyl-CoA. Since coenzymes are in effect cosubstrates that react with the substrate in stoichiometric proportions, the question of which of the two forms predominates may be decisive in determining the direction of reactions occurring at or near equilibrium. Specific portions of some metabolic pathways may be controlled in this way, e.g. the conversion of pyruvate to lactate in muscles during physical exertion.

$$\text{Pyruvate + NADH + H}^+ \underset{}{\overset{\text{Lactate dehydrogenase}}{\rightleftharpoons}} \text{Lactate + NAD}^+$$

Pyruvate dehydrogenase, the multienzyme complex responsible for the oxidation of pyruvate to acetyl-CoA and CO_2 and hence for a major part of aerobic energy production, is sensitive to both the CoA/acetyl-CoA and $NAD^+/NADH$ ratios. If these are high the reaction is speeded up and energy production is promoted. On the other hand, if the ratios are low this indicates that energy available in excess of the immediate requirements and the pyruvate is conserved by diverting it into storage products such as glycogen or fat. Pyruvate dehydrogenase is also subject to control by covalent modification (page 342).

Adenosine phosphate ratios

The proportions of the various adenosine phosphates (ATP, ADP and AMP) within a cell or cell compartment is a measure of its co-called *energy charge*, which may be defined as follows:

$$\text{Energy charge} = \frac{[ATP] + \frac{1}{2}[ADP]}{[ATP] + [ADP] + [AMP]}$$

The effect of the ATP:ADP ratio on oxidative phosphorylation, described on page 220, may be considered as an example of a controlling effect of the energy charge of the cell.

Activators and inhibitors

Obligatory activators

Some enzymes have an obligatory requirement for a particular activator, i.e. they have no measurable activity if the activator is absent. In such cases, the activators effectively change the V_{max} of the enzyme rather than the substrate dependence. An example of such an enzyme is *carbamoyl phosphate synthetase* which is involved in the conversion of ammonia to urea (page 283). This enzyme is completely inactive in the absence of *N*-acetylglutamate, which increases the activity at all substrate concentrations.

A further example is the enzyme *pyruvate carboxylase* which is involved both in gluconeogenesis and in maintaining the level of citrate cycle intermediates and requires acetyl-CoA as an obligatory activator.

Allosteric regulators

These have already been mentioned briefly on page 83.

Covalent modification

These latter two methods of enzyme activation and inhibition are of profound importance in the control and integration of metabolism and are dealt with in Chapter 23.

Compartmentation effects

The division of the cell into compartments by a variety of intracellular membranes (Chapter 15) is clearly of great metabolic significance but as yet this is poorly understood. Each membrane appears to possess a different selective permeability and each compartment has a characteristic composition with respect to both enzymes and substrate.

Moreover, as a result of the operation of various 'ion pumps' present in the membranes of the cell, ions may be very unevenly distributed within the various compartments and any factor that modifies the movement of ions through membranes may have an appreciable influence on metabolic processes. For example, Na^+ and K^+ ions are required by the membrane ATPase which is believed to be involved in active transport processes, and movements of Ca^{2+} are becoming increasingly implicated in the control of reactions, for example the breakdown of glycogen.

Attempts to unravel the problems posed by cell compartmentation are hampered by the extreme difficulty of determining the exact intracellular location of many enzymes, let alone the distribution of metabolites. Even within a compartment distribution may not be uniform. For example, the existence of multienzyme systems, in which each enzyme is adjacent to the next one in the metabolic pathway, limits the diffusion of metabolites from the site of their production. This inequality of distribution of metabolites within the cell makes it difficult to demonstrate *in vitro* control processes which may occur *in vivo*.

The various methods by which enzyme activity may be controlled are summarized in Figure 6.10.

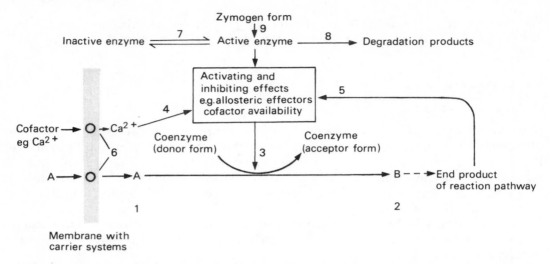

Figure 6.10 Summary of methods by which enzyme activity may be controlled. 1, Substrate concentration; 2, product concentration, 3, coenzyme ratios; 4, cofactor availability; 5, allosteric effectors; 6, membrane permeability; 7, phosphorylation/dephosphorylation; 8, enzyme degradation; 9, zymogen activation

Enzyme mechanisms

The amino acid sequence of a large number of enzymes is now known. In a number of cases the three-dimensional structure of the enzyme molecule has also been determined using X-ray crystallography, and the active site has been located. This information allows a description of the enzyme mechanism at the molecular level.

Chymotrypsin is a proteolytic enzyme which hydrolyses peptide bonds which lie on the *C*-terminal side of an aromatic amino acid. Chymotrypsin has a serine residue at the active site and this can be labelled by reaction with di-isopropyl fluorophosphate. Other proteolytic enzymes such as trypsin, subtilisin and thrombin have a similar serine residue at their active sites and these enzymes are termed *serine proteases*.

In the three-dimensional structure of chymotrypsin, the serine residue (which is residue 195 from the *N*-terminus of the chain and is hence termed serine-195) is located in close proximity to the residues histidine-57 and aspartate-102. The negatively charged aspartate-102 tends to withdraw a proton from the imidazole ring of histidine-57 adjacent to it. The imidazole ring then attracts a proton from serine-195. The effect of this *charge relay system* is to lower the effective p*K* of serine-195 and thus make it more reactive

$$Asp_{(102)}-\overset{\overset{O}{\|}}{C}-O^-\text{---}H-N\overset{\diagup\ C\ \diagdown}{\underset{HC=C-}{\diagdown\ \ \ \ \diagup}}N\text{---}H-O-Ser_{(195)}$$

$$His_{(57)}$$

A simplified reaction mechanism for chymotrypsin is shown in Figure 6.11. The carbonyl carbon atom of the peptide bond to be hydrolysed is subject to attack by the polarized oxygen atom of serine-195. An acylenzyme intermediate is formed. A water molecule then enters and is polarized by the charge relay system. The hydroxyl residue attacks the carbonyl carbon of the acyl group attached to serine-195, with the hydrolysis of the acylenzyme intermediate and release of the product.

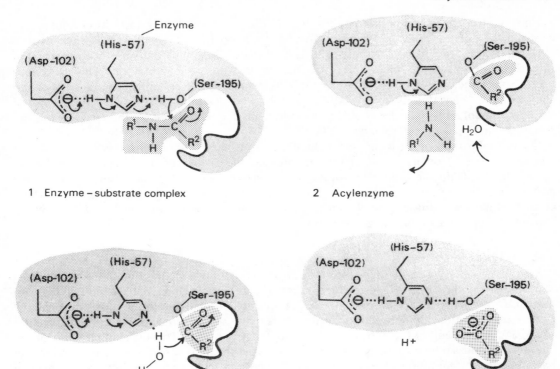

Figure 6.11 The mechanism of hydrolysis of a peptide bond by chymotrypsin

The specificity of chymotrypsin can also be explained from a knowledge of its three-dimensional structure. The enzyme molecule contains a hydrophobic cleft near the active site. This cleft accommodates only aromatic side chains. The enzyme trypsin hydrolyses peptide bonds in which the –CO– group is contributed by either lysine or arginine. The arrangement of amino acids at the active site of trypsin is similar to that in chymotrypsin and a similar charge relay system is involved in the catalytic mechanism but there is a pocket near the active site which contains a preponderance of negatively charged residues rather than hydrophobic residues, and these serve to bind the positively charged lysine or arginine group.

Carboxypeptidase (page 275), which splits peptide bonds to remove single amino acids from the *C*-terminus of peptide chains, has a pit into which the end of the chain can fit so that the terminal peptide bond is held in position at the catalytic site. Carboxypeptidase is, however, not a serine protease and breaks the peptide bond by a different mechanism.

Immobilized enzymes

Considerable interest has centred on the possibility of immobilizing enzymes on insoluble supporting materials and using these to carry out reactions in systems where substrates are continuously supplied and the products are continuously removed. Such reactions are of potential commercial importance since the enzyme is retained at the end of the process.

Enzymes have been immobilized by covalent binding to polymeric supports, by entrapment in cross-linked polymer gels or by physical adsorption on to suitable materials such as ion-exchangers, with retention of activity. The first example of an industrially useful application of this technique was in the separation of L-amino acids from racemic mixtures. This procedure used the enzyme aminoacylase which is immobilized in suitable columns. The racemic amino acid mixture is acylated chemically to form α-*N*-acetyl-DL-amino acids. When this is passed through the column, only the *N*-acetyl-L-amino acids are deacylated by the enzyme and the resulting L-amino acids can then be purified.

Other applications of the technique include the use of immobilized glucose isomerase for the enrichment in fructose of corn starch hydrolysates and the use of immobilized pectinases for the clarification of fruit juice and wine. Immobilized enzymes have also been used as sensors for particular substrates. For example, a glucose-specific electrode has been developed which consists of glucose oxidase (page 94) entrapped in a polyacrylamide gel which is layered over a conventional polarographic oxygen electrode.

Enzyme polymorphisms

Various reasons have been suggested for the discrepancy in molecular size between enzymes and most substrates. The first is the length of chain required to fold the molecule so as to achieve the exact spatial relationship between its various parts that is needed to maintain the configuration of the active site, and of the allosteric site or sites when present. This means that many of the amino acids must play a more or less passive role and this may afford protection against the harmful effects of mutations. If every amino acid played an active part in the enzyme mechanism a single alteration in its primary structure might well be lethal but, if proteins contain a large proportion of amino acids which play no part in the reaction, they can be replaced by other amino acids without any serious effect. Other suggestions are that large molecules are more readily retained at specific locations and that size gives some protection against proteolytic enzymes.

Indications of the structural features which are essential for a particular type of activity may be obtained by comparing the structure of different proteins which perform the same or similar functions. The characteristics which have remained unchanged during the course of evolution can thus be established. Such studies confirm that, as with the haemoglobins, there is considerable tolerance for replacement, deletion or insertion of amino acids in certain regions of the protein molecule.

In the course of electrophoretic studies it has been found that some enzymes exist in several distinct forms in a single organism and that the distribution patterns of the various forms may vary not only from tissue to tissue but also in the same tissue at different stages of development. Such multiple enzymes which catalyse the same reaction but which vary in their detailed structure and reactivity are known as *isoenzymes*. Perhaps the best known example is *lactate dehydrogenase* which is composed of four subunits of two different types, H and M. Five different forms of lactate dehydrogenase have been identified, having the constitution H_4, H_3M, H_2M_2, HM_3 and M_4 respectively. All five catalyse the reaction

$$
\begin{array}{ccc}
\text{CH}_3 & \quad \text{NAD}^+ \quad\quad \text{NADH} \quad & \text{CH}_3 \\
| & \qquad\qquad +\text{H}^+ & | \\
\text{CHOH} & \xrightleftharpoons[\text{Lactate dehydrogenase}]{} & \text{CO} \\
| & & | \\
\text{COOH} & & \text{COOH} \\
\text{Lactate} & & \text{Pyruvate}
\end{array}
$$

but show graded differences in their amino acid composition, electrophoretic behaviour and allosteric and immunological properties which are related to their subunit composition.

There is a steadily growing list of known isoenzymes. Their physiological significance is still uncertain but they provide a versatility which may relate to differing metabolic requirements, and they have some clinical significance as an aid to diagnosis.

Isoenzymes are *enzyme variants* found in all members of a species and their occurrence and distribution depend on such factors as the phase of development, the tissue in question and sometimes even the season of the year. The latter is instanced by the rainbow trout which produces summer and winter forms of brain cholinesterase while, at intermediate temperatures, both forms are produced.

Variants also undoubtedly occur in the enzymes and other proteins of individuals within a species. However, unless like haemoglobin pure samples of these proteins are readily obtainable, and unless there are easily recognizable differences in their properties such *protein polymorphisms* will only be detected in very special circumstances. They will, however, help to determine the inherited characteristics of the individual not only in terms of physical attributes but also susceptibility to disease, nutritional and drug intolerances and even perhaps such ill-defined qualities as intellectual and musical ability.

Chapter 7
Carbohydrates

In sheer amount carbohydrates make up the bulk of organic matter on the earth. They are predominantly of plant origin, one of the most abundant forms being the structural carbohydrate cellulose. In higher animals, however, protein rather than carbohydrate is the principal structural material although special types of carbohydrate, namely the glycosaminoglycans, are important constituents of skeletal and other connective tissues. Other types of polysaccharide play a structural role in the cell walls of bacteria. These may act as antigens so that, when invaded, the body is able to defend itself by producing specific antibodies that will lead to destruction of the bacteria.

Apart from their structural importance, carbohydrates provide energy for synthetic processes and other work undertaken by cells and also provide many of the simple starting materials that are required for the synthesis of more complex substances. Furthermore, certain sugars and their phosphate esters act as key compounds in the storage and transfer of energy. Sugars are also constituents of many coenzymes as well as of the nucleic acids.

The carbohydrates of the diet are of special interest to the dental profession since, as discussed later, their type and quality is an important factor affecting the health of the oral tissues.

A carbohydrate may be defined as a polyhydroxyaldehyde, polyhydroxyketone or a substance that can be hydrolysed to give these compounds. The carbohydrates are usually classified as follows:

1. *Monosaccharides*: simple sugars such as glucose, fructose and ribose which cannot be broken down into smaller units by mild hydrolysis.
2. *Oligosaccharides*: short chain compounds which on hydrolysis yield a limited number of monosaccharide units.
3. *Polysaccharides*: complex polymers which contain large numbers of monosaccharide units. They may be composed of only one type of monosaccharide, as in the case of starch, glycogen, cellulose and dextran, or of two or more different monosaccharides as in the glycosaminoglycans.

In addition, carbohydrate-containing polymers are known which contain an appreciable amount of non-carbohydrate material. These include glycoproteins, glycopeptides, glycolipids and nucleic acids.

The sugars, of which the most important are the mono- and di-saccharides, have been given trivial names characteristically ending in the suffix -ose. They are crystalline substances which are soluble in water and dilute ethanol but insoluble in most organic solvents. Usually they have a sweet taste.

Monosaccharides

The monosaccharides contain between three and seven carbon atoms and are given group names which indicate the number as shown below:

$$\text{trioses (C}_3) \qquad \text{hexoses (C}_6)$$
$$\text{tetroses (C}_4) \qquad \text{heptoses (C}_7)$$
$$\text{pentoses (C}_5)$$

Sugars differ from the polyalcohols from which they are theoretically derived in that one of the alcohol groups is oxidized to a carbonyl group. Thus removal of two H atoms from glycerol results in either an aldehyde or a ketone according to the position of the carbonyl group formed as shown below:

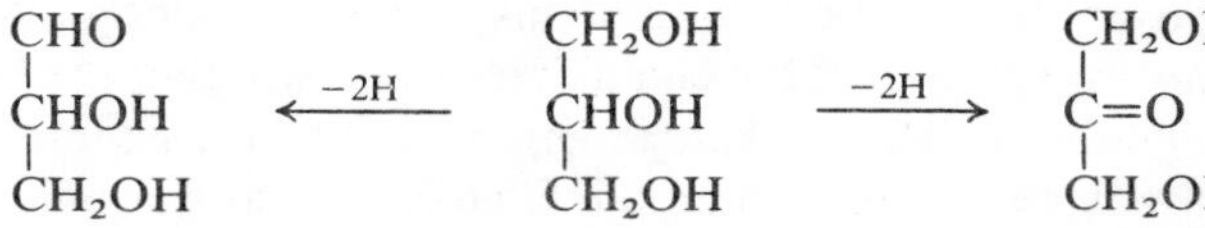

$$
\begin{array}{ccccc}
\text{CHO} & & \text{CH}_2\text{OH} & & \text{CH}_2\text{OH} \\
| & & | & & | \\
\text{CHOH} & \xleftarrow{-2\text{H}} & \text{CHOH} & \xrightarrow{-2\text{H}} & \text{C=O} \\
| & & | & & | \\
\text{CH}_2\text{OH} & & \text{CH}_2\text{OH} & & \text{CH}_2\text{OH}
\end{array}
$$

Glyceraldehyde   Glycerol   Dihydroxyacetone
(an aldotriose)   (polyhydric   (a ketotriose)
    alcohol)

Sugars that contain an aldehyde grouping are known as *aldoses* and those with a ketone grouping as *ketoses*. Thus the best known of the monosaccharides, glucose, which contains six carbon atoms and an aldehyde group, is an *aldohexose* whereas fructose is a *ketohexose*. Since the sugars possess one or more asymmetric carbon atoms they exist in various stereoisomeric forms. As with the amino acids the L and D forms of glyceraldehyde are used as reference compounds. Their molecular asymmetry, which is best appreciated by examining solid models, can be represented by projection formulae

$$
\begin{array}{cc}
\text{CHO} & \text{CHO} \\
| & | \\
\text{HO}-\text{C}-\text{H} & \text{H}-\text{C}-\text{OH} \\
| & | \\
\text{CH}_2\text{OH} & \text{CH}_2\text{OH}
\end{array}
$$

L-Glyceraldehyde   D-Glyceraldehyde

or more simply by

$$
\begin{array}{cc}
\text{O} & \text{O} \\
\dashv & \vdash \\
\text{X} & \text{X}
\end{array}
$$

where O = CHO
⊢ = the orientation of the OH group
X = CH$_2$OH

If the carbon chain is lengthened by the addition of another –CHOH unit between the asymmetric carbon atom and the aldehyde group this extra carbon atom will also be asymmetric and two new isomeric compounds will be formed. Thus the number of possible aldose sugars increases by a factor of 2 with each additional C atom so that the number of possible aldose sugars is 2^n where $n = $ the number of asymmetric C atoms in the molecule. It follows that there are four different aldotetroses and eight aldopentoses. In each case half the sugars belong to the D-series and half to the L-series.

Of the eight aldopentoses D-*ribose* is the most important from the biochemical point of view. It is a component of various coenzymes as well as the ribonucleic acids. Closely related to it is D-2-*deoxyribose* which differs only in the absence of an O atom from the second carbon of the sugar chain.

H O
\\ //
C
|
H—C—OH
|
H—C—OH
|
H—C—OH
|
CH₂OH

D-Ribose

H O
\\ //
C
|
H—C—H
|
H—C—OH
|
H—C—OH
|
CH₂OH

D-2-Deoxyribose

The naturally occurring sugars almost always belong to the D-series of compounds.

When sugars are represented by linear projection formulae the aldehyde, or other more highly oxidized group, is shown at the top and this C atom is designated C-1, while the asymmetric C atom nearest the bottom of the chain determines whether the sugar belongs to the D or L series. Such formulae clearly demonstrate the presence of any asymmetric C atoms but are misleading in suggesting that the bonds joining the C atoms are at an angle of 180°. When the bond angles of a pentose sugar are correctly shown at 110° the aldehyde group involving C-1 and the hydroxyl group in C-5 can be seen to be situated quite close together.

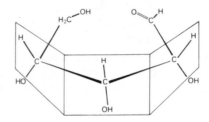

Figure 7.1 The angular structure of a pentose sugar

This proximity facilitates the formation of an oxygen-containing intramolecular ring which may be either a five-membered ($C_4 + O$) *furanose ring* or a six-membered ($C_5 + O$) *pyranose ring*. Compounds of this type which result from the condensation of an aldehyde group and a hydroxyl group are known as *hemiacetals* (page 10). Projection formulae such as the following, may be

D-Ribofuranose   D-Ribose   D-Ribopyranose

drawn showing these ring structures but they give a very distorted picture of the molecule and Haworth suggested that they should be replaced by *perspective formulae*. The perspective formulae for the pyranose and furanose forms of ribose are shown below with D-glucopyranose included for comparison:

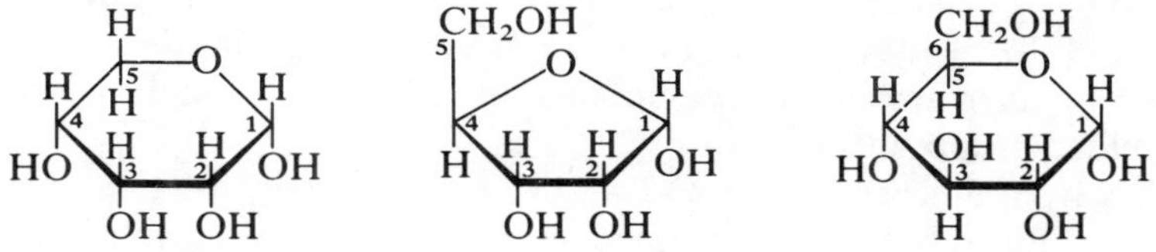

D-Ribopyranose   D-Ribofuranose   D-Glucopyranose

The five-membered furanose ring is an unstable structure. It is not found in the simple sugars but only when they exist in combination with other sugars or other types of compound. Some properties of sugars that cannot be explained by straight chain formulae can be accounted for on the basis of their existence as ring compounds.

It can be seen from the ring formulae for the sugars that, during the formation of the hemiacetal compounds, C-1, the 'carbonyl' carbon atom, becomes attached to four different groupings, i.e. it becomes asymmetric. D-Glucose (and other ring-forming sugars) can therefore exist in two distinct crystalline forms or *anomers* designated α-D-glucose and β-D-glucose. The designation α implies that the –OH group attached to C-1 lies below the plane of the ring and β that it lies above the plane of the ring. The anomers are interconvertible through the open chain aldehyde form:

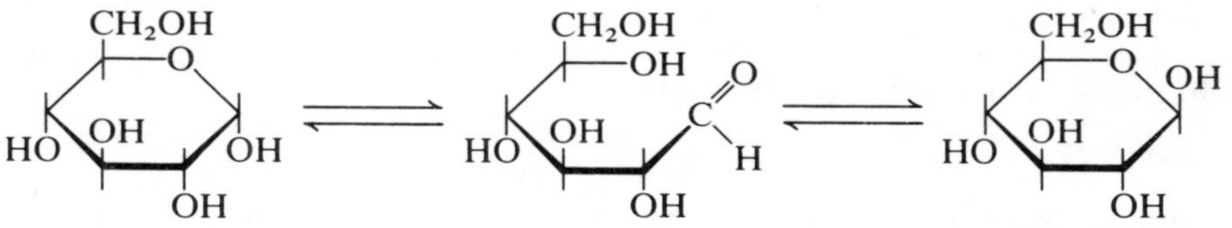

α-D-Glucopyranose β-D-Glucopyranose

All three forms are believed to be present in solutions of glucose, but the open chain aldehyde form is very unstable and present only in traces.

Hexose sugars

The most important and widely distributed of the hexose sugars is *D-glucose* or *dextrose*. The other naturally occurring hexoses of physiological importance are galactose and mannose, which are aldohexoses, and fructose which is the only commonly occurring ketohexose. All belong to the D-series, the differences between them being shown in the following simplified projection formulae:

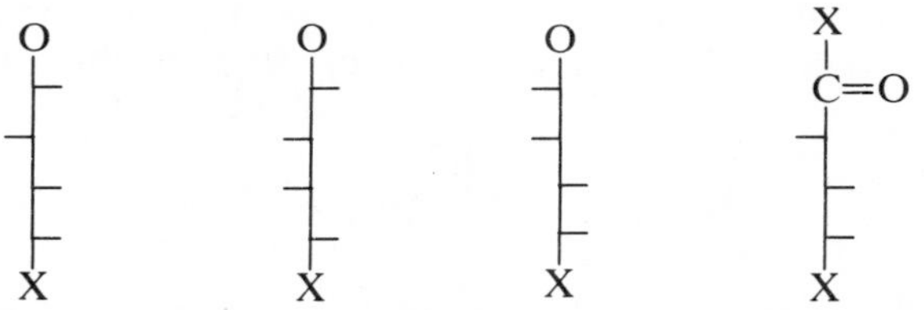

D-Glucose   D-Galactose   D-Mannose   D-Fructose

O = –CHO
X = –CH$_2$OH
⊣ and ⊢ indicate the orientation of the –OH groups

Aldoses   Ketose

It can be seen that galactose differs from glucose only in the steric configuration at C-4 while mannose differs only at C-2. The configuration at C-3, C-4 and C-5 of fructose is the same as for glucose.

Galactose is found primarily as a component of lactose, a disaccharide present in the milk of mammals, and in the galactolipids or cerebrosides, which occur in large amounts in the white matter of brain and the myelin sheath of nerves. *Mannose* occurs widely in plants and is also found in small amounts in animals as a component of such complex materials as glycoproteins, glycolipids and blood group substances.

Fructose differs from glucose only at C-1 and C-2. When free, fructose occurs in the more stable pyranose ring form, but when combined, as in sucrose or its phosphate esters, it assumes the five-membered furanose ring structure.

β-D-Fructopyranose   β-D-Fructofuranose

The presence of a ketone group in a sugar is usually indicated by the ending -ulose, e.g. sedoheptulose, a sugar containing seven carbon atoms and a ketone group. This is formed as an intermediate in the pentose phosphate pathway of carbohydrate metabolism (Figure 17.2).

Some biochemically important sugar derivatives

Oxidation products

Mild oxidation of the aldose sugars *in vitro* causes the ring structure to break down and a monobasic acid to be produced. Such acids are named by substituting the suffix -onic acid for -ose in the name of the sugar. Thus glucose is converted to *gluconic acid*. This reaction occurs readily *in vitro* but not in the body. It is, however, catalysed by a fungal enzyme known as *glucose oxidase*, which is highly specific and is used for estimating glucose. On the other hand, 6-phosphogluconic acid is formed in the pentose phosphate pathway of glucose metabolism (page 232).

Uronic acids

A second series of acids, the *uronic acids*, that cannot be prepared by direct oxidation of the aldoses *in vitro* are found as constituents of the glycosaminoglycans (page 407). They are also involved in the conversion of various aromatic compounds into conjugated derivatives, the *glucuronides*, which are suitable for excretion by the kidneys. In the uronic acids the primary

α-D-Glucuronic acid   β-D-Glucuronic acid

alcohol group (C-6) of the sugar has been oxidized to a –COOH group, the aldehyde group and hence the ring structure remaining unchanged. Individual members of the group are named by adding the suffix -uronic acid to the root of the name of the corresponding monosaccharide, e.g. *glucuronic acid* and *galacturonic acid*.

Glycosides

The glucose molecule contains three different types of hydroxyl group: (1) a primary alcohol group involving C-6; (2) three secondary alcohol groups involving C-2, C-3 and C-4; (3) the –OH group attached to C-1 which is different from the others and more reactive since it is attached to a C atom which is directly united to another O atom. Its configuration, i.e. whether it is in the α or β position, is fixed only as long as the pyranose ring is intact. In solution the α and β forms of glucose are interconvertible, although if the –OH group is substituted, e.g. by reaction with a phenolic or alcoholic grouping and the elimination of water, the ring structure is stabilized and the configuration becomes fixed. The resulting compound is known as a *glucoside* and belongs to the class of compounds known as *glycosides*.

α-D-Glucopyranose α-Methyl-D-glucoside

Glycosides of other sugars are known as *galactosides*, *ribosides*, etc., according to the particular sugar from which they are derived. Both α- and β-glycosides exist but they are not directly interconvertible.

The glycosidic linkage is very important and plays a role in carbohydrate chemistry analogous to that of the peptide bond in protein chemistry and the phosphate ester linkage in nucleic acids, since they each participate in forming polymeric compounds. The glycosidic linkage not only joins sugar units to other sugar units, as in the case of the oligo- and poly-saccharides, but it can link monosaccharides to non-sugar compounds. Glycosides containing non-sugar moieties include such compounds as digitalin, the cardiac glycoside obtained from foxglove leaves, and the drug phlorrhizin, which is used to induce experimental diabetes.

A variety of *glycosidases* which hydrolyse glycosidic bonds are found in plant and animal tissues and also in microorganisms. They are highly specific in their occurrence and action and have been used extensively in the elucidation of carbohydrate structures.

Amino sugars

Amino sugars are formed by the replacement of one of the hydroxyl groups of a sugar by an amino group or substituted amino group, e.g. –NHCOCH$_3$. Three amino sugars are of

Glucosamine   Galactosamine

physiological importance, namely glucosamine, galactosamine and neuraminic acid. Glucosamine and galactosamine are derived from glucose and galactose respectively, the amino group in each case replacing the hydroxyl group on C-2.

Neuraminic acid is more complex. It is a nine-carbon amino sugar formed by the condensation of mannosamine 6-phosphate and phosphoenolpyruvate (PEP). It is the parent substance of the *sialic acids* which are acyl derivatives of neuraminic acid, e.g. *N*-acetylneuraminic acid. Sialic acids are found as constituents of glycoproteins and glycolipids and are believed to have an important bearing on the formation of the acquired integuments of the teeth (Chapter 34).

$$
\begin{array}{c}
\text{COOH} \\
| \\
\text{CO} \\
| \\
\text{CH}_2 \\
| \\
\text{H}-\text{C}-\text{OH} \\
| \\
\text{HOCH}_2\cdot\text{CO}\cdot\text{NH}-\text{C}-\text{H} \\
| \\
\text{HO}-\text{C}-\text{H} \\
| \\
\text{H}-\text{C}-\text{OH} \\
| \\
\text{H}-\text{C}-\text{OH} \\
| \\
\text{CH}_2\text{OH}
\end{array}
$$

N-Glycolylneuraminic acid

Sugar phosphates

Phosphoric acid esters of sugars take part in many metabolic reactions. Their importance as intermediates was first recognized as a result of Man's long-standing interest in alcoholic fermentation, to which biochemistry owes a major debt!

Different esters of the same sugar, e.g. glucose 1-phosphate and glucose 6-phosphate, behave quite differently in biochemical reactions.

Glucose 6-phosphate   Glucose 1-phosphate

$-\text{(P)} = -\text{PO}_3\text{H}_2$

Oligosaccharides

In the formation of the disaccharides and other oligosaccharides the hydroxyl group derived from the reactive carbonyl group of one sugar combines with an alcohol group of another sugar molecule with the elimination of H_2O, forming a glycosidic bond. In some of the disaccharides, e.g. sucrose, the reducing groups of both constituent monosaccharides are involved in the linkage so that the disaccharide is non-reducing. In other disaccharides, e.g. maltose and lactose, only one reducing group is involved and the other remains free.

Maltose is best known as the main product of the breakdown of starch by enzymes. It is composed of two glucose units, C-1 of the first being joined by an α-glycosidic linkage to C-4 of the second glucose molecule.

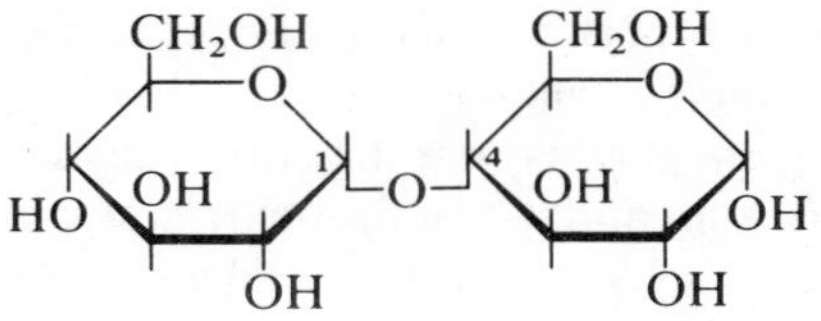

CH$_2$OH   CH$_2$OH

Maltose
(4-α-glucosidoglucose)

Lactose is found solely in the animal kingdom and is present in the milk of all mammals. It is composed of glucose and galactose, C-1 of the galactose being joined to C-4 of the glucose by a linkage of the β-type.

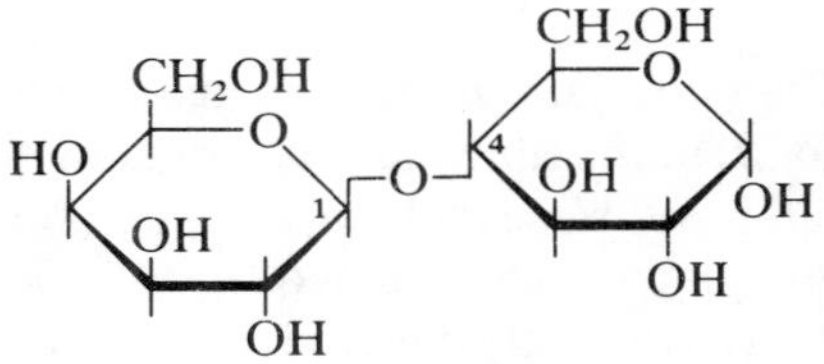

CH$_2$OH

CH$_2$OH

Lactose
(4-β-galactosidoglucose)

Sucrose is widely distributed in plants and is obtained commercially from sugar cane or sugar beet. It is also present in honey. Sucrose is one of the few foodstuffs that is used in crystalline form. It is composed of glucose and fructose and is a non-reducing sugar, since the carbonyl group (C-1) of the glucose is linked to the carbonyl group (C-2) of the fructose, the linkage being of the α-type with respect to the glucose and the β-type with respect to the fructose. The fructose is present in the furanose ring form. Sucrose is very readily hydrolysed, and, owing to the unusual nature of the linkage, the ΔG^0 of its hydrolysis is greater than that of the other disaccharides (page 213).

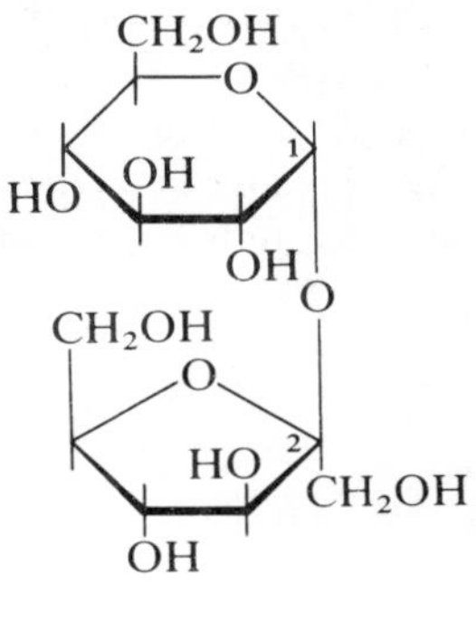

CH$_2$OH

CH$_2$OH

Sucrose
(α-D-glucopyranoside
β-D-fructofuranoside)

Polysaccharides

The polysaccharides are less complex than proteins and less specific in their reactions and functions. They can be broadly divided into those like starch and glycogen that act as food reserves and a more varied group of compounds that play a structural role and include cellulose, the glycosaminoglycans and bacterial cell wall constituents. Since glucose is a major source of energy for living cells, it is not surprising that polymeric forms of glucose, namely starch and glycogen, are found as storage materials. What is perhaps more surprising is that although plants contain large amounts of starch in their seeds and tubers, the amount of glycogen present in the adult human body is only about 500 g in a 70 kg man. This is because fat is the chief energy store in mammals.

The natural polymers are built up of long chains of sugar units which may be straight or branched. They show a wide variety of sizes, properties and functions which depend both on the constituent monosaccharide units and on the linkages which join them together. In starch, glycogen and cellulose, which are *homopolymers*, glucose is the only sugar present and the main type of linkage is between C-1 of one glucose unit and C-4 of the next. In starch and glycogen this is an α-glycosidic linkage, which can be readily hydrolysed by enzymes found in the digestive tract but in cellulose it is a β-linkage which is only broken by microbial enzymes.

Storage polysaccharides

Starch

Although starch occurs almost as widely as cellulose, it is found in much smaller quantities. It is the main source of dietary carbohydrate and occurs as characteristic granules in seeds, roots and certain fruits. It is a mixture of two compounds, *amylose* and *amylopectin*. Amylose consists of a single unbranched chain of about 250–300 glucose units joined by α-1,4-glycoside linkages giving it a molecular weight of 40 000–50 000. There is only one free reducing group in each chain so that amylose is in effect non-reducing. X-ray diffraction studies suggest that the molecule tends to coil up to give a spiral structure like a wide hollow tube in which there are six glucose units per turn.

In most starches amylose constitutes only about 20% of the total and amylopectin is the major constituent. The amylopectin molecule is very large and differs from amylose in its greater size and also in being highly branched, which gives it a tree-like shape. Values obtained for its molecular weight range from 50 000 to several millions. Like other macromolecules starch tends to be degraded during isolation and purification so the higher values are likely to be correct.

The branches of the amylopectin molecule consist of straight chain segments made up of about 20–30 glucose units joined by α-1 : 4 linkages. At the branch points are α-1 : 6 linkages, as shown in Figure 7.2. When starch is acted upon by amylases (page 224) a whole range of low molecular weight poly- and oligo-saccharides known as *dextrins* are produced as intermediate products and maltose is the major end product. Little or no free glucose is formed. The dextrins react with iodine to give colours that change from dark blue through purple to reddish brown and then colourless as the chains become shorter.

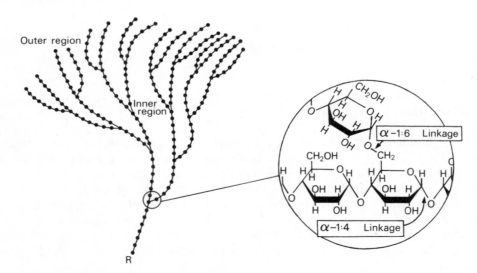

Figure 7.2 The structure of glycogen showing (inset) the structure of a branch point

Both amylose and amylopectin are hydrolysed completely when boiled with acid giving glucose as the only product.

Glycogen

This is the form in which animals store D-glucose and it is found chiefly in the liver and muscles. Its structure is very similar to that of amylopectin but the molecule is even more highly branched, since branching occurs on average after every 12 α-1 : 4-linked residues. Although its molecular weight is very high (1–5 million) it dissolves in water to give a colloidal solution.

The isolation of glycogen requires special precautions since, after removal of the tissues from the body, it is rapidly acted upon by enzymes which convert it to lactic acid.

Dextrans

Dextrans are bacterial polysaccharides which are formed chiefly from sucrose but also from dextrins. They are branched chain polymers of glucose having a slimy consistency and high viscosity. On this account they were used as plasma substitutes in the Second World War. Although dextran is soluble in water it can be converted into insoluble hydrophilic gels of varying porosity by cross-linking the chains to give a three-dimensional network. Dextrans are constituents of dental plaque and may be of considerable significance in the development of dental caries.

Structural polysaccharides

Glycosaminoglycans

These substances have a high viscosity and gel-like consistency which enable them to play a part in controlling the movement of materials through tissues. The same viscous quality is made use of in their role as biological lubricants. The mucous secretions of numerous tissues including those of the salivary glands owe their 'slimy' consistency to various *mucosubstances* which are combinations of carbohydrate and protein (Chapter 27). Mucosubstances are important constituents of connective tissues.

Cellulose

Although, like starch and glycogen, cellulose is constructed solely from glucose units, these are joined by β-1 : 4 linkages and this causes its structure and properties to be very different. The β-linkage allows the molecules of cellulose to pack together closely and enables hydrogen bonding to occur between adjacent chains which are flat and ribbon-like. Thus cellulose occurs as strong fibrous molecular bundles which are inert and very insoluble and are not attacked by the α-glycosidases produced by vertebrates. However, certain bacteria commonly found in the stomach of ruminants possess β-glycosidases which digest cellulose and allow it to be utilized by the animal.

Chapter 8
Lipids

The term 'lipid' covers a miscellaneous collection of compounds having a predominantly hydrocarbon nature. They are consequently insoluble in water and readily soluble in most organic solvents. Apart from solubility considerations, inclusion of a compound in the group usually depends on its content of long chain fatty acids.

Lipids may be subdivided into

1. *Simple lipids*. These consist of long chain *fatty acids* which may be either free or combined with an alcohol by an ester linkage. They include the *triglycerides* (*triacylglycerols*) and the *waxes*.
2. *Compound lipids* which contain additional groupings such as phosphoric acid, sugars, nitrogenous bases or proteins. Included in this group are the *phospholipids*, *glycolipids* and *lipoproteins*.
3. *Steroids*. Although they do not often contain fatty acids the steroids are frequently classed as lipids on account of their occurrence in natural fats and their solubility characteristics. They include *cholesterol* and the *sex* and *adrenocortical hormones*.

Lipids are widely distributed throughout both plant and animal kingdoms and are essential constituents of cell membranes; the phospholipids and cholesterol are particularly significant in this respect. Quantitatively the triglycerides are the most abundant of the lipids and form the chief energy reserve of animals. They also protect the body from heat loss and mechanical injury. In plants triglycerides occur in quantity only in seeds.

The waxes have a protective function. In animals they keep feathers, skin and hair soft, pliable and water repellant, while the cuticle waxes of plants protect them both from dehydration and from invasion by harmful organisms.

Simple lipids

Naturally occurring fatty acids

These are mainly straight chain aliphatic monocarboxylic acids containing an even number of carbon atoms. The series ranges from acetic acid (C_2) to members containing twenty or more carbon atoms which may be either saturated or unsaturated. The saturated fatty acids containing up to eight carbon atoms are liquid at room temperature but those with longer chains are solids. The introduction of a double bond renders even the long chain acids liquid, thus the 18-carbon saturated *stearic acid* has a melting point of 70°C whereas *oleic acid*, which contains 18 carbon atoms and one double bond, has a melting point of only 14°C.

The fatty acids were originally given Greek names indicating their source but their systematic names based on Greek numbers indicate not only the length of the chain but also the degree of saturation. The suffix *-anoic* indicates that the acid is saturated and *-enoic* that it is unsaturated. If there are two or three double bonds the suffix becomes *-dienoic* and *-trienoic* respectively. The carbon atoms are numbered along the chain, beginning with C-1, the carboxyl group. Alternatively the carbon atom adjacent to the –COOH group is known as the α-carbon atom and the one furthest from the –COOH group as the ω-carbon atom. The position of the double bond may be indicated by inserting the lower of the numbers of the two carbon atoms involved in the bond. Thus the systematic name for oleic acid which has 18 carbon atoms and a double bond between carbons 9 and 10 is 9-octadecenoic acid while that of linoleic acid which contains 18 carbon atoms and double bonds between carbon atoms 9 and 10 and between 12 and 13 is 9,12-octadecadienoic acid (Tables 8.1 and 8.2).

The general type of acid may be more simply represented by stating merely the number of C atoms and double bonds which it contains. Thus the type specifications for palmitic, oleic and linoleic acids are 16 : 0, 18 : 1 and 18 : 2 respectively.

The short and medium chain saturated acids are steam volatile and have unpleasant smells, that of butyric acid (C_4) present in rancid butter being well known.

Free fatty acids dissociate in water and in most cases the pK_a lies in the range 4·7–5·0. However, because of their negligible solubility in water, the acid properties of the higher members of the series cannot readily be measured.

Table 8.1 Naturally occurring straight chain saturated fatty acids

No. of C atoms	Common name		Systematic name
2	Acetic		n-Ethanoic
3	Propionic	Short chain	n-Propanoic
4	Butyric		n-Butanoic
8	Caprylic	Medium chain	n-Octanoic
10	Capric		n-Decanoic
12	Lauric		n-Dodecanoic
14	Myristic		n-Tetradecanoic
16	Palmitic	Long chain	n-Hexadecanoic
18	Stearic		n-Octadecanoic
20	Arachidic		n-Eicosanoic

The presence of both the non-polar hydrophobic hydrocarbon chain and the polar hydrophilic –COOH group is reflected in their physical characteristics. Thus fatty acids may be spread on the surface of water as monomolecular films or *monolayers* in which the molecules are orientated so that the polar –COOH group penetrates the surface and the hydrocarbon chain projects away from it. This property is even more pronounced in the case of the phospholipids.

The fatty acids that occur in greatest amount in natural fats are the saturated 16 : 0 *palmitic acid*, the 18 : 0 *stearic acid* and the unsaturated 18 : 1 *oleic acid*. Branched chain fatty acids and fatty acids containing an uneven number of C atoms are rarely found.

Unsaturated fatty acids

Oleic acid which contains a single double bond in the middle of a C_{18} chain is one of the most abundant fatty acids. Other members of the series are found in smaller amounts as are a number of *polyunsaturated fatty acids* containing more than one double bond (Table 8.2). These include *linoleic acid* and *arachidonic acid* which, although present in relatively small amounts, are physiologically important. They cannot be synthesized in the body and must therefore be supplied in the diet (page 123). Hence they are known as *essential fatty acids*.

Table 8.2 Some naturally occurring unsaturated fatty acids

No. of C atoms	No. of double bonds	Common name	Systematic name
16	1	Palmitoleic	*cis*-9-Hexadecanoic
18	1	Oleic	*cis*-9-Octadecenoic
18	2	Linoleic*	*cis*,*cis*-9,12-Octadecadienoic
18	3	γ-Linolenic*	*all-cis*-6,9,12-Octadecatrienoic
20	4	Arachidonic*	*all*-cis-5,8,11,14-Eicosatetraenoic

* Polyunsaturated fatty acids (PUFA)

The presence of every double bond introduces the possibility of *cis–trans isomerism*. Free rotation about a double bond is not possible, so there are two stereoisomers

Cis isomer   *Trans* isomer

The hydrocarbon chains of saturated fatty acids (and unsaturated fatty acids in which the configuration is *all trans*) assume a zigzag configuration with the C–C bonds forming a bond angle of 109°; if there is a *cis* double bond present, the zigzag alters course at this point. Since the naturally occurring unsaturated fatty acids usually have a *cis* configuration about their double bonds their chains tend to be less compact than those of saturated acids, which can fit into smaller spaces (Figure 8.1). This is a significant consideration in membrane structure (page 194) for, whereas saturated fatty acid chains are flexible, the unsaturated ones are kinked and relatively rigid.

As a result of the different relationships and distances between their component groups, *geometrical isomers* such as oleic and elaidic acids and maleic and fumaric acids, unlike optical isomers, have different properties and reactions:

Oleic acid   Elaidic acid

Maleic acid   Fumaric acid

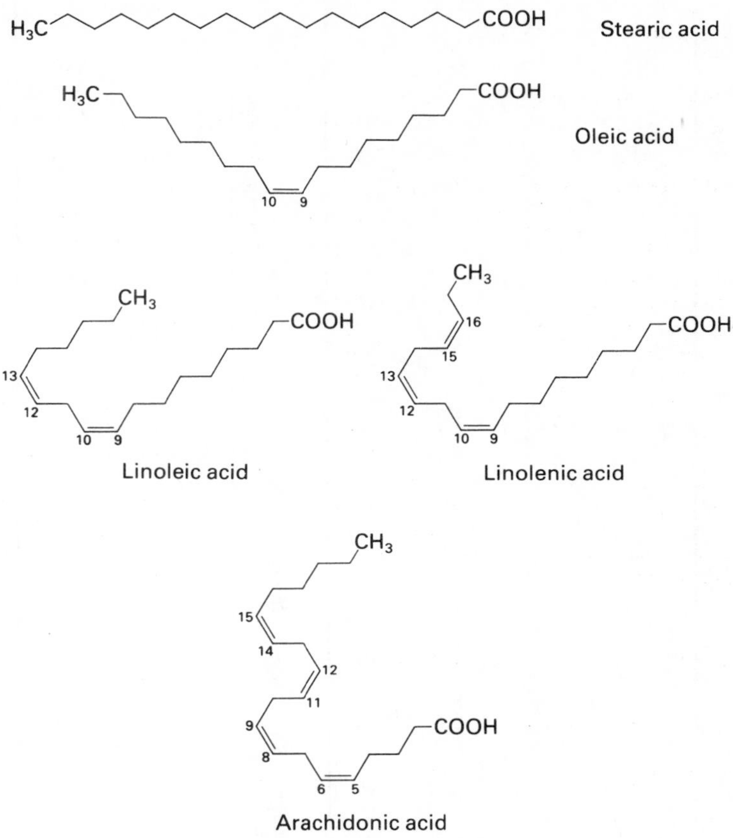

Figure 8.1 Naturally occurring saturated and unsaturated fatty acids

Since in living systems enzymes are highly specific and irregularly shaped it is usual to find only one of the forms occurring naturally.

The unsaturated fatty acids are considerably more reactive than the saturated ones. They tend to decompose at high temperatures and can be oxidized at the double bond.

The *prostaglandins* (page 364) are derived from arachidonic acid.

Esters of fatty acids

Although fatty acids are abundant in the body, only a small fraction is present as *free fatty acids* (FFA); by far the greater amount is found in the form of esters. The simple fatty acid esters are the glycerides and the waxes. In the waxes the fatty acids are esterified with long chain fatty alcohols containing from 12 to 34 C atoms, for example beeswax is composed chiefly of palmitic acid esterified with myricyl (C_{14}) alcohol.

The glycerides (acylglycerols)

These are esters of the trihydric alcohol *glycerol* which on oxidation yields glyceraldehyde, the simplest of the aldose sugars.

Table 8.3 The fatty acid composition of some plant oils

Fatty acid		Coconut	Corn (maize)	Cottonseed	Groundnut	Olive	Palm	Peanut	Sesame	Soya	Green leaf	Margarine Hard	Margarine Soft
Short chain (C_4–C_{10})		14										3	2
Medium chain (C_{12}–C_{14})		58		1·5			3			0·4		5	1
Palmitic	16:0	11	13	11	14	14	41	11	8	12	13	25	12
Stearic	18:0	3	2	2	4	3	5	3	4	4		10	8
Oleic	18:1	7	31	16	40	74	42	52	38	24	7	30	22
Linoleic	18:2	2	53	60	36	7	7	28	42	51	16	9	52
Linolenic	18:3		1	0·5		1				9	56	1	1

N.B. (i) Most seed oils contain palmitic, oleic and linoleic acids as their major constituents
(ii) Variations in the composition of oil samples of similar origin are determined more by environmental factors than the variety of plant

Table 8.4 The fatty acid composition of some animal fats

Fatty acid		Human	Beef	Sheep	Pig	Chicken	Rabbit	Beef muscle	Cod	Herring	Mackerel	Pilchard	Salmon	Milk Human	Milk Cow	Cod liver oil
Short chain (C_4–C_{10})														2	16	
Medium chain (C_{12}–C_{14})		5	3	3	1	1	7	3	2	8	5	10	7	17	12	3
Palmitic	16:0	25	25	25	25	27	32	13	33	18	28	19	14	23	21	11
Stearic	18:0	7	26	28	13	5	5	16	4	4	4			9	11	4
Oleic	18:1	47	40	37	51	46	28	21	12	17	19	17	26	34	31	24
Linoleic	18:2	6	2	4	8	14	19	20	1					7	5	1·5
Linolenic	18:3							2	1							1
Arachidonic	20:4							19			4					

N.B. (i) Fats of land animals are solid or semi-solid and are composed almost entirely of C_{16} and C_{18} acids. Fats of ruminants contain nearly 60% of saturated acids
(ii) Fats of aquatic origin are usually liquid and contain 20 or more different acids varying in chain length from C_{14} to C_{24}

$$\alpha\ CH_2OH$$
$$\beta\ CHOH$$
$$\alpha\ CH_2OH$$
Glycerol

$$CHO$$
$$CHOH$$
$$CH_2OH$$
Glyceraldehyde

Like the sugars, glycerol has a sweet taste and is completely soluble in water. Because it has three alcohol groups, one molecule of glycerol can combine with one, two or three molecules of fatty acid to yield *mono-*, *di-* and *tri-glycerides*.

$$CH_2O \cdot OCR^1$$
$$CHOH$$
$$CH_2OH$$
α-Monoglyceride

$$CH_2O \cdot OCR^1$$
$$CHO \cdot OCR^2$$
$$CH_2OH$$
α,β-Diglyceride

$$CH_2O \cdot OCR^1$$
$$CHO \cdot OCR^2$$
$$CH_2O \cdot OCR^3$$
Triglyceride

The mono- and di-glycerides occur in small amounts in the body, chiefly as intermediates in fat digestion and metabolism, but most of the fatty material present in the adipose tissue is in the form of triglycerides. In these the fatty acids may all be of the same kind as in *tristearin* or *triolein*, but usually more than one kind is present, i.e. they are *mixed triglycerides* such as *oleostearopalmitin* or *dioleostearin*. Since natural fats are mixtures of a number of different mixed triglycerides complete characterization is difficult if not virtually impossible. A mixture of six different fatty acids might occur as 6^3, i.e. 216 different triglycerides! It is, however, relatively easy to determine the nature and proportions of the various fatty acids present. Most plant fats are liquids since they contain a large proportion of unsaturated fatty acids with low melting points (Table 8.3). Animal fats, on the other hand, contain a high proportion of palmitic and stearic acids, and are solid or semi-solid at room temperature (Table 8.4). The depot fats of cattle and sheep are particularly low in polyunsaturated fatty acids since those present in their diet are hydrogenated by microorganisms in the rumen. Milk fat is unusual in containing a high proportion of shorter chain (C_4–C_{14}) fatty acids.

Compound lipids

Phospholipids

These represent a large and diffuse group of compounds. Among the most important are the *phospholipids* which contain a phosphate group as an integral part of their structure. This part of the molecule is highly polar and water soluble, while the part incorporating the bulky hydrocarbon chains of the fatty acids is non-polar and lipid soluble. As a result, phospholipids can bridge lipid–water interfaces, the polar region being associated with the aqueous phase and the remainder with the lipid or other non-polar milieu (Figure 8.2a). Thus when dispersed in water, phospholipid molecules, which may be regarded as two-pronged structures with a polar head and two hydrophobic tails, tend to form a double layer, with the hydrophobic hydrocarbon chains facing each other, and the hydrophilic polar groupings projecting outwards (Figure 8.2b). Alternatively, the molecules may form spherical micelles again with their hydrophobic groups projecting inwards and their polar groups outwards (Figure 8.2c). In a non-polar solvent the orientation tends to be reversed, polar groups projecting inwards and the hydrophobic groups outwards (Figure 8.2d). The inherent properties of the different parts of phospholipid molecules are highly significant in relation to the strucural organization of cell membranes (Chapter 15).

Typical examples of the class are the *lecithins* (*phosphatidylcholines*). These contain a

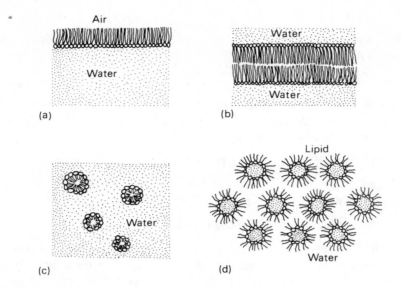

Figure 8.2 Association of phospholipid molecules. (a) As a monomolecular film at an air–water interface; (b) as a bilayer in water; (c) as a micelle in water; (d) as a micelle in a non-polar solvent

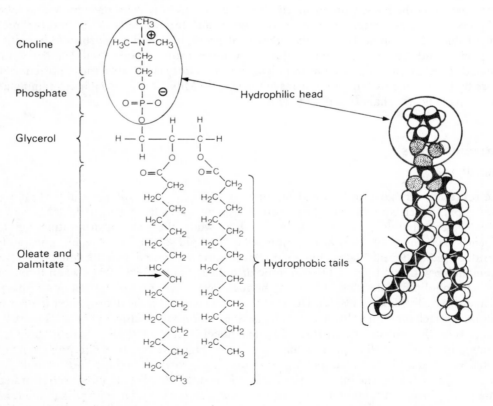

Figure 8.3 The structure of lecithin

backbone of *α-glycerophosphate* in which one of the α-CH_2OH groups of glycerol is esterified with phosphoric acid. If the remaining hydroxyl groups on the α and β carbon atoms are each esterified with a fatty acid residue the compound is known as a *phosphatidic acid*; usually the fatty acid in the β-position is unsaturated (Figure 8.3). The lecithins are derived from the phosphatidic acids by further esterification of the phosphate group with the nitrogenous base *choline*. Choline may be considered as being derived from ammonium hydroxide by substitution of three of its H atoms with methyl groups and the fourth with ethyl alcohol.

α-Glycerophosphate   Phosphatidic acid   Lecithin (phosphatidylcholine)

Ammonium hydroxide   Choline

At physiological pH values the quaternary nitrogen of choline carries a positive charge while the phosphate group is negatively charged, so that lecithin usually exists in the form of a dipolar ion.

In other types of phospholipid known as the *kephalins* the phosphatidic acid may be bound to β-ethanolamine or serine in place of choline:

Choline   β-Ethanolamine   Serine

Phospholipids are not generally soluble in water although they readily form emulsions. They are less soluble in acetone than are other lipids, and may be separated from them on this basis.

Phospholipids have a detergent action and are essential for the normal functioning of the lungs because the walls of the alveoli are not strong enough to maintain their shape against the surface tension of water. This is normally reduced by the secretion of an unusual form of lecithin which allows the alveoli to expand. Premature infants may not secrete enough of this *lung surfactant* and if so will suffer from respiratory distress which may be fatal.

Other compound lipids

Other compound lipids include the *sphingolipids* or *sphingomyelins* and the *glycolipids* or *cerebrosides*, which are found chiefly in the nervous system. The *plasmalogens* comprise a considerable proportion of the total phospholipids of muscle.

Lipoproteins are loose complexes of lipid and protein in which the components are held together by secondary forces rather than by covalent bonds. In blood plasma much of the lipid is found in this form, consisting mainly of phospholipids and esters of cholesterol. The class also includes the *chylomicrons* which appear in the blood after a fatty meal and are composed essentially of triglycerides surrounded by a protein envelope. The various membrane structures of the cell may be considered as lipoprotein complexes.

Steroids

Although the steroids are structurally very different from the other lipids they show typical solubility characteristics and like the phospholipids are important constituents of membranes. They all have a common ring structure derived from *phenanthrene*

<table>
<tr><td style="text-align:center">Phenanthrene</td><td style="text-align:center">The steroid ring structure</td></tr>
</table>

Of the four fused rings, three are six-membered and the fourth contains five carbon atoms. Although, as represented, the ring system appears flat it is, in fact, buckled. All the steroids have a side chain or an –OH or =O group on C-17 and most have methyl groups attached to C-10 and C-13. Many of the steroids also have an alcoholic hydroxyl group attached to the ring system and they are then known as *sterols*. The commonest member of the class is *cholesterol* (Figure 8.4) which is present in most animal tissues.

Cholesterol is readily synthesized from acetyl-CoA (page 231) and is the parent substance for the other natural steroids; these include *cholic acid* which is a constituent of the bile salts, the sex hormones and the adrenocortical hormones. In addition, a derivative of cholesterol, namely *7-dehydrocholesterol*, is present in the skin and this, on irradiation with ultraviolet light, is converted to vitamin D which is a steroid derivative (page 156).

A variety of steroids has been synthesized and many valuable drugs produced by slightly modifying the structure of the natural hormones. These products may be more soluble in water or less readily attacked by enzymes than the original and thus their activity may be enhanced or prolonged. Synthetic derivatives of the female sex hormones, which prevent ovulation, are widely used as contraceptives ('the Pill'). Relatively small structural changes have made them suitable for oral administration which the forms produced in the body are not.

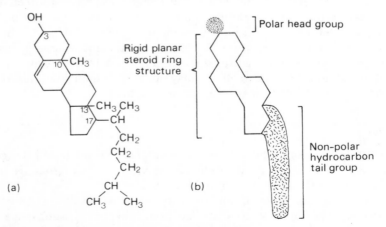

Figure 8.4 The structure of cholesterol. (a) Formula; (b) molecular outline

Chapter 9
Nucleotides and nucleic acids

The nucleotides which consist of three parts, namely a nitrogenous base, a pentose sugar and a phosphate radical, are a very important group of compounds since one or more of them is involved in virtually every biochemical process. The *adenosine di-* and *tri-phosphates* which play an essential part in cellular energy exchanges have a nucleotide-type structure as do many of the *coenzymes*. Furthermore, nucleotides constitute the monomeric units of which the nucleic acids are composed; that is to say nucleic acids are *polynucleotides*. The nucleic acids which are of two types, *deoxyribonucleic acid* (DNA) and *ribonucleic acid* (RNA), are responsible for directing the synthesis of proteins. They specify the unique sequence of amino acids in any particular protein and consequently should be regarded as primordial molecules on whose existence that of the proteins depends. However, since the synthesis of the nucleic acids depends on enzymes which are themselves proteins, this poses the fundamental evolutionary question as to which came first – the biochemical version of the problem of the chicken and the egg!

In addition to their role in protein synthesis nucleic acids transmit genetic information from parent to offspring and the entire range of inherited characteristics of any organism is believed to be defined in terms of the deoxyribonucleic acid that its cells contain.

Nucleic acid components

Nucleic acids may be broken down into their constituents by acid hydrolysis which produces a mixture of nitrogenous bases, pentose sugars and inorganic phosphate.

The *nitrogenous bases* are planar aromatic heterocyclic ring compounds which absorb ultraviolet light. They are of two different types, derived from *pyrimidine* and *purine* respectively.

The structure of pyrimidine is shown below. It is a six-membered unsaturated ring compound containing four carbon and two nitrogen atoms.

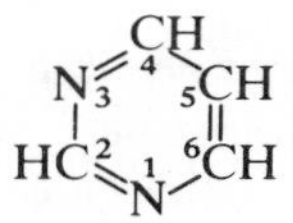

$$
\begin{array}{c}
\text{CH} \\
\text{N}_3 \overset{4}{\diagup} \overset{5}{\diagdown} \text{CH} \\
\| \qquad \| \\
\text{HC}_2 \diagdown \underset{\text{N}}{\overset{1}{\diagup}} \overset{6}{} \text{CH}
\end{array}
$$

Three different substituted pyrimidines are found in the nucleic acids, namely *cytosine* (2-oxy-4-aminopyrimidine) which is present in both DNA and RNA, *uracil* (2,4-dioxypyrimidine) which is present in RNA but not in DNA and *thymine* (5-methyluracil) which is present in DNA but not in RNA. They all exhibit keto-enol tautomerism.

| Cytosine | Uracil | Thymine |

Purine has a double ring structure in which one of the rings is similar to that of pyrimidine (although it is numbered differently!) and shares two of its carbon atoms with the second five-membered ring which also contains two nitrogen atoms and is similar to the imidazole ring of histidine.

DNA and RNA both contain the two substituted purines *adenine* (6-aminopurine) and *guanine* (2-amino-6-oxypurine). Small amounts of other bases including hypoxanthine and a variety of methylated purines and pyrimidines are found in certain types of RNA (page 299).

| Adenine | Guanine |

The *pentose sugars* obtained by complete hydrolysis of the nucleic acids are of two types. The pentose derived from RNA is *D-ribose* and that from DNA is *D-2-deoxyribose*. When present in nucleotide combination they are found in the furanose form, i.e. as D-ribofuranose and D-2-deoxyribofuranose respectively.

| D-Ribofuranose | D-2-Deoxyribofuranose |

Phosphoric acid is released on acid hydrolysis of both DNA and RNA.

Nucleosides and nucleotides

Compounds in which a purine or pyrimidine base is combined with a sugar are known as *nucleosides* and addition of a phosphoric acid moiety converts them into *nucleotides*. Deoxyribonucleosides and deoxyribonucleotides are of less general occurrence in the body than

Table 9.1 Some nitrogenous bases and their derivatives

Nitrogenous base	Type	Substituents	Nucleoside	Nucleotide
Adenine	Purine	6-amino	Adenosine	Adenylic acid
Guanine	Purine	2-amino-6-hydroxy	Guanosine	Guanylic acid
Hypoxanthine	Purine	6-hydroxy	Inosine	Inosinic acid
Cytosine	Pyrimidine	2-hydroxy-4-amino	Cytidine	Cytidylic acid
Thymine	Pyrimidine	2,4-dihydroxy-5-methyl	Thymidine	Thymidylic acid
Uracil	Pyrimidine	2,4-dihydroxy	Uridine	Uridylic acid

the corresponding ribose derivatives and in order to distinguish them it is usual to prefix the normal abbreviation for the ribonucleosides and ribonucleotides with d. Thus dA, dG, dC and dT specify the deoxyribonucleosides of adenine, guanine, cytosine and thymine and dAMP, dGMP, dCMP and TMP the corresponding deoxyribonucleotides. (No prefix is necessary to TMP because it does not exist in the ribonucleotide form.) A list of the most common nucleosides and nucleotides is given in Table 9.1.

Cautious hydrolysis of nucleic acids by alkali or enzymes produces a mixture of *nucleotides*. In these the base is linked through a nitrogen atom directly to C-1, which carries the reducing group of the pentose sugar. This is analogous to a glycosidic link, but it does not contain oxygen. The base–pentose linkage occurs between N-9 and C-1′ in the case of the purine nucleotides and between N-1 and C-1′ in the pyrimidine nucleotides. The configuration of the *N*-glycosidic linkage is β in all naturally occurring nucleosides.

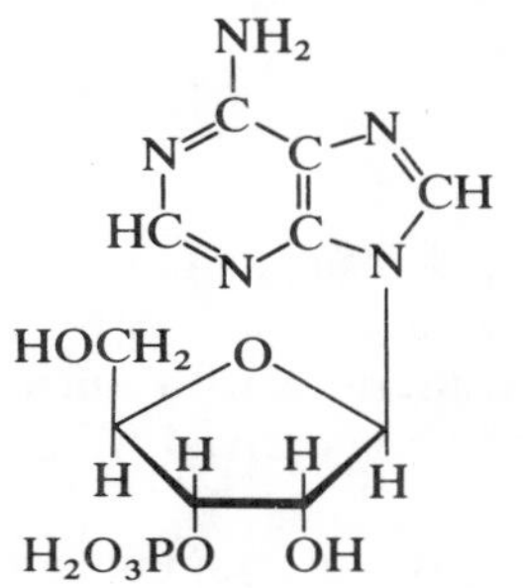

Adenosine
3′-phosphate
(Hydrolysis product)

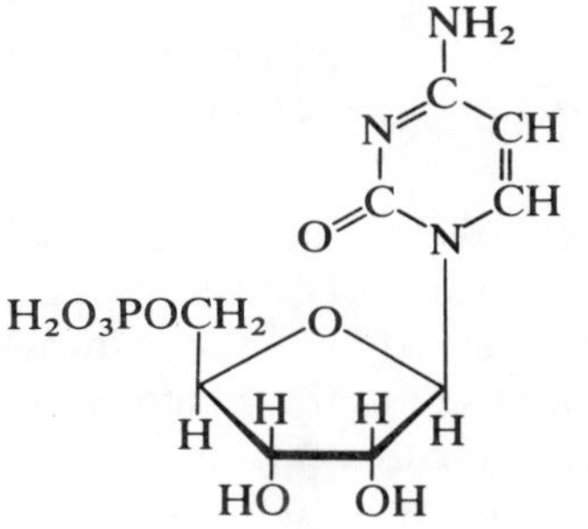

Cytidine
5′-phosphate
(Building unit)

The nucleotides from which DNA and RNA are built and which are present in coenzymes are phosphorylated in the 5′ position. In cyclic AMP (cAMP) and GMP (cGMP), which play an important role in the regulation of metabolism, the phosphate group is joined in diester linkage to both C-3′ and C-5′.

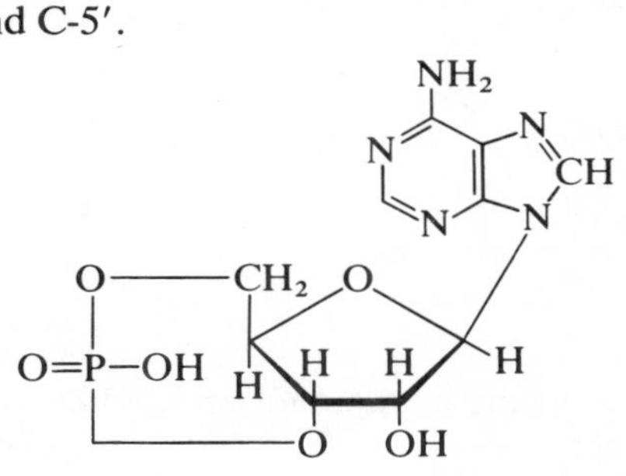

Adenosine 3′,5′-phosphate
(Cyclic AMP)

The 5′ phosphate group of the nucleoside 5′-phosphates may be further phosphorylated to yield the all important *di-* and *tri*-phosphates, e.g. ADP, CDP, ATP and CTP (page 211). The phosphate group of a nucleotide may be removed enzymically to yield a nucleoside.

Origin and fate of the bases

Synthesis

Both the pyrimidines and the purines are built up from small precursor molecules which are readily available in the metabolic pool (page 185). The free bases are not synthesized as such but, while being assembled, the partially constructed ring structure reacts with a special phosphorylated pentose known as PRPP (5-phosphoribosyl-1-pyrophosphate) and forms a ribonucleotide. The deoxyribonucleotides, with the exception of TMP which is formed by methylation of deoxyuridylate, are formed by reduction of the corresponding ribonucleoside diphosphate. The conversion is precisely controlled by allosteric effects which ensure that all four deoxyribonucleotides are available in amounts appropriate for nucleic acid synthesis.

The pyrimidine ring is synthesized from carbamoyl phosphate and aspartate which contribute ring atoms as shown. The carbamoyl phosphate has a high transfer potential because of its anhydride bond.

The purine ring, on the other hand, is synthesized from metabolic fragments from five different sources. The carbon atoms at positions 2 and 8 are derived from formate via tetrahydrofolate (page 165). Folic acid antagonists interfere with nucleic acid biosynthesis and are sometimes used in the treatment of cancer. C-6 is derived from carbon dioxide with biotin (page 166) acting as a carrier.

Purines may also be derived from the nucleic acids present in animal and plant foods. After liberation in the course of digestion they are absorbed and react with PRPP from which they receive the ribose phosphate moiety.

The pentose sugars originate from glucose during its metabolism by the pentose phosphate pathway (page 232).

Breakdown

Although DNA is one of the most stable compounds in the body, RNA is subject to continuous breakdown and synthesis even in the adult, There is considerable uncertainty regarding the pathway of pyrimidine catabolism but it appears that the ring is first reduced and then opened, the final products being carbon dioxide and ammonia; some of the latter appears as urea.

Unlike the pyrimidine ring the purine ring is not readily degraded and, after modification, is excreted in the form of uric acid (page 397).

Polynucleotides

The nucleic acids are unevenly distributed within the cell. DNA, which is the genetic material (page 289), is located in the nuclear chromatin in the resting cell and in the chromosomes in the dividing eukaryotic cell. Small amounts are also found in the mitochondria (page 200) and in the plasmids of bacterial cells.

Unlike DNA, RNA is found mainly in the cytoplasm where it is present in three different forms. The nucleus contains about 5% of the total RNA. Most of this is found in the nucleolus, although small amounts are found associated with the chromatin.

Structure of DNA

The molecular weights of DNA molecules are difficult to determine accurately by chemical methods because they are so high. Physicochemical methods are more reliable but, even with them, the results may be open to question owing to the difficulty of preparing intact molecules. This is because the very large molecules are susceptible to hydrodynamic shearing and also to the action of *nucleases* which are commonly present in the tissues. Their molecular weights are believed to range from about one million (10^6) to a thousand million (10^9) or even higher. Just as the amino acid composition and sequence varies from one protein molecule to another so the nucleotide composition and sequence varies from one nucleic acid molecule to another and, since the sugar and phosphate groups are the same for each nucleotide component, the variation only concerns the base composition and sequence.

Early studies by Chargaff (1950–1) on the base composition of DNA from various sources gave very striking results, the significance of which was not fully appreciated at the time. He observed that (1) the sum of the purines (adenine + guanine) present was equal to the sum of the pyrimidines (cytosine + thymine); (2) the sum of the amino bases (adenine + cytosine) was equal to the sum of the oxo bases (guanine + thymine); (3) adenine and thymine were present in equal amounts as were guanine and cytosine.

Molecular architecture of DNA

The way in which the nucleotides are linked together in a polynucleotide chain is shown in Figure 9.1. It can be seen that the sugar of one nucleotide is joined at C-3' to the phosphate group attached to C-5' of the sugar of the next nucleotide, i.e. nucleotides are joined by 3'–5' phosphodiester bonds. This gives a structure in which there is a backbone of alternating sugar and phosphate residues with the bases projecting laterally from the sugar residues in linear sequence. This may be considered as the primary structure of the polynucleotides but it gives little indication of the form taken up by the long chain-like molecule in the cell. Only by using

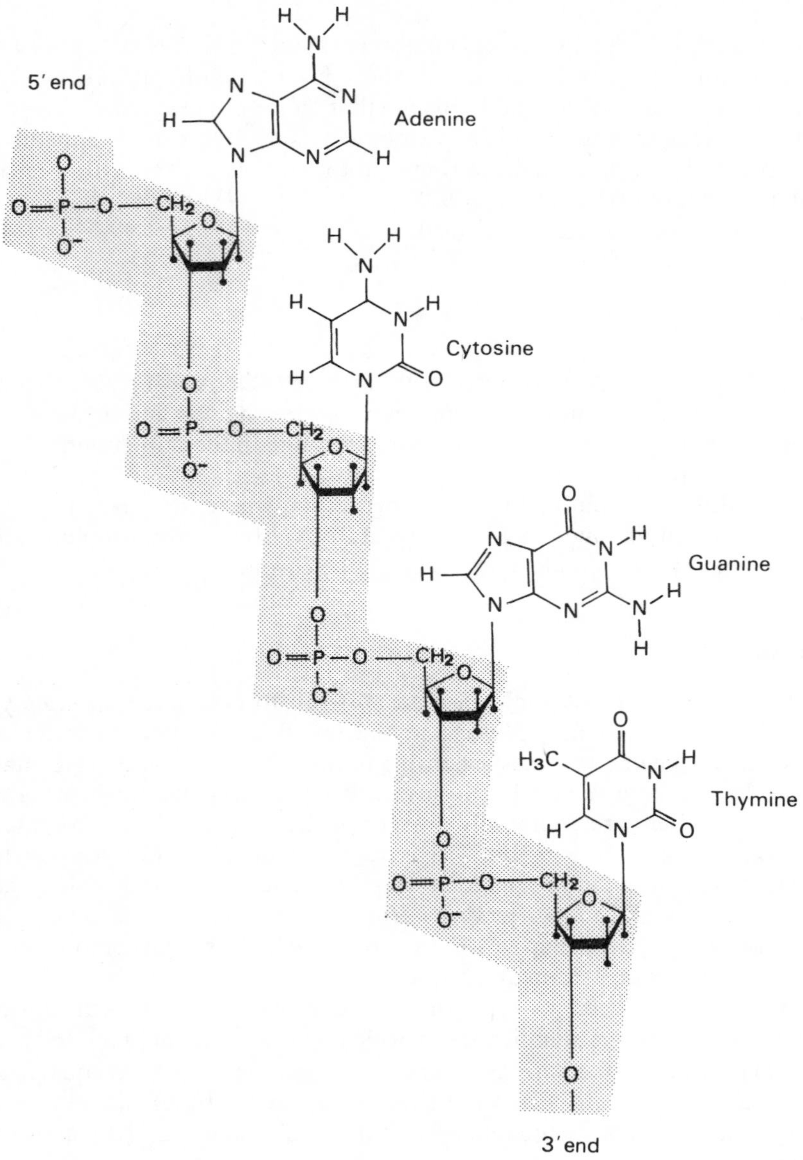

Figure 9.1 Structure of a single strand of DNA

X-ray diffraction methods is it possible to determine the spatial arrangement of the atoms within macromolecules and the interpretation of X-ray diffraction patterns requires many calculations and great skill. As regards DNA, the breakthrough came in 1953 when Watson and Crick proposed a model for its structure based on X-ray crystallographic data obtained by Wilkins and Rosalind Franklin. Watson and Crick proposed that a molecule of DNA consists of not one but two polynucleotide chains wound around each other to form a regular *double helix*. The strands, which run in opposite directions, are held together by hydrogen bonding between the bases which project laterally from the sugar–phosphate backbone (Figure 9.2). The dimensions of the

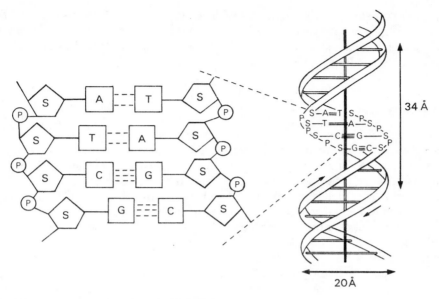

Figure 9.2 Schematic representation of the double helix

DNA molecule allow a purine base in one chain to be paired only with a pyrimidine base in the other. Two purines paired together would not permit a regular helix to be formed as they would occupy too much space; conversely two pyrimidines would occupy too little. Base-pairing is limited even further by the chemical structures of the individual purines and pyrimidines with the result that adenine always pairs with thymine with the formation of two hydrogen bonds and guanine always pairs with cytosine with the formation of three hydrogen bonds (Figure 9.3). These suggestions are entirely consistent with the regularities of composition noticed by Chargaff.

The strictness with which the base-pairing occurs means that a complementary relationship exists between the two strands of each DNA molecule. Consequently, if the base sequence of one strand is known, the sequence of bases in the complementary strand can be predicted.

$$5' \ldots \text{T-G-C-A-T-T-C-G-G-T-C-C-A} \ldots 3'$$
$$3' \ldots \text{A-C-G-T-A-A-G-C-C-A-G-G-T} \ldots 5'$$

Although hydrogen bonding between specific pairs of bases is largely responsible for the stability of the double helix, hydrophobic forces generate l between the stacked purines and pyrimidines also help to maintain the relatively rigid two-stranded structure. If, as suggested,

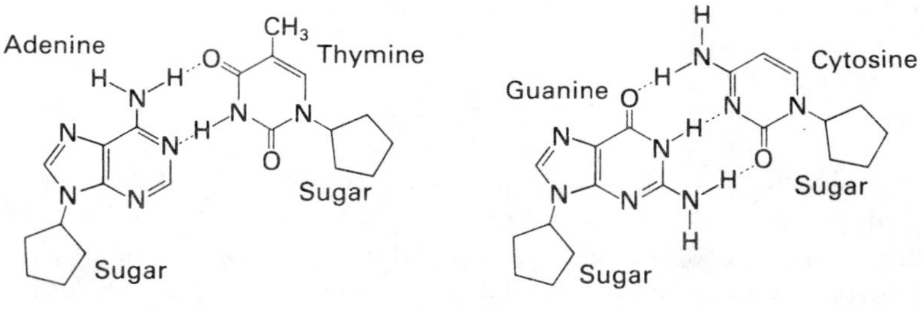

Figure 9.3 Base-pairing arrangements

DNA molecules take the form of extended double helices, a molecule of eukaryotic DNA would be about 5 cm long. Since they exist within cells, either dispersed as chromatin or compacted into chromosomes, they must, in fact, be extensively folded. The organization of DNA within eukaryotic cells is considered in Chapter 21.

Denaturation of DNA

The normal stable double helical form of DNA can be converted into a denatured form in which the strands unwind, separate and assume the properties of random coils. Denaturation is achieved by destroying the hydrogen bonds between the base pairs usually by heat or titration with alkali. The change from the double-stranded to the single-stranded form occurs abruptly and the helix → coil transition is accompanied by changes in the physical and chemical properties of the polynucleotide. *The helix → coil transition*, which is sometimes referred to as the 'melting' of DNA, is reversible and, if the original conditions are restored very gradually, the separated strands will recombine as a result of hydrogen bonding between the base pairs of the complementary strands so that the double helical form is regained. The ability to cause two polynucleotide strands, whether of DNA or RNA, which bear complementary sequences of bases to anneal together to form a double helix, has proved to be of great value in various areas of nucleic acid research and technology.

DNA sequencing

It is now relatively easy to determine the sequence of bases in DNA. A preparation of identical single-stranded fragments of the DNA is labelled with ^{32}P at their 5′ ends and divided into four samples. The first sample is treated with a reagent that destroys one of the bases, e.g. adenine, and cleaves the chain at these positions releasing a series of ^{32}P-labelled fragments of different lengths. The process is repeated with the other samples using reagents which cleave the DNA at positions occupied by one of the other three bases. In this way four DNA digests are prepared each of which contains labelled fragments of various sizes ending at a point originally occupied by a specific base. The digestion products are then separated according to their sizes by high-voltage electrophoresis on thin sheets of polyacrylamide gel. The position and hence the exact length of the fragments can be detected by autoradiography which produces an irregular 'ladder' effect. The four digests are run in parallel and give four separate base-specific tracks (Figure 9.4) from which the positions occupied by each of the bases can be directly read.

The method allows the sequence of up to 1000 base pairs to be determined in a day and, because it is so rapid and efficient, it is now also being used for determining the amino acid sequence of proteins. This is achieved by isolating and cloning the gene for the protein (page 308) and determining its base sequence. The base sequence is then translated into terms of amino acid sequence using the genetic code (page 300).

Structure of RNA

Ribonucleic acid molecules are single stranded and vary in size according to their type (page 297) but they are usually much smaller than those of DNA. They differ from DNA in the replacement of thymine by uracil and in containing ribose instead of deoxyribose. Although C-2′, C-3′ and C-5′ all carry hydroxyl groups that are available for esterification, the nucleotides are joined together through the sugar, as in DNA, by 3′–5′ phosphodiester bonds.

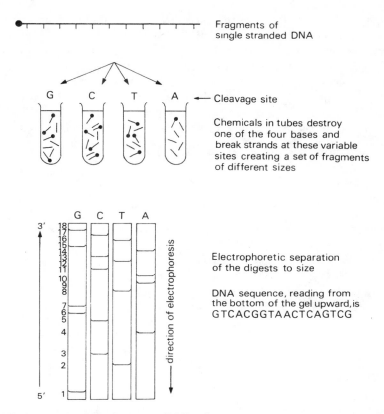

Fragments of single stranded DNA
G
C
T
A
Cleavage site
Chemicals in tubes destroy one of the four bases and break strands at these variable sites creating a set of fragments of different sizes
G C T A
3′
5′
18 17 16 15 14 13 12 11 10 9 8 7 6 5 4 3 2 1
direction of electrophoresis
Electrophoretic separation of the digests to size
DNA sequence, reading from the bottom of the gel upward, is GTCACGGTAACTCAGTCG

Figure 9.4 Method of sequencing DNA (Maxam and Gilbert)

HOCH2
O
R1
H
H
H
O
OH
O=P—OH
O
CH2
R2
CH2
R3
OH
R1 R2 R3
3′
5′
P
P
P
R1pR2pR3p

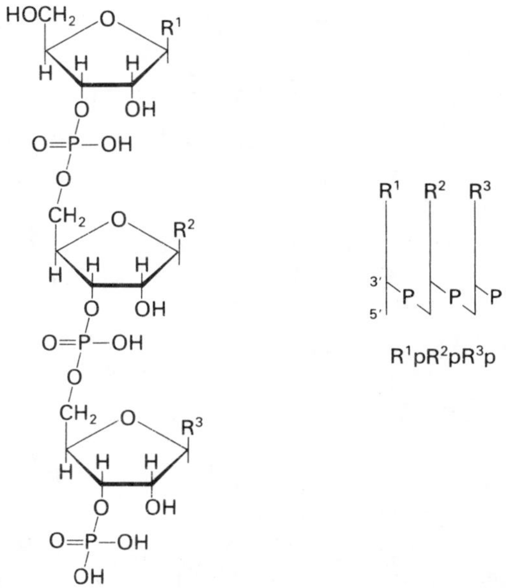

Figure 9.5 The primary structure of RNA. Shorthand representation shown on the right

A convenient method of representing the polynucleotides is shown on the right in Figure 9.5. The vertical line denotes the carbon chain of the sugar with the base attached at C-1′, and the diagonal line, the phosphate link which joins C-3′ of one nucleotide to C-5′ of the next.

Although they are single-stranded, RNA molecules may be folded in such a way as to give them a secondary structure. This results from the pairing of A and U and of G and C residues situated at different points along the same polynucleotide chain which becomes folded back on itself to give loops consisting of short regions of imperfect double helix (Figure 20.11). The hydrogen bonds between the base pairs are disrupted by heat which causes the molecule to unfold.

Section 3

Nutrition – sources of energy and materials

Chapter 10
General principles of nutrition

In the field of human nutrition there are few hard facts, and clearcut conclusions are almost impossible. Apart from the difficulty of performing experiments on human subjects there is the problem of their biological variability. Every individual has his own 'personalized' genetic constitution and, correspondingly, his own unique pattern of enzymes which render him/her more or less susceptible to particular external influences. These include the food he/she eats, the diseases to which he/she is exposed and the drugs he/she may take. However, although it is not possible to predict the requirements and reactions of any particular person certain nutritional principles have been established which are valid for populations taken as a whole. This was successfully demonstrated in World War II when, as a result of prudent food imports, rationing and such measures as the fortification of margarine with vitamins and bread with calcium, the general standard of nutrition was better than it has ever been before or since. This was the result of it being virtually impossible to eat any food in excess, so that the national diet, though restricted, was well-balanced.

Broadly speaking food is required to provide:

1. *Energy* without which no living structure can be built or maintained. This is derived mainly from carbohydrate and fat, although proteins also contribute.
2. *Structural materials* which are required for the growth and maintenance of the tissues. The main materials falling in this category are proteins, although minerals, notably calcium and phosphorus, also fulfil a structural role.
3. *Regulatory substances*. A variety of minerals and the vitamins fall most readily into this category.
4. *Water*. This is of over-riding importance in both structural and regulatory roles but its nutritional functions are often taken for granted. Death from lack of water occurs within 4–5 days, whereas starvation results in death only after 30 days or more.

It is easy to state that in order to sustain life and health the body requires carbohydrate, fat, protein, minerals, vitamins and water but very difficult to determine how much of these nutrients is required. Many factors need to be considered including the types of carbohydrate, fat and protein, the age and sex of the individual, the nature and extent of his activities and the climatic conditions. Furthermore a diet should be considered as a whole and should be balanced with respect to its various constituents.

Table 10.1 Recommended daily amounts of food energy and various specific nutrients

Age range (years)		Energy* (MJ)	Energy* (kcal)	Protein (g)	Thiamin (mg)	Riboflavin (mg)
Boys						
1		5·0	1200	30	0·5	0·6
3–4		6·5	1560	39	0·6	0·8
7–8		8·25	1980	49	0·8	1·0
9–11		9·5	2280	57	0·9	1·2
15–17		12·0	2880	72	1·2	1·7
Girls						
1		4·5	1100	27	0·4	0·6
3–4		6·25	1500	37	0·6	0·8
7–8		8·0	1900	47	0·8	1·0
9–11		8·5	2050	51	0·8	1·2
15–17		9·0	2150	53	0·9	1·7
Men						
18–34	Sedentary	10·5	2510	63	1·0	1·6
	Moderately active	12·0	2900	72	1·2	1·6
	Very active	14·0	3350	84	1·3	1·6
35–64	Sedentary	10·0	2400	60	1·0	1·6
	Moderately active	11·5	2750	69	1·1	1·6
	Very active	14·0	3350	84	1·3	1·6
65–74 ⎤	Assuming a	10·0	2400	60	1·0	1·6
75+ ⎦	sedentary life	9·0	2150	54	0·9	1·6
Women						
18–54	Most occupations	9·0	2150	54	0·9	1·3
	Very active	10·5	2500	62	1·0	1·3
55–74 ⎤	Assuming a	8·0	1900	47	0·8	1·3
75+ ⎦	sedentary life	7·0	1680	42	0·7	1·3
Pregnancy		10·0	2400	60	1·0	1·6
Lactation		11·5	2750	69	1·1	1.8

* Megajoules (10^6 joules) calculated from the relation 1 kcal = 4·184 kJ that is to say, 1 MJ = 240 kcal.
† 1 nicotinic acid equivalent = 1 mg available nicotinic acid or 60 mg tryptophan.
‡ 1 retinol equivalent = 1 μg retinol or 6 μg β-carotene or 12 μg other biologically active carotenoids.
§ No dietary sources may be necessary for children and adults who are sufficiently exposed to sunlight, but during the winter children and adolescents should receive 10 μg (400 i.u.) daily by supplementation. Adults with inadequate exposure to sunlight, for example those who are housebound, may also need a supplement of 10 μg daily.

The recommended daily amount (RDA) of a nutrient has been defined as 'the average amount which should be provided per head in a group of people if the needs of practically all members (sic) of the group are to be met'. From this it can be seen that individual variations are recognized and, since in any group there will be some people who require substantially more of the nutrient than others, the recommended amount should include a considerable safety margin to allow for this. The RDA for energy and for various specific nutrients for males and females of different ages living in the United Kingdom is given in Table 10.1. The figures are taken from the *Report of the Committee on Medical Aspects of Food Policy* published by the Department of Health and Social Security in 1979.

Nicotinic acid equivalents (mg)†	Ascorbic acid (mg)	Vitamin A retinol equivalents (μg)‡	Vitamin D cholecalciferol (μg)§	Calcium (mg)	Iron (mg)
7	20	300	10	600	7
9	20	300	10	600	8
11	20	400	—	600	10
14	25	575	—	700	12
19	30	750	—	600	12
7	20	300	10	600	7
9	20	300	10	600	8
11	20	400	—	600	10
14	25	575	—	700	12
19	30	750	—	600	12
18	30	750	—	500	10
18	30	750	—	500	10
18	30	750	—	500	10
18	30	750	—	500	10
18	30	750	—	500	10
18	30	750	—	500	10
18	30	750	—	500	10
18	30	750	—	500	10
15	30	750	—	500	12
15	30	750	—	500	12
15	30	750	—	500	10
15	30	750	—	500	10
18	60	750	10	1200	13
21	60	1200	10	1200	15

Energy sources

The main energy sources are carbohydrates from plants and fats of animal or vegetable origin. The use of protein as a source of energy is normally incidental to the continuous turnover of body protein which occurs throughout life (page 185). However, if insufficient carbohydrate and fat are available to cover essential energy requirements, protein will be called upon for this purpose instead of being used for the synthesis of nitrogenous compounds.

The energy used by all living creatures is ultimately derived from the sun. Photosynthetic *autotrophs* (self-feeders) use carbon dioxide as their sole source of carbon, and solar energy to convert it into glucose according to the overall equation:

$$6CO_2 + 6H_2O \xrightarrow{\text{energy}} C_6H_{12}O_6 + 6O_2$$

Energy derived from the breakdown of glucose is used for all their other energy-requiring reactions. The *heterotrophs* (feeding on others), which include animals and most micro-organisms, are only able to use chemical energy, stored in the form of organic compounds, which also provide the carbon required for synthetic purposes. Consequently the heterotrophs are totally dependent on the autotrophs. In fact, photosynthetic and heterotrophic organisms are interdependent, since while the former use carbon dioxide and produce organic compounds and oxygen, the latter utilize organic compounds and oxygen and produce carbon dioxide. This results in a *cycle of food materials* and a *flow of energy* that is derived externally.

The quantity of carbon used annually in the photosynthetic production of glucose is enormous, being estimated at some 150×10^9 tons, requiring about 5×10^{19} calories of solar energy. This conversion is achieved largely in forests, which are consequently responsible for controlling the level of oxygen and carbon dioxide in the atmosphere.

Energy equivalents of different nutrients

Average values for the amounts of energy released on oxidation of the various types of nutrient in the body are

1 g carbohydrate*	16 kJ (3·75 kcal)
1 g protein	17 kJ (4 kcal)
1 g fat	37 kJ (9 kcal)
1 g ethanol	29 kJ (7 kcal)

(* available carbohydrate expressed as monosaccharides)

Weight for weight fat provides more than twice as much energy as either carbohydrate or protein and alcohol produces nearly as much energy as fat.

Although good health may be maintained on diets of widely varying composition, in the adequately nourished western world protein usually supplies between 10 and 13% of the total energy. This value appears to be independent of income because, where there is a greater consumption of expensive protein-rich animal foods, there is also an increase in the consumption of fats and refined sugars.

Dietary carbohydrate

Dietary carbohydrate is derived almost entirely from plant sources mainly as starch and sucrose. Carbohydrate-rich foods are mostly relatively cheap and are readily digested and absorbed. Cereals and root crops give the highest yields of consumable energy per unit of land and contain appreciable amounts of protein (wheat 8–13%, rice 6% and maize 9%) as well as minerals and vitamins.

In the developing countries, large amounts of cereals and cereal products are consumed and carbohydrate supplies up to 75% of the total energy. However, in high income countries, where only 50–60% of the energy is obtained from carbohydrate, starchy foods tend to be replaced by sucrose, widely used for sweetening. This trend, now also beginning in the developing countries, is detrimental because while refined sugar provides energy it contains none of the 'protective' nutrients, i.e. protein, minerals and vitamins, hence the expression 'empty calories'. According to the British nutritionist Yudkin, sugar and sugar-containing foods are nutritionally disastrous, contributing not only to obesity, dental caries and diabetes but also to coronary thrombosis and ischaemic heart disease. The truth of these latter claims has not been fully established.

Dietary fat

Fat is important because of its high energy content. Diets containing little fat are bulky and unpalatable; since fat reduces the motility of the stomach and delays the secretion of gastric juice, fat-free diets tend to lack 'staying power'. Natural fats also supply essential fatty acids, fat-soluble vitamins and choline in the form of lecithin.

Fat may contribute from 10% to 40% of the total energy and well-fed families in Britain consume 80–100 g per day (3·0–3·7 MJ or 720–900 kcal). Although diets in which fat supplies less than 20% of the total energy tend to be unappetizing, low-fat diets have no ill-effects provided that the requirements for essential fatty acids and fat-soluble vitamins are met. An excessive intake of fat, e.g. more than 150 g per day, may result in ketosis (page 262). However, in cold climates the natural tendency to increase fat consumption is accompanied by adaptation to the higher intake. The importance of dietary fat in relation to coronary heart disease is discussed on page 267 and the problem of energy balance and obesity on page 268.

Essential fatty acids

It has been found that, when rats are fed on a diet completely devoid of fat, they fail to thrive and develop characteristic skin lesions; when fat is restored to the diet the lesions heal and normal growth is resumed. The factors present in fat that are essential for rat growth are certain polyunsaturated fatty acids. Linoleic (18 : 2) and arachidonic (20 : 4) acids have the highest biological activity and are able both to restore growth and to cure the skin lesions; linolenic acid (18 : 3), only does the former. The *polyunsaturated fatty acids* (PUFA) whose structure is shown in Figure 10.1 must be supplied in the diet because there is no system in the body for introducing double bonds between the central double bond of oleic acid and the methyl end of the fatty acid chain. Linoleic acid is present in large amounts in many vegetable oils (Table 10·2), while arachidonic acid is found only in animal fats and in small amounts. Human milk fat contains about 8% of linolenic acid but cow's milk is a very poor source.

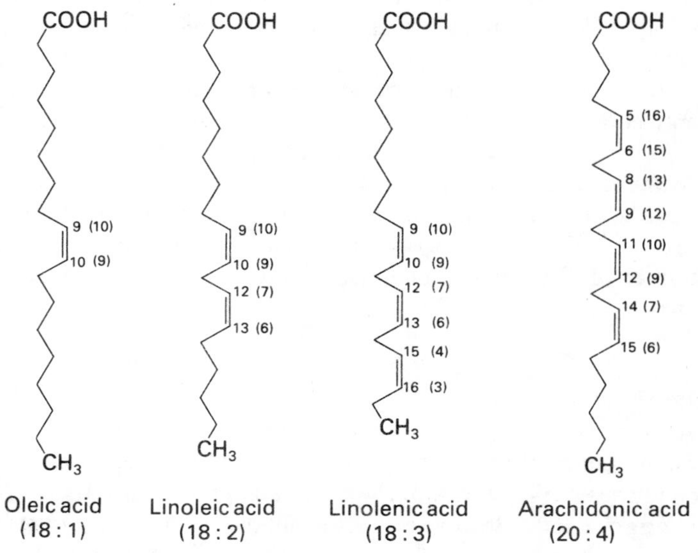

Figure 10.1 The relationship of the polyunsaturated fatty acids to oleic acid

Table 10.2 The linoleic acid content of some animal fats and plant oils (as an approximate percentage of total fatty acids)

Animal fats	Linoleic acid	Other polyunsaturated fatty acids
Butter, milk and cream	2	1
Beef	2	1
Pork	7	1
Chicken	18	2
Fish	7	43
Plant oils		
Margarine	12	1
Margarine (enriched)	52	1
Coconut	2	—
Olive	11	1
Rapeseed	15	10
Groundnut	30	1
Cottonseed	50	1
Corn	53	2
Soya bean	53	7
Sunflower	58	—

Until recently the essential fatty acids were considered to be of little practical importance in human nutrition and their function was largely unknown. The discovery of the prostaglandins (page 364) suggested that their role as precursors of this group of compounds might explain why they must be supplied in the diet. However, estimation of the amounts required for prostaglandin synthesis showed that they were some orders of magnitude lower than the estimated overall dietary requirement of 2–10 g linoleic acid per day for humans. Moreover, since inhibitors of *prostaglandin synthetase* do not induce symptoms of essential fatty acid deficiency other functions are implied.

Deficiency states seem to induce membrane disorders such as abnormalities of the erythrocytes, increased skin permeability and mitochondrial damage resulting in an increased metabolic rate. The essential fatty acids also play a part in the transport and metabolism of cholesterol (page 267). Recently, evidence has been obtained that the various esential fatty acids may not have identical functions and it is suggested that linolenic acid and the ω-3 fatty acids may be required in their own right. The polyunsaturated fatty acids are protected against peroxidation by vitamin E (page 158).

In normal circumstances an outright dietary deficiency of essential fatty acids is unlikely to occur but currently there is considerable speculation as to the role of subclinical deficiency in the aetiology of a number of diseases including ischaemic heart disease (page 267), cystic fibrosis and multiple sclerosis.

Dietary protein

Protein requirements depend on the nature of the proteins and their composition. Strictly speaking the need for protein is a need for *the essential amino acids* (page 277) which the body is unable to synthesize for itself. However, the so-called 'dispensable' amino acids also fulfil an important nutritional role, since not only are they directly incorporated into proteins but they also provide a non-specific source of nitrogen for the synthesis of a great variety of compounds.

If they were not available, the essential amino acids would be used for this purpose and the requirements for these would be greatly increased. However, since every protein contains large amounts of the non-essential amino acids, consideration need only be given to the supply of essential amino acids which have a more restricted distribution. Animal proteins are relatively rich in the essential amino acids and are normally considered to be nutritionally more desirable than plant proteins which tend to be deficient in tryptophan, lysine and the sulphur-containing amino acids and may contain other amino acids in excess. Major imbalances with respect to leucine and glutamic acid can have harmful effects. Notable exceptions to the general rule that animal proteins are nutritionally superior to plant proteins are collagen and its derivative, gelatin, which are almost totally deficient in tryptophan, tyrosine and the sulphur-containing amino acids. The amino acid composition of some representative proteins is given in Table 10·3.

Table 10.3 The essential amino acid contents of various foods (g per 16 g N)

	Arg	His	Leu	Ile	Lys	Met	Phe	Thr	Trp	Val	Met + Cys	Phe + Tyr
Cow's milk	3·7	2·7	10·0	6·5	8·2	2·5	4·9	4·7	1·4	7·0	3·4	9·0
Whole hen's egg	6·6	2·4	8·8	4·6	6·4	3·1	5·8	5·0	1·7	7·4	5·4	10·2
Beef	6·1	3·9	8·2	4·5	9·1	2·7	4·2	4·6	1·2	4·8	3·9	7·7
Chicken	6·0	2·4	6·9	5·2	7·2	2·5	3·7	3·9	1·1	4·5	3·5	6·8
Herring	7·0	3·5	9·1	4·9	9·8	1·9	4·5	5·1	1·4	5·7	3·3	8·4
Cod	5·8	1·8	8·1	5·5	8·5	3·1	3·7	4·5	0·9	5·6	4·0	7·0
Gelatin	6·8	0·6	2·9	1·4	3·2	0·8	0·8	1·8	—	2·4	0·9	1·3
Maize	4·5	2·4	11·4	3·7	2·7	2·0	4·6	3·2	0·5	4·2	4·0	7·5
Millet	3·2	1·8	11·1	3·4	1·6	2·3	5·2	2·8	1·5	4·3	4·0	7·2
Rice	7·8	2·5	7·2	6·8	3·8	2·0	6·6	3·5	1·2	6·6	2·7	11·2
Wheat	4·2	2·1	6·8	3·5	2·5	1·3	4·2	2·8	1·4	4·2	3·6	7·0
Cassava	12·5	1·4	3·7	2·4	4·9	0·5	2·6	2·3	1·6	3·3	0·9	4·1
Potato	5·4	1·9	6·2	7·0	6·0	1·6	4·4	4·0	1·4	5·4	2·4	8·4
Beans (*Phaseolus vulgaris*)	6·1	3·1	8·7	5·4	6·8	1·2	6·0	4·5	1·0	6·0	2·5	9·7
Peas	9·3	1·8	7·1	4·4	6·0	0·8	4·5	3·8	1·0	4·9	2·1	7·6
Soya bean	8·1	2·7	7·9	5·0	6·3	1·6	5·1	3·9	1·3	5·1	3·2	8·7

Since there are appreciable variations in the values obtained by different workers on different food samples these values must be taken as approximate. From D. Harvey, *Tables of Amino Acids in Foods and Feeding Stuffs*, 2nd edn., Technical Communication No. 19 of the Commonwealth Bureau of Animal Nutrition, Farnham Royal, Bucks, England, 1970

The concept of *protein quality* arose from early experiments in which single proteins were fed as the sole source of nitrogen to young growing animals. If the protein was an animal protein such as casein, the animals grew well and thrived, but if it came from a plant source, growth was often diminished or might cease altogether with the animal going into a decline. If, however, these poor quality proteins were supplemented with the amino acid(s) in which they were deficient, or fed in combination with other proteins containing them, growth was resumed. For supplementation to be effective it is necessary that all the essential amino acids should be simultaneously available. Even an hour's delay between the administration of a protein and its missing amino acid(s) will cause a significant decrease in effectiveness.

The nutritional value of a protein also depends on its digestibility; here again, plant proteins tend to be inferior to animal proteins. Their poor digestibility results from (1) the presence of peptide bonds which are relatively resistant to the digestive enzymes, (2) the presence of enzyme inhibitors such as the trypsin inhibitor present in soya beans (page 177), and (3) the presence of fibre which hinders the access of proteolytic enzymes (page 130).

Assessment of protein quality

Biological methods

The best methods of evaluating the nutritional value of a protein involve feeding it to experimental animals under carefully controlled conditions. A commonly used procedure is to determine the *net protein utilization* (NPU). This is a combined measure of the digestibility of the protein and the efficiency with which the absorbed amino acids are utilized. It is defined as the proportion of ingested nitrogen that is retained in the body under specified conditions. Egg protein which is almost completely digested and utilized is used as a control. Nitrogen retention is measured either directly from carcass analysis or derived from the urinary and faecal excretion of nitrogen.

When digestibility and the retention of absorbed nitrogen are separately determined the latter is known as the *biological value* (BV) of the protein.

Chemical scoring

Biological evaluation is costly and time-consuming so a chemical method is often used based on a comparison of the amino acid composition of the protein with a Provisional Reference or Scoring Pattern (Table 10.4). A score is obtained for each of the essential amino acids, e.g.

$$\text{Methionine score} = \frac{\text{mg of methionine in 1 g test protein}}{\text{mg of methionine in Reference Pattern}} \times 100$$

When the scores for all the essential amino acids have been calculated it is possible to pick out the amino acid with the lowest score and this is known as the *limiting amino acid* (see Table 13·2) for that protein since it presumably limits the extent to which the rest of the amino acids can be utilized in the body. The *chemical (or protein) score* is given by the score of its first limiting amino acid, but when a protein is notably deficient in more than one essential amino acid its second and third amino acids should also be specified.

Table 10.4 Provisional reference pattern of amino acids

Amino acid	Suggested level	
	mg per g protein	mg per g N
Isoleucine	40	250
Leucine	70	440
Lysine	55	340
Methionine + cystine	35	220
Phenylalanine + tyrosine	60	380
Threonine	40	250
Tryptophan	10	60
Valine	50	310

Protein requirements

As explained on page 273, the nitrogen intake of a normal healthy adult is balanced by his nitrogen output. To achieve balance, an adult requires an average of 77 mg of nitrogen per kg body weight per day when receiving egg, milk, purified casein or mixed diets containing appreciable amounts of animal protein, while an average of 93 mg per kg are needed when the nitrogen is derived solely from plant sources. Since proteins contain about 16% of nitrogen the *minimal daily requirements* appear to be as in Table 10·5.

Table 10.5 Minimal protein requirements for adults

Protein source	N (mg kg^{-1})	Protein (g kg^{-1})	Protein (g) required for:	
			Man	Woman
Animal or mixed protein	77	0·48	31	26·5
Vegetable protein	93	0·58	38	32

These minimum protein requirements throw little light on the optimal level of intake. After an initial period of adjustment, an adult can be kept in balance on daily protein intakes ranging from 30 to 150 g or even more. The average intake of adults in the West, some 80–100 g per day, including about 50% of animal protein, is probably higher than necessary. An arbitrary 'safe level' of intake, 60% greater than the minimum necessary to maintain nitrogen balance, provides a safety margin and allows for variation between individuals. When calculating the safe level of intake adjustments must also be made for protein quality (Table 10.6). A useful rough guide is that the protein intake should be about 1 g kg^{-1} body weight and should include some animal protein.

Table 10.6 Safe levels of daily protein intake for proteins of varying quality

Age	Body weight (kg)	Safe level of intake of egg protein		Adjusted level for proteins of different quality		
		Score 100 (g kg^{-1})	(g)	Score 80 (g)	Score 70 (g)	Score 60 (g)
9 months	9·0	1·53	14	17	20	23
2 years	13·4	1·19	16	20	23	27
5 years	20·2	1·01	20	26	29	34
8 years	28·1	0·88	25	31	35	41
11 years	36·9 (38·0)	0·81 (0·76)	30 (29)	37 (36)	43 (41)	50 (48)
14 years	51·3 (49·9)	0·72 (0·63)	37 (31)	46 (39)	53 (45)	62 (52)
17 years	62·9 (54·4)	0·60 (0·55)	38 (30)	47 (37)	54 (43)	63 (50)
Adult	65·0 (55)	0·57 (0·52)	37 (29)	46 (36)	53 (41)	62 (48)
Pregnancy (latter half)			(+9)	(+11)	(+13)	(+15)
Lactation (first 6 months)			(+17)	(+21)	(+24)	(+28)

Figures for women given in parentheses

Whether very high protein intakes in humans are desirable or harmful is uncertain. Normal adults, including Arctic explorers, who have lived for long periods mainly on meat, appear to tolerate protein intakes far in excess of what is believed to be necessary but this is not true for infants. Some animal experiments suggest that high protein intakes shorten life.

Protein deficiency

In many developing countries the total quantity of protein consumed per head is much lower than in the Western world and may include little, if any, animal protein; consequently there is a risk of protein deficiency. In rural Africa nutritional deficiency is often manifest in the form of *kwashiorkor*, which usually occurs in children of 2–4 years after they have been weaned, when they are fed on plant foods containing a high proportion of starch. The condition is characterized by growth failure and muscular wasting, but this is masked by oedema and the presence of subcutaneous fat which gives the child an unhealthy bloated appearance. Biochemical changes are apparent in the blood and it has been accepted that the condition results from an adequate intake of energy but an inadequate intake of protein.

After World War II the belief grew up that kwashiorkor was the most widespread nutritional disorder and that the main problem in feeding the expanding world population was to produce enough protein. In other words, it was held that whereas, except in localized disaster areas, overall energy requirements could be relatively easily met, there was for the immediate and foreseeable future a 'protein gap' between global production and needs. This view has been challenged. Even more common than kwashiorkor is the condition of *marasmus* in which there is severe wasting of the muscles but no oedema. The blood is normal in composition and although the child has a wizened appearance its condition is less serious than that of one suffering from kwashiorkor. Marasmus is believed to be due to lack of food in general rather than lack of protein, and, since the child has been 'living on its own flesh', its tissues, though reduced in amount, have been receiving a balance of nutrients. It is now believed that kwashiorkor and marasmus represent the extremes of a whole spectrum of clinical conditions resulting from *protein–energy malnutrition*.

The energy and protein requirements like those of any other nutrient vary considerably from individual to individual and in India no difference was found in the diet of children who developed kwashiorkor and those who became marasmic. Consequently it has been suggested that the form of protein–energy malnutrition seen in children may be determined as much by their individual requirements and response to stress as to the amount and type of food that they consume. A child with a high protein and low energy requirement will tend to develop kwashiorkor and one with a low protein and high energy requirement will tend to become marasmic.

The estimated protein requirement of 1-year-old children fell from $3 \cdot 3$ g kg^{-1} body weight in 1948 to $1 \cdot 27$ g kg^{-1} in 1973, while the estimated requirement for energy remained at 420 kJ (100 kcal) kg^{-1}. As a result it now appears that the deficit in energy intake is greater than the deficit in protein intake and this is supported by field studies in various countries. The need for energy is always paramount and if the intake of carbohydrate and fat is inadequate, protein will be used for energy production rather than for tissue maintenance and growth. Clearly then it is useless to increase the protein intake while the overall energy intake is insufficient and it is no longer protein that is considered to be the weakest point in the world's nutritional defences. This being so, priorities are changing and emphasis is veering away from the search for new sources of protein to finding further means of increasing the production of cereal and other plant foods.

A recent reappraisal of the nutritive value of cereals suggests that, if available in sufficient quantity, they should be able to provide sufficient protein for most children. This view is based partly on experience and partly on calculations of their *protein/energy (P/E) ratios* which relate the energy derived from protein to the total energy provided by the food.

$$\text{P/E ratio} = \frac{\text{g protein} \times \text{energy equivalent}^*}{\text{total energy of food in kJ (or kcal)}} \qquad * \ 17 \, kJ \, g^{-1} \, (4 \, kcal \, g^{-1})$$

Table 10.7 The protein content and protein–energy ratios of various foods

Foodstuff	Protein content (g/100 g)	Total energy content per 100 g		P/E ratio†	NPU	Chemical score	Adjusted* P/E ratio
		(kJ)	(kcal)				
Good sources							
Whole egg	11·9	662	158	30·2	100	100	30·2
Lean beef	14·8	1311	313	38·4	78	77	30·0
Fat fish (herring)	16·0	796	190	33·7	83	75	28·0
Soya flour	40·3	1820	433	37·2	56	70	20·8
Peas	5·0	205	49	40·8	44	60	18·0
Cow's milk	3·3	272	65	21·6	75	60	16·2
Beans	7·2	289	69	25·6	48	68	12·3
Human milk	2·0	286	68	11·8	94	100	11·1
Pork	12·0	1710	408	11·8	84	80	9·9
Groundnut flour	8·0	720	171	18·8	48	70	9·0
Adequate sources							
White flour	10·0	1458	348	11·5	52	50	6·0
Maize	10·3	1650	392	10·5	55	45	5·6
Potatoes	1·4	331	79	7·6	71	70	5·4
Rice	7·5	1508	360	8·0	63	75	5·2
Millet	9·7	1540	367	11·6	56	60	5·0
Poor sources							
Sweet potatoes	1·1	336	80	4·4	72	75	3·2
Cassava	0·4	1504	359	3·3	—	40	1·3

* Adjusted to allow for the net protein utilization (or chemical score)
† Protein content expressed as its percentage contribution to the energy provided by that food

When this value is adjusted to allow for the net protein utilization or chemical score of the protein it is found that wheat, maize, rice and millet all give values that lie within what is believed to be the 'safe' P/E level of between 5·0 and 6·5% (Table 10.7). It is now suggested that only about 5% of the world's malnourished who subsist largely on starchy roots such as cassava or yams are likely to suffer from a specific deficiency of protein rather than from general undernutrition. The main disadvantage of cereals is that they are very bulky when cooked, i.e. they have a low *nutrient density*, and, even when plentiful, it is not always easy for young children to eat enough to fulfil their energy needs. This is even more the case with root crops and for this reason the inclusion in the diet of more concentrated foods and better sources of protein such as fish or beans is always desirable. The best diets are always mixed diets but appropriate mixtures of plant proteins can be adequate.

Dietary fibre

The relative merits of white versus brown bread have been disputed since the time of Hippocrates. The subject was once again brought to the fore in the early 1970s as the result of work by Cleave, Burkitt and others who suggested that dietary fibre, or rather its lack, is implicated in a great variety of diseases.

Dietary fibre is not easy to define. In general the term denotes the supporting structures of plant cell walls. These are composed of a mixture of many different substances, present in varying combinations and proportions in different plants and in different parts of the plant at different phases of growth. *Cellulose*, a β-glycan, the best known constituent, makes up only 10–25% of the mixture. Other β-glycans and heteroglycans such as the *pectin substances* and *hemicelluloses* are also present as well as the non-carbohydrate compound *lignin*. The physical characteristics of dietary fibre are correspondingly diverse and pectic substances, for example, may not be fibrous but have a gel-like quality. Dietary fibre is a complex spongy material which retains water and binds acidic materials and metals by its cation exchange capacity. It cannot be digested by mammalian enzymes, but extensive degradation may occur as a result of microbial action in the colon, the amount varying with the individual and the time taken for the food residues to pass through the large bowel.

Wheat bran cellulose is much less well digested than that of fruit and vegetables and this has been attributed to its lignin content. The chief products of the anaerobic fermentation of fibre are volatile fatty acids (acetate, propionate and butyrate), gas (CO_2, H_2 and methane) and energy. Gas production is a normal part of colonic metabolism but may be one of the reasons why people in the West have tended to maintain a relatively low fibre intake.

Sources and intakes of dietary fibre

The main sources of fibre in human diets are cereals and cereal products but all natural plant foods contain some. Because of their high water content vegetables and fruits have a much lower content than cereals, nuts, pulses and dried fruits. This can be seen from Table 10.8. The best source is bran which is produced during the refining of flour and makes up 10–16% of the whole wheat grain. Bran itself contains 40–50% of fibre as well as some starch, sugars, protein, fatty acids, minerals and vitamins.

As can be seen from Table 10.9, the fibre intake in different countries varies widely and reflects the type of diet consumed.

Physiological effects of dietary fibre

In the mouth

Fibre-rich foods usually require considerably more mastication than ones which have a low fibre content and experiments suggest that when a food is hard to eat, less of it is eaten. It is suggested, therefore, that a fibre-rich diet may lead to a reduction in the amount of food consumed and hence may be useful in the control of obesity. The chewing which is needed when the fibre content of the food is high also promotes a greater flow of saliva and tends to prevent stagnation of food in the mouth and consequent dental troubles. A high level of periodontal disease is found to occur when the diet consists mainly of soft foods and when oral hygiene is poor. Furthermore, water-soluble factors present in dietary fibre, especially in wheat bran, oat husks, peanuts and crude sugar cane, have been found to reduce the solubility of the surface enamel of teeth incubated in saliva. The factors responsible are believed to consist mainly of phytates extracted during mastication.

In the stomach and small intestine

When foods contain relatively large amounts of fibre gastric emptying is delayed. This, together with the fact that digestion takes place more slowly when fibrous material hinders access of the digestive juices to the digestible material, means that sugar absorption is spread over a longer period which is an advantage for sufferers from *diabetes*. Diabetes also tends to be associated

Table 10.8 The fibre content of various foods (g/100 g)

Cereals and cereal products		Fruit	
Bran (wheat)	44·0	Apples – flesh only	2·0
Bread – wholemeal	8·5	Apples – stewed	2·0
Bread – brown (85% extraction)	5·1	Apricots – flesh only	2·1
Bread – white (72% extraction)	2·7	Apricots – dried and stewed	8·7
Porridge	0·8	Bananas – skinned	3·4
Rice – polished, boiled	0·8	Blackberries – fresh	7·3
		Blackberries – stewed	6·0
Breakfast cereals		Blackcurrants – stewed	7·0
All-Bran	26·7	Gooseberries – stewed	2·6
Cornflakes	11·0	Grape – flesh only	0·4
Muesli	7·4	Grapefruit	0·6
Rice Krispies	4·5	Oranges – flesh only	2·0
Weetabix	12·7	Peaches	1·4
		Pears	2·3
Biscuits, cakes, etc.		Plums	2·1
Cream crackers	3·0	Raspberries	7·4
Digestive	5·5	Rhubarb – stewed	2·3
Oatcakes	4·0	Canned fruit	0·3–2·0
Ryvita	11·7		
Semi-sweet	2·3	*Cooked vegetables*	
Chocolate	3·1	Beans – baked	7·3
Cakes – sponge	1·0	Beans – broad	4·2
Cakes – fruit	3·5	Beans – runner	3·4
Pastry	1·3–2·4	Brussel sprouts	2·9
		Cabbage – boiled	2·2
Dried fruit		Cabbage – raw	3·4
Apricots	24·0	Carrots	3·0
Figs	18·5	Cauliflower	1·8
Prunes	16·1	Lentils	3·7
Raisins	6·8	Lettuce	1·5
Sultanas	7·0	Parsnips	2·5
		Pes	5·2
Nuts (shelled)		Potatoes – crisps	11·9
Almonds	14·3	Potatoes – new	2·0
Brazil nuts	9·0	Potatoes – old	1·0
Coconut – fresh	13·6	Spinach	6·3
Coconut – desiccated	23·5	Spring greens	3·8
Peanuts – roasted and salted	8·1	Swedes	2·8
Walnuts	5·2	Sweet corn	4·7
		Tomatoes – raw	1·5
		Tomatoes – fried	3·0
		Turnips	2·2

with high food intakes and obesity so that if the high-fibre diet also results in a reduced food intake this is a further recommendation.

Fibre increases the volume of the intestinal contents due to its water-retaining capacity and also perhaps to an increased secretion of digestive juices. This reduces the transit time through the small intestine and hence the absorption of nutrients. More fat and nitrogen are found in the faeces when the intake of dietary fibre is increased.

In the large intestine

The stools produced on high-fibre diets are soft and bulky. This leads to a reduction in the colonic pressure and, whereas transit times of material through the alimentary canal of British

Table 10.9 Dietary fibre in various countries (g per person per day)

Country	Cereal	Vegetable	Fruit and nut	Total
USA	8	15	4	27
Great Britain	8	10	2	20
Germany	12	8	4	24
Sweden	6	—	—	14
Yugoslavia	13	9	4	26
Kenya				
(Kikiyu)	79	54	—	130
(Masai warriors)	0	0	0	0
Swaziland	40	19	1	60
Uganda (Buganda)	0	147	3	150
India				
Hos tribe (Behar)	26	12	—	38

—, Not known

schoolboys were found to average 70 hours, those of schoolchildren in rural Africa averaged only 33 hours.

These effects of dietary fibre are relevant to various functional disorders of the colon namely constipation, diarrhoea and the irritable bowel syndrome.

Other abnormal conditions of the large bowel to which lack of dietary fibre is said to be a contributory cause are *cancer of the large bowel* and *diverticular disease*. It is believed that the faeces contain carcinogenic substances of bacterial origin and the high incidence of cancer of the large bowel in the wealthier countries runs parallel with a high intake of fat, meat and cholesterol and low intake of fibre. Small stools with a low residue content will have a relatively high concentration of carcinogens and, the longer transit time, will provide a greater opportunity for their absorption.

It has also been suggested that ischaemic heart disease, appendicitis, haemorrhoids, hiatus hernia, gall stones and varicose veins which occur more commonly in technological than primitive societies are associated with a low fibre intake but the evidence is not conclusive.

Adverse effects of high-fibre diets

The refining of cereals leads to an appreciable fall in their mineral content but, on the other hand, dietary fibre decreases the absorption of minerals such as calcium and iron. It has been suggested that in Britain the consumption of wholemeal chapattis may be a factor in causing rickets and osteomalacia in immigrants from the Indian subcontinent. These subjects tend to be deficient in vitamin D (page 156) and therefore to absorb and metabolize the available calcium less efficiently.

Where there is any question of strictures of the intestine or where diets are restricted and marginal in their mineral content, high intakes of dietary fibre may be inadvisable. In practice, however, when the diet is restricted, low mineral and high fibre contents often go together.

In conclusion it may be said that claims for the beneficial effects of high intakes of dietary fibre are largely based on circumstantial evidence and are almost certainly overstated. At the same time many people could, with advantage, increase their intake of fibre by eating more unrefined cereals, fruit and vegetables. The *Report of the National Advisory Committee on Nutritional Education* (NACNE) in 1983 recommended that the intake in this country should be increased from 20 to 25 g per day.

Nutrition and dental disease

As a result of the introduction of more refined foods and dietary trends which accompany affluence in modern society, teeth are more vulnerable to decay than ever before. There is little evidence of caries in the teeth of prehistoric man and the disease is of rare occurrence in India, Africa and Indo-China but is found in 98% of the populations of Europe and North America. Although many features of diet contribute to the prevalence of caries, Nizel has summarized present-day views as follows: (1) the major cariogenic foodstuff is sucrose; (2) the major physical factor in caries is retention of sucrose on the tooth surface; (3) the major cariogenic food habit is frequency of eating.

Dietary factors appear to be of less importance in periodontal disease which results from gingivitis, an inflammatory condition produced by local irritants. The dietary consistency is, however, of some importance since foods that have a firm consistency increase the gingival circulation and promote keratinization of the epithelium. The formation of a thick horny layer provides protection against chemical and bacterial irritants, but if the diet is excessively coarse and granular it can have an adverse effect by causing inflammation through over-use or actual injury to the periodontal tissue.

A diet that requires to be chewed also promotes the formation of a dense strong periodontal ligament. Studies have shown that the width of the ligament is directly related to the intensity of mastication while soft foods may cause atrophy from disuse.

Effect of dietary carbohydrates on caries

Most dietary carbohydrate consists of starch or sucrose. Starch unlike sucrose is not immediately available as a substrate for microorganisms. For this and other reasons sucrose is much more cariogenic than starch. Rats and hamsters fed on diets containing 70% uncooked starch remain virtually free from caries, whereas similar diets containing 70% of sucrose are highly cariogenic. Other sugars such as glucose, fructose, maltose and lactose, although more cariogenic than starch, are less cariogenic than sucrose.

These findings agree well with observations made in World War II in Britain, Scandinavia and Japan where there were qualitative changes in carbohydrate consumption; more potatoes, vegetables and flour of high extraction rate (page 175) were eaten, while the consumption of sugar and highly refined flour was reduced. These dietary changes were accompanied by a progressive decrease in the incidence of caries in young children which was reversed in the post-war period. Dietary factors other than the consumption of refined carbohydrate, e.g. the intake of 'protective foods', could also have contributed to these findings but such foods are plentiful nowadays and caries is still rife. The average consumption of sucrose in 1969 reached the incredible level of 50 kg per head per year, i.e. nearly 2 lb per head per week.

Because this and much other evidence put forward for a relationship between sugar intake and dental caries in Man is circumstantial and the applicability of the results of animal experiments to humans was open to question, there was a need for a prolonged and well-controlled experiment on humans. Such an experiment was carried out in Sweden shortly after World War II over a period of 6 years on patients in a mental hospital at Vipeholm, where careful dietary supervision was possible. More than 400 subjects were fed on a nutritionally adequate basic diet which was rich in vitamins and other protective foods, contained 130 g carbohydrate and provided 7·5 MJ (1800 kcal). Groups of patients were then fed various supplements which raised their total calorie intake to 11·3 MJ (2700 kcal). The form of the supplements and the times at which they were provided were varied. Some groups were given extra bread or a sugar solution at meal times while others were provided with chocolate or toffees between meals. A summary of the

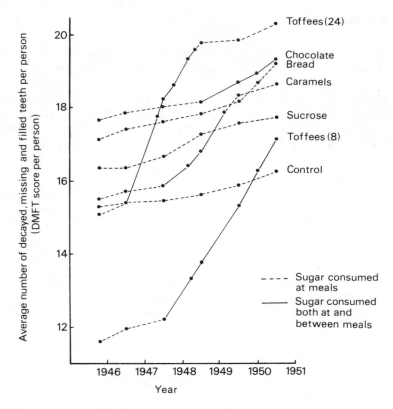

Figure 10.2 Summary of the results of the Vipeholm experiment

results is given in Figure 10.2. In all groups there was an increase in the incidence of caries, but for those given extra bread or a sugar solution at meal times this was only slight. By far the greatest increase occurred when sugar was given between meals in a sticky form, i.e. as toffees, which tend to adhere to the surface of the teeth.

The question whether sucrose is the most damaging of the sugars solely because it is consumed in the largest amounts or whether it has specific properties that render it more harmful than other sugars is considered in Chapter 34.

Is sucrose so harmful?

Sucrose has been labelled by an eminent nutritionist as 'pure white and deadly' but as with so many nutritional pronouncements this is a gross overstatement. Sucrose is naturally occurring, cheap, rich in energy, easy to digest and pleasing to the palate; it has a protein-sparing effect and protects against ketosis; it helps to blend flavours and provides bulk and texture to baked foods; it keeps indefinitely without preservatives and acts as a preservative itself. Finally it may be added that more food energy per unit of fertile land can be obtained by growing sugar cane and sugar beet than from any other crop. What needs to be clearly stated is that it should be eaten in moderation as part of a balanced diet. The faults lie not in sucrose but in our excessive appetite for it and the frequency with which sugar-containing items tend to be consumed. The relationship between diet and dental disease is discussed further in Chapter 36.

Alternative sweeteners

Substitutes for glucose and sucrose have for some time been sought for use by diabetics who have problems in metabolizing glucose and by people who wish to reduce their energy intake. More recently dental researchers and food and confectionery manufacturers, disturbed by the cariogenicity of sucrose-containing products, have been interested in alternatives.

A great many substances are known to produce the sensation of sweetness but, although this quality must stem from particular features of their chemical structure, it has not, so far, been possible to determine what these are. Most sugars and sugar derivatives have a sweet taste but so do many other totally unrelated compounds. Since the chemical basis of sweetness is unknown it is not possible to measure the property by scientific means and methods of sweetness measurement are necessarily subjective and include (1) *equal sweetness matches* in which the concentration that produces a sensation equivalent to that of a standard solution, usually sucrose, is determined and (2) *threshold measurements*, which involve finding the lowest detectable concentration of sweetener. Approximate relative sweetness values are given in Table 10.10 but there are, in addition, certain qualities of sweetness that are not easy to define. Some sweeteners lack the clean clear taste of sucrose and some have an unpleasant aftertaste.

Table 10.10 The relative sweetness of various compounds (approximate values only)

Ultrasüss	4100
Monellin	3000
Thaumatin	2000
Sucralose	650
Saccharin	550
Saccharin sodium	300
Aspartame	200
Chloroform	40
Sodium cyclamate	30
Fructose	1·35
DL-Alanine	1·30
Xylitol	1·23
Glycerol	1·08
Sucrose	*1·00*
Glycine	0·80
Glucose	0·75
Sorbitol	0·54
Maltose	0·45
Palatinose	0·42
Lactose	0·3

For a sweetener to be accepted by the authorities and by the consuming public it must:

1. Have an adequate and pleasing sweetening power.
2. Be non-toxic.
3. Be reasonably stable.
4. Be reasonably inexpensive in terms of cost per unit of sweetness.

Various categories of sweetener may be distinguished, e.g. nutritive (energy producing) and non-nutritive as well as natural and synthetic. If a nutritive sweetener is intensely sweet the amount of energy derived from it will, in fact, be negligible.

Nutritive sweeteners

These include a whole range of sugars and carbohydrate-related polyalcohols or *polyols*. Considerable scepticism exists about the advantage for diabetics of replacing inexpensive glucose and sucrose by any other sugar or sugar derivative because, (1) if they are metabolized, although insulin may not be required in the initial stages, once they have been drawn into the normal metabolic pathways for carbohydrate they will be subject to normal hormonal influences and requirements and (2) if they are not metabolized they are liable to cause osmotic diarrhoea. This does not, of course, apply to intensely sweet proteins and aspartame which come in this class, but are required in such relatively small amounts that their metabolic effects need not normally be taken into account.

Fructose

This is the sweetest sugar known and is less cariogenic than sucrose. Although it is a normal metabolite, fructose is not utilized as such by muscle, heart or brain and is largely converted to glucose by the liver on which large doses given intravenously have a potentially toxic effect. The large-scale replacement of sucrose by fructose even if economically practicable would seem to be physiologically undesirable.

Palatinose

Palatinose is a sweet-tasting disaccharide of glucose and fructose found in honey and sugar cane extract. It has similar properties to sucrose and can be used to provide bulk and texture in baked foods. Although it is hydrolysed less readily than sucrose due to the stability of its α-1 : 6-glycosidic link, it does not cause diarrhoea since the intestinal α-1 : 6-glycosidase converts it into glucose and fructose which are absorbed. Palatinose is readily available and because its low acidogenicity makes it non-cariogenic it is possible that, even though it is only about half as sweet as sucrose, it will be used as a non-cariogenic substitute.

Chlorinated sugars

Substitution of one or more of the –OH groups of sucrose by a –Cl atom has a profound effect on its taste; thus it may greatly increase the intensity of its sweetness or abolish it altogether. The most promising of these chlorinated sugars as an alternative sweetener is *Sucralose* which has a Cl atom substituted on carbon atoms 4, 1' and 6'. It is 650 times sweeter than sucrose itself, lacks the unpleasant aftertaste of saccharin and gives no evidence of any adverse effects. It will be interesting to see if it becomes a commercial success.

Sorbitol

Sorbitol is the polyalcohol corresponding to D-glucose, from which it can be prepared by hydrogenation.

$$
\begin{array}{c}
CH_2OH \\
| \\
H-C-OH \\
| \\
HO-C-H \\
| \\
H-C-OH \\
| \\
H-C-OH \\
| \\
CH_2OH
\end{array}
\qquad \text{Sorbitol (D-glucitol)}
$$

It has been used as a sweetener for many years and about one-third of the annual production is consumed in foods. Sorbitol is a normal intermediate in the conversion of glucose to fructose and is found in brain, nerve, kidney, aorta and red blood corpuscles. It is efficiently metabolized in the body.

Xylitol

Xylitol is obtained by hydrogenation of the pentose sugar xylose. It is as sweet as sucrose, and new relatively inexpensive methods have been devised for its production. Xylulose occurs naturally on the pathway by which breakdown products of gluconic acid (page 232) are fed into the pentose phosphate shunt. When administered, xylitol is readily metabolized but differs from glucose in the initial steps prior to the point at which it enters the glycolytic pathway.

$$
\begin{array}{cc}
\mathrm{CH_2OH} & \mathrm{CHO} \\
\mathrm{H-C-OH} & \mathrm{H-C-OH} \\
\mathrm{HO-C-H} & \mathrm{HO-C-H} \\
\mathrm{H-C-OH} & \mathrm{H-C-OH} \\
\mathrm{CH_2OH} & \mathrm{CH_2OH} \\
\text{Xylitol} & \text{Xylose}
\end{array}
$$

Recently xylitol has aroused considerable interest following reports that, while the addition of 10% sorbitol or mannitol to a cariogenic diet reduced the incidence of caries in rats by one-half to one-third, xylitol caused caries to be virtually eliminated. Other experiments showed that cariogenic streptococci will not grow on xylitol alone although they grew when sucrose was also present in the medium. These preliminary experiments have led to the suggestion that replacement of sucrose by xylitol might have a beneficial effect on caries incidence in humans. The Turku study on humans, in which all added sucrose was replaced by xylitol in one group of subjects, showed that caries was completely eliminated over a two-year period.

Oral ingestion of xylitol by diabetics in place of sugar was proposed by the WHO/FAO Joint Foods Programme (1960) and long-term studies on rats gave no indication of any ill effects; nor did relatively short studies in monkeys and humans. However, certain evidence suggests that the accumulation of sugar alcohols may be responsible for cataract development in experimental animals and diabetics. In the circumstances long-term administration of large amounts of these substances, even if proved to reduce caries, should probably be undertaken with caution.

Sweet proteins

Certain proteins have been found to have an intensely sweet taste. *Monellin* is found in the fruit of the serendipity berry (*Dioscoreophyllum cumminsii*) and *thaumatin* in the plant ketemfe (*Thaumatococcus daniellii*) both of which grow in West Africa. The proteins are each about 3000 times as sweet as sucrose. Thaumatin is slow acting, it clings to the tongue and has a lingering licorice-like aftertaste which may have restricted its use.

Aspartame

Aspartame is a relatively new sweetener which is readily available and known commercially as *Canderel*. It is the methyl ester of the dipeptide L-aspartyl-L-phenylalanine and has a natural sugar-like taste. It is about 200 times as sweet as sucrose and, in addition, has flavour-enhancing properties. In the body the methyl group is removed and most of it is cleaved into its constituent amino acids which are then metabolized in the usual way. Its chief disadvantage is that it is not very stable especially in alkaline solutions. When it decomposes the dipeptide tends to lose water and form its diketopiperazine and small amounts of this compound may be formed in the body. In normal subjects there is no evidence that either aspartame or the diketopiperazine give rise to any adverse effects but, since they produce phenylalanine when they decompose, aspartame is not recommended for phenylketonuric subjects (page 325). Aspartame is useful for reducing sugar consumption in obese and diabetic subjects and in people who are predisposed to dental caries. It can be used as a 'table top sweetener' and in jellies and fruit drinks but not in baked products or in liquids that are neutral in reaction and have to be stored for relatively long periods.

Non-nutritive sweeteners

Saccharin

For many years saccharin has been used by diabetics and slimmers. It has no food value and, since it is excreted unchanged in the urine, the continued use of small amounts is probably harmless. Saccharin is about 550 times as sweet as sucrose and a daily intake of up to 5 mg per kg body weight is considered to be acceptable. The sodium salt is preferable to saccharin itself since it is more soluble and comparatively free from the unpleasant aftertaste of saccharin. Although some people do not like saccharin few toxic symptoms have been reported, but on rare occasions photosensitization has been observed.

o-Benzoic sulphimide

Saccharin sodium

Cyclamates

Until 1970 cyclamates were used not only by individuals with a clear need to restrict their sugar or energy intake but also as a general sweetener. The sodium and calcium salts have advantages over saccharin since they leave no bitter aftertaste and, because they are stable to heat and acid, can be added to processed foods. When introduced it was believed that cyclamates were not metabolized, but subsequently cyclohexylamine, a compound about whose long-term toxicity little is known, was found in the urine of people consuming cyclamates. Furthermore, feeding experiments in which large doses of cyclamates were given to animals showed that, in such circumstances, they might be carcinogenic. Thus, while it is not certain that the continued ingestion of small amounts for special dietary purposes is harmful, no safe limit can be set and their use in many countries, including the UK and the USA, is no longer permitted.

Sodium cyclamate
(sodium cyclohexane sulphamate)

Cyclohexylamine

Chapter 11
Mineral nutrition and metabolism

Although carbon, hydrogen, oxygen and nitrogen together account for 96% of the body weight (Table 11.1), at least 24 other elements are present and, since calcium and phosphorus account for about 2·5%, the rest must be present in very small amounts. However, the quantity in which an element is present gives no indication of its biochemical importance, nor does it bear any close relationship to dietary requirements.

The functions of the mineral elements are many and various. Some act as essential structural components, others fulfil a catalytic or regulatory role, while some do both. Calcium and phosphorus are notable examples. Most proteins contain sulphur, some contain phosphorus, some iron and one, thyroglobulin, contains iodine. Other elements, notably sodium, potassium, chlorine and phosphorus, play an essential part in the maintenance of osmotic and acid/base balance and many ions are components of enzyme systems.

Table 11.1 Elementary composition of the adult body

	%	Amount per 70 kg
Oxygen	65·0	45·5 kg
Carbon	18·0	12·6 kg
Hydrogen	10·0	7·0 kg
Nitrogen	3·0	2·1 kg
Calcium	1·5	1·04 kg
Phosphorus	1·0	0·70 kg
Potassium	0·3	0·210 kg
Sulphur	0·25	0·175 kg
Sodium	0·15	0·105 kg
Chlorine	0·15	0·105 kg
Magnesium	0·05	35·0 g
Iron	0·006	4·2 g
Zinc	0·003	2·1 g
Manganese	0·0003	0·21 g
Copper	0·00015	0·105 g
Iodine	0·00004	0·028 g

Of the 26 elements known or claimed to be essential for animal organisms, 11 are considered as major elements, namely: C, H, O, N, S, P, Ca, K, Na, Mg, Cl. Two others, namely iron and zinc, are present in small but appreciable amounts. The remaining 13 elements are found only in trace amounts and some of these have not been conclusively shown to be essential. These 13 elements are: I, Cu, Mn, Co, Mb, Se, Cr, Ni, Sn, Si, Vd, As and F.

Evidence of a requirement for the last six rests on the effects on the growth and reproductive ability of experimental animals fed purified diets and reared in conditions in which atmospheric contamination by these elements was minimized.

Minerals are constantly being lost from the body, chiefly in the urine, and must continually be replaced. The approximate amounts of the seven principal minerals that are required daily to keep the adult human body in balance are:

Sodium 6·0 g	Chlorine 9·0 g
Potassium 4·0 g	Phosphorus 0·8 g
Calcium 0·6 g	Sulphur 1·0 g
Magnesium 0·35 g	

A good average diet should supply these without difficulty but some mineral constituents are inefficiently absorbed. The minerals which are nutritionally of most importance because their intake may be less than the requirements are calcium, iron, iodine and fluorine. However, defective absorption, resulting from general malnutrition or a variety of other causes, may be responsible for secondary deficiences of substances present in the diet in adequate amounts.

The nutritionally important minerals

Salt intake, hypertension and cerebrovascular disease

Salt, i.e. sodium chloride, an indispensable body constituent, is present in most natural foods but whether humans get enough from these sources or need additional amounts is a matter of dispute. Certain primitive tribes survive on what is naturally present in their food but, on the other hand, wars have been fought over sources of salt, and for centuries its trade was more important than that of any other commodity. Efficient mechanisms exist within the body of normal subjects both for the conservation and for the excretion of salt and a wide range of intakes is compatible with the health of such individuals. There is undoubtedly a minimum requirement for salt for the maintenance of electrolyte balance because, although its excretion in the urine can be reduced to an almost negligible amount, salt is also lost in sweat. At the other extreme, provided it is accompanied by an adequate intake of water, large amounts of salt can be excreted by normal subjects so that how much, if any, extra salt one adds to one's food resolves itself into a matter of taste.

The current suggestion that a high salt intake leads to hypertension and cerebrovascular disease is largely based on epidemiological evidence. Any such relationship is complicated by the fact that blood pressure is known to be influenced by many other factors, e.g. body weight, temperament, physical activity, stress, external temperature and smoking habits. Nevertheless, comparisons of populations show a general correlation between the average salt intake and the blood pressure level. The Japanese consume more salt than any other nation and have the highest incidence of hypertension and cerebrovascular disease, although not of ischaemic heart disease. However, within the various populations some individuals are much more sensitive to salt than others. This is also true for rats, some, but not all of which, develop hypertension in response to a high-salt diet. Salt sensitivity and essential hypertension in humans are believed to be caused by an inherited renal abnormality that makes it difficult for the kidneys to excrete Na^+

and this difficulty is compounded as the salt intake rises. Restriction of the sodium intake significantly reduced the arterial blood pressure of about 60% of people suffering from essential hypertension suggesting that a high salt intake does not always account for the development of this condition. It seems possible that, at least in some instances, hypertension may result from a deficiency of the newly discovered *natriuretic hormones*. These are a series of peptides which have been isolated from the atria of the heart and which cause a marked increase in sodium and water excretion. In the rat the predominant peptide contains 28 amino acid residues and is known as *cardionatrin I*. The human form differs from this by only one amino acid.

Whereas a high intake of sodium seems in some subjects to promote the development of high blood pressure, a high intake of potassium has the reverse effect and it is now thought that the Na/K ratio may be of greater significance than the Na intake alone.

According to the NACNE Report (1983) the average intake of sodium chloride in the UK is about 12 g per day which is in excess of the requirement even of people who undertake strenuous physical exercise and lose large quantities by sweating. The Report recommends that the average intake should be reduced to half or even a quarter of this amount since a high salt intake has not been shown to be of any benefit. There seems little doubt that hypertensive subjects should reduce their salt intake but whether it is necessary or desirable for others to do so is open to question. If an individual likes salty food, has no reason to believe he or she is at risk of hypertension and maintains an adequate water intake, there is no compelling evidence to suggest that he or she would benefit from a reduction in salt intake. An increased consumption of fruit and vegetables and the sparing use of foods and manufactured products which have a high sodium content would, however, result in a decrease in the Na/K ratio of the diet which might have a health-promoting effect. (It is important to distinguish between the salt (NaCl) intake and the sodium (Na) intake: 12 g of NaCl = 4·7 g of Na.)

Calcium

The importance of calcium in body structure and as a participant in and regulator of body processes can hardly be overestimated. Calcium is no less important from the nutritional point of view. Because of (1) the large reserve of calcium in the bones and its ability to maintain a long-term buffering effect against calcium loss, (2) the difficulties inherent in calcium absorption which are discussed below, and (3) the ability of the body to adapt to a low calcium intake, there is considerable controversy regarding calcium requirements. On the basis of balance studies in which the dietary intake was compared with the amount of calcium lost via the kidneys, intestine and skin, the recommended daily intake was for many years given as 1 g. However, as a consequence of global surveys the World Health Organization reduced this figure to 0·5–0·6 g for adults, infants and older children and recommended an intake of 1·0–1·2 g during pregnancy and lactation.

Special attention needs to be given to the requirements of child-bearing women, since the mother's skeleton yields up the calcium that the fetus and young infant require and the effect of repeated pregnancies on a woman receiving inadequate amounts of calcium and vitamin D can lead to *osteomalacia* (page 157). There is, however, no convincing support for the view that in normal well-fed women the teeth tend to become decalcified during pregnancy and lactation or that they are more prone to dental decay. Thus the maxim 'for every child a tooth' is not well founded.

A puzzling feature of calcium metabolism is that adaptation to much lower dietary calcium intakes than those which are generally believed to be desirable seems to be possible. Thus growing children in Sri Lanka were found to maintain a positive calcium balance on intakes of about 200 mg per day. Furthermore, experiments in animals have shown that, on a low calcium

Table 11.2 Approximate calcium content of various uncooked foods

	mg/100 g
Cheese (hard)	800
Cheese (soft)	80
Milk (cow's)	120
Milk (human)	30
Shelled nuts	13–250
Dried pulses	40–200
Root vegetables	20–100
Green vegetables	25–250
Eggs	56
Oatmeal	55
Wholemeal bread (100% extraction)	25
White bread (70% extraction fortified)	100
Millet	35
Fish	20–120
Meat	14
Maize	12
Rice	6
Potatoes	8

diet, calcium is absorbed more efficiently and the concentration of intestinal calcium-binding protein (page 445) increases. Whether, at the same time, calcium excretion is reduced has not been established.

Few foods are rich sources of calcium although fish such as whitebait and sardines, the backbones of which can be eaten, may provide up to 400 mg/100 g. Otherwise the best sources are milk and milk products such as cheese (Table 11.2). Green vegetables, cereals and pulses also contain appreciable amounts, but their calcium is less well utilized than that of milk. Since cow's milk contains about 0·12 g of calcium per 100 ml, half a litre or 1 pint (568 ml) should provide the daily requirement. Calcium deficiency is thus mainly a hazard in countries where milk and cheese are not regularly consumed.

Elderly people, particularly women, tend to develop the condition of *osteoporosis* in which complete loss of bone tissue occurs in small areas within the bones which become porous and brittle. There is no clear-cut evidence of a relationship between the calcium intake and the rate of bone loss in humans. Nevertheless, it would be unwise to let the calcium intake fall below the recommended level. The practice of adding calcium salts to flour to minimize the likelihood of calcium deficiency would seem to be a sound one, particularly in view of the negative association between the hardness of water and mortality from cardiovascular disease.

Phosphorus is closely bound up with calcium from both metabolic and nutritional viewpoints. Phosphorus occurs abundantly in plant and animal tissues and, if the other nutritional requirements are satisfied, the diet should contain adequate amounts. Meat, eggs, dairy products and cereals are all good sources.

The absorption of calcium and phosphorus

The absorption of calcium from the gut is always far from complete. About 70% of that ingested is excreted in the faeces. Many calcium salts are insoluble at physiological pH values and tend to be precipitated in the gut lumen. Spinach and rhubarb, although they contain appreciable amounts of calcium, may have an adverse effect on the calcium balance since their excess oxalate may precipitate calcium derived from other foods.

Phytic acid, which is present in cereal grains and is rich in phosphate, also tends to form insoluble salts with calcium, magnesium and iron and to render them unavailable. Since it is concentrated in the outer husk of the grain, high extraction flours (page 175) contain more phytate than those of lower extraction. People eating brown bread therefore absorb substantially less calcium, magnesium and iron than people eating white flour products.

Phytic acid
(inositol hexaphosphate)

The addition of phytic acid to white flour markedly reduced the absorption of these minerals in short-term studies. With prolonged ingestion, the body can adapt to a high phytate intake apparently as a result of the action of enzymes which release the phosphate from soluble phytates. *Phytases* may be derived from the food, the digestive secretions or the intestinal bacteria.

Calcium absorption is also affected by pH. Calcium compounds are readily soluble in the stomach and proximal duodenum where the contents are acid but, from there onwards, there is a steady increase in pH. Thus calcium absorption occurs chiefly in the duodenum and proximal jejunum.

Certain organic compounds also affect the absorption of calcium. Amino acids, notably arginine and lysine, facilitate its absorption, and lactose and other sugars as well as polyalcohols, such as sorbitol and mannitol, have a similar effect. These substances may act by chelating or otherwise complexing the calcium, converting it into a more readily absorbable form. On the other hand, long chain fatty acids react with calcium to form insoluble soaps, and if fat absorption is defective, as in biliary obstruction or coeliac disease, calcium absorption may be reduced. However, the effects of all these substances is slight in comparison with those exerted by vitamin D which promotes the synthesis of calcium-binding protein within the cells of the intestinal epithelium (page 445).

Iron

Iron performs a wide range of biological functions, many of which are connected with oxidation reactions and processes by which energy is conserved in the body. In haemoglobin and myoglobin, iron is responsible for oxygen uptake and in the cytochromes and iron–sulphur proteins, e.g. ferridoxins, for electron transport (page 216). Iron is also involved in the activation of oxygen by a variety of oxidases and oxygenases and of nitrogen by nitrogenases which take part in the nitrogen-fixing activities of bacteria.

The adult human body contains 4–5 g of iron of which about 70% is present in haemoglobin, 5% in myoglobin, 20% in storage and transport forms and 5% in iron-containing enzymes. These latter include enzymes such as cytochrome oxidase, catalase and peroxidase which contain iron in the form of haem compounds and others containing non-haem iron, e.g. succinate dehydrogenase and mitochondrial NADH dehydrogenase (Chapter 16).

Iron is one of the few nutrients where balance is maintained by alterations in its absorption rather than by regulation of its excretion. Its absorption is difficult and is affected both by the form in which it is ingested and by interaction with other dietary constituents. Although only a small proportion of ingested iron is absorbed, most of the iron released in the body by breakdown of iron-containing molecules is returned to the plasma for re-use, little being lost in the urine, faeces and sweat. Losses occur by desquamation of surface cells, in secretions and as a result of blood loss, but the total loss from the body of a normal adult male is only about 1 mg per day. In women, considerable losses occur during menstruation and reproduction and, since the safety margin between the dietary content and requirements is narrow, iron-deficiency anaemia is by no means uncommon in women. Recommendations for iron intake are difficult to make. Allowing for a loss of up to 1 mg per day and an absorption efficiency of 10% the dietary requirement for a man has been estimated as about 10 mg per day and that of a woman of child-bearing age as 15 mg.

Dietary sources of iron

Iron is probably the most difficult nutrient to obtain in sufficient amounts. The best sources are meat, especially liver, fish and eggs but milk is a poor source and babies rely on iron stored in their liver before birth. Bread, flour and other cereal products contain significant amounts, as do potatoes and green vegetables. Cocoa and chocolate have a surprisingly high content; drinking chocolate contains 12 mg/100 g and cocoa powder 15 mg/100 g compared with 0·1 mg/100 g for milk. Iron may also be obtained from the drinking water and from iron utensils.

The iron present in animal foods is more readily available than that of plant products. Not only is haem iron more easily absorbed than inorganic iron but, in addition, the amino acids derived from the proteins form soluble complexes with the inorganic iron. In contrast the iron in cereals and vegetables is bound with proteins, phytates, other phosphates, oxalates and carbonates as insoluble ferric complexes and is poorly absorbed.

Ferrous salts are absorbed more efficiently than ferric salts and are given in the treatment of iron-deficiency anaemia. They are not, however, always well tolerated and it is sometimes necessary to give special preparations, e.g. iron–dextran or iron–sorbitol parenterally.

Many factors that affect calcium absorption have a similar effect on the absorption of iron. Absorption is promoted by ascorbic acid possibly because it reduces ferric to ferrous iron. Absorption is augmented in iron deficiency and depressed when stores are increased. Thus when, after a haemorrhage, erthyropoiesis is accelerated, iron absorption is enhanced and, under conditions in which erythropoiesis is reduced, e.g. starvation or descent from a high altitude, absorption is reduced.

Iron released from the intestinal mucosa enters the portal blood where it combines with an iron-transporting β-globulin known as *transferrin* which distributes the iron throughout the body. Most of it is taken up by the reticulocytes for haemoglobin formation.

At the end of their life-span the red blood corpuscles are broken down by reticuloendothelial cells and their iron is released into the plasma in the ferrous state but it is oxidized to the ferric form before combining with transferrin once again.

Storage of iron

Iron is stored in the body as *ferritin* and *haemosiderin*. These give protection from the effects of sudden loss as, for example, after a haemorrhage. In women they provide for the needs of the developing fetus and newborn infant. Ferritin is a reddish brown high molecular weight water-soluble protein which contains variable amounts of ferric iron and is found in greatest amount in the liver, spleen and bone marrow.

If iron accumulates in large amounts it is deposited in the liver as insoluble intracellular granules of haemosiderin. Haemosiderin is less active metabolically than ferritin and serves as a longer term reserve. Excessive accumulation leads to *siderosis* in which there may be severe liver damage.

Zinc

Zinc has long been recognized as an essential body constituent but its dietary importance has only recently been established. Zinc is a component of more than 120 enzymes and it is indispensable for normal cellular growth and differentation. Zinc and protein are associated in foods and it is now believed that it is not possible to have a protein deficiency without a deficiency of zinc. The recommended dietary intake for Zn for adults is 15 mg which is as great as that for Fe. The body has no functional store of Zn and the mechanism of its absorption is probably similar to that of Fe.

Zinc deficiency is thought to be common in human populations living on restricted diets and to be one of the factors responsible for their poor general health. If the Zn intake is low, whether or not it is adequate will depend on other components of the diet. The endemic Zn deficiency encountered in Iran may be connected with the high phytate content of the rural diet which interferes with Zn absorption.

A wide range of adverse effects have been reported in Zn deficiency. They include *anorexia* (loss of appetite), diarrhoea, stunting, wasting, skin ulceration and an increased susceptibility to infection. Many of the features of deficiency are compatible with impairment of nucleic acid metabolism and protein synthesis and many of the enzymes involved in these processes contain Zn. Of special interest is the finding of an immunodeficiency particularly of the cell-mediated immune system. Zn deficiency also leads to abnormalities of taste perception. These are thought to be secondary to a decrease in *gustin*, the major Zn-containing protein in parotid saliva. The effects of Zn deficiency are clearly seen in the rare congenital disease *acrodermatitis enteropathica* which results from a defect in Zn absorption.

Topically applied zinc in the form of calamine has long been used to promote healing and it has been shown that Zn is absorbed through the skin. Administration of Zn to patients with ulcers whose serum Zn level was low was found to promote healing. Zinc deficiency has been found to cause *alopecia* (loss of hair) in both humans and animals.

Trace elements

Many of the elements listed on page 139 are present in the body in such small amounts that it is difficult to establish whether they are present by chance or whether they fulfil some special function and are essential dietary constituents. Cu, Mn, Mo, Co and Se have all been identified as constituents of enzyme systems but, apart from iodine, the role of the other elements, if any, has not been defined.

With the arbitrary exception of fluorine, trace element deficiences rarely occur in Man although deficiencies of Cu, Co, Mn and Se occur in grazing animals as a result of a deficiency of these elements in the soil and herbage. It is possible, however, that marginal states of deficiency may be responsible for some cases of non-specific indisposition and malaise.

Apart from a low dietary intake, deficiencies of trace elements may arise from defects in absorption or utilization. Trace element absorption can be greatly influenced by other dietary components both organic, such as phytates, and inorganic, such as metals. Only those elements which are of practical importance will be discussed.

Iodine

Iodine is an essential constituent of the two hormones, thyroxine (T_4) and tri-iodothyronine (T_3), produced by the thyroid gland. Dietary iodine is largely converted to iodide in the gastrointestinal tract and in this form is rapidly and completely absorbed. It is removed from the blood by the thyroid gland, salivary glands and gastric mucosa, which have the ability to concentrate it, although only the thyroid gland is able to use it for hormone synthesis. Iodine is readily excreted by the kidneys.

The richest sources of iodine are sea foods but it is also found in vegetables, meat, eggs, dairy products and cereals. However, the iodine content of a particular food varies widely according to the geographical location, type of soil and use of fertilizers. Iodine deficiency is most common in inland mountainous areas and it was once held responsible for all cases of goitre in such areas. However, although iodine administration reduces the incidence of goitre it does not completely abolish it. Genetic factors, infectious agents and dietary goitrogens may all be implicated and iodine deficiency may 'uncover' border-line biochemical defects. The foods that contain goitrogens are mainly members of the cabbage family.

The daily requirement of normal adults for iodine is given as $100 \mu g$. The body contains a total of 20–50 mg of iodine of which about 8 mg are found in the thyroid gland. It is now recommended that small amounts of iodine, as potassium iodide, should be added to cooking and table salt. This recommendation has never been adopted by the British Government, although experience elsewhere has shown that the addition of 20 parts per million is beneficial and has no harmful effects.

Fluoride – essential nutrient or health hazard?

When sufficiently sensitive methods are used fluorine is detectable in every bone and tooth and it has even been suggested that the formation of biological apatites may not be possible in the complete absence of fluoride. This, together with the finding that optimal concentrations of fluoride in the drinking water significantly reduce the number of carious lesions that develop in children's teeth, suggests that fluoride may be an essential nutrient. However, owing to the difficulty of preparing a diet from which fluoride is altogether absent yet which is otherwise adequate, it is virtually impossible to substantiate this claim. Fluorine is the most electronegative element and is highly reactive. Various fluorine-containing salts, most commonly calcium fluoride (fluorspar), are widely distributed in rocks and soils. Mineral apatites which are present in igneous rocks act as fluoride carriers, and salt deposits of marine origin also contain significant amounts.

Fluorine in the form of fluorides is present in most soils in amounts ranging from 10 to 7000 mg kg^{-1} (parts per million) with an average of 250 ppm. No appreciable increase has been found in the fluoride content of vegetables grown on soils rich in fluoride, although some plants, particularly broad-leaved varieties like cabbage and lettuce, absorb airborne fluorides from industrial processes, sprays and fertilizers.

Fluoride ingestion

Natural waters almost always contain some fluoride, the concentration depending on the fluoride-containing minerals with which the water is in contact. Most fluoride-containing minerals are only sparingly soluble in water so that, except in unusual circumstances, surface waters have levels of less than 1 mg per litre and sometimes contain less than $0 \cdot 1$ mg per litre. Underground or subsoil waters, which have greater contact with fluoride-bearing minerals, may contain considerably higher concentrations and a value of 2800 mg per litre has been reported for lake water in Kenya!

Thus most people, wherever they live, are likely to ingest some fluoride in their drinking water. Fluoride is also present in the diet; most foodstuffs contain small amounts and a few are relatively rich sources. These include mackerel, salmon, sardines, some mineral waters, wines and tea. This latter is important since its fluoride content may be as much as 100 mg kg^{-1} of which up to 90% is extracted during infusion, and quite large volumes of tea may be drunk each day.

Fluorides in the body

Some inorganic fluorides have a high solubility; for example, sodium fluoride (NaF) is about 4% soluble at room temperature, sodium monofluorophosphate (Na_2PO_3F) 25%, stannous fluoride (SnF_2)>10% and stannous hexafluorozirconate ($SnZrF_6$)>24%. Other fluorides are virtually insoluble, e.g. calcium fluoride (CaF_2) 0·0016%. The soluble fluorides are rapidly and almost completely absorbed from the gastrointestinal tract and insoluble fluorides less completely and at a slower rate. Absorption probably occurs by simple diffusion through the gut wall; it is reduced by the presence of large amounts of Ca^{2+} and Mg^{2+}.

Blood contains about 0·1–0·2 mg F per litre but only a small part of this is in ionic form. The level shows only a transient rise after the ingestion of fluoride and the range is not exceeded in subjects consuming up to 4 mg per litre in drinking water. Thus it seems that the plasma fluoride level in Man is effectively regulated. The fluoride content of the soft tissues seem to be of the same order as that of the plasma, although the intracellular concentration of ionic fluoride is probably less. Two mechanisms, namely excretion and deposition in the calcified tissues, operate to keep the fluoride content of the body fluids and soft tissues at a low level.

1. Fluoride excretion. About half of the soluble fluoride ingested is rapidly excreted mainly via the urine.
2. Uptake by the calcified tissues. The remainder of the fluoride is removed by the calcified tissues which take it up with great avidity. However, certain experiments indicate that, as with most other body constituents, a steady state is eventually established.

Deposition of fluoride in the bones is not completely irreversible and a person who moves from a region where the concentration in the drinking water is high, e.g. 8 mg per litre, to one where it is appreciably lower excretes increased amounts of fluoride in his urine for some time afterwards. Presumably this is due to loss of physicochemically exchangeable fluoride and also to osteoclastic activity.

Fluoride toxicity

Like most substances, fluoride is toxic if taken into the body in sufficient amounts. Acute fluoride poisoning, either by ingestion or inhalation, is very rare, the fatal dose being about 5·0 g of sodium fluoride. Fluoride is an irritant poison which inhibits many enzymes. There is early involvement of the alimentary, cardiovascular, respiratory and central nervous systems and death occurs in 2–3 days.

Chronic fluoride intoxication is more common and, since fluoride is concentrated in the hard tissues, the bones and teeth show the most obvious effects of *fluorosis*. Intake of excessive amounts of fluoride during tooth development results in *mottled enamel* which is characterized by the presence of scattered irregular white flecks. The permanent teeth are particularly susceptible. Towards the end of the last century this condition was found to be of common occurrence among people living near Naples where drinking water was contaminated by volcanic fumes. Their newly erupted permanent teeth had a mottled appearance; in addition the enamel was sometimes found to be pitted and later developed an unsightly brown stain. At that time, various observations suggested that mottling of the enamel, which in its mild form is not disfiguring, was associated with a lowered incidence of dental caries. These findings were confirmed by the classic studies of Dean who, while working for the US Public Health Service in the 1930s, carried out an extensive survey of certain parts of the USA where the water contained higher than average levels of fluoride. He concluded that in a temperate climate when the fluoride content of the water was about 2 mg per litre, the teeth of about 50% of the population showed a mild degree of mottling but staining, when it occurred, was only faint. At a level of 4 mg per litre, however, *endemic dental fluorosis* of a moderate degree (Table 11.3) occurred in 90% of children. They concluded that at levels of 4 mg per litre and above children suffered from low-grade fluorine poisoning. Thus ingestion of excess fluoride during the development of the enamel organ adversely affects both the organic and inorganic phases of enamel, resulting in hypoplasia of the permanent teeth.

Table 11.3 Classification of degree of fluorosis

Grade of fluorosis	*Description of fluorosis*	*Dental fluorosis index (DFI)*
Normal	None	0
Questionable	A few white flecks or white spots	0·5
Very mild	Small opaque, paper-white areas involving less than 25% of the surface	1·0
Mild	White opacities are more extensive but do not involve more than 50% of the surface	2·0
Moderate	Distinct brown stain, all enamel surfaces affected	3·0
Severe	Besides brown staining, the tooth is worn and hypoplastic. All enamel surfaces affected	4·0

It is interesting to compare human with shark's teeth, where the outermost layer which is of mesodermal and not of epithelial origin contains apatite crystals similar to those of human enamel. This layer contains more than 100 times as much fluoride as mottled human enamel but shows no mineralization defects. It appears that the enamel organ has a specific sensitivity to fluoride.

Mottling and discoloration of the teeth may occur for reasons other than an excessive fluoride intake. The broad-spectrum antibiotic tetracycline, probably as a result of its calcium-binding properties, is specifically deposited in growing bones and teeth which become discoloured.

Whereas dental fluorosis is easily recognizable, *skeletal fluorosis* is not obvious until the condition has advanced to a stage at which it may become crippling. However, since fluorosis is characterized by increased density of the bones, radiological examination allows it to be diagnosed at an early stage. The condition was first described as an industrial disease in workers handling powdered cryolite and inhaling as dust 20–80 mg of fluoride per day for 10–20 years. It also occurs in areas of India, where large quantities of water, containing 10 mg per litre or more of fluoride, are drunk as a result of the hot climate.

Apart from causing a stimulation of osteoblastic activity the ingestion of excessive amounts of fluoride over long periods may lead to calcification of tendons, ligaments and occasionally muscles. The vertebrae, ribs and pelvis are more prone to the development of non-malignant swellings or growths known as exostoses than the long bones. Although the toxic effects of fluoride are mainly confined to the hard tissues, in crippling fluorosis the nervous system may be secondarily affected. High fluoride intakes may affect the thyroid and the kidney but no clinically obvious disturbance in their function has been reported in endemic fluorosis. Reports that mongolism (Down's syndrome) is more frequent where the water contains more than 1 mg per litre have not been substantiated.

The pros and cons of water fluoridation

It was shown by Dean that, where the level of fluoride in the water was about 1 mg per litre (1 ppm), the incidence of mottled enamel was slight while the incidence of caries was 50% lower than in places where the water contained 0·2 mg of fluoride per litre or less. Where the level of fluoride was 2 mg per litre there was a slight further decrease in the incidence of caries but an increase in the degree of mottling. As a result of this and many other studies, it was concluded that the optimal level of fluoride in the water supply in temperate climates is about 1 mg per litre. From 1945 onwards, studies on the effects of raising the fluoride level of the communal water supply to approximately 1 mg per litre were made in various parts of the world.

Investigations of the efficacy of fluoridation carried out in Canada, the Netherlands, Finland, Ireland, New Zealand, the USSR, Puerto Rico and South America, as well as in the UK and USA, have all shown that fluoridation reduces the incidence of caries. A comparison of the number of decayed, missing and filled teeth (DMFT) in 15-year-old children in control and fluoridated towns in various parts of the world is shown in Table 11.4. From this it can be seen that fluoridation consistently caused a reduction of about 50% in spite of the fact that the DMFT indices of the control group varied from 8·04 to 16·80.

The effect of fluoridation is not equal at all ages. The greatest benefit is derived when optimal amounts of fluoride are ingested during tooth formation and, since most of the fluoride deposited in early life is retained in the teeth, the effect persists in adults. Between the ages of 8 and 11 years fluoridation may appear to be of little benefit. At this period less than half the permanent teeth have erupted and the occlusal pits and fissures of newly erupted molars and premolars are more susceptible to caries than the smooth surfaces on which fluoride has a greater protective action, so that limited comparisons of this sort can be misleading. Furthermore, fluoridation affords less protection to deciduous than to permanent teeth. This may be because the fluoride content of milk is low and consequently the intake during the

Table 11.4 Number of decayed, missing and filled teeth (DMFT) in 15-year-old children from control (C) and fluoridated (F) towns

	Muskegon (C) *Grand Rapids (F)* *USA*	*Hastings*[a] *Hastings*[b] *(F)* *NZ*	*Sarnia (C)* *Brantford (F)* *Canada*[c]	*Oak Park(C)* *Evanston (F)* *USA*[d]	*Culemborg (C)* *Tiel (F)* *Netherlands*
Control group	12·38	16·80	8·04	11·35	13·9
Test group	6·22	8·52	3·90	5·95	6·8
Difference (number)	6·16	8·28	4·14	5·40	7·1
Difference (%)	49·8	49·3	51·4	47·6	51·1

From O. Backer Dirks (1974). The benefits of water fluoridation. *Caries Research*, Vol. 8, Suppl. 1, 2–15
[a] Hastings before water fluoridation
[b] Hastings after 15 years of fluoridation
[c] Children aged 14 and 15
[d] Children aged 14

formation and maturation of the enamel is restricted. There is also a relatively short time between eruption and the shedding of the teeth during which the enamel can take up fluoride from its surroundings. Sometimes an apparent decrease in effectiveness results from loss of teeth from periodontal disease rather than dental decay.

Although experience has shown that in temperate zones and western living conditions a concentration of fluoride of about 1 mg per litre produces the best results, variations in normal fluoride and water intakes should be taken into account when determining fluoridation levels. Thus in Japan dental fluorosis occurred at lower water fluoride concentrations than elsewhere because both sea food and tea are staple articles of diet. The consumption of fluoride in the food is said to be 1·0–2·0 mg per day higher in Japan than in North America, where the average intake is 0·2–0·4 mg per day. In those parts of Japan where water supplies have been fluoridated, it was found that after 10 years a level of 0·6 mg per litre gave a reduction in dental decay comparable with that obtained with a level of 1 mg per litre elsewhere.

The question of whether water should be artificially fluoridated remains a matter of considerable public debate. In 1970 the European Organization for Caries Research (ORCA) gave firm support to the view that, where the fluoride content of the natural supply was low, fluoridation was the most effective public health measure for reducing the incidence of tooth decay. The opponents of fluoridation are, however, concerned about the addition of a dose-dependent toxic substance to the public water supply. They argue that it is not possible to ensure that individuals such as stokers, athletes and sufferers from incipient diabetes or kidney complaints who have a high fluid intake, and also people who for one reason or another consistently ingest higher than average amounts of fluoride from food, do not exceed the safe intake. There is, in fact, no way of knowing how much fluoride any particular individual may be absorbing and damaging effects on small sections of the population may not be apparent from statistical analyses. However, as Ericsson states in *Reports of ORCA on Water Fluoridation* (1974):

> While nobody can guarantee the safety of any human measure under all circumstances, the safety of the adjustment of drinking water fluoride to about 1 ppm is supported by so large and so manifold scientific material and clinical data that any health hazard with this measure is extremely improbable. Specific claims of such hazards have been few and inadequately supported.

A report by the Royal College of Physicians (1978) endorsed this view and recommended the fluoridation of water supplies in the United Kingdom where the fluoride level is appreciably below 1 mg per litre.

Another major point of attack by the antifluoride campaigners concerns the principle of mass medication. They fear that if 'the authorities' are allowed to dose the public with substances that they believe to be good for them, a dangerous precedent is set which could have far-reaching effects. This argument is countered by the supporters of fluoridation who emphasize that water supplies are commonly chlorinated to make them safe and that there is little difference in principle between fluoridation to prevent dental decay and chlorination to prevent bacterial infection. They point out, moreover, that it would be possible for a household to install a fluoride filter containing, for example hydroxyapatite, which would remove the fluoride from their personal supply. The use of such filters should probably be recommended for patients undergoing regular haemodialysis.

Although it is understandable that some people may still have reservations about water fluoridation the measure is supported by the World Health Organization and by the majority of dentists, who recognize it not only as an efficient means of reducing caries but also as a highly economic measure. The costs involved in fluoridation are economically outweighed by the

Footnote   It is interesting to note that the incidence of *osteoporosis* has been reported to be lower in areas where the natural fluoride content of the water is high.

saving in time for both dentist and patient and should allow dentists to provide a better overall standard of treatment.

Alternative methods of fluoride administration

Fluoridation of the communal water supply is not the only way in which fluoride may be administered although it seems that ingestion of soluble fluoride, which ensures that the ion is obtainable from the blood during tooth development, is the best way of obtaining full benefit from it. On this basis it has been suggested that fluoride might be included in some regular article of diet such as milk, flour or salt; but fortification of staple articles of diet is open to one of the same objections as water fluoridation, namely that it is impossible to regulate the fluoride intake of particular individuals. It would, however, allow the consumer the choice of using the supplemented or unsupplemented article according to preference. Iodine-enriched salt is already available in areas where there is a risk of iodine deficiency and additional enrichment with fluoride has been tried in Switzerland with encouraging results. However, the problem of dosage in different regions still needs to be solved and the clinical effectiveness of the procedure established. Another method that has been adopted in low-fluoride areas by some people, including dentists, for their own children, is the daily administration of fluoride tablets. When these are given regularly from an early age, the results are said to be as good as those obtained by water fluoridation.

Once teeth have erupted the effectiveness of systemically derived fluoride is questionable and it is then necessary to ensure that the fluoride comes in contact with the external surface of the tooth. Various methods of topical application have been tried but they provide relatively poor caries protection and require a large expenditure in terms of organization and time. Fluoride-containing toothpastes are now widely available and if used regularly have an appreciable effect (Chapter 36).

While water fluoridation may be the most effective public health measure for inhibiting dental decay it would, at the same time, seem obvious that much more should be done to discourage the consumption of refined sugar which is so largely responsible for the high incidence of the disease in Western societies (page 133).

Selenium

It has long been known that Se deficiency results in a form of muscular dystrophy in lambs and calves and it has been shown that a complex relationship exists between the metabolism of Se, vitamin E and the polyunsaturated fatty acids. Until recently, however, no evidence had been obtained of Se deficiency in humans. Now a disease known as *Keshan disease*, which is responsive to Se, has been found in certain areas of China. It takes the form of a patchy necrosis of the heart muscle and is regarded as a geochemical disease resulting from a deficiency of Se in the soil and hence in the staple diet.

Vanadium

Vanadium is a ubiquitous element which is an excellent catalyst *in vitro* and readily forms chelates. Its concentration in the body is homoeostatically controlled. Evidence has been obtained that vanadate may control the response of the Na^+ pump to K^+ and that vanadium deficiency may explain the retention of salt and water in nutritional oedema. The concentration of vanadium in children with kwashiorkor (page 128) is low compared with normal controls.

Chapter 12
The vitamins

Evidence for the existence of 'accessory food factors', later to be known as 'vitamins', was obtained from the study of deficiency diseases such as scurvy, beriberi, pellagra and rickets, which were suspected to be of dietary origin, and also from experiments in which highly purified diets were fed to rats and mice. From these two independent lines of investigation the idea emerged that natural foodstuffs contain small quantities of substances, other than proteins, carbohydrates, fats and minerals, that are essential for normal growth and health. The nature of these substances was unknown, but that there was more than one was soon recognized because both fat-soluble and water-soluble factors were required. Initially the vitamins were designated by letters of the alphabet but as their structure and functions were determined most of them were given specific names. However, since in various instances several closely related compounds have similar biological effects, it is convenient to use a generic term for a group of substances, e.g. vitamin D to include both cholecalciferol and ergocalciferol (page 156).

A vitamin is an organic substance present in natural foodstuffs which the body requires in very small amounts but is not able to make for itself in sufficient quantity. This rather clumsy definition is necessary to cover what is now known about this very varied collection of nutrients.

From the dietary point of view the vitamins may be divided into 'major' and 'minor' vitamins. Lack of any of the so-called major vitamins, which include vitamins A, D and C and three or four members of the vitamin B complex, leads to a recognizable deficiency disease. The requirement for the remaining vitamins is much less; they are very widely distributed and many of them are synthesized by microorganisms that inhabit the gut so that deficiency rarely occurs.

Other important points are that a vitamin may be an essential dietary constituent for one animal species but unnecessary for another, and that in certain instances the body may have a limited ability to synthesize a particular vitamin but be unable to meet its requirements in all circumstances. Furthermore, even though the diet may contain what is normally regarded as an adequate supply of a vitamin for one reason or another the body may not be able to use it.

The fat-soluble vitamins

The fat-soluble vitamins include vitamins A, D, E and K and their distribution is as varied as their functions. Their absorption is closely tied to that of fat and, if for any reason the intake or absorption of fat is inadequate, a secondary deficiency may occur. Furthermore, they tend to be stored in body fats, notably in the liver and an excessive intake of vitamin A or D produces toxic effects.

Vitamin A – retinol

Vitamin A is a colourless substance that is present in animal fats, e.g. liver, milk, butter and eggs, although the richest sources are fish liver oils. Margarines are fortified to bring their content up to that of butter. Because of its specific effects in the visual process and the fact that it is an alcohol, the alternative name for vitamin A is *retinol*.

all-*trans*-Retinol
(Vitamin A)

Plants do not contain vitamin A as such, although many of them include a variety of highly pigmented *carotenoids*. Some of these, namely the α-, β- and γ-carotenes, can be converted into vitamin A in the body and hence are *provitamins*. *β-carotene* is the most active of these. It is a symmetrical compound and can be converted into two molecules of vitamin A in the intestinal wall and in the liver, but since β-carotene is poorly absorbed and only partially converted, its utilization efficiency is only about one-sixth. Unchanged carotene is found in the plasma and in the body fat. Vitamin A and carotene are both fairly stable and not much affected by cooking, although some activity may be lost if fats become rancid. The recommended daily intake for adults is 750 μg (5000 International Units) of retinol, 6 × 750 μg of β-carotene or 12 × 750 μg of α- and γ-carotene.

β-Carotene

Vitamin A deficiency

Apart from its specific function in the visual process (page 155), vitamin A is needed for growth, reproduction and the maintenance of the integrity of epithelial cells. Since retinol is stored in the liver, signs of its deficiency develop very slowly. In Man the earliest noticeable effect is *night-blindness*, i.e. the inability to see in dim light, and this is readily cured by administration of the vitamin. Later, *xerophthalmia* develops, the eyes become dry and susceptible to infection and the conjunctiva and cornea become keratinized. This is followed by *keratomalacia* or softening of the cornea which leads to permanent blindness. Even today vitamin A deficiency is the commonest cause of blindness in Africa, India and the Far East in spite of the fact that carotene can be obtained from green leaves, maize and other vegetables. Carotene is poorly absorbed even in normal subjects and, where nutrition is inadequate, not only may the diet be deficient in fat but the gastrointestinal tract may be abnormal so that the fat-soluble vitamins are very poorly absorbed.

Experimental animals which are deficient in vitamin A fail to breed. Spermatogenesis is affected and female rats, if they conceive, resorb the fetuses or produce malformed offspring. In both animals and Man there are widespread generalized changes in the epithelial tissues which, whatever their normal type, become increasingly stratified, squamous and keratinized. Glandular epithelium is affected before the acinal cells so that the ducts become blocked by desquamating cells, and secretion, e.g. of the lachrymal and sweat glands, is impaired. This results in dryness of the eyes and *hyperkeratosis* of the skin. Nevertheless the basal cells appear not to be affected since, when the vitamin is administered, the epithelium promptly reverts to the normal type. The epithelial changes which result from deficiency reduce the local resistance to infection, and death often results from secondary infections. The general defence mechanisms of the body appear to be impaired.

Metabolism

Retinol is nearly always present in the food in the form of esters which are hydrolysed in the lumen of the intestine. The retinol released is quite readily absorbed into the mucosal cells where it is re-esterified, chiefly with palmitic acid. The retinyl esters are then transported via the lymphatic system into the portal circulation from which they are removed and stored in the liver. Release of the vitamin from the liver depends on the production by the liver of a special *retinol-binding protein* (RBP). Production of the retinol-binding protein may be disturbed in diseases of the liver or kidneys or in protein/energy malnutrition. In such circumstances retinol cannot be mobilized from the stores and a secondary deficiency may result. Thus it can be seen that the level of retinol in the general circulation is normally highly regulated and is more or less independent of the body's reserves.

In the liver a small proportion of the retinol is oxidized to *retinoic acid* for which the liver has no storage capacity so that it is released into the bloodstream, where it is carried directly by serum albumin with which the retinol–RBP complex also combines. Some retinoic acid may be taken up by the tissues but it is constantly eliminated through the bile as glucuronide so that no accumulation occurs.

The biochemical significance of retinoic acid is under debate. Rats deficient in vitamin A, when given retinoic acid as the sole source of vitamin A activity, grew normally and showed no epithelial irregularities but were both blind and sterile, whereas, if given the corresponding aldehyde, *retinal*, they were normal in all respects. Retinoic acid cannot, however, be dismissed as a mere by-product because there are intracellular binding proteins for both retinol and retinoic acid. The existence of the latter suggests that retinoic acid may have a specific role in metabolism.

Cellular effects

From the effects of its deficiency it appears that vitamin A is required for the controlled division and differentiation of cells. Retinol is delivered to specific sites on the cell surface that recognize the RBP and cause it to release the retinol. Once inside the cell the retinol combines with the *cellular retinol-binding protein* and retinoic acid with *cellular retinoic acid-binding protein* and each is delivered to nuclear binding sites which may be important in gene expression. Thus their mode of action resembles that of the steroid hormones (page 349).

Apart from effects on the nucleus, retinol has been found to have a stabilizing effect on cell membranes. More specifically retinol seems to take part in glycosyl-transfer reactions and the synthesis of various glycoconjugates (page 407). Effects on cell surface components may mediate changes in intracellular recognition and interactions and also in the process of cell adhesion and aggregation.

Vitamin A and vision

Normally after exposure to a bright light it takes several minutes before a person is able to perceive dimly lit objects. Vision then slowly improves over the next 30 min or so. This process of *dark adaptation* is associated with the regeneration in the rod cells of the retina of a pigment known as *visual purple* or *rhodopsin* which is bleached by strong light. Rhodopsin consists of a protein *opsin* combined with a stereoisomer of retinal, the aldehyde of vitamin A, Δ^{11}-*cis*-retinal. During the visual process, i.e. the conversion of the energy of the light falling on the

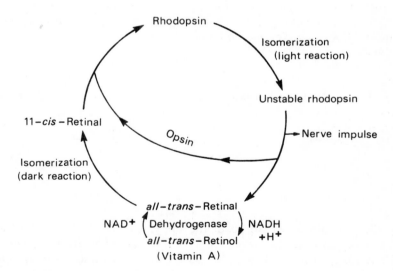

11-*cis*-Retinal   all-*trans*-Retinal

retina to nerve impulses, the *cis*-retinal undergoes a molecular rearrangement to form all-*trans*-retinal which is more stable. This change in configuration causes the rhodopsin to dissociate into its constituents, opsin and all-*trans*-retinal. Rhodopsin can then only be regenerated after the retinal has been rearranged to the 11-*cis* form and this can only occur in dim light. Reutilization of the retinal is never complete since an appreciable fraction of the all-*trans*-retinal is reduced to retinol by alcohol dehydro-genase and NADH and some may be lost into the blood. The visual cycle is shown in Figure 12·1.

Rhodopsin

Isomerization
(light reaction)

Unstable rhodopsin

Nerve impulse

Opsin

11–*cis* – Retinal

Isomerization
(dark reaction)

all–*trans*– Retinal

NAD⁺ (Dehydrogenase) NADH
all–*trans*–Retinol +H⁺
(Vitamin A)

Figure 12.1 The visual cycle

It is not clear why scotopic vision is so much more readily affected by vitamin A deficiency than photopic vision since retinal is a constituent of the three cone pigments as well as of rhodopsin. Normal vision requires the presence of 11-*cis*-retinal and the synthesis of four different opsins.

Hypervitaminosis A

If the rate of uptake of retinol from the intestine consistently exceeds the capacity of the liver to dispose of it, significant amounts of retinol, mainly in the form of retinyl palmitate, appear in the general circulation and may give rise to toxic effects. The effects of hypervitaminosis A are many and varied. They include increased intracranial pressure, severe headache, hyperirritability, vomiting, diarrhoea, bone decalcification and skin lesions. The condition can be fatal. It has in the past been caused by over-zealous administration of concentrated sources of the vitamin such as halibut liver oil. This may contain several hundred times as much vitamin A and 40 times as much vitamin D as cod liver oil. It has also occurred in people who have eaten polar bear or husky dog liver which contain massive amounts of vitamin A.

Vitamin D – the calciferols

Recent work has undermined the status of vitamin D as a true vitamin (which was always dubious) but certainly not its biochemical significance. That it is not an essential nutrient for people whose skin is sufficiently exposed to sunlight has been known for many years, but it has now been shown that vitamin D can claim to be a hormone precursor.

The deficiency disease that results from a lack of vitamin D is *rickets*, a condition that used to be common in the smoky cities of the Northern hemisphere and for which even in the nineteenth century cod liver oil and sunshine were recognized treatments.

Like the other fat-soluble vitamins, vitamin D is found in more than one form and of these the two most important are *cholecalciferol* (vitamin D_3) and *ergocalciferol* (vitamin D_2). They occur largely as inactive provitamins which are converted into the active forms on exposure to ultraviolet light. The provitamins are both sterols and the effect of irradiation is to open the B ring; this means that the vitamins themselves are not sterols. Provitamin D_3 or 7-dehydro-cholesterol is present in the unsaponifiable fraction of animal fats. It is always present in the skin and is converted to vitamin D_3 on exposure to sunlight.

7-Dehydrocholesterol   Vitamin D_3

Vitamin D, like vitamin A, is stored in the body, chiefly in the liver. It is not readily metabolized or excreted and excessive amounts have a toxic effect. *Hypervitaminosis D* produces a variety of symptoms including increased resorption of the bones. In children there is a loss of appetite, nausea, vomiting, diarrhoea and eventually stupor; fatal cases have shown calcification of the arteries, renal tubules, heart and lungs. Since the consequences of an overdose are so damaging it is important that the body should not produce too much vitamin D and the need for protection against overproduction may have been a major factor in determining the selection and distribution of races of different skin colour. Penetration of the solar rays to the site of provitamin activation is determined by the pigmentation and degree of keratinization of the stratum corneum.

Alternatively vitamin D may be obtained from the diet. The only rich sources are the liver oils of fish; few other foods contain significant amounts. In recognition of the risk of deficiency in Britain, where sunshine cannot be relied upon, margarine, dried milk and infant foods are fortified by the addition of vitamin D, while in the USA foods such as milk and yeast are irradiated in order to increase their content. A dietary intake of 10 μg cholecalciferol per day is sufficient to protect a child against rickets without fear of causing hypervitaminosis, while the adult requirement is 2·5 μg.

The metabolism of vitamin D is discussed in Chapter 30.

Vitamin D deficiency

This is responsible for the clinical condition of rickets which in infants and children is characterized by abnormal endochondral calcification. The degenerating hypertrophic cellular zone in the epiphyseal cartilaginous plate fails to calcify. The epiphyseal plate increases in width and deforming cartilaginous swellings form at the ends of the long bones and at the junctions of the ribs with the sternum, giving them a knobbly appearance. The bones are soft because they are hypocalcified and consequently the legs are unable to support the weight of the body and become bowed. In rickets there is usually a fall in the levels of both calcium and inorganic phosphate in the serum, although the most consistent feature is an increase in the serum alkaline phosphatase.

Rickets does not often occur in adults although an adult counterpart, *osteomalacia*, now mercifully rare, may occur in women living mostly indoors and consuming a diet containing inadequate amounts of calcium and vitamin D, and subjected to frequent childbearing. Demineralization of the bones, resulting from these circumstances, may cause gross deformities.

Dental changes in vitamin D deficiency

During tooth development in vitamin D-deficient animals, the enamel and dentine become hypoplastic and, since the ameloblasts are unable to function properly, the enamel calcifies poorly. The dentine matrix may also remain uncalcified with the result that interglobular spaces are formed.

No clear-cut relationship has been established between vitamin D intake and the incidence of dental caries. If ameloblast formation is interrupted and the enamel matrix is defective it will become inadequately mineralized and the enamel will be pitted. While the enamel itself does not appear to be more susceptible to caries than usual, the rough surface may favour plaque formation.

Vitamin E – the tocopherols

Vitamin E was discovered in 1922 by Evans and Bishop who found that a fat-soluble factor present in vegetable oils prevented the abnormalities in reproduction that occurred in rats fed on a diet containing rancid lard. This led to the discovery of a group of alcohols known as *tocopherols* which differ from each other in the number and position of methyl groups attached to the tocol ring. The most active of these is α-tocopherol whose structure is shown. Tocopherols are present in almost every food, and particularly in vegetable fats and the germ of cereal grains, so that a dietary deficiency of vitamin E is rare in normal subjects. Deficiency may, however, result from conditions in which there is prolonged malabsorption of fat. These include the rare inherited condition of *abetalipoproteinaemia* in which chylomicron formation is prevented by

α-Tocopherol
(Vitamin E)

the absence of apoprotein B. Under such circumstances the serum tocopherol level falls and the fragility of the red blood corpuscle membrane is increased. Vitamin E deficiency also occurs in premature and low-birth-weight babies in which it may be responsible for haemolytic normocytic anaemia, blindness and intraventricular haemorrhage.

Vitamin E deficiency can be induced in animals but the symptoms vary very widely according to the species: they include interference with reproduction (rats); muscular dystrophy (sheep and cattle); hepatic necrosis (rats and pigs); and loss of brain substance (chicks). Clearly therefore, vitamin E has some important physiological functions which seem to be related to its antioxidant properties. This is supported by the finding that certain other antioxidants and also selenium are able to replace dietary vitamin E. Furthermore, if the intake of polyunsaturated fatty acids is increased, so is the requirement for vitamin E. This can be explained on the basis that vitamin E protects the body against lipid peroxidation to which polyunsaturated fats, and hence phospholipids, are particularly susceptible. It is uncertain whether the tocopherols have any other function or whether they have any clinical value other than in the conditions mentioned earlier. It has been suggested that the structure of their side chain allows the tocopherols to interact specifically with the polyunsaturated fatty acids of membrane phospholipids and to act as membrane stabilizers. Their principal function, however, seems to be that of scavenging singlet oxygen and protecting the tissues against the damaging effects of *free radicals* (molecules which possess an unpaired electron).

Free radical production

Although the oxygen molecule is normally completely reduced to water by the addition of four electrons in the terminal reactions of the electron-transport chain, reduced components of the mitochondrial and microsomal electron-transport systems lose a small proportion of single electrons in side reactions with oxygen forming significant amounts of the *superoxide anion* ($O_2^{-\cdot}$) and hydrogen peroxide. These may initiate a chain of reactions in which a variety of free radicals are produced that may damage the cells.

The superoxide radical is formed by the reduction of molecular oxygen with one electron.

$$O_2 + e \rightarrow O_2^{-\cdot}$$

Two superoxide anions may then interact in a reaction catalysed by the enzyme *superoxide dismutase*, which is present in nearly all aerobic cells, to form molecular oxygen and hydrogen peroxide.

$$O_2^{-\cdot} + O_2^{-\cdot} \xrightarrow{2H^+} O_2 + H_2O_2$$

This dismutation of oxygen occurs at an appreciable rate even in the absence of the enzyme.

The H_2O_2 produced can subsequently react with a further superoxide radical to produce the highly reactive hydroxyl radical ($OH^\cdot$) in a reaction which is catalysed by iron or copper ions.

$$O_2^{-\cdot} + H_2O_2 \xrightarrow{Fe^{2-}} O_2 + OH^- + OH^\cdot$$

This hydroxyl radical can react with almost every organic molecule and cause damage not only to cell lipids but also to proteins and even nucleic acids. The particular susceptibility of phospholipids to peroxide attack results in damage to the cell membranes. The products of free radical attack are usually free radicals themselves so that a chain reaction may be set up. Oxidative damage of this kind may be a factor in carcinogenesis as well as in the ageing process and certain inflammatory diseases such as gout and rheumatoid arthritis. Such oxidative stress may be exacerbated by physical exercise and over-exposure to sunlight.

Protection against free radical damage

The body possesses at least two means by which damage by free radicals may be limited.

1. Certain compounds are able to react with free radicals to form a stable compound which is harmless. Vitamin E is especially effective in this respect and its antioxidant activity is promoted by vitamin C, β-carotene and certain other lipid-soluble antioxidants. On the other hand, iron and copper salts have a deleterious effect. The ability of β-carotene to scavenge free radical intermediates is not related to its role as provitamin A but depends on the large number of double bonds in the molecule.

2. Certain defensive enzymes are able to destroy the peroxides which appear to be so damaging to the tissues. These are:

(a) *Catalase.* This is one of the most active enzymes known. It is present in all cells and is responsible for the destruction of H_2O_2

$$2H_2O_2 \xrightarrow{\text{Catalase}} 2H_2O + O_2$$

(b) *Glutathione peroxidase.* This too is present in all animal cells in high concentration. It is a metalloenzyme which contains selenium as an integral part of its active site. Not only can glutathione peroxidase destroy H_2O_2 but it is also able to destroy any other toxic peroxides which may have been formed. In the course of the reaction reduced glutathione (GSH) (page 287) is oxidized (GSSG).

$$H_2O_2 + 2GSH \xrightarrow{\text{Glutathione peroxidase}} 2H_2O + GSSG$$

Superoxide production and neutrophil activation

The production of superoxides is not always disadvantageous to the body. Infecting microbes stimulate the phagocytic activity of the neutrophils, eosinophils and macrophages. The neutrophils become activated so that they adhere more readily to endothelial surfaces while the specialized electron-transport system present in the leucocyte membrane produces a *respiratory burst* during which oxygen is taken up very rapidly to produce a mixture of highly toxic oxygen radicals. This activated oxygen is necessary for efficient killing of the engulfed microbes. In the rare genetic disorder, *chronic granulomatous disease*, the phagocytic leucocytes are unable to produce these oxygen radicals and consequently the patients suffer from chronic infections. Interestingly, it has been reported that the administration of large doses of vitamin E, which can terminate free radical reactions, impairs the bactericidal capacity of the neutrophils.

Vitamin E requirements

Because it seems to be part of a complex system the requirement for vitamin E is difficult to ascertain. For example, work has shown that it can be replaced by selenium in the prevention of liver necrosis in rats while, for farm animals, the requirement is increased when the diet contains large amounts of polyunsaturated fatty acids. The animal's mineral status also seems to be important, depending on the presence of adequate amounts of Zn, Cu and Mn in addition to Se. Inter-relationships of vitamin E metabolism with that of vitamin C and iron salts may also be relevant. However, in normal circumstances vitamin E does not present a dietary problem.

Vitamin K

In 1934 the Danish scientist Dam discovered that a nutritional disease of chicks, which was characterized by severe bleeding, could be cured by a variety of foodstuffs, including alfalfa (lucerne grass) and putrefying fishmeal. The active principle was isolated and given the name Koagulations Vitamin or vitamin K.

Vitamin K occurs in various forms. *Vitamin K$_1$* (phylloquinone) is synthesized by plants while vitamins of the K$_2$ group (the menaquinones) are synthesized by bacteria. The substituted naphthoquinone ring cannot be synthesized by animals, but synthetic compounds such as

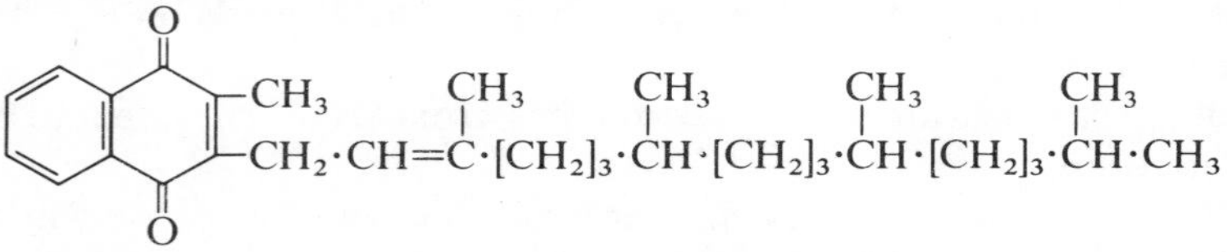

Vitamin K$_1$; (phylloquinone; 2-methyl-3-phytyl-1,4-naphthoquinone)

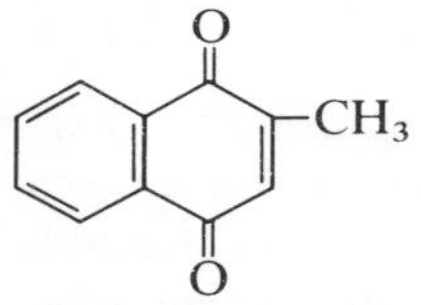

Menadione (2-methyl-1,4-
naphthoquinone

menadione, which has no side chain, are biologically active. The natural forms are fat-soluble but some of the synthetic analogues are water-soluble, which is therapeutically advantageous, since deficiency is most likely to occur when fat absorption is defective.

Vitamin K is not stored in the body. It is required in the synthesis of several of the blood-clotting factors and its deficiency is characterized by *hypoprothrombinaemia* and a tendency to haemorrhage. It acts as a cofactor in the post-translational modification (page 316) of the precursor forms of Factors II (prothrombin), VII, IX and X. This modification involves a carboxylation reaction which converts particular glutamate residues into *γ-carboxyglutamate* (Gla) and thereby activates the precursor proteins. The presence of two adjacent –COOH groups on these Gla residues confers characteristic calcium- and phospholipid-binding properties on the proteins which relate to their role in the clotting process (page 391).

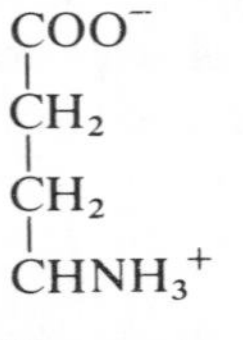

Glutamate
(Glu)

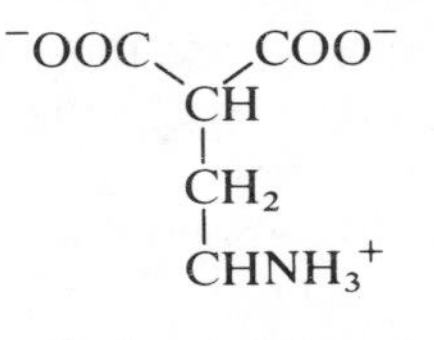

γ-Carboxyglutamate
(Gla)

Proteins containing Gla have also been found in other tissues known to transport and concentrate Ca^{2+} ions, e.g. bone and dentine. *Osteocalcin*, the Gla-containing protein of bone matrix, constitutes 1–2% of the total protein (10–20% of non-collagenous protein), but its function has not been established. Similar proteins are present in kidney cortex, lung, spleen, liver and placenta. Their presence in tissues of such widely diverse properties and functions suggests that they may have a broader role than mere calcium binding.

The body derives the vitamin K it requires from food or following synthesis by bacteria in the gut. Consequently normal human beings are largely independent of a dietary supply and deficiency rarely occurs. It may occur, however, in newborn infants or when growth of the gut microorganisms is prevented, e.g. during treatment with antibiotics or bacteriostatic drugs such as *neomycin*, which are not significantly absorbed and are given specifically to suppress the intestinal flora. It may also occur when fat absorption is defective as in obstructive jaundice, coeliac disease and ulcerative colitis. It is very important, therefore, in patients whose digestion is impaired or who are undergoing treatment with antibiotics, to test the clotting ability of their blood before undertaking any form of surgery, including tooth extractions.

Antivitamins K

The chance finding of a haemorrhagic disease in cattle feeding on spoiled sweet clover led to the discovery of *dicoumarol* (*bis*-hydroxycoumarin), which acts as an antivitamin K. This opened up a whole new field of treatment for conditions such as thrombosis, in which it is necessary to reduce the ability of the blood to clot. Dicoumarol and other drugs of the coumarin class, such as phenindione, are well absorbed after oral administration, but a synthetic analogue, *warfarin*, is the only form that is suitable for injection. After administration of anticoagulants of this type, lowering of the plasma prothrombin level only occurs slowly since time is needed for the disappearance of the prothrombin already synthesized. Conversely, if patients under treatment with these drugs show a tendency to haemorrhage, administration of vitamin K will only allow a gradual restoration of the prothrombin level. To obtain an immediate increase in coagulability prothrombin itself must be given.

The water-soluble vitamins

Water-soluble vitamins include the various members of the vitamin B complex and vitamin C. There are eight clearly recognized members of the vitamin B group (Table 12.1) and one or two other substances that are sometimes included. Although structurally unrelated there is some reason for classifying them together because they tend to occur together in natural foods. Deficiencies of single members of the group are therefore unlikely to occur and, if a person appears to be deficient in one member of the vitamin B complex, it is advisable that the intake of all should be increased. Except in cases of acute deficiency, a general improvement in the diet is much to be preferred to the administration of vitamin pills. Nearly all the members of the vitamin B complex have been found to act as, or be constituents of, coenzymes and the only water-soluble vitamins for which no clear-cut coenzyme activity has been established are vitamin B_{12} and vitamin C. Except for vitamin B_{12}, problems of absorption are not often encountered and, since water-soluble vitamins are readily excreted in the urine, hypervitaminoses do not occur. Deficiencies of several water-soluble vitamins have specific and diagnostically important effects on oral structures.

Table 12.1 The vitamin B complex

Vitamin	Alternative designation	Deficiency disease	Corresponding coenzyme	Function	Notes
Major components					
1. Thiamine	B_1	Beriberi	TPP	a. Oxidative decarboxylation b. Pentose phosphate pathway	
2. Riboflavin	B_2	Ariboflavinosis	FAD	Hydrogen carrier	
3. Nicotinamide	Niacin	Pellagra	NAD and NADP	Hydrogen carrier	Can be synthesized from tryptophan
Nutritionally less important members					
4. Pyridoxine	B_6		Pyridoxal phosphate	Amino group transfer and other aspects of amino acid metabolism	
5. Pantothenic acid			Coenzyme A	Acyl group transfer	
6. Folic acid		Macrocytic anaemia	THFA (tetrahydro-folic acid)	Metabolism of single carbon fragments	Required for the synthesis of purines and pyrimidines
7. Cobalamin	B_{12}	Pernicious anaemia		In various reactions	Deficiency usually results from inadequate absorption
8. Biotin	These factors are of little nutritional importance in Man but have a role in metabolism and have been found to be growth factors for certain microorganisms			CO_2 transfer	
9. *p*-Aminobenzoic acid				In bacterial metabolism	Metabolically antagonized by sulphonamide drugs
10. Lipoic acid				Oxidative decarboxylation	

Vitamin B₁ – thiamine

In 1897 Eijkman, a Dutch doctor in Java, noticed that domestic fowls fed on scraps from the food of prisoners which consisted mainly of polished rice developed symptoms of polyneuritis. This condition in which there is inflammation of the peripheral nerves was very similar to *beriberi*, a disease from which some of the prisoners suffered. When whole grain instead of polished rice was given the birds recovered. Eijkman then showed that a substance was present in very small amounts in the husk and germ of the rice that protected the birds. These and other findings led to the discovery of vitamin B₁:

Thiamine

Vitamin B₁ or thiamine is a white water-soluble crystalline solid which is destroyed by heat in neutral and alkaline conditions. Consequently losses during food preparation can be high since they result both from leaching of the vitamin into the cooking water and from heat destruction.

Thiamine was the first vitamin to have its precise biochemical functions determined. In the form of its pyrophosphate, thiamine participates in several very important enzyme systems namely: (1) pyruvate dehydrogenase (page 232) which converts pyruvate to acetyl-CoA and carbon dioxide in the course of carbohydrate breakdown; (2) the reaction of the citrate cycle in which oxoglutarate is oxidatively decarboxylated to succinyl-CoA (page 242); (3) the transketolase reaction of the pentose phosphate pathway of glucose breakdown (page 233).

These findings explain why deficiency is most readily induced in animals fed on diets rich in carbohydrate and also why the nervous system, which is almost entirely dependent on glucose for its supply of energy, is particularly affected. Interference with oxidative metabolism also explains the effects on the heart, which has a high energy requirement.

In beriberi, which is less common in the East now that its aetiology has been established, local accumulation of pyruvate and lactate may cause vasodilatation and oedema. The wet form of the disease is characterized by oedema and heart failure and the dry form by polyneuritis and paralysis but no oedema.

Since all animal and plant tissues contain thiamine, the vitamin is widely distributed in foods but usually in small amounts. The germs of cereals and pulses are good sources as are yeast, pork products and offal.

The requirement for thiamine is related to the amount of carbohydrate in the diet but is usually given as between 1·0 and 1·5 mg per day. In the UK, Government regulations specify that all flours must contain a minimum of 0·24 mg thiamine per 100 g. Enrichment procedures are also carried out in the USA.

Vitamin B₂ – riboflavin

Riboflavin is a yellow compound with a green fluorescence which is found in liver, milk, egg yolk, green vegetables and legumes. It is much more stable to heat than thiamine and is not destroyed by cooking.

The monophosphate derivative of riboflavin, flavin mononucleotide and flavin adenine dinucleotide (Chapter 16), are constituents of the flavoproteins of which thirty or more are now

Riboflavin
(Vitamin B$_2$)

known. They all appear to function in hydrogen transfer reactions and are involved in the metabolism of all types of energy-producing material.

Deficiency of riboflavin causes a variety of symptoms both in animals and in Man. These include *glossitis* or inflammation of the tongue, which becomes magenta red, *cheilosis (angular stomatitis)*, i.e. a fissuring at the corners of the mouth, *photophobia* and *corneal vascularization*, invasion of the cornea by capillaries. The symptoms of deficiency are surprisingly mild in view of the metabolic importance of the flavoproteins. Deficiency is associated with general poverty of the diet and has been seen in China, Ceylon and the Southern States of the USA. When the intake of animal products is low the riboflavin intake needs watching, but yeast and yeast extracts are good sources. The requirement is about 1·3 mg per day for women and 1·7 mg per day for men.

Nicotinic acid

The vitamin activity of nicotinic acid was discovered as a result of work on *pellagra*, a disease particularly prevalent in maize-eating populations and characterized by the '3 Ds'–dermatitis, diarrhoea and dementia. The 'pellagra-preventing' factor found to be present in yeast was identified as nicotinic acid.

Pellagrous dermatitis is particularly noticeable on parts of the body that are exposed to sunlight or are subject to mechanical irritation or contact with body secretions. Oral lesions are of diagnostic importance and the lesion of the gastrointestinal tract responsible for the diarrhoea in the mouth which is swollen and painful, the tongue being smooth, sore and bright red. Mental symptoms include irritability, headaches, sleeplessness and loss of memory advancing to confusion and delirium.

Nicotinic acid is readily converted to nicotinamide, the physiologically active form. The term *niacin* is sometimes used to include both compounds which are only distantly related to nicotine, the alkaloid in tobacco.

Nicotinic acid   Nicotinamide

Nicotinamide is a constituent of nicotinamide adenine dinucleotide (NAD) and nicotinamide adenine dinucleotide phosphate (NADP) (page 214) which act as hydrogen carriers in many important oxidation–reduction reactions. As such it is widely distributed in both plants and animals.

Pellagra is now recognized as a multifactorial disease and the vitamin status of nicotinic acid is questionable. The body is able to synthesize nicotinic acid from tryptophan so that nicotinic acid only becomes a dietary essential when the tryptophan content of the diet is low. The fact that maize proteins are relatively poor in tryptophan, and that the nicotinic acid it contains is in a form which is not readily available, would seem to explain the association of pellagra and the use of maize as a staple foodstuff. For nutritional purposes 60 mg tryptophan are believed to be equivalent to 1 mg of nicotinic acid and the recommended intake for an adult male is given as 18 mg of nicotinic acid or its equivalent. Primary nicotinic acid deficiency is unlikely to occur in this country where appreciable amounts of animal products are consumed and where flour must, by law, contain 1·6 mg nicotinamide per 100 g.

Vitamin B$_6$ – pyridoxine

Vitamin B$_6$ occurs in the three forms shown below. In the form of pyridoxal phosphate the vitamin acts as a coenzyme for more than sixty enzymes concerned with amino acid metabolism, e.g. aminotransferases, decarboxylases, deaminases and desulphurases. It also plays a role in the absorption of amino acids and is a constituent of glycogen phosphorylase.

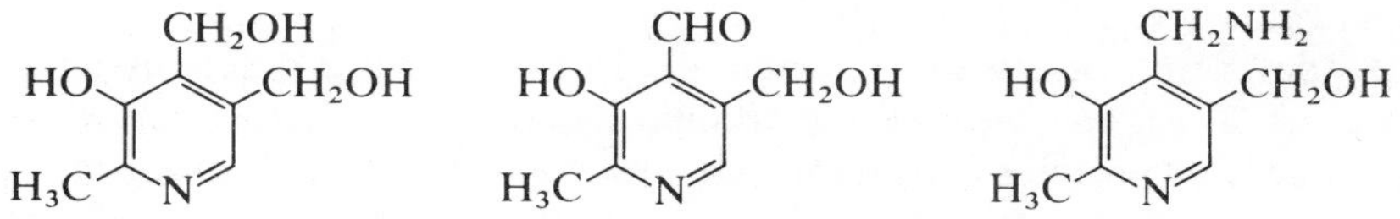

Pyridoxine   Pyridoxal   Pyridoxamine

In animals deficiency of vitamin B$_6$ has effects on the nervous system, the convulsions of acute deficiency probably resulting from a shortage of γ-aminobutyrate (GABA) which acts as an inhibitor of nervous transmission. Deficiency also causes a special form of dermatitis and a microcytic anaemia. In monkeys deficiency was found to cause atherosclerosis and dental caries. Since vitamin B$_6$ is more uniformly distributed than most other members of the vitamin B complex, nutritional deficiency in humans is rare, but some forms of iron-resistant hypochromic anaemia respond to vitamin B$_6$ therapy.

The lesser members of the vitamin B complex

Dietary deficiency of these compounds rarely occurs but they have important metabolic roles and some, e.g. folic acid and cobalamin, are of clinical importance. *Pantothenic acid* derives its name from its universal distribution. It is an essential constituent of coenzyme A, which plays a key role in the metabolism of compounds containing two carbon atoms. Three other members of the vitamin B complex, namely *biotin*, *folic acid* and *cobalamin* (vitamin B$_{12}$), together with the essential amino acid methionine are concerned in the metabolism of units containing single C atoms. The nature of the substance used to carry these units depends on the degree of oxidation or reduction of the C atom. In the reduced form, i.e. CH$_3$– groups, single carbon atoms are carried by 'active methionine' or *S-adenosylmethionine* while hydroxymethyl (–CH$_2$OH), formyl (–CHO) and formate (–COOH) groups are carried by a reduced form of folic acid known as *tetrahydrofolic acid* (THFA). Such compounds are important in the synthesis of purines and hence of nucleotides and nucleic acids (page 112).

Folic acid deficiency, when it occurs, results more commonly from a failure of utilization than from an inadequate dietary intake. It is manifested by macrocytic anaemia and leucopenia. As the name suggests, green leaves are good sources; so is yeast.

The most highly oxidized form of a single C atom is carbon dioxide and in certain reactions involving its assimilation, for example the formation of malonyl-CoA (page 255) and oxaloacetate (page 248), *biotin* acts as a carrier. Biotin deficiency has been found to occur in people who eat raw eggs in quantity. It results from the presence in egg white of *avidin*, a small protein that binds biotin. This property is lost on heating.

Vitamin B_{12} also seems to function in the metabolism of single carbon units, probably in a coenzyme capacity. It may play a part in the conversion of ribonucleotides to the deoxyribonucleotides required for the synthesis of DNA. Vitamin B_{12} acts synergistically with folic acid in haemopoiesis and its deficiency causes *pernicious anaemia*, a macrocytic type of anaemia accompanied by characteristic lesions of the nervous system. Folic acid is able to cure the anaemia but only vitamin B_{12}, which comprises a group of related compounds known as *cobalamins*, is able to correct both disorders. The cobalamins are red crystalline compounds that contain a tetrapyrrole ring which bears a superficial resemblance to a porphyrin and which surrounds a cobalt atom. The cobalamins are only synthesized by microorganisms. Plants other than legumes, which contain symbiotic bacteria, do not contain them. Since vitamin B_{12} is present only in foods of animal origin, strict vegetarians may develop a deficiency. This is of insidious onset and may take decades to appear since there is an enterohepatic circulation of vitamin B_{12} and almost total conservation.

Vitamin B_{12} deficiency results more commonly from a stomach defect than from a dietary deficiency. Before it can be absorbed the vitamin B_{12} (extrinsic factor) that is released from associated peptides and proteins in the stomach must combine with the '*intrinsic factor*', a small glycoprotein secreted by the parietal cells. Subjects who suffer from pernicious anaemia fail to produce intrinsic factor with the result that the vitamin is not absorbed and must be given by injection. Vitamin B_{12} produced by microbes in the lower reaches of the intestine is of no use to the body.

Vitamin C – ascorbic acid

In the sixteenth century, in Newfoundland, the French explorer Jacques Cartier, on the advice of the native Indians, cured scurvy, the disease that bedevilled early voyages of discovery, by giving his crew an extract of the needles of an evergreen tree. Much of the credit for finding a cure for the disease, however, goes to James Lind, a Scottish naval surgeon who in 1753, in a controlled study carried out at sea, demonstrated that lemons and oranges were an effective treatment. Thereafter scurvy was eliminated from the British Navy and, on account of their daily ration of lemon juice, British sailors became known as 'limeys'. Even so in 1912 Captain Scott omitted to include any source of vitamin C in the rations that his expedition took to the South Pole and perished as a result.

Ascorbic acid was identified in 1932 as the antiscorbutic vitamin. Chemically L-ascorbic acid is related to the hexose sugars from which it can be synthesized by most animal species. The chief exceptions are primates and guinea-pigs. L-Ascorbic acid is very soluble in water and, although when dry it is stable in light and air, it is readily oxidized in solution, particularly in the presence of metals such as copper. On oxidation it is converted first to dehydroascorbic acid but although the ascorbic acid–dehydroascorbic acid conversion is reversible, subsequent stages of oxidation are irreversible and the oxidation products have no vitamin activity.

$$O=C$$
$$HOC$$
$$HOC \quad O$$
$$HC$$
$$HOCH$$
$$CH_2OH$$

L-Ascorbic
acid

$$\rightleftharpoons$$

$$O=C$$
$$O=C$$
$$O=C \quad O$$
$$HC$$
$$HOCH$$
$$CH_2OH$$

L-Dehydroascorbic
acid

Vitamin C deficiency

Vitamin C deficiency causes widespread connective tissue abnormalities and the matrix of bone, cartilage, dentine, fibrous tissue and intercellular cement are affected. Symptoms usually appear within 1–2 months. They include swelling of the gums which become soft, spongy and bluish-red in colour, particularly in the region of the papillae between the teeth. The gums tend to bleed spontaneously and often become secondarily infected. Finally, as a result of lack of periodontal support, the teeth become loose and may fall out. In guinea-pigs the odontoblasts of the developing incisors atrophy with the result that irregular dentine, or no dentine at all, is produced.

Apart from effects on the oral tissues, the joints become swollen and painful and, since lack of intercellular cement makes the walls of the capillaries fragile, tiny haemorrhages (*petechiae*) appear under the skin. The bones too become fragile and wounds fail to heal properly. Since the scar tissue consists mainly of amorphous material with few collagen fibres, it lacks tensile strength and readily breaks down. A secondary anaemia may also develop.

Scurvy, which results from the prolonged consumption of a diet devoid of fresh fruit and vegetables, is no longer widespread but may occur at the two extremes of age, in old people living alone on a restricted diet and in infants whose mothers are ignorant or uncaring. Two facts that make it relatively easy for a deficiency to occur are (1) that fresh fruits and vegetables are often expensive and scarce and (2) that extensive losses of the vitamin occur during the storage and preparation of food. It is reasonable to assume that only 50% of that originally present is available.

Function in the body

Ascorbic acid plays a part in many body processes. It is the strongest reducing agent found in living tissues and protects the body against many damaging oxidative effects. It is required for a number of hydroxylation reactions in the body and is involved in the synthesis of collagen, glycosaminoglycans, bile acids, various steroid hormones and neurotransmitters (adrenaline, noradrenaline and serotonin). It also inactivates histamine, facilitates the absorption of iron (page 144) and other heavy metals, enhances the immunological defence system and also the liver microsomal system which is involved in the detoxication of drugs and environmental chemicals. It is not surprising therefore that many claims have been made for its beneficial effects. What is surprising is that primates have lost one of the genes required for its synthesis and have become dependent on external sources of supply.

Requirements

It is always difficult to formulate a recommended intake for a nutrient, and for ascorbic acid for adult humans these have ranged from 30 mg to 4 g per day. The latter recommendation was made by the distinguished chemist Linus Pauling on the basis of the amount consumed by primates living in the wild. The amount currently recommended by WHO is 30 mg per day, whereas in the USA it is 45 mg. However, a number of nutritionists believe that an intake of 100–150 mg is desirable. There is no reliable evidence to suggest that a daily intake of several grams is necessary and there is evidence that, in some people, a high intake maintained over long periods may be deleterious and lead to gastrointestinal disturbances and kidney stones. At the same time it has been shown that in conditions of biochemical stress there is a marked fall in the level of ascorbic acid in the plasma and in the leucocytes in which it is concentrated. It has also been found that animals able to synthesize ascorbic acid increased their output by as much as 10 times when exposed to certain drugs. For this reason, the taking of extra amounts after injuries, before and after operations and during infections may well be beneficial although under normal circumstances enough of the vitamin should be available from a good varied diet containing plenty of fruit and vegetables.

Vitamin C and the common cold

Citrus fruits as well as ascorbic acid itself have long been claimed to be valuable for colds but the amounts required and the degree of their effectiveness have been a matter of dispute. There seems to be little evidence that a high ascorbic acid intake reduces the incidence of colds but an intake of 4–5 g per day for the duration of the cold often seems to reduce the severity and duration of the symptoms. It has been shown *in vitro* that ascorbic acid causes depolymerization of glycosaminoglycans. Such a mucolytic effect, which would only occur if greater than physiological concentrations are achieved, might be responsible for a reduction in the unpleasant catarrhal symptoms. On the other hand, high concentrations of the vitamin might also promote its normal physiological functions such as maintenance of the integrity and functions of the mucous membranes, its non-specific antiviral and antibacterial effects and the inactivation of histamine.

Vitamins and cancer

Cancer is a multifactorial disease with a major genetic element and there is evidence that it may be promoted by such factors as oxidative stresses, ionizing radiations, certain dietary constituents, environmental pollutants and drugs. The transformation of normal into malignant cells appears to occur in at least two stages. In the early stage which is known as *initiation* there is a partial alteration of the normal cell which is irreversible and this may or may not be followed by the later stage which is known as *promotion*. Both stages are required in order to transform a normal cell into a fully neoplastic cell which then proliferates. Many substances including vitamins A, C and E may act as modifiers of carcinogenesis and studies on tumour cells in culture have shown that all three vitamins can exert antiproliferative effects. Retinoids, in particular, have been shown to influence the development of epithelial cancers, and epidemiological studies have provided evidence that human cancer risks are inversely correlated with the level of blood retinol and the dietary intake of carotene.

The correlation is of particular interest in view of the evidence that retinoids may bind to chromatin and modulate the expression of genes that control and direct the differentiation of epithelial tissue (page 154). The retinoids appear to inhibit the later rather than the earlier processes of carcinogenesis and their effect seems to be explicable in terms of an increase in the latent period before tumour growth becomes exponential, i.e. tumour growth is delayed rather than prevented altogether.

Apart from the role of vitamin A in controlling cellular differentiation, it is possible that the vitamins exert their protective effect by some other unrelated means. It is known, for example, that both carotene and tocopherol may inhibit the formation of toxic products by quenching singlet oxygen (page 159) and if this is so β-carotene may have an effect which is independent of the effect of the retinol which may be derived from it. A further suggestion is that the vitamins may enhance the body's immunological competence. Furthermore vitamins C and E are known to inhibit the formation of nitrosamines which may be derived from the nitrites and nitrates added to meat products as preservatives. Nitrosamines have been found to be carcinogenic to animals, but not, so far, to humans. Combinations of vitamins are more effective anticancer agents than any one singly.

As a result of these findings considerable effort is being put into the question of whether vitamins and notably vitamin A might be used therapeutically as anticancer agents, but various difficulties have been encountered. Firstly, the level of retinol in the blood is controlled by the amount of retinol-binding protein available and is largely independent of the dietary intake. On the other hand, the level of β-carotene in the blood is dependent on the dietary intake and as already mentioned β-carotene may have an independent anticancer effect. More work is needed in this field. Secondly, while pharmacological doses of vitamin A appear to enhance the control mechanisms that normally prevent cancer, the doses found to be effective in experimental animals are so high that they carry the risk of inducing hypervitaminosis. For these reasons a search is being made for retinol analogues which are therapeutically active but, at the same time, less toxic than retinol and retinoic acid. Results with some of these, e.g. 13-*cis*-retinoic acid, are encouraging and this compound has, in addition, been used successfully in the treatment of various skin diseases including psoriasis and acne.

As regards the use of vitamins in cancer prevention, as distinct from cancer treatment, there is no evidence that a vitamin intake above that required for normal nutrition provides extra protection. However, since vegetables contain β-carotene, tocopherols, ascorbic acid and also considerable amounts of fibre, all of which are credited with beneficial effects, a high vegetable diet would seem to have much to recommend it. A list of some of the dietary factors currently believed to have either cancer-preventing or cancer-promoting effects is given in Table 12.2.

Table 12.2 Dietary factors suggested as affecting carcinogenesis

Cancer promoting	*Cancer preventing*
High fat intake	Vitamin A
Alcoholism	Vitamin C
Smoked meat and fish	Vitamin E
Nitrates/nitrites	Carotenoids (as such)
Fungal toxins	Selenium
Low-fibre diet	High fibre intake
	High vegetable intake

Chapter 13
The composition and choice of foods

The range of materials that can be used as food is very great. More than 100 different animal species and 300 plant species are used regularly as human food. Even so the major part of the world's total food supply is furnished by a mere 20 plant species, namely:

Cereals: rice, wheat, maize, sorghum, rye, barley and buckwheat.
Legumes: peas, beans and lentils.
Root crops: potatoes, sweet potatoes, yams, cassava and sugar beet.
Miscellaneous: coconuts, groundnuts, bananas, plaintains and sugar cane.

The approximate composition of the more common foodstuffs and many of the foods prepared from them can be obtained from food tables such as those of McCance and Widdowson (Table 13.4). Such tables, though extremely useful, can serve merely as guidelines since they only give average values. Apart from this, the actual amount of nutrients obtained from food will depend on the efficiency of the consumer's digestive processes, how fresh the food was, how it was cooked and how much was wasted.

Animal foods

Dairy produce

This includes milk, cheese, eggs, cream and butter. The first three are chiefly sources of protein and the latter two sources of fat, but many of their other constituents are also of nutritional importance.

Milk

If any single article of diet can be considered as a near perfect food it is milk that provides for the nutrition of young mammals. Milk contains reasonable amounts of protein, carbohydrate and fat, as well as significant quantities of minerals and vitamins. As shown in Table 13.1, its composition per 100 ml varies appreciably in different mammalian species.

Three types of protein occur in milk, namely *caseinogen*, *lactalbumin* and *lactoglobulin*. Caseinogen, the chief protein, is a phosphoprotein and is responsible for the clotting that occurs

Table 13.1 The composition of human and cow's milk

	Energy		Protein (g)	Lactose (g)	Fat (g)	Calcium (mg)
	kJ	kcal				
Human	285	68	1·5	6·8	4·0	30
Cow	275	66	3·5	4·8	3·8	120

Table 13.2 The protein content of various uncooked foods*

	Protein (g/100 g)	Limiting amino acid
Animal foods		
Whole hen's egg	12·4	
Cow's milk	3·5	S/C†
Cheese	18·0	S/C
Fresh fish (average)	18·8	Trp
Beef	17·7	{ Val, Trp
Chicken	20·0	Trp
Lamb	15·6	S/C
Pork	15·0	S/C
Cereals		
Barley	11·0	{ Ile, Lys
Maize	9·5	Lys
Millet	9·7	Lys
Oats	13·0	Ile
Rice	7·5	Ile
Rye	11·0	Trp
Sorghum	10·1	Lys
Wheat	12·2	Lys
Legumes		
Bean	22·1	S/C
Chick pea	20·1	S/C
Groundnut	25·6	S/C
Lentil	24·2	S/C
Pea	22·5	S/C
Soya bean	38·0	S/C
Nuts and seeds		
Coconut	6·6	Lys
Cotton seed	20·2	Ile
Starchy roots and tubers		
Cassava (dried)	1·6	{ Phe, Tyr
Potato	2·0	S/C
Sweet potato	1·3	S/C
Yam	2·4	S/C

* Appreciable alterations occur during cooking (Table 13.4)
† S/C, sulphur-containing amino acids

in the infant's stomach and delays the passage of milk through the gut. In the clotting process caseinogen is converted into casein by partial proteolysis, i.e. the removal of a peptide under the influence of the enzyme *rennin* which is secreted by the stomach of young mammals. Once formed, the casein is spontaneously precipitated as its calcium salt.

Caseinogen is relatively deficient in sulphur-containing amino acids but whole milk proteins give higher NPU values than other protein-containing foods except whole eggs, even though their chemical score (see Table 10.7, page 129) is not particularly high. Milk is not a concentrated source of protein and therefore it suits young children who, because of the poor concentrating powers of their kidneys, require relatively large volumes of fluid.

Milk fat, present as a fine stable emulsion which is readily digestible, differs from other dietary fats in containing an appreciable amount of short chain (C_4–C_8) fatty acids.

The carbohydrate present in milk is *lactose*, a compound sugar synthesized only in the mammary glands which promotes the absorption of calcium from the ileum.

Lactose intolerance

A few infants are unable to digest lactose because of a congenital deficiency of lactase. True congenital lactose intolerance in infants is rare but, when the gastrointestinal tract has been seriously damaged, e.g. in marasmus or kwashiorkor (page 128), lactase production may be inadequate and milk is then poorly tolerated. Under these circumstances a casein preparation containing glucose is a more effective aid to recovery than milk. Such preparations may also be of more value for the treatment of protein deficiency in older children and adults, since in people of many races although not in most Caucasians, production of lactase ceases 2–4 years after birth. This is an interesting example of the changes in enzyme pattern that occur with age and suggests that, contrary to earlier belief, milk is not a particularly suitable food for most adults.

The calcium content of human milk is only about 30 mg per 100 ml, but, provided that the volume produced by the mother is sufficient, the infant's need will be covered. Milk is low in iron but infants accumulate a store of iron during intrauterine life, and this is usually sufficient for the first 4–6 months of independent existence. After this time it is important to supplement the milk diet with iron-containing foods such as strained meat and vegetables. Milk is also relatively deficient in vitamins C and D. The vitamin C content of breast milk is usually adequate, but infants fed on cow's milk may need a supplementary source. Although fresh orange juice and rose hip syrup are good sources, it is undesirable to accustom children to sweet drinks at an early age since later on these can have disastrous effects on the teeth.

Milk products

Cheese

Cheese production is a traditional and effective method of preserving much of the food value of milk. There are at least 400 varieties of cheese but the process of cheese making always involves the clotting of milk by rennin at some stage.

Most cheeses contain 20–30% of protein and 25–35% of fat and are rich sources of calcium and vitamin A. The protein is of good quality although, because of the loss of some of the lactalbumin, it is not so good as that of whole milk. Cheese is a compact and highly nutritious food and it is said that 8 oz (227 g) of bread, 4 oz (114 g) of cheese and 2 oz (57 g) of watercress provide 4184 kJ (1000 kcal) and form a meal which contains a virtually complete ration of nutrients. From the dental viewpoint cheese, if eaten at the end of the meal, is particularly beneficial since it stimulates the flow of saliva and neutralizes acid present in the plaque.

Furthermore, the caseinogen may initiate the formation of a protective calcium–protein complex on the enamel surface.

A constituent of cheese which is sometimes of clinical importance is *tyramine*, which is normally destroyed by *monoamine oxidase* (MAO). However, where MAO inhibitors are prescribed as antidepressants it is essential that cheese and other foods such as chocolate, which contain pharmacologically active amines, be avoided since they may cause severe hypertensive reactions.

Cream and butter

Cream contains all the fat and usually from half to one-third of the protein and lactose of milk. Single cream must by regulation contain at least 18% by weight of milk fat, double cream not less than 48%, clotted cream having nearly 60%. Cream is a good source of calories but is less economical than butter, which is produced by churning cream. On average butter contains 82% of fat and 12–15% of water but little sugar or protein. It is low in essential fatty acids. There is no evidence that butter has any nutritional advantage over margarine. In fact, since in Britain margarine is largely derived from vegetable oils, is fortified with vitamins A and D and contains appreciable amounts of the essential fatty acids, it may well be nutritionally preferable to butter.

Eggs

Eggs contain the complete food supply for the embryo chick and consequently are rich in essential nutrients. Since they contain very little carbohydrate they cannot be considered as a complete food for humans. The white of eggs consists almost entirely of protein with *ovalbumin* constituting 70% of the total. The yolk contains the phosphoprotein *vitellin* and 21–33% of fat including phospholipids and cholesterol.

In addition to phosphorus, eggs are rich in sulphur and also contain appreciable amounts of minerals as well as most vitamins other than ascorbic acid. Eggs form an admirable combination with cereals which are rich in carbohydrate, but poor in fat and sulphur-containing amino acids.

Table 13.3 Percentage composition of hen's eggs

	Water	Protein	Fat	Minerals
Whole egg (edible portion)	73·7	13·4	10·5	1·0
White	86·2	12·3	0·2	0·6
Yolk	49·5	15·7	33·3	1·1

Meat

Humans have a natural appetite for meat but it is expensive and consumption is closely related to income. Flesh from different animals and different parts of the same animal varies considerably in its nutritional quality which is not always related to price.

The fat content may vary from about 5 to 50% with resultant major differences in energy content. In addition to muscle cells, meat contains considerable amounts of fibrous connective tissue which is both tougher and more plentiful in older animals. Although collagen is less readily digested than the muscle proteins, much of it is converted to gelatin during cooking. The characteristic flavour of meat is due to the presence of a variety of readily soluble substances known as *extractives*. They include various peptides, nucleotides, vitamins and salts. If removed by prolonged boiling, the meat becomes tasteless and insipid.

Meat contains between 15 and 30% of good quality protein but no carbohydrate, since after death any glycogen present is rapidly converted to lactic acid by the glycolytic enzymes. Meat is a good source of B vitamins and also of iron and phosphorus although, with the exception of tripe, it does not contain much calcium. In spite of the lack of carbohydrate, meat seems to be one of the few single articles of diet on which life can be supported indefinitely.

Offal

This term covers most of the viscera many of which are of good nutritional value. Liver, pancreas and kidney are richly cellular organs and have a high content of nucleic acids, which give rise to uric acid, so that persons who are susceptible to gout are advised not to eat them.

Fish

Fish is as useful a source of good quality protein as meat (Table 13.2) and is richer in vitamins A and D. Fish, however, vary considerably in their fat content. Lean white fish contain less than 1% and fat fish such as herrings and salmon up to 15%. Fish fat usually contains relatively high concentrations of polyunsaturated fatty acids. Both hard and soft roes are rich in both protein and nucleic acids. Fish supplies about the same amount of the nutritionally important members of the vitamin B complex as does meat.

Plant foods

While most people consume animal products if they have the opportunity, it is possible to live solely on plant foods. Vegetable diets, however, tend to be poorly digested and to cause distention of the gut by gas and residues. They increase the frequency of defecation and micturition and are likely to be low in protein, fat and calcium and devoid of vitamin B_{12}.

Cereals

Modern civilization with its high population densities was made possible by the development of a stable agriculture based on cereal production. In many parts of Asia and Africa cereals provide 70% or more of the energy requirement. The type of 'corn' that is grown in a particular region depends on the climate, soil, economic considerations and local custom. Cereal grains, of which wheat, rice, maize, millet, oats and rye are the most important, are the seeds of domesticated grasses. They all have a high carbohydrate content and the ranges of composition of their whole grains are: carbohydrate, 60–72%; proteins, 8–14%; fat, 1–6%. Cereals are good sources of energy and provide appreciable amounts of protein, although, when cooked, they take up large quantities of water. The mixture of proteins in the whole grains is of reasonably good quality (see Table 10.7, page 129). Owing to the presence of *phytic acid* (page 143), their calcium and other minerals may not always be well absorbed. They also contain useful amounts of the B vitamins but are lacking in ascorbic acid and vitamin A. Before cereals can be used as food it is usually necessary to remove their coarse outer husk. Where grains such as rice and wheat are polished or ground to a flour, appreciable quantities of their vitamins and minerals may be lost.

Wheat

Wheat is the most nutritious cereal, but can only be grown in temperate climates on relatively rich soils. One of the chief advantages of wheat results from the peculiar viscid properties of *gluten*, the mixture of proteins present, which enable wheat, unlike other cereals apart from rye, to be used for making bread. However, a few people who suffer from *coeliac disease* are sensitive to gluten and develop lesions of the small intestine which lead to malabsorption, notably of fat.

The outer husk (pericarp) of the wheat grain, making up about 13% of the total, is coarse and indigestible and is commonly removed from the flour as bran and used as food for domestic animals. According to the proportion of the grain that is removed, flours of varying *extraction rate* are produced. If the whole grain is used in making the flour it is said to be 100% extraction flour, whereas wholemeal flour which usually has only the coarsest bran particles removed, represents about 95% of the original wheat. White flours have extraction rates varying from 70 to 80% and consist of the endosperm and some of the germ. In the UK the Government has set minimum values of 1·65, 0·24 and 1·60 mg/100 g respectively, for the iron, thiamine and nicotinic acid contents of flour. If the flour does not reach these standards it has to be appropriately fortified. Furthermore, 14 oz of calcium carbonate per 280 lb must be added to all except true wholemeal flours.

Controversy has been raging for many years as to whether, from the nutritional point of view, white or brown bread is better. Brown bread made from high extraction flour contains more protein, calcium, iron, B vitamins and fibre than white bread but its nutrients tend to be less well digested and absorbed. The case for white bread is based on its more attractive appearance, finer texture, better baking and keeping qualities and also its lower content of fibre and phytic acid which are responsible for the poorer utilization of nutrients. In Britain, where bread is only one of many articles of diet, nutritional differences between wholemeal and fortified white flours are of little practical significance. However, such differences could become important if bread ever became the single staple food.

Rice

In hot damp climates rice, which is essentially a mud plant, is usually the principal cereal. Of all the cereals it has the lowest content of both protein and minerals but it is well absorbed and utilized and its protein is of good quality (see Table 10.7, page 129). Because of its low content of protein and fat, rice is best eaten with supplementary sources of these nutrients.

Polished rice has long been associated with beriberi caused by thiamine deficiency since the polishing process reduces the content from about 4·0 to 0·7 μg g^{-1}. This problem can be largely overcome if the rice is parboiled before removing the husk or by enrichment of the polished rice with thiamine.

Maize

Maize is hardy and easy to cultivate and is widely grown in Central and South America, South Africa and parts of Southern Europe. It may be boiled and made into a porridge or baked into tortillas. Cornflakes consist of maize cooked and treated with malt and honey and then dried, rolled and baked.

Maize protein has a higher biological value than was at one time thought, but the use of maize as a staple food is associated with pellagra (page 164).

Oats

These are a hardy crop now used mainly as animal fodder, although oatmeal used to be a staple article of diet in Scotland and is still used there. Among cereals oatmeal is particularly rich in fat and its protein is of quite good quality. It has a high content of phytic acid and, in view of the effects of this compound on calcium absorption, this used to be thought to account for the prevalence of dental caries among Scots. However, this is now considered most unlikely since phytate reduces caries in animals and is the 'protective factor' shown by test tube experiments to be present in unrefined cereals.

Oatmeal porridge contains about 90% water and a 200 g helping provides only about 380 kJ (90 kcal). As with cornflakes, its food value lies mainly in the milk or cream with which it is taken.

Millet

Millet forms the principal crop in many tropical regions where the soil is poor and water supply limited. It is the staple food of many people in Africa and in parts of Asia and Latin America. Although less tasty than wheat or rice, millet is nutritious, its protein being one of the few plant proteins that is rich in methionine (see Table 10.3, page 125).

Sorghum

This is a larger variety of millet widely grown in Africa and Asia. Its protein contains less of the S-containing amino acids and it has a high leucine content which may have an adverse effect when intakes of tryptophan and nicotinic acid are low.

Rye

Rye grows on poor soils and in cold climates and is commonly produced in Russia, Poland and Scandinavia. It has a low gluten content and the bread that is made from it is dense and moist. It is, however, tasty and rich in members of the vitamin B complex.

Pulses (legumes)

Pulses, i.e. peas, beans, lentils etc., are the seeds of the large Leguminosa family. Pulses are grown in almost every part of the world and most people regularly eat one type or another. When cooked they contain about 6% of protein but its content of the S-containing amino acids is low and its quality correspondingly poor. However, since pulses are usually relatively rich in lysine, they make a useful combination with cereals which though low in lysine contain valuable quantities of cysteine and methionine.

Pulses are also well supplied with carbohydrate but, except for soya beans and peanuts, do not contain much fat. They have a reputation for not being readily digested but, if properly cooked, are well utilized.

Pulses are good sources of most of the B vitamins and there is no question of losses during milling since the whole seed is eaten. They contain no vitamin C but, if allowed to germinate, large amounts are formed; therefore sprouting pulses will prevent scurvy.

The soya bean (Glycine hispada)

This bean contains about 40% of protein, more than double that of most other pulses, and 18% of fat. Its nutritional importance is now clearly recognized and it is widely grown, not only in China where it has been eaten in various forms for thousands of years, but also in other parts of the Far East, Central Europe and in the USA where it is grown mainly as cattle food.

Groundnuts

These are also known as 'peanuts' or 'monkey nuts' and are the seeds of *Arachis hypogaea*. They are even richer in fat than soya beans and are grown chiefly for their oil which is used in the manufacture of cooking oil, margarine and soap. The residue or 'cake' left after the oil has been expressed is a protein-rich product that forms excellent cattle fodder. But for its unpleasant taste it could be used for human nutrition and when used as a diluent of cereal flours it is well tolerated.

Toxins

A problem with the pulses is the presence of various types of toxin, some of which are only destroyed by prolonged heat. For example, soya beans contain a trypsin inhibitor. *Aflatoxins* produced by the mould *Aspergillus flavus*, which may contaminate groundnuts, have been found to damage the liver and cause carcinoma in various species. These substances have restricted the use of groundnuts both for human and animal nutrition. *Lathyrism* (page 419), which may produce permanent paralysis, results from the consumption of large quantities of the pea, *Lathyrus sativus*, usually when the main crops have failed.

Starchy roots and tubers

This class of food includes the potato, which is widely consumed in temperate climates, and cassava, sweet potatoes and yams grown in the tropics. They are easily cultivated and give high yields even on poor soils. Since they consist mainly of starch and are poor in proteins, minerals and vitamins their nutritional value tends to be low.

Potato

Potatoes are very important since they yield more energy per acre than any cereal crop. Furthermore, they are said to be the only cheap food which, when fed as the sole article of diet, can support life. This is surprising in view of their composition (Table 13.4).

Potatoes contain appreciable but variable amounts of vitamin C and, since they are consumed in fairly large amounts, may contribute a large proportion of the daily requirement.

Cassava

Cassava (tapioca or manioc) is the principal food of many people living in the tropics. The juice must be washed from the grated root before it is eaten, because many varities contain hydrocyanic acid. After drying, cassava still contains rather less than 2% of protein and understandably protein-energy malnutrition is common in all communities that depend on it for most of their food.

Table 13.4 The composition of selected foods (per 100 g foodstuff)

Foodstuff	Energy		Protein (g)	Fat (g)	Carbohydrate (g)	Calcium (mg)	Iron (mg)
	kJ	kcal					
Milk (cow)	276	66	3·4	3·7	4·8	120	0·08
Milk (human)	285	68	2·0	3·7	6·9	25	0·07
Cream (double)	1820	462	1·5	48·2	2·0	50	0·20
Cheese (Cheddar)	1780	425	25·4	34·5	tr.	810	0·57
Eggs, fresh whole	682	163	11·9	12·3	0	56	2·53
Egg white	155	37	9·0	tr.	0	5	0·10
Egg yolk	1470	350	16·2	30·5	0	131	6·13
Bacon, streaky fried	2200	526	24·0	46·0	0	52·3	3·2
Beef, roast, lean and fat	1620	385	21·3	32·1	0	5·8	4·6
Chicken, boiled, weighed with bone	851	203	26·2	10·3	0	10·7	2·1
Liver – calf, fried	1100	262	29·0	14·5	2·4	8·8	21·7
Cod, fried	590	140	20·7	4·7	2·9	49·6	1·0
Herring, baked in vinegar	759	189	16·9	12·9	0	58·2	1·6
Salmon, fresh steamed, no skin or bone	835	199	19·1	13·0	0	28·9	0·8
Flour (English 100%)	1400	333	8·9	2·2	73·4	35·5	3·05
Flour (Manitoba 100%)	1420	339	13·6	2·5	69·1	27·6	3·81
Bread (white)	1020	243	7·8	1·4	52·7	92	1·8
Bread (brown)	1010	242	8·7	2·1	49·9	95	2·44
Rice, polished, boiled	510	122	2·1	0·3	29·6	1·3	0·16
Cornflakes	1540	367	6·6	0·8	88·2	7·4	2·8
Oatmeal (porridge)	189	45	1·4	0·9	8·2	6·3	0·47
Beans, baked	390	93	6·0	0·4	17·3	61·6	2·05
Cabbage, spring, boiled	33	8	1·1	tr.	0·8	30·0	0·45
Carrots, old, boiled	80	19	0·6	tr.	4·3	36·9	0·37
Peas, fresh, boiled	210	49	5·0	tr.	7·7	12·6	1·22
Potatoes, old, mashed	505	120	1·5	5·0	18·0	11·7	0·45
Potatoes, new, boiled	315	75	1·6	tr.	18·3	5·0	0·46
Apples, English, eating	189	45	0·3	tr.	11·7	3·5	0·29
Bananas	324	77	1·1	tr.	19·2	6·8	0·41
Oranges, weighed with peel and pips	113	27	0·6	tr.	6·4	31·0	0·25
Lard	3850	920	tr.	99·0	0	0·8	0·1
Margarine	3340	795	0·2	85·3	0	4·1	0·3
Olive oil	3900	930	tr.	99·9	0	0·5	0·1
Boiled sweets	1379	327	tr.	tr.	87·3	4·8	0·43
Chocolate (plain)	2280	544	5·6	35·2	52·5	63·0	2·9
Icecream	820	196	4·1	11·3	19·8	137	0·27
Liquorice Allsorts	1320	315	3·9	2·2	74·1	62·9	8·05
Biscuits (cream crackers)	2335	557	8·5	33·0	57·5	96	1·48
Biscuits (sweet, mixed)	2330	556	5·5	30·7	66·5	83	1·2
Spaghetti	1530	365	9·9	1·0	84·0	22·6	1·21
Butter	3340	793	0·4	85·1	tr.	15	0·16
Ham, boiled, lean and fat	1820	435	16·3	39·6	0	12·7	2·5
Mutton, leg, roast	1225	292	25·0	20·4	0	4·3	4·3
Mutton chop, fried lean and fat (weighed with bone)	2150	512	12·6	49·0	2·1	11·4	2·1

Table 13.4 (*cont.*)

Foodstuff	Energy		Protein (g)	Fat (g)	Carbohydrate (g)	Calcium (mg)	Iron (mg)
	kJ	kcal					
Potatoes, old 'chips'	1000	239	3·8	9·0	37·3	13·8	1·35
Draught ale (bitter)	132	31	0·25	tr.	2·25	10·8	0·01
Cider (sweet)	176	42	tr.	0	4·28	7·9	0·49
Sherry (dry)	478	114	0·19	0	1·36	7·1	0·39
Champagne	311	74	0·25	0	1·40	3·4	0·50
Spirits (70% proof)	930	222	tr.	0	tr.	tr	tr.

All values given per 100 g foodstuff
Values selected from R. A. McCance and E. M. Widdowson (1960). *The Composition of Foods*, 3rd edn., Medical Research Council Special Report Series 297. HMSO London.

Vegetables

The botanical structure of vegetables is very varied. They include flowers, stalks, fruits, leaves and roots. As a result, although they possess certain common features, their composition is very varied. Usually they are not major sources of energy, but the presence of indigestible cellulose fibre makes them bulky and promotes a feeling of satiety.

Normally vegetables make little contribution to the protein requirements, although if the fibre is removed protein concentrates containing about 60% protein can be prepared from green leaves which, it is suggested, could form a valuable supplement in areas where protein is in short supply.

The value of vegetables lies mainly in the carotene and ascorbic acid which they contain as well as their calcium and iron contents.

Fruit

Fruits, like vegetables, make an important contribution to the ascorbic acid intake. Most fruits also contain small quantities of carotene, and B vitamins and considerable amounts of cellulose. They contain between 5 and 20% of carbohydrate but little or no protein or fat. In ripe fruits the carbohydrate is mainly fructose and glucose, although apricots and peaches contain sucrose. Fruits when unripe contain a variety of organic acids. As they ripen the concentration of the acids falls and that of the sugar rises. Since they are organic in nature the acids are readily oxidized in the body and do not cause acidosis. In fact, the consumption of large quantities of fruit and vegetables usually results in an alkaline urine partly because of their high potassium content.

Fruit is believed to be beneficial to the teeth on account of its cleansing action and effect in provoking salivation. However, the traditional apple removes plaque only from the smooth surfaces of the teeth which are not prone to caries and may be so acid that the saliva is unable to neutralize it. Cheese appears to have a greater protective effect (page 523).

Normal diets

Table 13.4 gives values for the composition of selected foods and Table 13.5 shows the percentage contribution of different foods to the nutrient content of the average household diet in the UK.

Table 13.5 Percentage contribution of different foods to the nutrient content of the average household diet in the UK

	Energy value	Protein	Fat	Calcium	Iron	Vitamin A	Thiamine	Riboflavin	Nicotinic acid	Vitamin C	Vitamin D
Milk, cream and cheese	12	23	17	57	4	15	13	41	4	8	8
Meat	15	25	30	2	27	21	22	19	36	1	2
Fish	1	4	1	2	2	—	—	2	4	—	27
Eggs	2	6	3	2	7	8	3	9	—	—	13
Fats	15	—	39	—	—	27	—	—	—	—	43
Sugar and jam	12	—	—	—	1	—	—	—	—	2	—
Vegetables	7	9	—	6	17	19	21	11	18	52	—
Fruit	2	1	—	2	4	6	4	2	3	36	—
Cereals and cereal products	33	31	9	28	35	3	36	8	32	—	7
Beverages, etc.	1	1	1	1	3	1	1	8	3	1	—
	100	100	100	100	100	100	100	100	100	100	100

From Ministry of Agriculture, Fisheries and Food (1970). *Manual of Nutrition*, HMSO, London.

Food choice

Human beings consume an enormous variety of different foods in an infinite number of combinations, and no single food pattern needs to be adhered to in order to ensure good nutrition. Human diets range from the almost completely carnivorous diet (meat and fish) of the traditional Eskimo to strictly vegetarian diets which do not include eggs, milk or cheese. The latter tend to be very bulky and low in protein but, provided they contain a variety of plant products including protein-rich pulses, they can be adequate. It is necessary, however, to see that people consuming such diets do not become deficient in vitamin B_{12} (page 166).

The chief factor determining what people eat is, of course, availability in both the physical and economic sense but food choice is also influenced by such factors as race, religion, social class and education. The question as to whether men and animals have any instinct for choosing the type and amounts of food that they need has never been satisfactorily answered. The results of experiments on food choice in animals have been inconclusive and, as far as humans are concerned, there is little evidence for the instinctive selection of appropriate types of food. The choice seems to depend more on the palatability of the food than on anything else. People eat what they like and hope that it will fulfil their nutritional needs. In the distant past Man's liking for sweet foods enabled him to select from his natural environment foods which were wholesome and palatable and provided him with energy, vitamins and minerals. In addition, most people seem to have a natural appetite for meat and eat it if it is available. It is interesting therefore that two of the foods said to be eaten in excess today are refined sugar and meat. The problem is to know what constitutes an excess of these or any other foodstuff.

In the past many, if not most, human societies were subject to seasonal food shortages. Under such circumstances those people who were able to store energy efficiently when food was plentiful had a greater chance of survival when food was in short supply. In the West where seasonal shortages no longer occur, major fat stores confer no advantage on the individual. In fact with the increase in average length of life and the fact that obesity has been found to predispose people to a variety of degenerative diseases they can be a positive disadvantage.

A person's life-span depends on both genetic and environmental factors of which nutrition is only one. Experiments showed that if the growth of rats was retarded by dietary restriction, their life-span was significantly increased. While it is not possible to dissociate nutritional from genetic factors and overall life-style, studies on longevity in human populations suggest that the life-span is longest and incidence of chronic disease lowest in people living a physically active life in a harsh environment where food is not abundant. The food consumed in most industrialized societies differs from that in such Third World countries in that it provides a continuous energy surplus and contains much more fat, much less fibre, large amounts of refined carbohydrate and a great variety of additives which are indispensable to modern food technology. The National Advisory Committee on Nutrition Education Report (NACNE) published in 1983 recommended as reasonable and modest the following aims for the 1980s:

1. Reduction of the average *total fat intake* by 10% (from 38% to 34% of the total energy intake).
2. Reduction of the average intake of *saturated fatty acids* by 15% (from 18% of total energy to 15%)
3. A small increase in the intake of *polyunsaturated fatty acids* (from 4% of total energy to 5%), thus raising the P/S ratio to 0·36 from 0·24.
4. Reduction of the sugar intake by 10% (from 14% of total energy to about 12%).
5. Maintenance of the overall energy intake by increasing the intake of low-fat foods and encouraging the taking of more exercise.

6. An increase in dietary fibre of about 25%.
7. Reduction of the salt intake by 10%.
8. Reduction of the average alcohol intake by 10% (from 6% of total energy intake to 5%).

Such objectives should be achieved if the diet contains plenty of fresh fruit and green vegetables, plenty of bread (preferably brown), cereals and root vegetables and some animal protein derived from poultry, fish, eggs and cheese rather than red meat. Fats such as butter, cream and lard should be restricted as well as sugar in the form of confectionery, soft drinks, cakes and biscuits.

Nutrition is a subject with more so-called experts than almost any other and is open to innumerable fads, fancies and fallacies. Food should be eaten sensibly and enjoyed remembering that '*a little* of what you fancy does you good'. Sound nutritional advice can, in fact, be given in a mere four words – variety and no excesses!

Section 4

Molecular organization and interactions

Chapter 14
General principles of metabolism

Once the food has been digested and absorbed, the various nutrients are distributed to the tissues via the blood and, having passed through the cell membranes, are exposed to the metabolic machinery of the cell. The purpose of this machinery is (1) to release some of the energy contained in the nutrients and convert it into a form that can be used for the various functions of the cell, and (2) to use the rest of the material for the synthesis of substances that the body needs for its growth and activities.

In order to do this the food materials are subjected to a variety of metabolic processes, each of which involves a well-defined sequence of reactions. Nearly every step is catalysed by a different enzyme, and results in a small but specific chemical change. This field of *intermediary metabolism* constitutes a major part of biochemistry. The main metabolic pathways have by now all been elucidated, and metabolic maps prepared, which show the possible origins and fates of all the major cellular constituents.

Broadly speaking, metabolism may be divided into three areas. (1) *Catabolism*. This deals with the breakdown of materials with the release of energy. In the process, carbon dioxide and water are produced, but these are essentially by-products since it is the energy liberated during their formation that the body requires, and rarely the carbon dioxide and water themselves. (2) *Anabolism* covers the processes by which complex substances are built up from simple precursors, and this utilizes much of the energy released during the course of catabolism. (3) Between the clearly defined anabolic and catabolic pathways lies a *central area of metabolism* in which various simple compounds are interconverted. The pathways are said to be *amphibolic* since they have a dual function (*amphi* = both) and provide material which may be used either for synthesis or for breakdown. All the metabolic pathways involve the uptake or release of energy. Energy is required for:

1. Chemical syntheses and the process of growth in which complex, highly organized molecules are built and assembled from small molecular precursors.
2. The maintenance of the highly ordered structure of the cell.
3. Transport and the movement of materials against a concentration gradient, i.e. from a region of lower to one of higher concentration.
4. Mechanical work, e.g. the contraction of muscles and movement of cilia.

Without the expenditure of energy, membranes and other cell structures would disintegrate and it is only by the constant expenditure of energy that living organisms are able to adapt continually to the prevailing conditions.

The study of energy exchanges is known as *thermodynamics*, and covers the fields of heat movement and overall energy exchange. The *First Law of Thermodynamics* is the Law of Conservation of Energy, which states that 'energy is neither created nor destroyed', although different forms of energy are often interconvertible. In everyday life it is seen that mechanical forms of energy can be converted into electrical energy by a generator and the kinetic energy of water into electricity by a suitable turbine. Moreover, since electrical energy can be stored in a battery and petrol provides the energy to drive internal combustion engines it is clear that energy can be conserved in the form of chemical compounds. Nevertheless, although many forms of energy are interconvertible, conversion is never quantitative, and a large proportion is always lost as heat.

According to the *Second Law of Thermodynamics*, any organized collection of matter tends towards a state of maximum randomness or disorder. It is this tendency that determines the direction in which energy will move within a system which is not already in equilibrium. For example, the ordered condition of a gas at high pressure in contact with a gas at low pressure will not persist; gas will flow from the high pressure region to the low pressure region thereby replacing an ordered state by a random one. As explained in Chapter 16, similar considerations govern the direction in which chemical reactions will proceed, the tendency which any given reactants have to form products being expressed by the *equilibrium constant* (K_{eq}). Reactions occur because the final state is more random than the initial state. This randomness is called *entropy*, and another way of expressing the Second Law of Thermodynamics is to say that all systems tend towards maximum entropy. Living systems are highly ordered, so that their development, at first sight, appears to be in direct conflict with this law. The localized ordering of living systems is achieved by increasing the randomness of their surroundings since a decrease in entropy (increase in orderliness) can occur provided that it is coupled with the release of energy and the overall ΔG^0 is negative. Consequently considerably more energy must always be removed from the environment than is incorporated into the living organism.

Extraction of energy from the environment

Cells consist of about 70% by weight of water, so that all cellular reactions take place in a predominantly aqueous environment. The conditions therefore are quite different from those under which man-made machines operate. Furthermore, living cells can only survive if both the temperature and the pressure are maintained within a narrow range. As in the case of heat engines, when fuel is burnt oxygen is used up and carbon dioxide is produced; but in the body the energy is released in a controlled manner which makes it possible for a large part of the energy to be utilized for the synthesis of the special carrier of free energy, *adenosine triphosphate* (ATP), from its precursor adenosine diphosphate (ADP). When 1 mole of glucose is oxidized to carbon dioxide and water, 2878 kJ (688 kcal) of energy are released, whereas only 29–38 kJ (7–9 kcal) are required to convert 1 mole of ADP to ATP. These two quantities of energy are altogether disproportionate but by breaking down the glucose in a large number of small steps, the amount of energy released during certain of the reactions is converted to the same order of magnitude as that required for the formation on one *high-energy bond* (page 211). Even so, only about half of the energy released during the breakdown of foodstuffs is conserved in the form of ATP, the remainder appearing as heat. However, since the body is equipped with efficient temperature-regulating mechanisms, the heat is transferred to the surroundings with no appreciable rise in body temperature.

A second important difference between living organisms and machines is that living systems are *open systems*. Whereas a closed system is isolated from its surroundings and reactions occurring within it will proceed only until equilibrium has been established, an open one is in constant interaction with its surroundings from which material (oxygen and food) is continually being withdrawn, whilst other substances (carbon dioxide, urea, heat) are being returned to them. Owing to the very sensitive control mechanisms that have been built into living organisms, and without which their existence would be impossible, they exist in a finely balanced *steady state* in which the intake of energy and materials is matched with the output. This *dynamic equilibrium* is maintained by controlling the passage of materials both into and out of the system. Thus, while innumerable reactions are occurring all the time, and each is progressing in a manner that will tend to establish equilibrium, equilibrium is never attained, since new substrates are continually entering the system and products are continually being removed from it.

Metabolic pools and the turnover of body constituents

The body may be regarded as being composed of pools of materials of different types, whose volume and rate of exchange of material may be very different. Thus, in some cases the pool itself may be large but the *turnover* quite small; this is so for the mineral elements of the skeleton. In other cases the amount of material in the pool is quite small but the turnover of material in the pool is very rapid. For example, ATP is present in quite low concentrations in cells (about $1 \cdot 5 \, \text{mg ml}^{-1}$ of cell water) but its turnover rate is such that the body produces its own weight (70 kg) of ATP from ADP every 24 hours.

Nearly every body constituent is subject to continuous breakdown and resynthesis, although the rate of turnover varies according to the nature of the compound and the type of cell in which it occurs and its physiological state. The turnover of liver cell protein is very rapid, whilst that of tissues such as bone and cartilage, which have a mainly structural role, is very much slower.

Two separate processes are involved in the maintenance of the dynamic equilibrium of the body constituents namely (1) the destruction and replacement of whole cells and (2) the destruction and replacement of intracellular and extracellular constituents.

With respect to the first process, cell turnover rates range from that of the intestinal epithelium which is very high, the cells being replaced in a matter of hours, to that of the neurons which, once formed, never divide or are replaced. However, although exempt from the first process, the cellular constituents of neurons, like those of all other cells, are subject to continuous breakdown and replacement.

The *dynamic state of the body constituents* was demonstrated by Schoenheimer and his colleagues in 1941 as the result of some of the first experiments in which isotopes were used. They fed amino acids labelled with ^{15}N to adult rats and showed that, even where there was no net synthesis of protein, the labelled amino acids were incorporated into the tissue proteins. They also fed fatty acids labelled with deuterium (^{2}H) to animals fed a restricted diet, so that they were losing weight, and found that even so the labelled fatty acids were incorporated into the adipose tissue triglycerides. This showed clearly that even when the fat reserves were being depleted, synthesis of triglycerides was taking place. It was this work that led to the concept of continual release and uptake of substances by the tissues to and from a *metabolic pool*. Two exceptions to this general rule of continuous metabolic exchange should be mentioned, namely DNA and collagen.

Catabolism and energy production

The breakdown of the energy-producing foods is outlined in Figure 14.1; it occurs in three stages.

Stage 1. In the first stage the carbohydrate, fat and protein are broken down to relatively simple products, that is, to monosaccharides, fatty acids, glycerol and amino acids. These changes are brought about by the digestive processes occurring in the gastrointestinal tract and are accompanied by relatively little loss of energy.

Stage 2. In the second stage the relatively numerous products of Stage 1 are converted into a relatively small number of intermediary metabolites that can be utilized in Stage 3. These are pyruvate, acetyl-CoA, which is the main fuel for the citrate cycle, and a number of citrate cycle intermediates. During this stage a small amount of ATP may be used in order to prime some of the reactions, while during the breakdown of the sugars and fatty acids there is a net synthesis of ATP, although the amounts formed at this stage are small.

Stage 3. This represents the final common pathway for the breakdown of carbon-containing compounds. It includes the reactions of *the citrate cycle* and the *respiratory chain* which are responsible for producing 90% or so of the ATP required by the body. The reactions of the citrate cycle (page 240) cause two carbon atoms to be oxidized to carbon dioxide, but molecular oxygen is not involved; instead oxidation results from a number of dehydrogenation reactions each of which causes a pair of hydrogen atoms to be released. These are picked up by special *hydrogen carriers* and passed along the respiratory chain (page 216), finally to be united with molecular oxygen so that water is produced. As the hydrogen atoms (or electrons) pass along

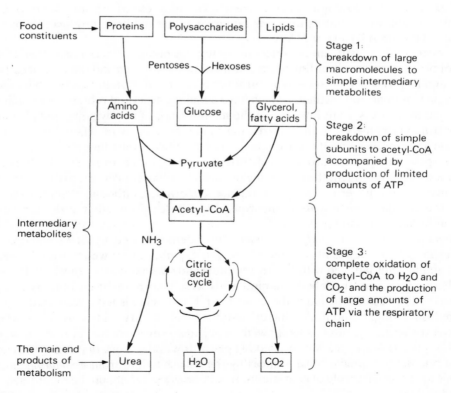

Figure 14.1 An outline of catabolism

the respiratory chain energy is released and this is utilized for the conversion of ADP to ATP, and thus for the synthesis of high-energy bonds (page 214). The inclusion of a large number of intermediates enables more efficient utilization of the energy of oxidation. It may be emphasized that it is the utilization of hydrogen and not the production of carbon dioxide which is the decisive energy-yielding process and the one which requires respiratory oxygen.

Anabolism

The term 'anabolism' encompasses the reactions concerned in the synthesis of the large complex molecules that are characteristic of living organisms. Compared with the relatively crude and unspecific reactions of catabolism, those of anabolism are far more delicate and precise. As a simple analogy, only crude apparatus and unskilled labourers are needed to demolish a house, whereas the building of a house requires many workmen skilled in a variety of specialized techniques. The construction of cells requires not only the production of a great variety of molecules both small and large, but also their organization and assembly into increasingly elaborate structures. For this a tremendously complex programme of events must be built into the system, based on patterns of integrated reactions, all of which are genetically determined.

The separation of anabolic and catabolic pathways

Most cells have alternative pathways by which a compound may either be degraded or synthesized although one direction may be favoured over the other; for example, in muscle cells glucose is broken down rather than synthesized and in adipose tissue fatty acids are synthesized rather than broken down.

In other cases the pathways by which a substance may be synthesized or degraded may be almost equally active although under one set of conditions the emphasis will be on synthesis and in another on degradation. If the same enzyme is used to catalyse a reaction which may proceed in either direction, the reaction is necessarily sensitive to Mass Action effects. Consequently if a metabolic pathway were to operate by a whole series of readily reversible reactions it would be subject to continuous fluctuations according to the relative concentrations of a large number of reactants. In such circumstances the existence of stable biological structures would be impossible and a state of metabolic confusion would result comparable to that occurring if people were to stream aimlessly up and down a staircase and to change directions from one moment to the next. For this reason it is essential that the anabolic and catabolic pathways are wholly or partially independent.

There are a number of ways in which the synthetic and degradative pathways are kept separate. Firstly, at least for some steps, different enzymes and coenzymes may be used. Of the 11 enzymes involved in the conversion of glycogen to lactate eight are identical with those used in the conversion of lactate to glycogen, i.e. three steps in the glycolytic pathway are irreversible. The anabolic pathway is longer than the catabolic pathway and involves a total of 15 steps. The extra steps required in the 'uphill' direction ensure that, taken as a whole, the pathway is exothermic and its overall ΔG^0 is negative. This is, of course, essential if synthesis is to occur. Similarly the pathway by which fatty acids are synthesized from acetyl-CoA is longer than the catabolic pathway; moreover, the two processes occur at different sites within the cell, fatty acid breakdown taking place in the mitochondria and fatty acid synthesis in the cytoplasm.

As will be seen in Chapter 23 the use of different enzymes to catalyse particular steps in the breakdown and synthesis of a compound means that the pathways can be independently and/or reciprocally controlled. In this way the system is made flexible and capable of rapid homoeostatic adjustments.

Biosynthetic pathways

Biosynthetic pathways show certain distinctive features.

1. They require ATP. Since many of the individual reactions are endergonic they require energy derived either directly or indirectly from ATP. For example, its terminal phosphate group may be transferred to a substrate converting it to a more reactive form as in the formation of glucose 6-phosphate by the hexokinase reaction. Glucose 6-phosphate is not a high-energy compound, but it is considerably more reactive than glucose and is a key compound in carbohydrate metabolism (Figure 17.3).

In other types of biosynthetic reaction the second high-energy bond of ATP is hydrolysed instead of the terminal one and a molecule of *pyrophosphate* is formed.

$$ATP \rightarrow AMP + P{\sim}P$$

Although the energy released is no greater than in the first method, the pyrophosphate is immediately acted upon by the enzyme *pyrophosphatase* which splits the high-energy bond of the pyrophosphate with the release of a further amount of energy. The apparently wasteful expenditure of this second quota of energy ensures that the reaction which is coupled with the ATP breakdown goes to completion. Both the fatty acids (page 252) and amino acids (page 299) are activated by this type of reaction and converted to high-energy compounds (fatty acyl $\sim$ CoA and aminoacyl $\sim$ tRNA compounds respectively) by linking the individual reactions in such a way that the overall reaction is exergonic since two high-energy bonds are expended in order to create one new covalent bond with a high-energy quality.

2. They are often reductive. Whereas the main energy-producing reactions are oxidative the main energy-storing reactions and certain other synthetic reactions are reductive in type.

This is notably so with the synthesis of fatty acids and steroids. Since the oxidation of pairs of hydrogen atoms proceeds with the evolution of large amounts of energy, pairs of hydrogen atoms attached to an appropriate *hydrogen carrier* (NAD^+ or $NADP^+$ (Chapter 16)) may be considered as a potential energy source. Hydrogens that are to be used for oxidation and energy production are mainly found in the mitochondria in the form of reduced NAD^+, whereas those that are to be used for storage of energy tend to be found in the cytoplasm in the form of reduced $NADP^+$. As will be seen later, this distinction between the two closely related hydrogen carriers and their locations within the cell is highly significant.

3. Macromolecules need to be constructed to a particular design and regardless of the nature and complexity of the product, the formation of a biopolymer involves three processes:

(*a*) Group activation, i.e. the conversion of the monomeric units into a reactive form.
(*b*) Chain elongation, i.e. the formation of covalent linkages between activated chain constituents.
(*c*) Molecular modelling. This is achieved either by the provision of a template (space pattern) or by using an assembly line process (time pattern).

Since the individual units from which the proteins and nucleic acids are built possess identical reactive groups, a common enzyme system may be used to link the various monomers together. The problem is to ensure that the dissimilar constituents, i.e. 20 amino acids or four nucleotides, are joined together in the correct sequence. The activated monomers are aligned according to instructions provided by a template in the form of one of the two strands of a segment of DNA during the synthesis of either DNA itself or of RNA, and by RNA for the synthesis of proteins (Chapter 20).

The *assembly line principle* is used in the synthesis of fatty acids, heteropolysaccharides and the carbohydrate side chains of glycoproteins. Here one unit is added after another according to the dictates of an *enzyme array*. In the carbohydrate-containing compounds the length of the chain and the numbers and types of sugar incorporated are generally related to the number of enzymes in the array and a unit can only be introduced after the preceding enzyme has operated.

Space and time patterning must also underlie the complex events involved in the assembly of molecules into subcellular structures and whole cells, as well as the processes of cell division, differentiation and morphogenesis.

Amphibolic pathways and the central area of metabolism

In the central area of metabolism pools of intermediary metabolites exist in a constant state of flux. The amphibolic pathways fill the gap between the catabolic pathways, which have clearly defined origins but no certain end, and the anabolic pathways, which have no certain beginnings but clearly defined end products. Small molecules derived either from the food or from the breakdown of cell constituents may be channelled into the terminal phases of oxidative metabolism with the production of urea, carbon dioxide, water and energy, or may be used to generate precursors for anabolic pathways. Notable among these amphibolic pathways is the citrate cycle, which can function not only as the final common pathway for the breakdown of carbon compounds, but also as an important source of carbon-containing material for the synthesis of glucose, fatty acids and amino acids, and hence for polysaccharides, triglycerides and proteins.

Apart from reactions involving constituents of the citrate cycle such as α-oxoglutarate, oxaloacetate, succinate and fumarate, reactions involving the triose phosphates and pyruvate from carbohydrate metabolism and acetyl-CoA and glycerol from fat metabolism also fall into this category. These compounds provide the carbon skeletons for more complex molecules, while in certain cases simple carbon groupings may be introduced into molecules in various ways, e.g. as methyl (CH_3) or formyl (–CHO) groups, or as carbon dioxide.

Where a nitrogenous compound is involved, the amphibolic pathways are centred around glutamate, aspartate and carbamoyl phosphate. These provide nitrogen which may be used either for the synthesis of nitrogenous compounds of many types, e.g. amino acids, proteins, nucleotides, nucleic acids, haem, or for conversion to urea or ammonium salts, in which form most of the nitrogen is excreted.

The integration of cellular activities

In order that the activities of the various cells and tissues of the body may be integrated, efficient communication must be maintained between them. This is mainly the function of the nervous and endocrine systems which are responsible for producing various types of chemical signal.

When cells differentiate they acquire a specific set of *receptor proteins* which enables them to bind and react to appropriate chemical stimuli. Cells of different types may be able to respond to the same signal but they may react to it in a different way. Most signals act by modifying the properties of particular proteins within the cell or by altering the rate of their synthesis.

At least three types of chemical signal are currently recognized.

Neurotransmitters

These are extracellular chemicals that are released during the transmission of impulses from one nerve cell to another or from a nerve cell to a muscle cell or gland. They include acetylcholine, adrenaline, noradrenaline, serotonin (5-hydroxytryptamine) and γ-aminobutyric acid (GABA). Neurotransmitters are rapidly removed or broken down as it is essential that the resting membrane potential should be restored so that further impulses may be transmitted.

Local chemical mediators

Histamine, prostaglandins and various growth factors may be included in this group. The distance over which they operate tends to be greater than that of the neurotransmitters and they are found in tissues other than the nervous system. They are readily taken up and destroyed by cells in their vicinity so that they only act on cells in their immediate environment.

Hormones

Hormones, for example insulin, parathormone, cortisol and testosterone, exert their effects on cells which may be widely distributed and a considerable distance from the endocrine gland where they are produced. They are carried in the blood and consequently are greatly diluted before they reach their target cells. Whether or not the cells of a tissue will be affected by any particular hormone depends on whether they are equipped with the necessary *hormone receptor*. The hormones may be divided into two categories, fat soluble and water soluble. The fat-soluble hormones include the steroid and thyroid hormones. Owing to their hydrophobicity they are able to pass through the cell membrane of their target cells and bind to specific receptor proteins inside the cell. Their effects are usually fairly prolonged. The water-soluble hormones are usually proteins, peptides or amino acid derivatives. Many of them bind to receptors on the cell surface and use either cyclic AMP or Ca^{2+} ions as *second messengers* (page 350). Others, such as insulin and growth hormone, are ingested and enter the cell by *receptor-mediated endocytosis* (page 198). Tehe effects of many of the water-soluble hormones are rapid and short-lived, e.g. insulin, glucagon and adrenaline.

Further signalling molecules act at extremes of distance, e.g. the pheromones. These topics are considered in more detail in Chapter 24.

Chapter 15
Cellular organization

All cells, regardless of the tissue or species from which they are derived, use broadly similar methods to perform such functions as the conversion of chemical bond energy into free energy for cellular processes, the transmission of information from one generation of cells to another and for the translation of this information into terms of protein structure.

Most cells fall within a fairly narrow size range. Thus the majority of cells have diameters ranging from 0·5 to 20 μm. At the lower end of the scale are the bacteria; their size is probably determined by the number of proteins required to perform the essential functions of the cell, and the quantity of DNA required to code for the synthesis of these proteins. The number of different types of protein that are needed has been estimated to be between 500 and 1000, and each of these will require for its specification about twenty times its own weight of DNA. The upper limit of cell size is probably determined by such physical factors as the ratios of the surface area of the cell membrane to the cytoplasmic volume and of the nuclear and cytoplasmic volumes.

In every cell provision must be made for the orderly flow within it of raw materials, energy and information, and for this membranes, enzymes and nucleic acids are required. For such flows to be effective they must be directional and the various intracellular systems must be precisely located. Coordinating mechanisms are required to regulate the activities of single cells both in relation to themselves and to their neighbours and the control of many cellular activities is believed to depend on the existence of various compartments within the cell which ensure that the components of a system are sometimes freely accessible to one another and, at other times, are effectively segregated.

Cells fall into two categories, namely *prokaryotes*, which comprise the bacteria and blue–green algae, and *eukaryotes*, which include protozoal, fungal, plant and animal cells. In eukaryotic cells there is a clearly defined *nucleus* set in what appears under the light microscope to be an amorphous gel, i.e. the *cytoplasm*. Electron microscopy has shown that, in fact, the cytoplasm is permeated by a network of protein filaments which constitute the *cytoskeleton* and that it also contains a variety of physically and chemically distinct membrane-bound *organelles*. These include the *endoplasmic reticulum, Golgi complex, mitochondria, lysosomes, secretory granules* and *peroxisomes*.

The endoplasmic reticulum, which is a prominent feature of the cytoplasm, is an extensive system of membranes which permeates it throughout and typically consitutes more than half the

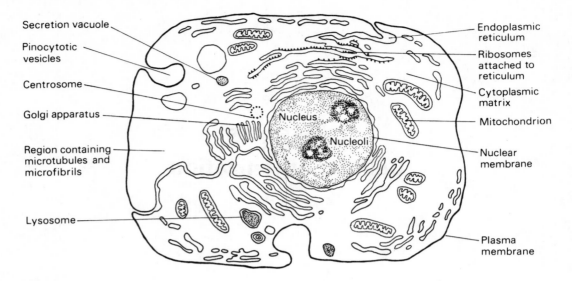

Figure 15.1 A generalized cell and its constituents

total membranes of the cell. It plays an important part in the biosynthesis of macromolecules which are required for the construction of the various cell components. The endoplasmic reticulum consists of sheets of thin paired membranes surrounding cavities or *cisternae* which divide the cytoplasm into an inner compartment which is enclosed by the membrane and the outer compartment which represents the cytoplasmic matrix or *cytosol*. Part of the membrane appears smooth while other parts are studded with a large number of granules known as *ribosomes* in which case it is known as *rough endoplasmic reticulum*. Ribosomes also occur free in the cytoplasm.

Although the various subcellular structures just described are present in most cells, the degree of their development shows considerable variation in different cell types. Since no single type of cell, e.g. liver, muscle or glandular, can be said to be more typical than another, the features of a hypothetical generalized cell are illustrated in Figure 15.1.

Cell fractionation

Various methods have been used in attempts to correlate the structure and function of the different cell components. Comparison of the fine structure of cells with differing functions shows that the number of mitochondria is correlated with metabolic activity and that the number of ribosomes relates to protein-synthesizing ability. Cytochemical techniques, including histochemistry, autoradiography and the use of fluorescent antibodies, have also contributed to our knowledge of the localization of particular enzymes, hormones and reactions. While these techniques have their limitations, they possess the great advantage that they cause little disturbance of the cell structure. On the other hand, cell fractionation techniques, which are widely used by biochemists, require the total disruption of cells. This is followed by the isolation and analysis of the released components.

Cells are usually disrupted by homogenization which breaks up the cell membrane, and liberates the contents which can be separated by differential centrifugation. By progressively increasing the speed of centrifugation the following sequence of fractions may be obtained: nuclei, mitochondria, lysosomes, a microsomal fraction, the cytosol.

The flow of materials

Membranes are the only structural elements that are found in all living organisms. They are essential for keeping the components of living systems together and preventing them from equilibrating with their environment. Biological membranes also control the passage of materials in and out of the system. They are sheath-like structures, composed of lipids and proteins held together by non-covalent forces.

In addition to the external or *plasma membrane* which bounds every cell there are various intracellular membranes including the endoplasmic reticulum and the membranes which surround the various organelles, e.g. the nucleus, mitochondria and lysosomes. It has been estimated that membranes may comprise up to 80% of the dry mass of certain cells.

It is becoming increasingly apparent that membranes are dynamic structures; they are rapidly and continually synthesized and degraded and are inherently implicated in vital processes. Membranes from different sources show wide variations in their composition and properties.

Membrane components

The main components of membranes are lipids and proteins although it is usual to find some carbohydrate as well. Lipids usually constitute about 25–50% of the dry weight of plasma membranes and consist mainly of phospholipids, glycolipids and cholesterol. The nature of the fatty acids does not seem to be fixed and may vary according to the temperature and other conditions. It appears to be essential that the fluidity of the membrane is maintained.

The lipid character of membranes explains their high electrical resistance, their ready destruction by lipolytic agents, and why they are permeable to lipid-soluble materials but have a low permeability for ions and most polar molecules. The presence of protein accounts for their mechanical strength, low surface tension and high specific conductance. The membrane proteins are also responsible for the specific properties of membranes and different types of protein are found in different membranes.

In aqueous solutions most phospholipids and glycolipids will assemble themselves into double layers in which the polar ends of the molecules are directed outwards and the long fatty acid chains are directed inwards as befits their amphiphilic nature (Figure 8.2b). Bimolecular lipid structures of this type are an essential feature of membrane structure.

Membranes also contain relatively large amounts of cholesterol which is thought to increase the mechanical stability and to help regulate the fluidity of the membrane. The relatively flat steroid ring is inserted between the phospholipid molecules with the polar –OH group adjacent to the polar heads of the phospholipids (Figure 15.2).

The most widely applicable model of membrane structure which allows for the physico-chemical properties of membrane lipids and proteins and accounts for the dynamic nature and versatility of membranes is the *fluid mosaic model* (Figure 15.3). According to this the membrane is composed of a two-dimensional array of phospholipid and globular protein molecules in which the protein molecules are floating in a phospholipid continuum. About 70–80% of the protein molecules are *integral proteins*, which are held in association with the lipid bilayer by hydrophobic interactions. They, like the lipids, are amphiphilic and form an essential part of the structure. Other proteins known as *peripheral* or *surface proteins* can be dissociated from the membrane by the addition of salts. From this it is concluded that they are

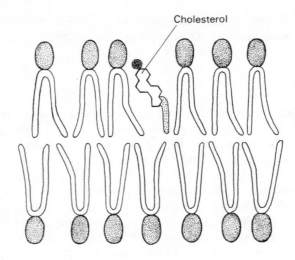

Figure 15.3 The fluid mosaic model of membrane structure

bound to the membrane surface by hydrogen bonds and salt linkages.

The functions of membrane proteins are many, varied and specific; they include transport, communication and energy transductions. Membranes are asymmetrical and the properties of their two surfaces are different.

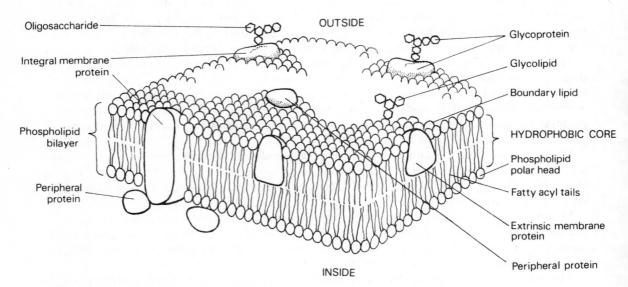

Figure 15.2 A phospholipid bilayer with an inserted cholesterol molecule

All eukaryotic cells have carbohydrate groupings on their external surface. These are mainly the oligosaccharide side chains of glycoproteins and glycolipids. In addition the 'cell coat' may contain secreted glycoproteins and proteoglycans (page 407). The cell surface carbohydrates contain mannose, fucose and sialic acid in addition to glucose, glucosamine, galactose and galactosamine. The sialic acid is usually found at the ends of the side chains which are often branched, and it is the sialic acid which is believed to be mainly responsible for the negative charge found on the surface of all eukaryotic cells. The cell surface carbohydrates play an important role in recognition processes and cellular interactions.

The structure of membrane proteins

Structural studies on integral proteins suggest that the portions of polypeptide chain which are located within the lipid bilayer take up an α-helical conformation. Thus the membrane-crossing regions of these proteins have a relatively rigid rod-like structure. Two structurally distinct classes of integral protein occur. In the first class, which could be described as *anchored proteins*, the active site of the protein is held in the aqueous environment at the membrane surface while a single helical segment of protein traverses the membrane anchoring the protein within it (Figure 15.4a). Examples of this type of protein are the intestinal hydrolases as well as hormone receptors and antigens such as the *histocompatibility antigens* on which recognition sites are presented at the membrane surface. The integral proteins which function in membrane transport and as 'gates' have a different type of structure. The part within the membrane which forms the transporting region is complex and is made up of a cluster of transmembrane helices (Figure 15.4b). The sodium pump and the calcium pump of muscle are proteins of this type.

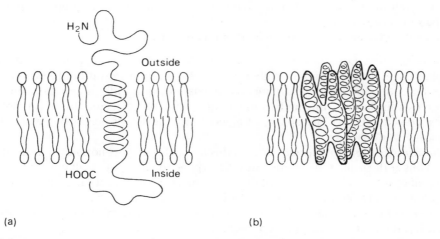

Figure 15.4 Types of integral membrane protein. (a) An anchored protein; (b) a transport protein

Membrane transport and membrane gates

Biological membranes are selectively permeable. They allow free diffusion of certain materials but act as a barrier towards others. In addition, they possess special pumping or active transport mechanisms which are responsible for the uptake or elimination of particular substances and which ensure that the composition of the enclosed compartment is closely controlled.

The physical forces responsible for the movement of materials across membranes, although based on diffusion and osmosis and the existence of electrochemical gradients, are extremely complex since they are affected not only by the composition of the membrane but also by such factors as the molecular size, lipid solubility, charge and degree of hydration of the penetrant as well as on its relative concentrations on the two sides of the membrane. Furthermore, many different substances are moving at the same time and the movement of one may have an effect on the movement of others.

The distribution of ions on the two sides of a membrane is also affected by the presence of large charged non-diffusible molecules, e.g. proteins and nucleic acids, which may themselves be unequally distributed.

Without considering in detail the factors mentioned above, it may be stated that most membranes will allow the passage of small uncharged molecules by simple diffusion and that the rate of their passage is related to their lipid solubility. The passage of other materials may occur as a result of the presence of pores, polar regions and gates over a small area of the membrane surface. Certain evidence suggests that the average pore is about 0·3–0·4 nm in diameter. A molecule that is larger than this will not cross the membrane passively, and for reasons given above neither will some smaller molecules.

Carrier-mediated transport processes

Whereas synthetic membranes such as cellophane are useful in the study of passive distribution processes resulting solely from physical effects, biological membranes are notably different in that they contain special in-built transport mechanisms. It appears that the transported molecule binds specifically and reversibly with a carrier molecule, present in the membrane, which operates between the two surfaces of the membrane, alternately picking up and releasing the transported substance.

Carrier-mediated transport can be divided into two types:

1. *Passive transport or facilitated diffusion*. In this form no energy is expended and movement only takes place from a region of higher to one of lower concentration. However, owing to the presence of the carrier, substances can pass more rapidly along the concentration gradient existing across the membrane than would be expected from simple physico-chemical considerations. The uptake of glucose into most cells occurs by passive transport of this sort.

2. *Active transport or 'pump' mechanisms*. In this form of transport not only is a specific carrier required but at the same time energy must be expended and, as a result of cellular metabolic activity, materials can be moved 'uphill', i.e. against a concentration gradient. The energy is provided by ATP and a specific ATPase is required for the process. If this enzyme is blocked or if there is a failure of ATP synthesis, e.g. by the inhibition of oxidative phosphorylation, then active transport is prevented.

The properties of the carriers involved in both active and passive transport suggest that they are proteins. Apart from the fact that no other type of molecule has the necessary ability for specific recognition of the substance to be carried, carrier-mediated transport mechanisms show features that are reminiscent of enzyme catalysis, i.e. they are pH dependent, can be competitively inhibited by structurally similar compounds and poisoned by other compounds. Moreover, they show a relationship to the concentration of transported material that is essentially similar to that of substrate concentration on enzyme activity. It appears therefore that passive carrier-mediated transport may be a catalysed permeability in which the equilibrium of the reaction is not affected although the rate of attainment of equilibrium is greatly enhanced while in the case of active transport, there is a modification of the diffusion equilibrium as a result of the coupling of the transport process to an energy-yielding reaction.

All cells have certain carrier-mediated directionally specific transport systems located within their membranes. Some of the transport proteins responsible for the process carry a single solute from one side of the membrane to the other, while others function as co-transport systems in which the carriage of one substance is obligatorily linked with the carriage of another either in

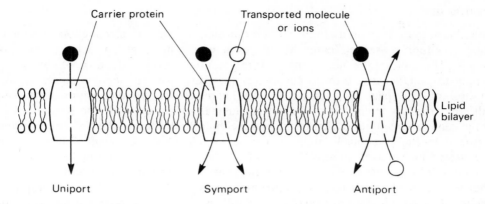

Figure 15.5 Diagram of different types of membrane transport system

the same (*symport*) or in the opposite (*antiport*) direction (Figure 15.5). The mechanisms are highly specific and directional transport is possible because the transport proteins are specifically orientated within the membrane.

If the penetrant is assumed to react with the 'active site' of an asymmetrical carrier which is specifically orientated, then the penetrant will also become specifically orientated and the reaction is given a directional or vectorial quality that is not possible when molecules are free in solution. Since the membrane is extremely thin, a reversible conformational change such as that illustrated in Figure 15.6 might be sufficient to account for the slight movement required to carry the penetrant across the membrane. In these '*gated pores*' the pores are substrate-conducting channels formed by the amino acid residues in the central core of a cluster of transmembrane α-helices such as that shown in Figure 15.4b. Although it is known that a 'gate' in such proteins provides specificity for the substrate being transported, as well as providing for unidirectional transport, it is not yet known how, in molecular terms, any of these transporters work.

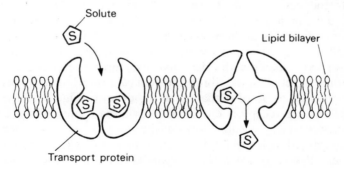

Figure 15.6 Suggested conformational change mechanism for the operation of transport proteins

Amino acids, glucose and certain other sugars are taken up by carrier-mediated mechanisms which may be either passive or active according to the type of cell. Active transport processes are particularly highly developed in the cells of the intestinal mucosa and kidney tubules which are specialized for the absorption of material and its transport across the cell. Most other types of cell, e.g. liver, muscle and erythrocytes, take up glucose and amino acids by facilitated diffusion rather than by active transport.

Ion transporters

Cell membranes also contain a number of *ion transporters* and the selective ionic permeability resulting from their presence creates differences in ionic concentration on the two sides of the membrane. This enables the membrane to store potential energy in the form of ionic gradients which may be used for active transport processes, the transmission of nerve impulses and also for the synthesis of ATP (page 221). It is well known that the electrolyte composition of intracellular fluid differs strikingly from that of the extracellular fluid; for example the K^+ concentration inside the cell is about 40 times that of the extracellular fluid whereas the Na^+ concentration of the extracellular fluid is about 12 times that inside the cell. This is the result of the presence of a *sodium pump* which actively pumps Na^+ out of the cell and K^+ in. The pump has been found to be an ATPase which consists of a transmembrane catalytic subunit of the type described above, together with a smaller associated glycoprotein of unknown function. The sodium pump not only maintains the ionic composition of the cell but also its volume and membrane potential. It can also drive the active transport of sugars and amino acids (page 213). The importance of the pump is indicated by the fact that it uses a large part of the cell's total energy output. In nerve cells the Na^+ channels are voltage gated, i.e. they open and close in response to changes in voltage across the membrane making the cells electrically excitable and enabling them to conduct axon potentials.

In addition to the sodium pump, there is a calcium pump which plays an important part in the regulation of muscular contraction. Calcium ions released during the passage of an impulse act as an intermediary between the nerve and the muscle. Although there is no doubt that these cations are actively transported, the concentrations of Cl^- and HCO_3^- within the cell seem to depend on ordinary electrochemical phenomena.

Endocytosis

Cells are able to ingest certain substances of low solubility as well as specific macromolecules by the process of endocytosis. This involves invagination of the plasma membrane and the formation of membrane-bound vesicles. This ensures that the material being ingested does not mix randomly with other cell constituents. Instead the membrane of the vesicle fuses with that of other organelles and the material is carried to the appropriate cell compartment (Figure 15.7).

In the process of endocytosis the substance to be ingested must be recognized by a specific receptor on the cell surface. Most eukaryotic cells possess specialized pits or vesicles which, because they appear to be coated with bristle-like structures, are known as *coated pits*. These contain several proteins including the fibrous protein *clathrin* which is highly conserved (page 67) and therefore thought to be of fundamental importance (Figure 15.3a). Substances that bind to specific cell-surface receptors enter the cell via the coated pits at a rapid rate. They include certain hormones, e.g. insulin, low-density lipoproteins, cholesterol and iron. The process may be considered as a specialized form of *pinocytosis* (cell drinking) in which fluid droplets are ingested. *Receptor-mediated endocytosis* occurs rapidly and allows cells to take in large amounts of specific ligands without simultaneously taking up fluid.

Exocytosis

A process that may, in many respects, be regarded as the reverse of endocytosis occurs when substances are released from the cell. This is known as *exocytosis* and is used when substances are secreted. Under appropriate conditions the membrane-bound secretory granules and/or lysosomes (page 203) work their way through the cytosol to the cell surface, their surrounding

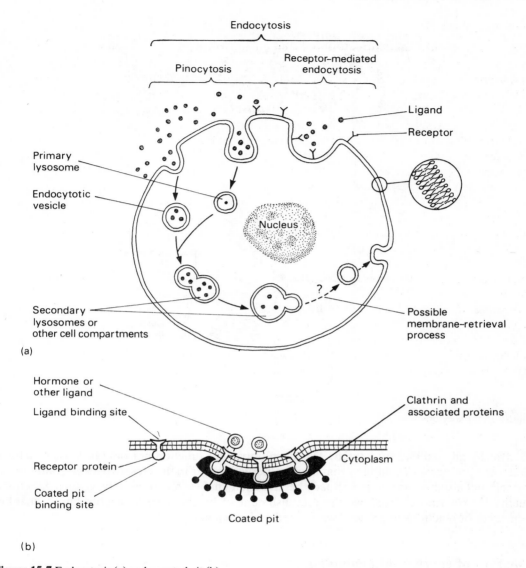

Figure 15.7 Endocytosis (a) and a coated pit (b)

membrane fuses with the plasma membrane and their contents are released to the exterior (Figure 15.8). During secretion large amounts of vesicular membrane components may be introduced into the plasma membrane. Since the area of the cell surface remains more or less constant a corresponding amount of constituents must be removed by endocytosis or some other process. Thus it appears that there is a continuous recycling of membrane components but it is not known how it is regulated.

Membranes as supporting structures

In addition to acting as containers of cell constituents and to controlling the flow of materials in and out of cells, membranes provide surfaces on which enzymes and coenzymes may be

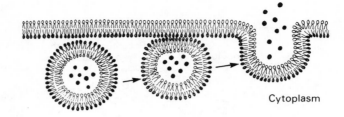

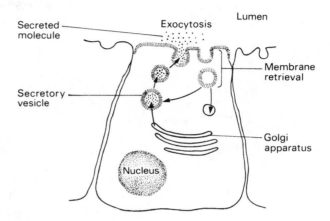

Figure 15.8 Exocytosis

specifically aligned and orientated. This is an important function not only because it helps to overcome problems of solubility that might otherwise occur in the closely packed conditions of the cell, but also because, as has already been seen, it enables reactions to be given a directional quality. Furthermore, it allows the establishment of biochemical 'assembly lines', enabling sequences of reactions to proceed with speed and efficiency.

The flow of energy: mitochondria

Although many of the reactions by which substances are broken down into smaller fragments occur in the cytoplasm and some of them result in the production of ATP, the terminal stages of catabolism, including the major oxidative reactions that produce about 95% of the total ATP, occur in the mitochondria. The mitochondria are small organelles that are frequently rod-shaped and about the same size as many bacteria, e.g. in liver cells they are about 2–3 μm long and about 1 μm in diameter. The number varies from 10 to 20 in some microorganisms to 100 000 or more in very large cells; a mammalian liver cell contains about 1000.

Mitochondria are enclosed by a double membrane; the outer membrane is smooth and permeable to substances of 1000 daltons or less but the inner one is highly specialized and has a series of shelf-like foldings known as *cristae* which greatly increase its surface area. The double membrane surrounds a semi-fluid matrix (Figure 15.9). Isolated mitochondria can operate as completely independent units and are able to oxidize intermediary metabolites such as pyruvate

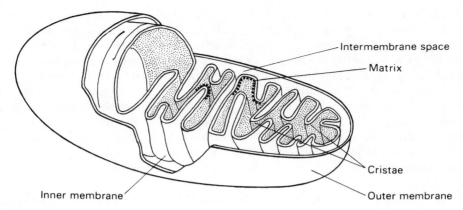

Figure 15.9 A mitochondrion

to CO_2 and H_2O while at the same time converting ADP to ATP. By the action of *pyruvate dehydrogenase* (page 232) the pyruvate is converted into aceyl-CoA which is then caught up into the reactions of the *citrate cycle* and the *respiratory chain* all of which take place within the mitochondria.

It has been established that whereas the enzymes and coenzymes of the citrate cycle are present in the mitochondrial matrix, pyruvate dehydrogenase and the enzymes and coenzymes of the respiratory chain are built into the inner mitochondrial membrane. Functioning of the respiratory chain is accompanied by changes in the permeability and dimensions of the membrane showing once again the closeness of the relationship between structure and function at the subcellular level.

New mitochondria, like chloroplasts in plant cells, arise by growth and division. Mitochondria possess their own DNA in the form of a small circular molecule which is able to (a) replicate, (b) be transcribed into RNA and (c) code for the synthesis of some of the mitochondrial proteins. Many of these are, however, encoded in the nuclear DNA and must be obtained via the cytoplasm. Mitochondria are now regarded as semi-autonomous entities which, while not entirely independent of nuclear genes, are able to replicate themselves by binary fission. This is of considerable interest in view of the hypothesis that mitochondria evolved from bacterial ancestors which, after entering the host cell, established a functional symbiotic relationship with it.

A further interesting feature of mitochondria is that their protein-translating system shows certain fundamental differences from those of bacteria and eukaryotes. Thus it operates with only 22 types of transfer RNA instead of 31 or more and four of the 64 codons have different meanings from those of the 'Universal' code (page 301).

The flow of information

The protein-synthesizing apparatus

Every living cell contains a set of instructions that dictates the amino acid composition of its proteins and is responsible for programming its development and structural organization. These instructions are readily passed from one generation of cells to another and are only modified in exceptional circumstances. The instructions are coded in molecules of deoxyribonucleic acid (DNA) which constitute the *genome* (defined as a complete set of hereditary factors). In eukaryotic cells this is made up of pairs of genes of many different sorts. A *gene* may be defined as a unit of heredity or, in biochemical terms, as a segment of DNA which specifies the sequence of amino acids in a particular type of polypeptide chain. (A few genes which code for ribosomal RNA and the various transfer RNAs are not translated into terms of polypeptides.) The DNA is located in the *chromatin* of the nucleus. In the resting nucleus it takes the form of a meshwork of long slender threads, but during nuclear division these threads condense to form the *chromosomes*. In the chromosomes the DNA is combined as a nucleohistone complex (page 312). Small amounts of acidic proteins and ribonucleic acid are also present.

As well as containing virtually all the DNA of the cell, the nucleus possesses the enzyme systems that are necessary for the synthesis of both DNA and RNA. It also contains a small highly refringent body or *nucleolus* which is particularly concerned with the synthesis of ribosomal RNA.

The nuclear DNA has two functions. Firstly, it must be able to replicate in order that when a cell divides each daughter cell may have a complete set of hereditary instructions. Secondly, it must be able to transmit to the protein-synthesizing machinery present in the cytoplasm information which will enable that machinery to synthesize particular proteins at the time and in the amounts required. For this purpose, constant two-way communication between the nucleus and the cytoplasm is essential. The DNA is confined to the nucleus but instructions are transmitted to the cytoplasm in the form of an RNA transcript of the gene or genes which is known as *messenger RNA*. This becomes attached to the ribosomes, which proceed to translate the coded instructions and string amino acids together to form the polypeptide, the sequence of which is prescribed by the RNA (page 299).

The flow of information within a cell can be summarized in general terms as follows:

$$\text{Replication} \; \overset{\frown}{\underset{\smile}{\text{DNA}}} \xrightarrow{\text{Transcription}} \text{RNA} \xrightarrow{\text{Translation}} \text{Protein}$$

This represents what Crick has called the 'central dogma' of molecular genetics.

As mentioned earlier, ribosomes may either be free in the cytoplasm or attached to the endoplasmic reticulum. If the protein to be synthesized is for export from the cell (e.g. a digestive enzyme produced by an acinar cell of the pancreas), it is synthesized by ribosomes attached to the endoplasmic reticulum and passes directly across the membrane of the endoplasmic reticulum into the cisternae formed by the membrane system which are in communication with the exterior of the cell. On the other hand, if the protein is to be retained within the cell it is synthesized by the ribosomes which lie free in the cytoplasm.

Many, if not most, of the proteins secreted by cells are glycoproteins and recent evidence suggests that the Golgi apparatus (see below) may be responsible for adding the carbohydrate moiety to the newly synthesized polypeptide chains. It may also be responsible for packaging the secretory proteins into membrane-bound vesicles or *secretion granules*.

In spite of the fact that in any differentiated cell many of the genes appear to be completely non-functional, all nuclei are equipotential. This was shown by some illuminating experiments carried out by Gurdon and his colleagues in 1966. They destroyed the nucleus of frogs ova by ultraviolet irradiation and introduced in its place a nucleus removed by microdissection from the columnar epithelium of the intestine of the same species (i.e. a diploid nucleus from a differentiated cell). Subsequently a number of these experimentally treated ova developed into normal adult frogs, some of which were shown to be fertile.

This experiment demonstrated that, during differentiation, the nuclei of the intestinal epithelial cells had retained their full complement of genes; thus even in specialized cells, in which some genes are expressed and others suppressed, there is no irreversible loss or inactivation of genes. Nevertheless, once a cell has become structurally and functionally specialized, its pattern of gene expression and suppression is normally retained in all its progeny. This points to a close and continuous functional interaction of nucleus and cytoplasm in every cell and the establishment of a permanent pattern of interactions, which is characteristic for each type of specialized cell.

These experiments were some of the first to point to the possibility of producing *clones* or carbon copy offspring of prize bulls, racehorses or even human beings. The necessary provisions are that

1. viable ova should be available;
2. techniques of nuclear transplantation which have been developed for amphibian eggs can be extended to the much smaller eggs of mammals;
3. after the nuclear transplants have been made, the modified ova can be successfully implanted into a corresponding mammalian uterus or reared *in vitro*.

Whether it is desirable or not, sooner or later it will almost certainly be done, at least with animals.

The Golgi apparatus

This is a system of flattened smooth-surfaced membranous sacs which lie stacked on top of one another near the nucleus. While the cisternae of the endoplasmic reticulum are thought to be connected together to form a single much folded sac, the Golgi apparatus is believed to consist of a number of discrete sets of cisternae. Not only does the Golgi apparatus modify the macromolecules which pass through it, e.g. by glycosylation and selective protein cleavage, it also concentrates them and packages those which are to be exported from the cell into membrane-bound secretory granules. It also somehow directs the various products to the appropriate site within the cell.

Other cell components

Lysosomes

Lysosomes are small bodies bounded by a single membrane that are formed by budding from the Golgi apparatus and contain a variety of hydrolytic enzymes. They play a role in intracellular digestion which may be either beneficial or detrimental to the cell. They are responsible for the destruction of worn-out portions of the cytoplasm or damaged organelles, which they remove by *autophagic digestion*. The damaged area is enclosed by a membrane which fuses with the lysosomal membrane so that it is then exposed to the hydrolytic enzymes, which proceed to destroy it. If, for any reason, instead of coalescing with another membrane, the lysosomal membrane ruptures and its contents are liberated into the cytoplasm, the whole cell may be digested. Thus it can be seen that lysosomes are potentially very dangerous and that the integrity of their membranes is of crucial importance.

Lysosomes may also be responsible for the digestion of extracellular material which may occur in two ways. In the first the material is ingested by phagocytosis or pinocytosis and an intracellular vesicle is formed. The membrane of the vesicle then fuses with that of a lysosome whose digestive enzymes convert the vesicular contents into smaller soluble products, which can diffuse through the membrane into the cytoplasm. Some indigestible material may remain in so-called *residual bodies*. Alternatively the lysosome may move to the surface of the cell where its membrane coalesces with the external cell membrane. The hydrolases are then discharged from the cell by this process of exocytosis and digestion of extracellular material will occur. This is the method used in the remodelling of bone by osteoclasts in the growing skeleton and in the resorption of tadpole tails and the disposal of damaged or senescent cells.

Although cell death and removal occur at all phases of life, pathological conditions may result if this process becomes uncontrolled; for example, in some cases, inflammation of the joints is believed to be the result of abnormal fragility of lysosomal membranes. Certain agents including vitamins A and D can decrease the stability of lysosomal membranes and, in excess, may act as *teratogens* disturbing the normal sequence of development and causing congenital defects. On the other hand, cortisone and the antimalarial drug chloroquine act as lysosome stabilizers.

A number of inherited disorders are known in which the lysosomes lack a specific hydrolase. As a result there is a massive accumulation of the substrate of the missing enzyme within them. This occurs in *Hurler's disease* in which an enzyme needed for the breakdown of glycosamino-glycans is missing and various complications, including bone deformities, occur.

Peroxisomes

These are small vesicles which are present in almost all eukaryotic cells. They contain a variety of oxidative enzymes and are a major site of O_2 utilization. Although hydrogen peroxide is produced, this is prevented from accumulating because catalase is present. Peroxisomes are believed to play an important part in detoxication reactions in the liver and kidney, e.g. in the conversion of alcohol to acetaldehyde.

The cytosol

This represents the ground substance or soluble fraction of the cell, formerly known as the cell sap. It contains a variety of enzymes including those of the glycolytic and pentose phosphate pathways and also transaminases, aminoacyl and fatty acyl-CoA synthetases and acetyl-CoA carboxylase.

One of the most characteristic properties of the cytosol is its ability to undergo sol–gel transformation. Calcium ions are necessary for maintaining the gel condition and liquefaction occurs in their absence.

Recently small fibrils known as *microtubules* have been shown to be present in the cytoplasm. During nuclear division these aggregate in parallel bundles radiating from the centriole and form the spindle fibres. Microtubules have also been isolated from cilia and flagella. They are composed of globular units having a molecular weight of 60 000 and an amino acid composition which resembles that of the muscle protein actin.

The cell surface

It is not always easy to determine whether material present on the surface of a cell is part of the membrane structure or merely associated material adsorbed on its surface. There is no doubt that many antigenic substances are present. These include the *blood group substances* that have been found to be glycoproteins containing carbohydrate and polypeptides and usually including sialic acid. Those antigens that are responsible for transplantation immunity and the rejection of foreign tissues are also associated with the cell surface. The remarkable specificity of the surface antigens is apparent when it is considered that immunologically detectable differences occur not only between those of cells of different species but also between those of different individuals of the same species and sometimes also between those of different organs in the same individual.

At physiological pH values all cells so far examined have a negative surface charge which causes them to move if an electric field is applied to a cell suspension. The charge appears to result largely from the presence of sialic acid residues, since it is greatly reduced if the cells are treated with the enzyme *neuraminidase*, which removes them. Tumour cells frequently carry an increased surface charge; for example, in leukaemia the normal myeloid cells are replaced by cells with a higher motility. This may be a general characteristic of malignant cells, an increased concentration of sialic acid on the surface reducing their adhesiveness and preventing them from making normal cell contacts. When two normal cells come into contact they react by ceasing to move and in some cases also by ceasing to divide, a phenomenon known as *contact inhibition*. The affinity of cells for each other, as shown by contact inhibition, is fairly specific. Thus, if cells of a certain tissue, e.g. liver, are isolated from each other by mild treatment with trypsin to break up the intercellular ground substance, and are then mixed with similarly isolated kidney cells, the two types of cell separate out, the liver cells aggregating with other liver cells and the kidney cells with other kidney cells. Hybrid aggregates do not occur. If, however, the experiment is repeated using cancer cells the ordinary cellular affinities are not apparent and mixed aggregates of, for example, normal kidney cells and malignant skin cancer cells have been found to result. Loss of normal cellular affinities may account for the way in which malignant cells invade a variety of normal tissues causing secondary growths.

Bacterial cells

Bacteria are prokaryotes and their cellular organization is much simpler than that of eukaryotic cells. They are spherical or rod-shaped and often possess a tough protective coat or cell wall. The only membrane that bacterial cells possess is the outer cell membrane or plasma membrane; they have no proper nucleus or other membrane-bound organelles, such as mitochondria. Instead of a nucleus they possess a single chromosome consisting of a circular molecule of double-stranded DNA. Bacteria normally reproduce by an asexual process in which the daughter cells each receive a genome which is identical with that of the parent cell. Their ribosomes are appreciably smaller than those of eukaryotes.

Bacterial cell walls

The outer cell wall which protects the delicate cell membrane also provides mechanical support and gives bacteria their characteristic shape. It has a *peptidoglycan* structure being made up of long polysaccharide chains which are linked together by short polypeptide chains to form a mesh-like bag which completely surrounds the organism. The unbranched polysaccharide chains consist of alternating *N*-acetyl-D-glucosamine and *N*-acetylmuramic acid units which are linked by β-1 : 4-glycosidic bonds. Each *N*-acetylmuramic acid unit has a small tetrapeptide attachment which is cross-linked via a pentapeptide unit to a neighbouring *N*-acetylmuramic acid unit (Figure 15.10). The amino acid residues of the pentapeptide differ from species to species.

In Gram-positive bacteria, so-called because they stain deeply with Crystal Violet (the Gram stain), the wall is composed of peptidoglycan together with a sugar phosphate compound, *teichoic acid*. In Gram-negative bacteria, which do not stain in this way, the peptidoglycan is covered by a complex layer of protein, lipid and lipopolysaccharide. Some antibiotics act by interfering with the synthesis of the bacterial cell wall, e.g. *penicillin* and *cephalosporin* inhibit the enzyme responsible for cross-linking the peptidoglycan strands.

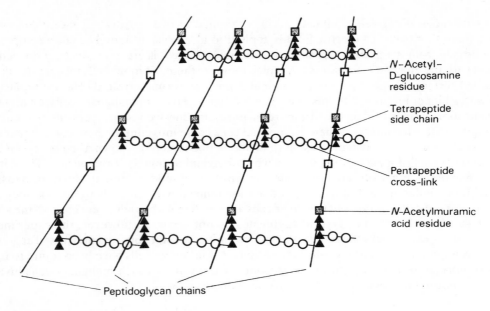

N–Acetyl–D-glucosamine residue

Tetrapeptide side chain

Pentapeptide cross-link

N–Acetylmuramic acid residue

Peptidoglycan chains

Figure 15.10 A bacterial cell-wall peptidoglycan

Viruses

Viruses are nucleoprotein particles that are much smaller than bacteria and cannot be classed as living organisms. They are, however, extremely important not only because they are implicated in a wide range of human and plant disease but also because they are used extensively for research in molecular biology.

Viruses act as self-reproducing intracellular parasites. Although they have no metabolic machinery of their own and are unable to generate ATP or synthesize proteins, they are able to penetrate living cells and put the cell's metabolic machinery to their own use, causing it to manufacture new virus particles instead of normal cell products. Viruses contain either DNA or RNA but not usually both. The nucleic acid that carries the information that instructs the host cell to produce new virus particles is enclosed by a protein coat which protects it from mechanical breakage and enzymic attack. The coat also determines the specificity of the virus, i.e. the nature of the cell that the virus can infect. Bacteria may be infected by viruses known as *bacteriophages*.

The viruses range from very simple forms containing only three genes to others that may contain as many as 250 genes. Among the viruses that have been most extensively studied are the RNA-containing *tobacco mosaic virus* (TMV), which is a relatively simple plant virus, and the more complex *T-4 bacteriophage*, which contains double-stranded DNA and attacks *Escherichia coli*, a small bacterium normally resident in the lower reaches of the gastrointestinal tract. It is not usually pathogenic and is readily grown under laboratory conditions. Another virus that has received considerable attention is bacteriophage ϕX 174 which contains single-stranded DNA.

Lysogeny

Not all viruses are so virulent that they kill the infected cell. The so-called 'temperate' viruses may enter a cell and exist in a latent state in which their genome remains inactive and no progeny is produced. The integration of the nucleic acid of a bacteriophage with that of the host is known as *lysogeny*. After they have become incorporated in this way, the phage genes are inherited together with those of the host in the form of *prophage*.

Most of the prophage genes are repressed and their lytic functions remain dormant, but certain agents that interfere with DNA replication in the host may, at a later date, cause the viral DNA to be excised from the bacterial chromosome. It can then become virulent, reproduce and cause lysis of the cell.

Lysogeny allows temperate viruses to survive and replicate within a limited population of cells that are protected from further infection. On the other hand, the survival of virulent bacteriophages depends on the continuous availability of susceptible bacteria, e.g. in sewage.

The use of microorganisms in biochemical research

Owing to the fact that the major metabolic pathways are common to most, if not all, living forms, microorganisms are widely used in biochemical research. The use of bacteria and viruses has many advantages since

1. their organization is relatively simple;
2. they provide uniform populations which are free from the complications that result from the interaction of cells of different types;
3. they are easily grown in cultures;
4. they reproduce rapidly;
5. they normally reproduce by an asexual process and are nearly always in a haploid state so that problems of dominance and recessiveness, which complicate studies of inheritance on diploid cells, are avoided;
6. they can be induced to mutate to give abnormal forms with which the normal form can be compared.

It is easy to assume that this basic biochemical unity extends further than it actually does and care must be taken not to make unwarranted extrapolations from microorganisms to higher organisms since major differences obviously exist.

Chapter 16
Bioenergetics

The properties of enzymes as catalysts for chemical reactions were considered in Chapter 6. This chapter now considers some of the associated energetic aspects of enzyme reactions in the cell.

Chemical equilibria

Considering the reaction:

$$A + B \rightleftharpoons C + D$$

if solutions of A and B are mixed and an appropriate enzyme is added C and D will be formed. Once this happens the back reaction will also take place with the re-conversion of $C + D$ to $A + B$. Net production of C and D proceeds until the concentrations of substrates and products have adjusted to values where the rate of the back reaction is equal to the rate of the forward reaction. At this point, there will be no further net formation of products and the reaction is said to have attained equilibrium.

The relative concentrations of reactants and products for a particular reaction at equilibrium is characteristic of that reaction and is defined by the *equilibrium constant* (K_{eq}). This is the product of the concentrations of products formed at equilibrium divided by the concentration of reactants remaining. Thus for the reaction given above:

$$K_{eq} = \frac{[C] \times [D]}{[A] \times [B]}$$

Reactions have widely differing values of K_{eq}. Where K_{eq} is very large, the reaction proceeds until virtually all the initial reactants have been converted to products. Such reactions are described as irreversible or effectively irreversible. Where K_{eq} is very small, equilibrium is reached when only a small proportion of the initial reactants have been converted to products. Finally, for reactants with a value of K_{eq} near to 1, the reactants and products are present in nearly equal proportions at equilibrium and the reaction will proceed in either direction depending on the initial concentration of products and reactants.

Biochemists find it useful to employ a thermodynamic function termed *Gibbs free energy* (abbreviated to free energy or the symbol G) in the consideration of enzyme reactions. For present purposes, the free energy of a system may be described as the potential of that system for doing work at constant temperature and pressure. The free energy of a system is not measurable, but the *free energy change (ΔG)* which occurs during the conversion of substrate to products in an enzyme reaction can be quantified. The free energy change which occurs during a reaction is characteristic of that reaction if the reactants and products are initially present at standard concentrations. This *standard free energy change (ΔG^0)* is defined as the free energy change which occurs when both substrate(s) and products(s) are initially present at a concentration of 1 M, and 1 mol of reactant is converted to 1 mol of product.

The standard free energy change of a reaction is related to the equilibrium constant as follows:

$$\Delta G^0 = -\boldsymbol{R}T \ln K_{eq}$$

where $\boldsymbol{R}$ is the gas constant and T is the absolute temperature.

Many reactions involve the production or removal of hydrogen ions. For this reason it is convenient to redefine the standard state to be at pH 7 rather than at pH 0 (i.e. 1 M H^+). The standard free energy change at pH 7 is written $\Delta G^{0'}$ and is related to the equilibrium constant at pH 7 (K_{eq}') by the equation:

$$\Delta G^{0'} = -\boldsymbol{R}T \ln K_{eq}'$$

Thus reactions with a high value of K_{eq}' have a large negative standard free energy change, while reactions with a low K_{eq}' have a large positive $\Delta G^{0'}$. For reactions with K_{eq}' near 1, the standard free energy change is near zero. Values of K_{eq}' together with the corresponding values of $\Delta G^{0'}$ are given in Table 16.1.

Table 16.1 The numerical relationship between K_{eq} and ΔG^0 at 25 °C

K_{eq}'	ΔG^0 (kJ mol^{-1})	
0·001	17·2	⎫
0·01	11·5	⎬ Endergonic
0·1	5·7	⎭
1·0	0	
10·0	−5·7	⎫ Exergonic
100·0	−11·5	⎬ (spontaneous)
1000·0	−17·2	⎭

Reactions will proceed only if the change in free energy, ΔG, is negative. The magnitude of the actual free energy change that occurs during a reaction is a function of the standard free energy change characteristic of that reaction and also of the initial concentrations of reactants and products:

$$\Delta G = \Delta G^{0'} + \boldsymbol{R}T \ln \frac{[\text{C}] \times [\text{D}]}{[\text{A}] \times [\text{B}]}$$

where [A], [B], [C] and [D] are the initial concentrations of reactants and products in the system. If the reactants and products are initially present at their equilibrium concentrations then the above equation reduces to $\Delta G = 0$ and no energy can be obtained from the system.

For reactions with a large negative $\Delta G^{0'}$, ΔG will always be negative and hence the reaction always proceeds in the forward direction unless the initial concentration ratio of products to reactants is extremely high. Where $\Delta G^{0'}$ is near zero, the sign of ΔG will depend on the initial concentration of products and reactants and the reaction can be made to proceed in either direction by manipulation of these concentrations. If, however, $\Delta G^{0'}$ is large and positive, ΔG will also be positive and such a reaction will not proceed. It is, however, often possible to couple a reaction with a positive free energy change to another with a numerically larger negative free energy change. Since free energy changes are additive, the combined overall reaction will have a negative free energy change and will then proceed.

It should be recalled at this point that enzymes alter the rate at which a reaction occurs, but do not affect the position of equilibrium. Enzymes likewise have no effect on the free energy change of a reaction or on the direction in which a reaction will proceed.

ATP (adenosine triphosphate)

ATP occurs in all cells and is a universal intermediate in cell energy metabolism. The structure of ATP is shown below. The base adenine is joined to C-1' of ribose, the 5' position of which is linked to a phosphate residue to form *adenosine monophosphate* (AMP). Addition of a second

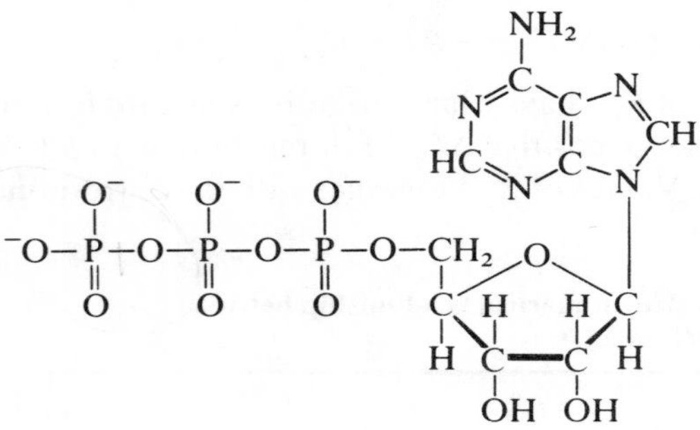

phosphate group to the first via an anhydride bond gives the compound *adenosine diphosphate* (ADP) while ATP is derived by the addition of a further phosphate again via an anhydride linkage. At pH 7·4 ATP bears four negative charges and forms a stable complex with Mg^{2+} ions.

ATP can be hydrolysed enzymically to ADP and inorganic phosphate:

$$ATP^{4-} + H_2O \rightleftharpoons ADP^{3-} + phosphate^{2-} + H^+$$

The standard free energy change ($\Delta G^{0'}$) of this reaction is approximately $-30\ \text{kJ mol}^{-1}$ and this is high relative to many other hydrolysis reactions (Table 16.2). The high standard free energy of

Table 16.2 The standard free energy change ($\Delta G^{0'}$) of hydrolysis of some phosphate-containing compounds

Compound	$\Delta G^{0'}$ (kJ mol^{-1})
Phosphoenolpyruvate	$-53\cdot5$
1,3-Diphosphoglycerate	$-49\cdot5$
Phosphocreatine	$-44\cdot0$
ATP	$-29\cdot4$
Glucose 1-phosphate	$-21\cdot0$
Fructose 6-phosphate	$-16\cdot0$
Glucose 6-phosphate	$-13\cdot8$
3-Phosphoglycerate	$-13\cdot0$
Glycerol 1-phosphate	$-9\cdot6$

hydrolysis of ATP arises in part from the fact that the products of the reaction, ADP and phosphate, both carry negative charges and hence tend to repel each other. Hydrolysis of the terminal phosphate–phosphate bond of ATP can be regarded as relieving some of the intramolecular strain caused by the presence of neighbouring negatively charged groups in the molecule.

ATP can also undergo hydrolysis as follows:

$$ATP \rightleftharpoons AMP + pyrophosphate$$

The value of $\Delta G^{0'}$ for this reaction is also $-30\,\text{kJ mol}^{-1}$. Where this reaction occurs, the pyrophosphate is rapidly hydrolysed to phosphate by the enzyme *pyrophosphatase*:

$$Pyrophosphate + H_2O \rightarrow 2\ phosphate \quad \Delta G^{0'} = -30 \text{ kJ mol}^{-1}$$

The overall effect of the combined reactions is the hydrolysis of the two terminal phosphate–phosphate bonds of ATP with the formation of AMP and two phosphate molecules. The value of $\Delta G^{0'}$ for the overall reaction is then -60 kJ mol^{-1}.

The other nucleoside triphosphates UTP, CTP and GTP are also involved in certain biosynthetic reactions. These triphosphates are regenerated by transfer of the terminal phosphate group from ATP by the following transferase reactions:

$$ATP + GDP \rightleftharpoons ADP + GTP$$
$$ATP + UDP \rightleftharpoons ADP + UTP$$
$$ATP + CDP \rightleftharpoons ADP + CTP$$

The value of $\Delta G^{0'}$ is approximately zero, i.e. the values of $\Delta G^{0'}$ for hydrolysis for all the nucleoside triphosphates are similar so that the direction of the reaction depends on the relative concentrations of the reactants.

Since the hydrolysis of the terminal phosphate bond of ATP proceeds with a large negative standard free energy change, ATP is sometimes referred to as a *high-energy compound*, or, in older texts, as possessing *high-energy bonds*. It is important to realize that the function of ATP as an intermediate in energy metabolism depends on the fact that the value of ΔG for ATP hydrolysis at the concentrations of ATP, ADP and phosphate present in the cell, is large and negative, and this is the only sense in which the 'high energy' terminology should be understood. For example consider conditions under which ATP, ADP and phosphate are mixed at their equilibrium concentrations. Then the value of ΔG is zero and no energy could be obtained from the system, although ATP is still present.

The ATP/ADP cycle

In the cell, ATP can be regarded as undergoing a continuous cycle of breakdown and resynthesis:

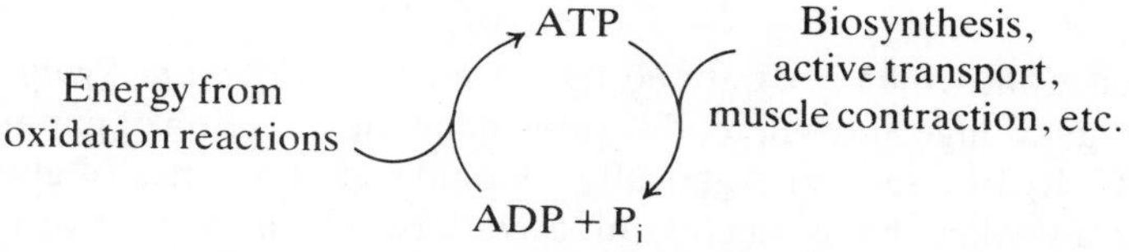

The free energy released by the hydrolysis of ATP is used to drive biosynthetic reactions and also to drive the active transport of metabolites across cell plasma membranes and the membranes of intracellular organelles. In some cells ATP is used for specialized purposes as in the case of muscle contraction. During these reactions ADP and phosphate are produced. In animal cells the ATP is resynthesized from ADP and phosphate by the process of *oxidative phosphorylation* which occurs in the mitochondria; this uses the free energy released by the oxidation of nutrients to drive the ATP hydrolysis reaction in reverse. Bacteria synthesize ATP by a similar process of oxidative phosphorylation. In plant cells the energy for ATP synthesis comes from the absorption of light and the process is termed *photosynthetic phosphorylation*.

ATP turns over rapidly in the cell although the total pool of adenine nucleotides (ATP + ADP + AMP) remains relatively constant. ATP can thus be regarded as an intermediate in the transfer of free energy from substrate oxidation to energy-utilizing processes. It is able to fulfil this role because, while the ΔG for ATP hydrolysis in the cell is high enough to drive synthetic reactions, it is also low enough to allow the hydrolytic reaction to be reversed by the input of free energy from oxidative reactions.

A number of other phosphate-containing compounds have standard free energy changes of hydrolysis even greater than that of ATP (Table 16.2). Reactions in which such molecules transfer their terminal phosphate groups to ADP to form ATP are therefore energetically favourable. ATP can be formed in this way from ADP plus phosphoenolpyruvate (page 229), ADP plus creatine phosphate (page 331) and ADP plus 1,3-diphosphoglycerate (page 228). All these are important so-called *substrate level phosphorylation reactions* although far more ATP is synthesized by oxidative phosphorylation and the respiratory chain.

Utilization of ATP

Biosynthetic reactions

Degradative and hydrolytic reactions in general have a large negative value of $\Delta G^{0'}$. Consider for example the hydrolysis of the amino acid glutamine to glutamate and ammonium ions which is catalysed by the enzyme *glutaminase*:

$$\text{Glutamine} \rightleftharpoons \text{glutamate} + \text{NH}_4^+$$

$\Delta G^{0'}$ for this reaction is $-14.3 \text{ kJ mol}^{-1}$, i.e. the equilibrium position of the reaction lies far to the right. From the previous discussion, the value of ΔG for this reaction will be negative at physiological concentrations of glutamine and glutamate and the reaction will proceed in the direction of glutamine hydrolysis.

Under certain conditions it is necessary to synthesize glutamine from glutamate and ammonia. Free energy changes are additive, and glutamine is synthesized by using the free energy of ATP hydrolysis to reverse the glutamine hydrolysis reaction:

$$\text{Glutamate} + \text{NH}_4^+ \rightleftharpoons \text{glutamine} \quad \Delta G^{0'} = +14.3 \text{ kJ mol}^{-1}$$
$$\text{ATP} \rightleftharpoons \text{ADP} + \text{P}_i \quad \Delta G^{0'} = -30 \text{ kJ mol}^{-1}$$

Add these reactions:

$$\text{Glutamate} + \text{NH}_4^+ + \text{ATP} \rightleftharpoons \text{glutamine} + \text{ADP} + \text{P}_i$$
$$\Delta G^{0'} = -15.7 \text{ kJ mol}^{-1}$$

The combined reaction, which is catalysed by the enzyme *glutamine synthase*, has a negative standard free energy change and will readily proceed in the direction of glutamine formation. In this example, ATP hydrolysis is energetically coupled to the reversal of glutamine hydrolysis. However, this must be done by using glutamine synthase which has ATP as one of its substrates instead of glutaminase.

Similarly glucose 6-phosphate, an important intermediate in glucose metabolism, is hydrolysed by the enzyme *glucose 6-phosphatase*:

$$\text{Glucose 6-phosphate} \rightleftharpoons \text{glucose} + \text{P}_i \quad \Delta G^{0'} = -13.8 \text{ kJ mol}^{-1}$$

At physiological concentrations of glucose 6-phosphate, glucose and P_i, ΔG will be negative and the reaction will proceed in the direction of glucose 6-phosphate hydrolysis. In other circumstances, however, glucose 6-phosphate is formed and this is in effect a reversal of the hydrolysis of glucose 6-phosphate which depends on the free energy of hydrolysis of ATP:

$$\text{Glucose} + P_i \rightleftharpoons \text{Glucose 6-P} \qquad \Delta G^{0'} = +13\cdot8 \text{ kJ mol}^{-1}$$
$$\text{ATP} \rightleftharpoons \text{ADP} + P_i \qquad \Delta G^{0'} = -30 \text{ kJ mol}^{-1}$$

Add:

$$\text{Glucose} + \text{ATP} \rightleftharpoons \text{Glucose 6-P} + \text{ADP} \qquad \Delta G^{0'} = -16\cdot2 \text{ kJ mol}^{-1}$$

The overall reaction is catalysed by the enzyme *hexokinase* which uses ATP as a cosubstrate. This enables the reaction to proceed since the value of $\Delta G^{0'}$ is relatively large and negative.

A third example of the use of ATP in biosynthesis is the synthesis of sucrose in plants. Sucrose has a relatively high $\Delta G^{0'}$ so that the *sucrase* reaction:

$$\text{Sucrose} \rightleftharpoons \text{glucose} + \text{fructose} \qquad \Delta G^{0'} = -28 \text{ kJ mol}^{-1}$$

proceeds in the direction of sucrose hydrolysis. For the synthesis of sucrose a number of different enzymes are involved and both ATP and UTP are required as substrates. The overall equation for the pathway of sucrose synthesis is:

$$\text{Fructose} + \text{glucose} + 2\text{ATP} + \text{UTP} \rightleftharpoons \text{sucrose} + 2\text{ADP} + \text{UDP} + 3P_i$$

Both ATP and UTP are broken down to provide sufficient energy to reverse the hydrolysis of sucrose.

These examples indicate the general principles of the role of ATP in biosynthetic reactions. An energetically unfavourable reaction is coupled to ATP hydrolysis which provides the energy necessary for its occurrence. This coupling is achieved by enzymes which use ATP as one of their substrates.

Active transport

Another general function of ATP is to provide energy for the transport of certain metabolites across cell membranes. In many cells, glucose and neutral amino acids are accumulated across the cell plasma membrane by specific transport systems so that the internal concentration is higher than the external concentration. This so-called *active transport* requires the input of energy.

The free energy change involved in transporting an uncharged solute such as glucose from an external concentration C_1 to an intracellular concentration C_2 is given by the relationship:

$$\Delta G = RT \ln (C_2/C_1)$$

If C_2 is greater than C_1 then ΔG is positive, and the process will not occur spontaneously. For a tenfold concentration difference the free energy change is $+11\cdot3$ kJ mol^{-1} of glucose transported.

Energy for active transport is again provided by ATP hydrolysis, although the coupling is somewhat indirect. The transport of glucose is linked to the inward transport of sodium ions which are present at a concentration of approximately 150 mM in the plasma but only 5–20 mM in the cell. The Na^+ ion gradient is maintained by the Na^+/K^+-*ATPase* or sodium pump, a membrane-associated enzyme which uses the energy of ATP hydrolysis to pump Na^+ out of the cell against a concentration gradient and at the same time to pump K^+ ions in, also against a gradient (Figure 16.1). In this way Na^+ ion concentration gradients are used to couple the hydrolysis of ATP to the transport of glucose against a gradient. Similar active transport systems exist for neutral amino acids, and these are discussed further in Chapter 19.

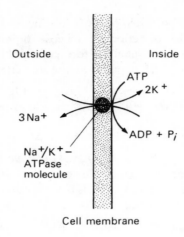

Figure 16.1 The sodium pump

Synthesis of ATP

After discussing the utilization of ATP in the cell it is necessary to consider the other part of the ATP/ADP cycle, i.e. the energetics and mechanism of ATP synthesis. ATP synthesis from ADP and phosphate requires the input of a considerable amount of free energy. Sufficient free energy to reverse ATP hydrolysis may be derived from the oxidation of nutrients such as carbohydrates and fats.

In considering biological oxidation reactions it is necessary first of all to outline the structure and function of *nicotinamide adenine dinucleotide* (NAD) which is the major coenzyme involved in such reactions.

Nicotinamide adenine dinucleotide – structure and function

The structure of the oxidized form of NAD is shown below:

The nicotinamide ring is attached through an *N*-glycosidic linkage to ribose. This ribose is linked via a phosphate group to a second ribose which is linked in turn to adenine. The nicotinamide ring of NAD in the oxidized form bears a positive charge on the nitrogen atom, and oxidized NAD is therefore correctly written as NAD^+.

NAD^+ is a coenzyme for many dehydrogenases. These enzymes catalyse the removal of two hydrogen atoms from their substrates, with the reduction of the NAD^+. The nicotinamide ring takes up one proton and two electrons, the nitrogen atom loses its charge and one proton is released:

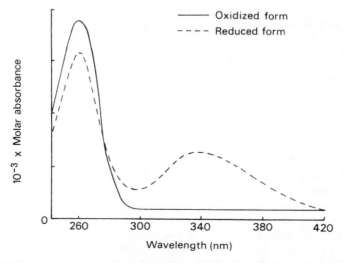

The reduced form of NAD^+ is thus written as NADH and the general dehydrogenase reaction as:

$$SH_2 + NAD^+ \rightleftharpoons S + NADH + H^+$$

where S and SH_2 are the oxidized and reduced forms of the substrate respectively.

The change in structure when NAD^+ is reduced or oxidized is reflected in an alteration of its ultraviolet spectrum. The reduced form has an absorption maximum at 340 nm, while the oxidized form has little absorption at this wavelength (Figure 16.2). This forms the basis for assays of biological oxidation/reduction reactions where alteration in the absorption at 340 nm can be related to changes in the concentration of NADH.

NAD^+ is not the only hydrogen acceptor in cells. Another important compound is *nicotinamide adenine dinucleotide phosphate* ($NADP^+$) which consists of NAD^+ with an additional phosphate group attached to the C-2 position of the ribose linked to the adenine. This compound is oxidized and reduced in exactly the same way as NAD^+. However, whereas NAD^+ is involved mainly in degradative reactions such as the citrate cycle, fatty acid oxidation and

Figure 16.2 Absorption spectra of the oxidized and reduced forms of the nicotinamide adenine nucleotides (NAD and NADP)

glycolysis, $NADP^+$ is important in biosynthetic pathways such as fatty acid and steroid synthesis and the pentose phosphate pathway.

Mitochondrial oxidation of NADH – the respiratory chain

Oxidation of metabolites in the cell leads to the generation of reduced NAD^+ in the mitochondria. The mitochondrial inner membrane contains a series of hydrogen and electron carriers which together constitute *the respiratory chain*. This catalyses the overall reaction:

$$NADH + H^+ + \tfrac{1}{2}O_2 \rightleftharpoons NAD^+ + H_2O$$

A major function of the mitochondria is to couple the free energy released by the oxidation of NADH to the synthesis of ATP from ADP plus inorganic phosphate. This coupled process is known as *oxidative phosphorylation* and is catalysed by a specific ATPase which, like the components of the respiratory chain, is situated in the mitochondrial inner membrane.

The respiratory chain consists of a number of proteins containing specific prosthetic groups which are involved in the linear transfer of electrons or hydrogen atoms from NADH to oxygen. The sequence of reactions is as follows:

NADH is first oxidized to NAD^+ by the enzyme *NADH–ubiquinone reductase*. This enzyme consists of at least 16 polypeptide chains. The electrons obtained from the oxidation of NADH are then transferred to the oxidized form of the prosthetic group of the enzyme which is the compound *flavin mononucleotide* (page 244).

$$NADH + H^+ + FMN \rightleftharpoons NAD^+ + FMNH_2$$

The $FMNH_2$ is reoxidized by the transfer of electrons to further prosthetic groups known as *iron–sulphur* (FeS) *centres*. The iron atom in these complexes alternates between the ferric and ferrous states and is bound to sulphur atoms which may be inorganic or derived from cysteine residues. Such centres are also referred to as *non-haem iron residues*. Since the oxidation of $FMNH_2$ produces H atoms while the FeS centres accept only electrons, $2H^+$ ions are also produced:

$$FMNH_2 + 2FeS(III) \rightleftharpoons FMN + 2FeS(II) + 2H^+$$

The iron–sulphur centres then pass electrons to *ubiquinone* (UQ). Ubiquinone (otherwise known as *Coenzyme Q*) is a substituted quinone which can be readily oxidized and reduced:

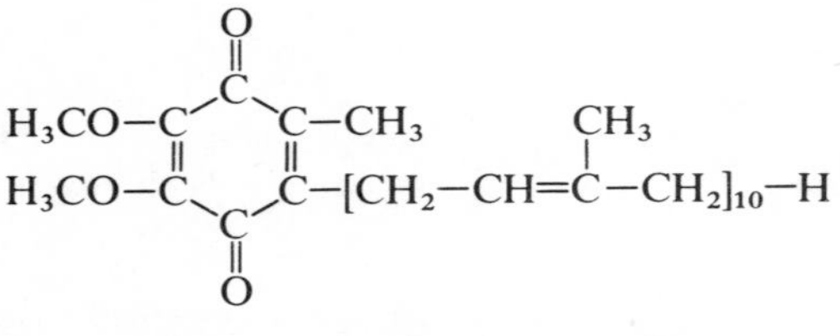

Oxidized form of coenzyme Q 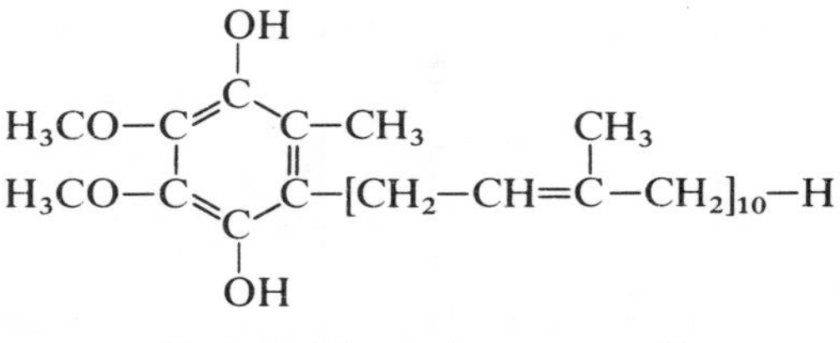   Reduced form of coenzyme Q

Ubiquinone is a hydrogen atom acceptor and $2H^+$ are therefore taken up during its reduction by the reduced iron–sulphur centres:

$$UQ + 2FeS(II) + 2H^+ \rightleftharpoons UQH_2 + 2FeS(III)$$

From ubiquinone to oxygen, electron transfer is effected by the *cytochrome system*. Cytochromes are proteins containing a haem (page 371) prosthetic group, the iron atom in the haem group being alternately oxidized and reduced by the transfer of electrons. Each cytochrome is reduced by the addition of only one electron ($Fe^{3+} \rightarrow Fe^{2+}$). Cytochromes *b*, *c* and c_1 contain the same form of haem as that found in haemoglobin, while cytochromes a and a_3 contain a slightly modified haem. Cytochrome a_3 also contains a copper atom which undergoes oxidation and reduction during electron transfer. The various cytochromes can be distinguished by their different absorption spectra. Electrons from ubiquinone are passed first to cytochrome b, then sequentially to cytochromes c_1, c, and on to an enzyme complex called *cytochrome oxidase* which contains two cytochromes, namely a and a_3. Reduced cytochrome oxidase is reoxidized by molecular oxygen with the formation of water. The reduction of one molecule of oxygen requires four electrons:

$$O_2 + 4e + 4H^+ \rightleftharpoons 2H_2O$$

Although most electrons are fed into the respiratory chain via NAD^+ some dehydrogenases by-pass NAD^+ and feed them in at the level of ubiquinone. The membrane-bound enzyme *succinate dehydrogenase* which catalyses the oxidation of succinate to fumarate in the citrate cycle contains flavin adenine dinucleotide (FAD) (page 244) as its prosthetic group and operates in this way.

The flow of electrons from NADH to oxygen in the respiratory chain can be represented as follows:

$$NADH \rightarrow FMN \rightarrow FeS \rightarrow UQ \rightarrow b \rightarrow c_1 \rightarrow c \rightarrow aa_3 \rightarrow \tfrac{1}{2}O_2$$
$$\uparrow$$
$$\text{Succinate dehydrogenase (FAD)}$$

The respiratory chain can be separated by various techniques into three *multienzyme complexes* (Figure 16.3). Complex I is NADH–ubiquinone reductase. Complex III is known as *ubiquinone–cytochrome c reductase* and contains cytochromes b and c_1. Complex IV is cytochrome oxidase. (Succinate dehydrogenase is referred to as Complex II). Ubiquinone and cytochrome c are small molecules which do not form part of these complexes. Reconstitution of the isolated Complexes I–IV with cytochrome c and ubiquinone leads to recovery of the activity of the respiratory chain.

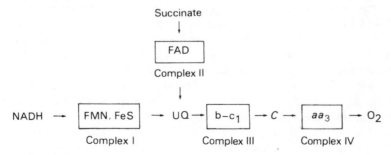

Figure 16.3 The respiratory chain

Certain compounds inhibit the activity of the respiratory chain by blocking the transfer of electrons at certain points. *Rotenone* and *amytal* inhibit electron transfer through Complex I. *Antimycin A* inhibits at the level of Complex III. Cytochrome oxidase activity is inhibited by carbon monoxide, cyanide and hydrogen sulphide. The prevention of electron transport by cyanide which is very rapidly absorbed is responsible for the high toxicity of this compound.

Energetic aspects of NADH oxidation via the respiratory chain

Oxidation/reduction or *redox reactions* such as those described above involve the transfer of an electron or electrons from the reduced form of an electron donor to the oxidized form of an electron acceptor. The oxidized and reduced forms of a compound which undergoes such reactions are called *a redox couple* and each redox couple has a characteristic tendency to donate electrons. This tendency can be quantified by a function called the *standard redox potential* (E_o). This is the electromotive force generated between a solution containing a mixture of the oxidized and reduced forms of the compound, in which each is present at a concentration of 1 M, and a reference solution. The reference taken is a solution containing 1 M hydrogen ions in equilibrium with H_2 gas (the reduced form of H^+) at 1 atm pressure. The redox potential of this reference is defined as zero. Thus, if a compound has a greater tendency to give up electrons than does H_2, it will have a negative standard redox potential while if it has a greater tendency than H_2 to accept electrons, its standard redox potential will be positive.

Table 16.3 Standard oxidation–reduction potentials (E_0') of some reactions

Reduced form	Oxidized form	E_0' (V)
Pyruvate	Acetate + CO_2	−0·70
α-Oxoglutarate	Succinate + CO_2	−0·67
NADH + H^+	NAD^+	−0·32
NADPH + H^+	$NADP^+$	−0·32
Lactate	Pyruvate	−0·19
Malate	Oxaloacetate	−0·17
$FADH_2$-protein	FAD-protein	−0·05
Succinate	Fumarate	+0·03
Ubiquinone-H_2	Ubiquinone	+0·10
Cytochrome b (Fe^{2+})	Cytochrome b (Fe^{3+})	+0·12
Cytochrome c (Fe^{2+})	Cytochrome c (Fe^{3+})	+0·22
Cytochrome a (Fe^{2+})	Cytochrome a (Fe^{3+})	+0·29
H_2O	$\frac{1}{2}O_2 + 2H^+$	+0·82

In the same way as for free energy changes, it is convenient to redefine the standard state to refer to pH 7 and the standard redox potential at pH 7 is written E_o'. The value of E_o' for hydrogen is −0·42 V. Therefore compounds with a lower affinity for electrons than hydrogen have a value of E_o' more negative than −0·42 V while those with a higher affinity for electrons will have a value of E_o' more positive than −0·42 V. The values of E_o' for a number of redox couples are shown in Table 16.3. The standard redox potential for the NADH/NAD couple is −0·32 V, and the E_o' values for the components of the respiratory chain become sequentially more positive. The standard redox potential of the O_2/H_2O couple is +0·82 V.

Any redox reaction can be divided into two partial reactions, each associated with a characteristic standard redox potential. By convention, the oxidized form of the electron acceptor is written on the left, e.g. the overall oxidation of NADH by the respiratory chain can be written:

$$NAD^+ + H^+ + 2e \rightleftharpoons NADH \quad E_o' = -0·32 \text{ V} \tag{16.1}$$

$$\tfrac{1}{2}O_2 + 2H^+ + 2e \rightleftharpoons H_2O \quad E_o' = +0·82 \text{ V} \tag{16.2}$$

Reversing (16.1) gives:

$$NADH \rightleftharpoons NAD^+ + H^+ + 2e \quad E_o' = +0·32 \text{ V} \tag{16.3}$$

Adding (16.2) and (16.3)

$$NADH + H^+ + \tfrac{1}{2}O_2 \rightleftharpoons NAD + H_2O \quad E_o' = +1·14 \text{ V}$$

The difference in standard redox potential at pH 7 (E_o') of the two partial reactions is 1·14 V.

For a redox reaction, the standard free energy change is related to the standard free energy change at pH 7 by the equation:

$$\Delta G^{0\prime} = -nF\, E_{o}{}'$$

where n is the number of electrons transferred and F is the Faraday, a factor converting volts into joules ($F = 96 \cdot 5\,\mathrm{kJ\,V^{-1}}$). Using this relationship, the standard free energy change $\Delta G^{0\prime}$ for the overall transfer of two electrons from NADH to $\frac{1}{2}O_2$ by the respiratory chain is $-2 \times 96 \cdot 5 \times 1 \cdot 14 = -220\,\mathrm{kJ\,mol^{-1}}$. This may be compared with $\Delta G^{0\prime}$ for ATP synthesis which is $+30\,\mathrm{kJ\,mol^{-1}}$; it is clear that the free energy available from NADH oxidation is sufficient to synthesize a number of molecules of ATP under standard conditions.

Figure 16.4 shows the flow of energy during the passage of electrons down the respiratory chain. Starting from NADH there are three steps in the respiratory chain where the change in standard redox potential $\Delta E_{o}{}'$ is large enough to provide sufficient energy for ATP synthesis. These steps are (1) between NADH and ubiquinone, (2) between cytochrome b and cytochrome c and (3) between cytochrome oxidase and oxygen. When two electrons from a molecule of NADH pass down the respiratory chain, sufficient energy is available to drive the synthesis of a molecule of ATP at each of these steps which are known as *coupling sites* so that three molecules of ATP are formed per NADH oxidized.

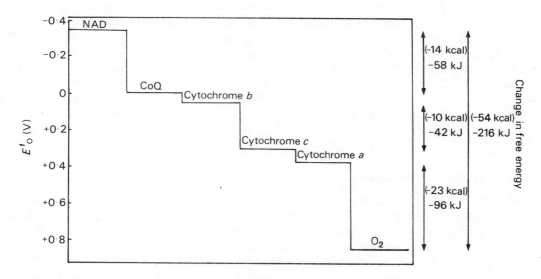

Figure 16.4 The flow of energy during the passage of electrons along the respiratory chain

The number of molecules of phosphate esterified (or ATP molecules synthesized from ADP and P_i) per atom of oxygen consumed is called the *P/O ratio*. The P/O ratio for NADH oxidation is therefore 3. However for the oxidation of succinate via succinate dehydrogenase, since the part of the respiratory chain between NADH and ubiquinone is by-passed (page 217) only two coupling sites are traversed and the P/O ratio for succinate is 2. Similarly, if isolated mitochondria are presented with ascorbic acid which reacts directly with cytochrome c, the first two coupling sites are by-passed and the P/O ratio for the oxidation of ascorbic acid is 1. These considerations will be applied later to calculate the number of ATP molecules that can be synthesized during the oxidation of a molecule of glucose or of fatty acids.

Mitochondrial organization

Mitochondria can be isolated from many tissues by disintegration of the tissue mechanically so that the cells are disrupted. The homogenate is subjected to differential centrifugation and a mitochondrial fraction is obtained. If such a preparation is performed carefully, the mitochondrial fraction will contain intact and undamaged mitochondria that will oxidize substrates and synthesize ATP. Since 1950 a great deal of work has been performed on isolated mitochondria, and a considerable amount is now known about their properties.

Mitochondria have two membranes (Figure 15.9). The outer membrane is freely permeable to molecules as large as cytochrome *c* (molecular weight 13 000); the function of this membrane is not yet clear. The inner membrane contains folds or *cristae* and has a number of distinctive properties. The protein/lipid ratio of this membrane is high. It contains the phospholipid *cardiolipin* which is found nowhere else in mammalian organisms. The unique composition and structure of this membrane give it a very low permeability even to small charged molecules.

The inner membrane contains the respiratory chain, succinate dehydrogenase, and the ATPase enzyme which is responsible for mitochondrial ATP synthesis. The space enclosed by the inner membrane, which is known as the *matrix space*, contains the other enzymes of the citrate cycle, and also many enzymes involved in the metabolism of amino acids and fatty acids.

The permeability properties of the inner mitochondrial membrane were elucidated in the late 1960s. The membrane has a low intrinsic permeability to all ions including H^+ ions. Nevertheless, for metabolic pathways to operate, ions such as pyruvate and phosphate must cross the membrane which contains a number of *specific transport proteins*. These carriers, with one or two exceptions, catalyse the exchange of equally charged molecules in opposite directions across the membrane so that there is no net alteration of charge distribution. NADH from the cytoplasm is not transported into the mitochondria, but the reducing equivalents from cytoplasmic NADH are transferred to the intramitochondrial pool of NADH by a system known as the *malate/aspartate shuttle* which is described later (page 230).

The mechanism of ATP synthesis

With this background, it is now possible to describe briefly present views on the mechanism of ATP synthesis in mitochondria. This problem is best illustrated by reference to a classical experiment first performed on isolated mitochondria some thirty years ago (Figure 16.5). A suspension of isolated mitochondria is placed in an oxygen electrode which measures the concentration of oxygen in the suspension. The mitochondria are incubated with a substrate such as succinate plus phosphate. The rate of oxygen consumption is slow until a small amount of ADP is added, when the rate increases sharply. When the ADP has all been converted to ATP, the rate of oxygen uptake reverts to the original slow rate, but increases again on further addition of ADP.

This experiment demonstrates that oxygen uptake in mitochondria is coupled to the synthesis of ATP, in that in the absence of ADP little oxygen uptake will occur even in the presence of excess respiratory substrate. This is called *respiratory control*. Certain compounds, of which 2,4-dinitrophenol is a well-known example, act as *uncouplers* of oxidative phosphorylation. On adding such a compound to mitochondria in the presence of substrate, a rapid rate of oxygen uptake is observed with no synthesis of ATP.

The molecular mechanism by which the passage of electrons along the respiratory chain is coupled to the phosphorylation of ATP has been the object of an immense amount of investigation since the phenomenon of respiratory control was first observed. At various times a

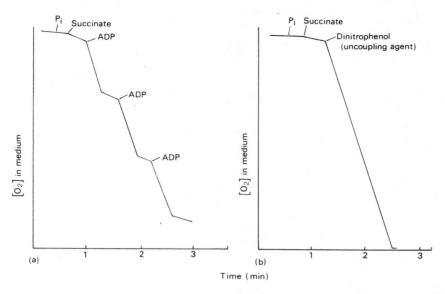

Figure 16.5 Respiratory control. (a) Oxygen consumption is shown to be linked to ATP synthesis. (b) Oxygen consumption uncoupled from ATP synthesis by addition of 2,4-dinitrophenol

number of different hypotheses have been proposed, but the presently accepted theory is known as the *chemiosmotic theory*. This was first set out in detail in 1965 by Mitchell who was later awarded the Nobel prize for his work.

The chemiosmotic theory

The main features of the theory are summarized in Figure 16.6. As discussed above, the passage of electrons from NADH to oxygen along the respiratory chain leads to the production of hydrogen ions at some stages and the uptake of hydrogen ions at others. In the chemiosmotic theory, the components of the respiratory chain are physically orientated across the inner membrane so that, during the passage of electrons, hydrogen ions are produced at the outer surface and taken up at the inner surface. This results in the *pumping of protons* out of the mitochondria and the establishment of an electrical potential of about 0.22 V and a pH gradient of 0.3 pH units across the inner mitochondrial membrane. The membrane is considered to be impermeable to protons.

It was further proposed that the ATPase, i.e. the ATP-synthesizing enzyme, is orientated in the inner membrane in such a way that protons could return across the membrane only by passing through this large protein molecule, part of which forms a channel through the membrane. During the passage of two protons through the ATPase, one molecule of ATP is synthesized from ADP and phosphate. The different P/O ratios were explained by the pumping of a certain number of protons at each coupling site. Thus from an energetic point of view, the free energy released by the passage of electrons from NADH to oxygen is conserved in the form of an electric potential and pH gradient across the mitochondrial membrane. The energy for the reversal of the ATPase reaction is derived from the movement of protons back across the membrane down their electrical and concentration gradients.

The experiment shown in Figure 16.5(a) is then explained as follows. In the absence of ADP, the protons pumped out by the respiratory chain cannot return across the membrane. The

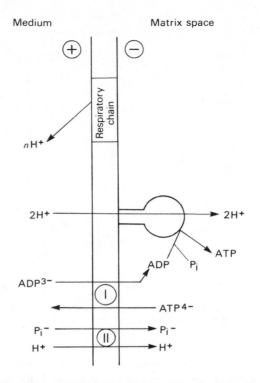

Figure 16.6 Simplified outline of ATP synthesis in mitochondria according to the chemiosmotic theory. Passage of electrons along the respiratory chain is associated with ejection of protons from the mitochondria, producing a large membrane potential (negative inside) and a relatively small pH gradient (alkaline inside). One molecule of ATP is synthesized from ADP plus phosphate during the inward passage of $2H^+$ ions through the ATPase system. ATP synthesis requires the inward transport of ADP^{3-} in exchange for ATP^{4-} on the adenine nucleotide carrier (I) and the inward movement of phosphate together with one H^+ ion on the phosphate carrier (II).

membrane potential set up opposes the ejection of more protons and hence respiration is slow. On addition of ADP, the protons can return through the ATPase with the synthesis of ATP and respiration therefore increases until the ADP is used up. Uncoupling agents such as dinitrophenol are considered to make the membrane permeable to protons at all points and thus to dissipate the driving force for ATP synthesis. In the presence of an uncoupler, protons re-equilibrate rapidly and respiration can proceed at a maximum rate (Figure 16.5b). It is noteworthy that the theory predicted the impermeability of the membrane to protons, the existence of electroneutral substrate-transporting systems and the mechanism of action of uncoupling agents before any of these facts had been established experimentally.

A considerable amount of evidence has now accummulated which is consistent with the predictions of this theory. The establishment of a potential across the membrane of respiring mitochondria has been measured by various indirect methods and been found to be of a magnitude consistent with that predicted. It has also been shown that the artificial creation of an electrical potential and pH gradient across the membrane of mitochondria can lead to ATP synthesis even in the absence of respiration. Furthermore it has been shown that uncoupling agents do, in fact, make membranes specifically permeable to protons.

A particular point of interest is that the chemiosmotic theory predicts that no ATP synthesis can occur other than in membranes which form closed vesicles since no membrane potential can exist unless there is membrane continuity. Observation of ATP synthesis in the absence of such a closed vesicular system would immediately disprove the chemiosmotic theory, but no such observation has been made.

The above is a very simplified account of the chemiosmotic theory and a number of the details of oxidative phosphorylation remain to be elucidated, in particular the molecular mechanism of proton pumping and the exact mechanism of action of the ATPase. However, the basic principles of the theory are now widely accepted. This theory is also able to account for photosynthetic phosphorylation in chloroplasts and for the synthesis of ATP by bacteria.

Chapter 17
Carbohydrate metabolism

Carbohydrates occupy an important place in metabolism because of their roles in energy production and various biosynthetic pathways. Starch is the main source of energy in most populations (page 122) and before it can be absorbed it must be broken down. The hydrolysis of starch is catalysed by enzymes known as *amylases* which occur in the saliva and the pancreatic juice. The amylases of animal origin are called α-amylases in order to distinguish them from the β-amylases of plants, which differ in their point of attack on the starch molecule. The β-amylases are *exoamylases* which nip off maltose units from the ends of the amylose and amylopectin molecules, whereas the α-amylases are *endoamylases* and catalyse the breakdown of bonds occurring in the interior of the molecules. The first products of the action of the α-amylases are the *dextrins* (page 98) which are progressively degraded into smaller and smaller units. The final product consists mainly of maltose together with some small branched-chain oligosaccharides. A separate enzyme produced in the intestine is required to hydrolyse the α-1:6 bonds of amylopectin.

The amylase present in saliva is unlikely to have a significant digestive function in Man because of the short time during which the food is in the mouth and the fact that the gastric pH (1–2) is well below the optimum pH (6·8) of salivary amylase. It is likely, therefore, that the breakdown of starch is mainly effected in the small intestine by pancreatic amylase. The α-amylases require Cl^- as a cofactor whereas most ionic cofactors are cations.

The dietary carbohydrates also include sucrose and lactose. Specific *disaccharidases* which convert these sugars into their constituent monosaccharides are present in the brush border of the intestinal epithelial cells. Only monosaccharides can be absorbed and an active transport system ensures that glucose, galactose and other sugars having the structural features shown below

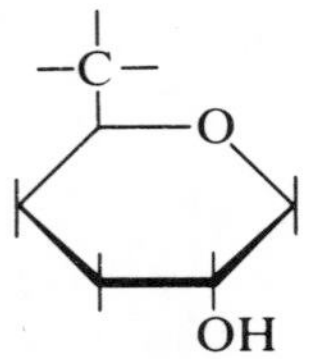

are absorbed even against a concentration gradient. The active transport of such sugars into the mucosal cells is linked with the transport of Na^+ in the same direction. Other monosaccharides including fructose and the pentoses are absorbed by passive means. The monosaccharides pass into the portal system and are transported to the liver, where they are converted into compounds that are normal intermediates of glucose metabolism.

Glucose breakdown

Three distinct but integrated pathways are responsible for the breakdown of glucose and its conversion to carbon dioxide, water and utilizable energy. They are: (1) the *glycolytic* or *Embden–Meyerhof pathway*; (2) *the citrate cycle* and *electron-transport chain* which provide the final common pathway for the products of carbohydrate, lipid and amino acid metabolism; (3) *the pentose phosphate pathway*.

The glycolytic or Embden–Meyerhof pathway

The process of glycolysis, whereby glucose is converted to pyruvate and a small amount of ATP is produced, occurs in the cytoplasm and is essentially the same in all living cells regardless of whether the organism is an aerobe or an anaerobe. Variations occur, however, in the subsequent metabolism of the pyruvate.

The intermediates in glycolysis are all phosphorylated derivatives of hexose (C_6) or triose (C_3) sugars and the first three steps in the pathway convert the glucose into a form that can be broken down into two triose phosphate units.

Reaction 1

The glucose is phosphorylated by ATP to give glucose 6-phosphate. This reaction, which is irreversible, is catalysed by *hexokinase* and requires Mg^{2+}. As its name suggests hexokinase is not very specific and is able to phosphorylate a variety of hexose sugars.

Glucose   Glucose 6-phosphate

Reaction 2

The next step is a reversible isomerization reaction in which the six-membered pyranose ring of glucose is converted into the five-membered furanose ring of fructose under the influence of *glucose 6-phosphate isomerase*.

Glucose 6-phosphate   Fructose 6-phosphate

Reaction 3

The fructose 6-phosphate is then converted into fructose 1,6-bisphosphate by a second phosphorylation with ATP which is catalysed by *phosphofructokinase*. Phosphofructokinase is an allosteric enzyme and the reaction, which is irreversible, is an important control point, i.e. rate-limiting step (page 337), for the glycolytic pathway.

Fructose 6-phosphate   Fructose 1,6-bisphosphate

Reaction 4

At this stage fructose 1,6-bisphosphate is cleaved to give two triose phosphate molecules, namely glyceraldehyde 3-phosphate and dihydroxyacetone phosphate in a reversible reaction which is catalysed by *aldolase*.

Fructose
1,6-bisphosphate   Dihydroxyacetone
phosphate   Glyceraldehyde
3-phosphate

Glyceraldehyde 3-phosphate   Dihydroxyacetone phosphate

Because of the presence of *triose phosphate isomerase* the glyceraldehyde 3-phosphate and dihydroxyacetone phosphate are interconvertible. Glyceraldehyde 3-phosphate is on the direct pathway of glycolysis (Figure 17.1) and is continuously removed with the result that dihydroxyacetone phosphate is continuously converted into glyceraldehyde 3-phosphate. Not all the dihydroxyacetone phosphate is used in this way; some is converted to α-glycerophosphate which takes place in the α-glycerophosphate shuttle (page 230) and some may be used in the synthesis of triglycerides. However, when considering the oxidation of glucose it may be assumed that each molecule will give rise to two molecules of glyceraldehyde 3-phosphate which will both participate in the subsequent reactions.

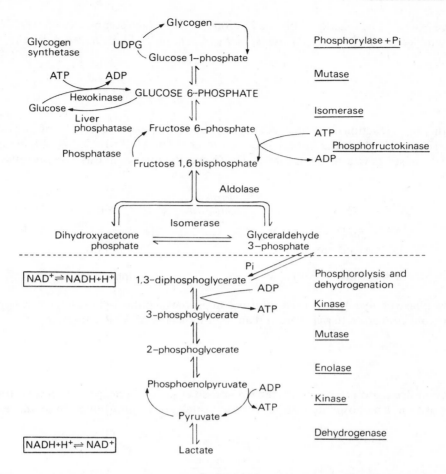

Figure 17.1 The glycolytic pathway. It should be noted that for every glucose unit metabolized the reactions shown below the dotted line occur twice

Reaction 5

Up to this point two molecules of ATP have been used in the reaction sequence and no energy has been extracted from it. The next reaction, however, involves an oxidation in which the aldehyde group of the glyceraldehyde 3-phosphate is both dehydrogenated and phosphorylated and converted into the high-energy compound 1,3-diphosphoglycerate which is a mixed anhydride of a carboxylic acid and phosphoric acid. The energy required for this conversion comes from the oxidation of the aldehyde group and enables inorganic phosphate to act as the donor. The hydrogen atoms that are removed are transferred to the hydrogen-carrying

Glyceraldehyde 3-phosphate   1,3-Diphosphoglycerate

coenzyme NAD^+. The reaction is blocked by iodoacetate which combines with an –SH group of the enzyme *glyceraldehyde 3-phosphate dehydrogenase* and interferes with the substrate binding.

Reaction 6

This is the first reaction in which ATP is produced. It is an example of *substrate level phosphorylation* in which the energy required to convert ADP to ATP is obtained from an energy-rich substrate in a reaction catalysed by a specific kinase, in this case *phosphoglycerate kinase*.

1,3-Diphosphoglycerate   3-Phosphoglycerate

The last phase of glycolysis consists of three steps in which the 3-phosphoglycerate produced in reaction 6 is converted to pyruvate and another molecule of ATP is formed.

Reaction 7

By an intramolecular rearrangement, the phosphate group of 3-phosphoglycerate is transferred to the 2-position in a phosphate transfer reaction catalysed by *phosphoglyceromutase*.

3-Phosphoglycerate   2-Phosphoglycerate

Reaction 8

The next step is a dehydration reaction whereby 2-phosphoglycerate is converted to phosphoenolpyruvate (PEP). The dehydration raises the group transfer potential of the phosphate group so that phosphoenolpyruvate is a high-energy compound. The reaction which is catalysed by *enolase* is dependent on Mg^{2+} and is inhibited by fluoride.

2-Phosphoglycerate   Phosphoenolpyruvate

Reaction 9

The high-energy phosphoenolpyruvate is used in a second substrate level phosphorylation catalysed by *pyruvate kinase* in which ADP is converted to ATP and pyruvate is produced. The reaction is irreversible under normal physiological conditions.

Phosphoenolpyruvate   Pyruvate

Energy production and the importance of glycolysis

During the conversion of one molecule of glucose to two molecules of pyruvate, two molecules of ATP are used to prime reactions 1 and 3 but, since reactions 5–9 occur twice over, for every molecule of glucose metabolized, a total of four molecules of ATP are produced, two each in reactions 6 and 9, giving a net synthesis of two molecules of ATP. Thus the overall reaction is

$$\text{Glucose} + 2P_i + 2ADP + 2NAD^+ \rightarrow 2\,\text{pyruvate} + 2ATP + 2NADH + 2H^+$$

Pyruvate is an important compound. After entering the mitochondria it may be converted to acetyl-CoA (page 232) which is then oxidized to carbon dioxide and water by the joint activities of the citrate cycle and electron-transport chain with the production of much greater quantities of ATP than are produced by glycolysis alone. It also has a role in amino acid synthesis as it may be transaminated to form alanine (page 281). Pyruvate is also an important intermediate in *gluconeogenesis* the process whereby glucose is synthesized from non-carbohydrate sources (page 237). In bacteria a variety of end products may be formed from pyruvate depending both on the nature of the bacterium and the environmental conditions. When oxygen is in short supply, muscle tissue converts pyruvate to lactate while yeasts ferment it to ethanol.

The three-dimensional structures of seven glycolytic enzymes, three dehydrogenases, three kinases and a mutase have been worked out. All of them, in spite of the diversity of the reactions they catalyse, contain a region which has a similar structural pattern in which 150 amino acids take part. This suggests that all these enzymes are derived from a common primeval gene and that the glycolytic pathway must have developed at a very early stage in evolution.

Aerobic and anaerobic glycolysis

During the oxidation of glyceraldehyde 3-phosphate to 1,3-diphosphoglycerate, which is the only oxidative step in the glycolytic pathway, NAD^+ is converted into its reduced form (NADH) and, unless there is a continuous supply of NAD^+, the oxidation of glyceraldehyde 3-phosphate will cease. Glycolysis takes place in the cytoplasm and it is here that NADH must be oxidized to NAD^+. However, the enzymes specifically responsible for this reaction are constituents of the electron-transport chain and are localized in the mitochondria. A simple solution would appear to be that NADH should pass into the mitochondria and, after oxidation to NAD^+ should return to the cytoplasm. The mitochondrial membrane is not, however, readily permeable to NADH and NAD^+; this complication is overcome by oxidizing NADH to NAD^+ at the expense of dihydroxyacetone phosphate which is reduced to glycerol 3-phosphate. The enzyme catalysing the reaction is *glycerol 3-phosphate dehydrogenase*. The glycerol 3-phosphate then passes into the mitochondria where it is reoxidized to dihydroxyacetone phosphate. The dehydrogenase which catalyses the conversion of glycerol 3-phosphate to dihydroxyacetone phosphate in the mitochondria is different from the NAD^+-linked glycerol 3-phosphate dehydrogenase present in the cytosol. It is linked to FAD instead of NAD^+ and transfers electrons to the respiratory chain at the level of coenzyme Q (page 216). Consequently only two molecules of ATP, instead of three, are formed when cytoplasmic NADH is oxidized in this way. The dihydroxyacetone phosphate returns from the mitochondria to the cytoplasm where it is once again available to participate in the oxidation of NADH, thus permitting the oxidative step in aerobic glycolysis to proceed. This is known as the *glycerophosphate shuttle*.

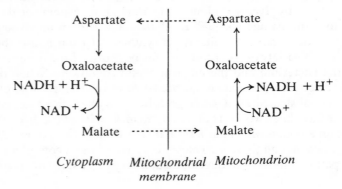

Another way in which reducing power may be transferred across the mitochondrial membrane is by means of the *malate–oxaloacetate shuttle*. The cytoplasmic NADH is used to reduce oxaloacetate to malate which, unlike oxaloacetate, is able to pass into the mitochondrion. Having done so it is reconverted to oxaloacetate with the formation of mitochondrial NADH. The oxaloacetate is returned to the cytoplasm in the form of aspartate.

Aspartate $\longleftarrow$ ------ Aspartate

Oxaloacetate   Oxaloacetate

$NADH + H^+$ $NADH + H^+$

NAD^+ NAD^+

Malate ------ $\longrightarrow$ Malate

Cytoplasm   *Mitochondrial* *Mitochondrion*
membrane

Anaerobic glycolysis in muscle

When glycolysis is occurring under aerobic conditions the hydrogen atoms released in the oxidative reaction take the pathway shown above and are oxidized to water via the reactions of the electron-transport chain. However, when, as in a muscle that is being strenuously exercised, there is a shortage of oxygen, the mitochondrial system, which is essentially aerobic, cannot operate effectively and an alternative method must be found to oxidize the NADH produced during glycolysis. Under these conditions, instead of the NADH being used to convert dihydroxyacetone phosphate into glycerophosphate, it is used to convert pyruvate into lactate by the following reaction which is catalysed by *lactate dehydrogenase*:

$$CH_3 \cdot CO \cdot COOH + NADH + H^+ \underset{\text{dehydrogenase}}{\overset{\text{Lactate}}{\rightleftharpoons}} CH_3 \cdot CHOH \cdot COOH + NAD^+$$

In this way NAD^+ is regenerated and the muscle cells can continue to produce small amounts of ATP glycolytically. ATP may also be derived from phosphocreatine and from the myokinase reaction.

Quite large amounts of lactate may be produced in muscle as a result of anaerobic glycolysis and its fate is considered later (page 239). It is mainly derived from muscle glycogen since, although when resting the muscles obtain their energy by metabolizing glucose and fatty acids obtained directly from the blood, during exercise the stored muscle glycogen is called upon. This has the advantage that, at a time when ATP is in short supply, one molecule is 'saved' for every glucosyl residue of glycogen used instead of glucose itself. This is because the glucosyl residues are in a higher energy state than free glucose and are phosphorylated by a low-energy phosphoryl donor, i.e. inorganic phosphate (page 234) rather than ATP, which is needed for the phosphorylation of glucose.

Anaerobic glycolysis in yeast

In yeast the enzyme *pyruvate decarboxylase* catalyses the decarboxylation of pyruvate to CO_2 and acetaldehyde. Pyruvate decarboxylase requires Mg^{2+} and thiamine pyrophosphate as a coenzyme. The acetaldehyde is then reduced to ethanol in a reaction catalysed by *alcohol dehydrogenase* in which the NADH produced during glycolysis is oxidized and NAD^+ is regenerated

$$CH_3 \cdot CO \cdot COOH \xrightarrow[Mg^{2+},\ TPP]{\text{Pyruvate decarboxylase}} CH_3 \cdot CHO + CO_2$$

$$\underset{\text{Acetaldehyde}}{CH_3 \cdot CHO} + NADH + H^+ \xrightarrow{\text{Alcohol dehydrogenase}} \underset{\text{Ethanol}}{CH_3 \cdot CH_2OH} + NAD^+$$

The net reaction for the fermentation of glucose is

$$\text{Glucose} + 2P_i + 2ADP \rightarrow 2\,\text{ethanol} + 2CO_2 + 2ATP$$

Other microorganisms have different ways of metabolizing pyruvate. End products include lactic acid, butyric acid and propionic acid as well as various alcohols. Some of the reactions are considered in more detail in connection with the metabolism of plaque.

Conversion of pyruvate to acetyl-CoA

Glycolysis is linked to the citrate cycle (page 240) by a series of reactions in which pyruvate is converted into the acetyl derivative of coenzyme A. Coenzyme A has a nucleotide-type

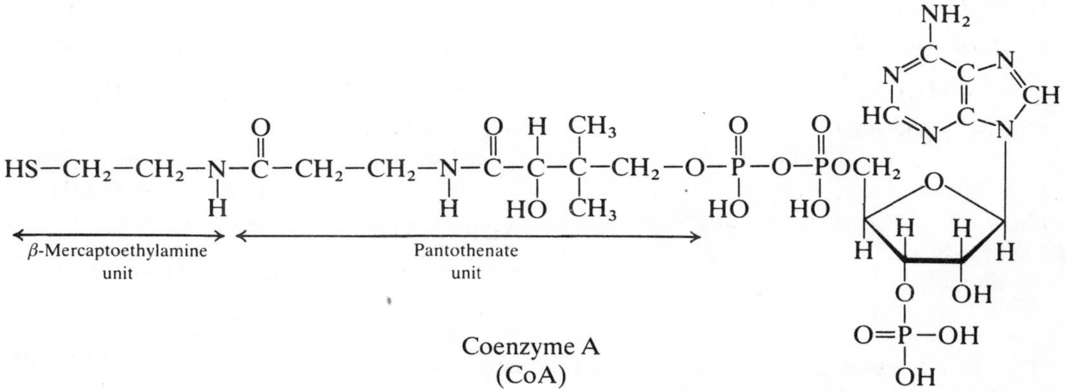

Coenzyme A
(CoA)

β-Mercaptoethylamine unit

Pantothenate unit

structure and bears a reactive –SH group that combines with acyl groups to form thiol esters. These are energy-rich compounds that can take part in reactions which would not be possible but for the favourable equilibrium established by cleavage of the thiol ester bond.

Formation of acetyl-CoA takes place in the mitochondrial matrix and is catalysed by *pyruvate dehydrogenase*. This is a multienzyme complex containing three enzymes which together are responsible for the oxidative decarboxylation of the pyruvate. Although the overall reaction may be represented quite simply as follows:

$$CH_3 \cdot CO \cdot COOH + CoA{-}SH + NAD^+ \rightarrow CH_3 \cdot CO \sim SCoA + CO_2 + NADH + H^+$$

four different steps and five different cofactors are required. In addition to the coenzyme A and NAD^+ indicated above, thiamine pyrophosphate, lipoic acid, and FAD are involved.

Coordination of the various reactions is ensured by the structural integration of the enzymes into the multienzyme complex. Their affinity is such that, if they are independently isolated and then mixed together again, they will associate spontaneously to form the original complex.

The reactions catalysed by the pyruvate dehydrogenase complex (PDH) irreversibly commit the carbon skeleton of glucose to ultimate oxidation by the reactions of the citrate cycle either directly or via the formation of fatty acids. It is not surprising therefore to find that such an important reaction is under close control. Thus it is subject to:

1. End product inhibition by increasing concentration ratios of acetyl-CoA/CoA and of NADH/ NAD^+.
2. Covalent modification by phosphorylation/dephosphorylation (page 341).
3. Metabolic activators and inhibitors of the kinase which phosphorylates pyruvate dehydrogenase and of the phosphatase that dephosphorylates it.

The citrate cycle to which the acetyl groups produced by the pyruvate dehydrogenase reaction are committed is described on pages 240–246.

The pentose phosphate pathway

This alternative pathway of glucose breakdown is sometimes referred to as the *phosphogluconate pathway* or *hexose monophosphate shunt*. Instead of generating ATP the main

The initial reactions of the pentose phosphate pathway catalysed by *glucose 6-phosphate dehydrogenase*

purpose of the pathway is: (1) to generate reducing power in the form of NADPH which can be used for biosynthetic purposes; (2) to produce ribose 5-phosphate which is needed for the synthesis of nucleotides, including the various coenzymes that have a nucleotide-type structure such as ATP, NAD^+, FAD and CoA, and also the nucleic acids.

Like those of glycolysis the reactions of the pentose phosphate pathway begin with glucose 6-phosphate and all take place in the cytoplasm. The initial reactions are shown below, from which it can be seen that carbon-1 of the glucose 6-phosphate is first dehydrogenated by *glucose 6-phosphate dehydrogenase* with $NADP^+$ acting as the H acceptor. The 6-phosphogluconate which is produced is oxidatively decarboxylated to ribulose 5-phosphate, with $NADP^+$ once again acting as the H acceptor. The ribulose 5-phosphate then undergoes isomerization to give ribose 5-phosphate. These initial reactions may be summarized:

$$\text{Glucose 6-phosphate} + 2NADP^+ + H_2O \rightarrow \text{ribose 5-phosphate} + CO_2 + 2NADPH$$

A simplified scheme of the remaining reactions is given in Figure 17.2 which shows how the monophosphates of various 3-, 4-, 5-, 6- and 7-carbon sugars are interconverted by a variety of non-oxidative reactions. The enzymes *transketolase* and *transaldolase* are responsible for

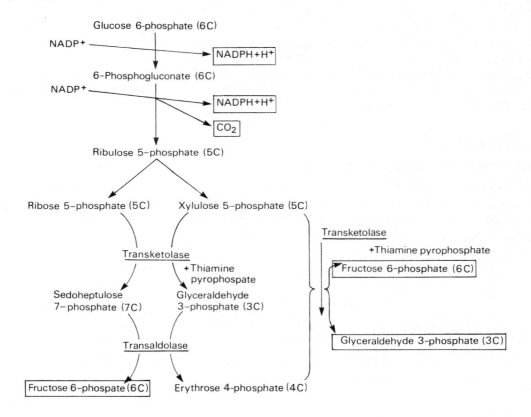

Summary

3 Glucose + 3NADP$^+$ ⟶ 2 fructose 6-phosphate + 2 glyceraldehyde 3-phospate + 3 CO$_2$ + 6 NADPH + 6H$^+$

Figure 17.2 An outline of the pentose phosphate pathway of glucose metabolism showing its relationship to the glycolytic pathway

reactions by which three molecules of pentose phosphate can be converted into two molecules of fructose 6-phosphate and one of glyceraldehyde 3-phosphate. In this way a reversible connection is established between the pentose phosphate and glycolytic pathways.

In order to produce the six molecules of CO_2 that represent the complete oxidation of one molecule of glucose, six molecules of glucose 6-phosphate must be oxidatively decarboxylated. The net result is

$$C_6H_{12}O_6 + ATP + 6H_2O + 12NADP^+ \rightarrow 6CO_2 + 12NADPH + ADP + P_i$$

The various tissues differ in their requirements both for NADPH and for ribose 5-phosphate and the activity of the pathway is much greater in tissues such as liver, adipose tissue and mammary gland than in others such as skeletal muscle and kidney.

Glycogen metabolism

Free glucose is present in the body fluids but only in small amounts. Appreciable quantities are, however, stored in the tissues, chiefly the liver and the muscles, in the form of glycogen granules in the cytoplasm. The liver glycogen, which may constitute 6% or more of the wet weight of the liver, is much more variable than the muscle glycogen. It is used to maintain the blood glucose concentration between meals and almost completely disappears on prolonged fasting. The muscle glycogen, on the other hand, remains relatively constant within the 0·5–1·0% range. It is used for 'home consumption' when the needs of the muscle are increased during exercise and it never appears as free glucose.

Glycogenolysis

Reaction 1: The phosphorylase reaction

In both liver and muscle, glycogen breakdown is initiated by the enzyme *phosphorylase* which catalyses the sequential removal of terminal glucosyl residues from the branches of the glycogen molecule by phosphorolytic cleavage. The presence of inorganic phosphate is essential and the glucosyl residues are released in the form of glucose 1-phosphate. Phosphorylase is unable to

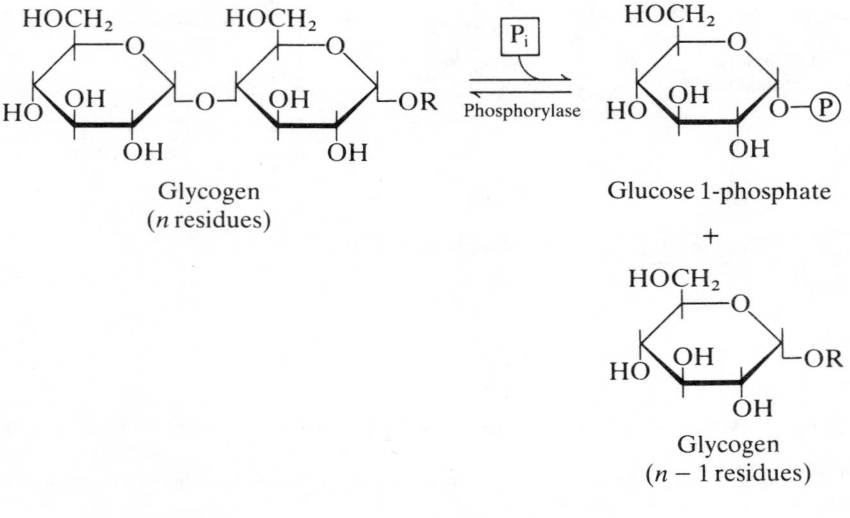

Glycogen
(*n* residues)

Glucose 1-phosphate

+

Glycogen
(*n* − 1 residues)

cleave the α-1 : 6 linkages which occur at the branch points of the molecule and two other enzymes are needed for the debranching process.

This initial reaction of glycogen breakdown is closely controlled by a complex process involving more than one phosphorylation/dephosphorylation reaction (page 343).

Reaction 2

The glucose 1-phosphate released by phosphorolysis is converted into glucose 6-phosphate by *phosphoglucomutase*. In muscle the glucose 6-phosphate enters the glycolytic sequence and is used for ATP production.

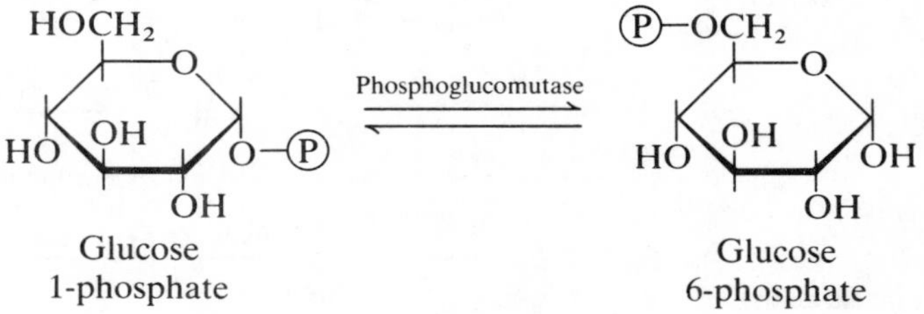

Glucose
1-phosphate

Phosphoglucomutase

Glucose
6-phosphate

Reaction 3: Glucose formation in the liver

In the liver, although some of the glucose 6-phosphate will be used for glycolysis and the production of ATP for use within the liver cell, a large proportion may be used to maintain the blood glucose concentration. Cell membranes are impermeable to the sugar phosphates but the liver contains a *glucose 6-phosphatase* which hydrolyses the glucose 6-phosphate to glucose and inorganic phosphate. The glucose is then able to leave the cell. Glucose 6-phosphatase is absent from muscle and brain which depend on a rapid rate of glycolysis for their normal activities. It is present in the kidneys and the intestine.

Glycogenesis

Glycogen is synthesized by adding glucose units one at a time to pre-existing glycogen molecules. The pathway is the same in both liver and muscle. Glucose enters the tissue cells by a process of facilitated diffusion which, in the case of muscle and many other tissues, but not the liver, is promoted by insulin. The uptake of glucose is a rate-limiting step in carbohydrate metabolism.

Reaction 1

Once inside the cells the glucose is converted into glucose 6-phosphate by *hexokinase*. Not only is glucose 6-phosphate more reactive than glucose itself but, once a sugar has been phosphorylated, it is unable to leave the cell. Glucose 6-phosphate, it will be realized, occupies a central position in carbohydrate metabolism (Figure 17.3).

Reaction 2

When it is to be used for glycogen formation the position of the phosphate group is switched from the C-6 to the C-1 position on the glucose molecule by *phosphoglucomutase*. This reaction, which is reversible, is comparable to the phosphoglyceromutase reaction in glycolysis.

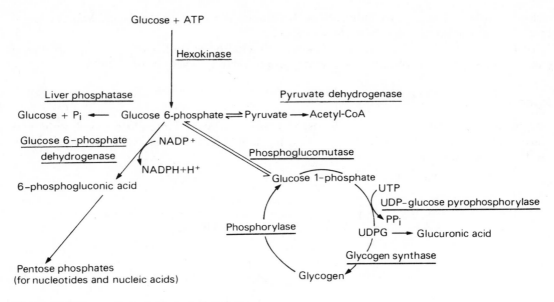

Figure 17.3 The reactions of glucose 6-phosphate

Reaction 3

The glucose 1-phosphate interacts with uridine triphosphate under the influence of *UDP-glucose pyrophosphorylase* to give uridine diphosphoglucose (UDPG) which is a high-energy derivative of glucose which acts as a glucose donor in glycogen synthesis and in the synthesis of complex polysaccharides and glycoproteins. During the reaction pyrophosphate is released and its subsequent hydrolysis ensures that the overall reaction is strongly exergonic and proceeds in the forward direction.

$$\text{UTP} + \text{glucose 1-phosphate} \xrightarrow{\substack{\text{UDP-glucose} \\ \text{pyrophosphorylase}}} \text{UDP-glucose} + \text{PP}_i$$

Reaction 4

$$\underset{(n \text{ glucosyl})}{\text{UDP-glucose} + \text{glycogen}} \xrightarrow{\substack{\text{Glycogen} \\ \text{synthase}}} \underset{(n+1 \text{ glucosyl})}{\text{UDP} + \text{glycogen}}$$

In this reaction the glucosyl residue of UDP-glucose is transferred to a terminal glucosyl unit present on a primer molecule. This must contain more than four glucosyl residues and ideally is glycogen itself. The reaction is catalysed by *glycogen synthase* and an α-1 : 4 linkage is formed.

UTP is regenerated from UDP by phosphoryl transfer from ATP

$$\text{UDP} + \text{ATP} \rightleftharpoons \text{UTP} + \text{ADP}$$

Glycogen synthase, like phosphorylase, exists in both an active and a relatively inactive form and, like phosphorylase, is subject to phosphorylation/dephosphorylation. Glycogen synthesis and breakdown are reciprocally controlled and the many different hormones and neuronal signals to which the processes are subject are integrated so as to give finely regulated changes in glycogen metabolism as required by the circumstances.

Reaction 5

In order to produce a tightly packed spherical glycogen molecule that is suitable for storage, it is necessary to rearrange the growing elongated glycosyl chains into a highly branched structure. Branching is also important in that it increases the solubility of the glycogen and enables breakdown and synthesis to occur more rapidly. A special *branching enzyme* transfers a block of seven or so α-1:4-linked glucose residues to another chain at a point which is at least four residues removed from a pre-existing branch point. The branch is formed by cleaving a 1:4 linkage and creating a new 1:6 linkage (Figure 17.4).

Consideration of the overall process shows that glycogen synthesis is a very efficient method of energy storage since only one ATP equivalent is expended during the conversion of a molecule of glucose 6-phosphate into a glucosyl residue of glycogen.

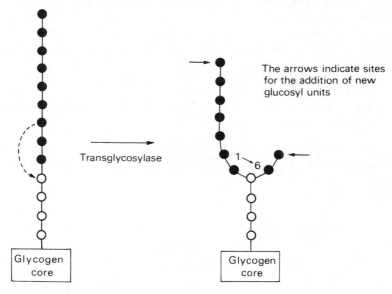

Figure 17.4 The role of the branching enzyme in glycogen synthesis

Gluconeogenesis

In mammals, synthesis of glucose from non-carbohydrate sources takes place only in the liver and kidney. The process which is known as *gluconeogenesis* is very important since, in starvation when the stores of liver glycogen have been used up, it is the only means by which the blood glucose level may be maintained. Substances that are capable of being converted to pyruvate or to oxaloacetate can serve as glucose precursors. The most important of these are lactate and those amino acids which give rise either to pyruvate or a citrate cycle intermediate in the course of their metabolism. Glycerol may also be used but not fatty acids.

Glucose is synthesized from pyruvate in a series of reactions some of which represent the direct reversal of reactions occurring during glycolysis. There are, however, three important distinctions.

1. The pyruvate kinase reaction (page 229) by which phosphoenolpyruvate is converted to pyruvate is virtually irreversible under physiological conditions because phosphoenolpyruvate formation is associated with a large change in free energy. Moreover, pyruvate kinase is inhibited by ATP and alanine so that wastage of energy which would occur if the reaction were to proceed in both directions simultaneously, i.e. *futile cycling*, is prevented. Consequently alternative pathways are needed for the conversion of pyruvate to phosphoenolpyruvate. One of the most important involves the carboxylation of pyruvate to oxaloacetate by the enzyme *pyruvate carboxylase*.

$$CH_3 \cdot CO \cdot COOH + CO_2 + ATP \xrightarrow[\substack{Mg^{2+}, \text{biotin,} \\ \text{acetyl-CoA}}]{\substack{\text{Pyruvate} \\ \text{carboxylase}}} COOH \cdot CH_2 \cdot CO \cdot COOH + ADP + P_i$$

Pyruvate carboxylase is a mitochondrial enzyme which requires Mg^{2+} and biotin as a carrier of activated carbon dioxide. In addition, it has an absolute requirement for acetyl-CoA, which acts as an allosteric activator (page 340). In this way the accumulation of acetyl-CoA normally triggers the formation of oxaloacetate. If ATP is in short supply, oxaloacetate will combine with some of the acetyl-CoA to form citrate, and so be drawn into the citrate cycle. On the other hand, if there is a surplus of ATP, both this and the oxaloacetate will be used for gluconeogenesis.

Whereas oxaloacetate is formed from pyruvate in the mitochondria, the other enzymes that take part in gluconeogenesis are found in the cytoplasm. However, the mitochondrial membrane is not permeable to oxaloacetate which, before it can pass into the cytoplasm, is reduced to malate at the expense of NADH (Figure 17.5):

$$\underset{\text{Oxaloacetate}}{COOH \cdot CH_2 \cdot CO \cdot COOH} + NADH + H^+ \underset{\text{dehydrogenase}}{\overset{\text{Malate}}{\rightleftharpoons}} \underset{\text{Malate}}{COOH \cdot CH_2 \cdot CHOH \cdot COOH} + NAD^+$$

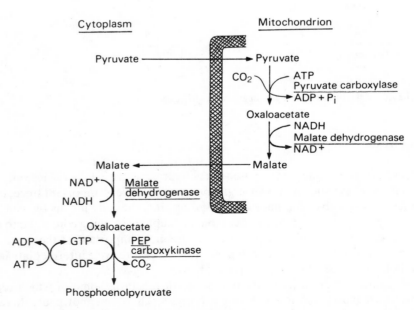

Figure 17.5 The formation of phosphoenolpyruvate from pyruvate

Thus as the malate passes into the cytoplasm it takes reducing potential with it. Once in the cytoplasm a different type of *malate dehydrogenase* releases the oxaloacetate and causes the reduction of cytoplasmic NAD^+. In this way not only oxaloacetate but surplus energy in the form of reducing potential is transferred from the mitochondria to the cytoplasm.

In the second part of the conversion the oxaloacetate is acted upon by *phosphoenolpyruvate (PEP) carboxykinase* which simultaneously causes its decarboxylation and phosphorylation at the expense of GTP.

$$COOH \cdot CH_2 \cdot CO \cdot COOH + GTP \xrightarrow[Mg^{2+}]{\substack{PEP \\ carboxykinase}} CH_2 {=} C \cdot COOH + GDP + CO_2$$

Oxaloacetate   Phosphoenolpyruvate

2. The phosphofructokinase reaction in which fructose 6-phosphate is phosphorylated to fructose 1,6-bisphosphate is also irreversible. Instead, fructose 1,6-bisphosphate is hydrolysed to fructose 6-phosphate and inorganic phosphate. The enzyme that catalyses this reaction is *fructose 1,6-bisphosphatase* and is exclusively present in those tissues that carry out gluconeogenesis. ATP, which inhibits the phosphofructokinase reaction, stimulates fructose 1,6-bisphosphatase activity and AMP inhibits it while favouring the phosphofructokinase reaction.

$$\text{Fructose 1,6-bisphosphate} \xrightarrow[Mg^{2+}]{\text{Fructose bisphosphatase}} \text{fructose 6-phosphate} + P_i$$

3. The phosphorylation of glucose to glucose 6-phosphate, which is catalysed by hexokinase, is also irreversible under physiological conditions. Glucose 6-phosphate, which is formed by the isomerization of fructose 6-phosphate, is converted to glucose in the last step of gluconeogenesis by a hydrolytic dephosphorylation reaction requiring *glucose 6-phosphatase*.

$$\text{Glucose 6-phosphate} + H_2O \xrightarrow{\text{Glucose 6-phosphatase}} \text{glucose} + P_i$$

The fasting blood glucose concentration remains remarkably constant and, even in starvation, it is not appreciably reduced. In these circumstances, while most tissues derive their energy from stored fat, blood glucose, which is essential for the normal functioning of the central nervous system, is mainly derived from amino acids released as a result of tissue breakdown. The glycerol released when the triglycerides are hydrolysed will have a sparing effect on the blood glucose. It is converted to glycerol 3-phosphate in the liver by *glycerol kinase* and ATP. The glycerol 3-phosphate can then be converted to dihydroxyacetone phosphate by dehydrogenation (page 252) and as such will enter the glycolytic pathway.

The importance of these reactions is shown by the fact that, if hepatectomized animals are starved, their blood glucose concentrations fall to a very low level. Little is known of the way in which the activity of glucose 6-phosphatase is controlled.

The Cori cycle

A major source of material for gluconeogenesis is the lactate that is produced anaerobically during muscular activity. Some of this may be reconverted to pyruvate in the muscles themselves when oxygen again becomes available, but most of it diffuses out into the bloodstream and passes to the liver. Here it is oxidized to pyruvate and converted to glucose. It then passes back

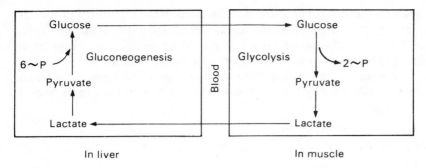

Figure 17.6 The Cori cycle. Lactate formed by active muscle is converted into glucose by the liver. This cycle shifts part of the metabolic burden of active muscle to the liver.

into the blood and once again becomes available to the muscles and other tissues. This recycling process is known as the Cori cycle (Figure 17.6) after its discoverers. It is stimulated by adrenaline.

Blood glucose

Glucose occurs in blood at a concentration that varies between 3·3 and 7·2 mmol l^{-1} (60–130 mg dl^{-1}) according to the temporal relationship to meals. Normal fasting individuals have a post-absorptive blood glucose concentration of 3·3–5 mmol l^{-1} (60–90 mg dl^{-1}) while after meals, in the absorptive phase, it may reach 7·2 mmol l^{-1} (130 mg dl^{-1}). The liver exerts a controlling influence on the blood glucose removing glucose when the level is high and releasing it when it is low. The blood glucose has three different origins. It may be (1) directly absorbed from the small intestine, (2) released from the liver as a result of glycogen breakdown, or (3) formed by gluconeogenesis chiefly in the liver. On the other hand, glucose is removed from blood by the tissues for oxidation and energy production, it may be diverted into glycogen synthesis in muscle and liver and may also be converted into fat, notably in adipose tissue. It is also used in pentose synthesis and in other synthetic pathways producing glycosaminoglycans, glycoproteins and proteoglycans. When the intake of glucose grossly exceeds the body's capacity to metabolize it as in *diabetes mellitus*, the blood glucose concentration rises to high levels and glucose is excreted in the urine. Under normal conditions the glucose that passes into the glomerular filtrate is quantitatively reabsorbed in the kidney tubules. But in the condition of *hyperglycaemia*, in which the concentration of glucose in the blood is abnormally high, the maximum absorptive capacity of the renal tubules (T_m) for glucose is exceeded and glucose appears in the urine. This loss of glucose in the urine is known as *glycosuria* and it is likely to occur when the blood glucose concentration rises to 10 mmol l^{-1} (180 mg dl^{-1}) or over.

Endocrine influences on carbohydrate metabolism are considered in Chapter 24.

The citrate cycle

The cyclic nature of the reactions involved in the oxidation of metabolic fragments containing two carbon atoms was established by Krebs in 1937. Since they involve the condensation of acetyl-CoA and oxaloacetate to form citrate, which is a tricarboxylic acid, the cycle is also known as the *tricarboxylic acid* or *Krebs cycle*. Although it only operates under aerobic conditions, molecular oxygen takes no direct part in the reactions of the cycle. The four oxidative reactions are dehydrogenation reactions in each of which a pair of hydrogen atoms is removed and transferred either to NAD^+ or to a flavoprotein. In addition to the highly exergonic oxidation reactions, the cycle contains several preparative reactions in which certain intermediates are converted to others, to facilitate their subsequent oxidation. The cycle can only function in the presence of oxygen which is required for the regeneration of NAD^+ and the oxidized form of the flavoprotein.

Reaction 1: The formation of citrate

The first step in the cycle is the formation of citrate by the condensation of acetyl groups derived from acetyl-CoA with oxaloacetate. The reaction is catalysed by the enzyme *citrate–oxaloacetate lyase*, commonly known as *citrate synthase*. The energy required for the synthesis is obtained from the acetyl-CoA which is an energy-rich compound.

Reaction 2: The conversion of citrate to isocitrate

Citrate, which is a symmetrical compound, is converted to asymmetrical isocitrate in an isomerization reaction catalysed by *aconitase*. It is accomplished by a dehydration followed by a hydration during which an –H and an –OH are interchanged.

Isocitrate is more readily oxidized than citrate because it possesses a secondary hydroxyl group. This reaction paves the way for the ensuing oxidative step.

Reaction 3: Oxidative decarboxylation of isocitrate to 2-oxoglutarate

This is the first oxidative step and is catalysed by *isocitrate dehydrogenase*. While the substrate is attached to the enzyme two hydrogen atoms are removed, and transferred to NAD^+, a molecule of CO_2 is also lost and the five-carbon dicarboxylic acid, 2-oxoglutarate, is formed.

The mechanism of this oxidative decarboxylation reaction is different from the oxidative decarboxylation of pyruvate. In particular there is no involvement of thiamine pyrophosphate or

$$
\begin{array}{ccc}
\underset{|}{\text{COO}^-} & & \underset{|}{\text{COO}^-} \\
\underset{|}{\text{CH}_2} & \text{Isocitrate} & \underset{|}{\text{CH}_2} \\
\underset{|}{\text{H}-\text{C}-\text{COO}^-} + \text{NAD}^+ \overset{\text{dehydrogenase}}{\rightleftharpoons} & & \underset{|}{\text{CH}_2} + \text{NADH} + \text{H}^+ + \text{CO}_2 \\
\underset{|}{\text{HO}-\text{CH}} & & \underset{|}{\text{CO}} \\
\text{COO}^- & & \text{COO}^-
\end{array}
$$

Isocitrate	2-Oxoglutarate

lipoic acid, and no high-energy derivative is produced. Isocitrate dehydrogenase is inhibited by high ratios of ATP/ADP and also of $NADH/NAD^+$, and this inhibition is considered to be important in the regulation of the citrate cycle.

The activity of isocitrate dehydrogenase is also subject to regulation by calcium ions. In the presence of a calcium chelating agent such as EGTA, the enzyme shows a sigmoidal dependence on isocitrate concentration and half-maximum activity is obtained at approximately 0.3 mM isocitrate. In the presence of 10μM Ca^{2+} ions, the isocitrate concentration dependence becomes hyperbolic. Half-maximum activity is obtained at $<50 \mu$M isocitrate while the maximum velocity is unchanged. A half-maximal effect of Ca^{2+} is obtained at a concentration of 1μM. As a result of this activation by Ca^{2+} ions, the activity of isocitrate dehydrogenase at low isocitrate concentrations changes severalfold as the concentration of Ca^{2+} increases in the range $0.1-10 \mu$M. Isocitrate dehydrogenase is located in the mitochondrial matrix, and the intramitochondrial concentration of Ca^{2+} is difficult to determine. Nevertheless, there is good evidence that this activation of isocitrate dehydrogenase by Ca^{2+} is important in the hormonal control of the citrate cycle.

Reaction 4: The oxidative decarboxylation of 2-oxoglutarate

This decarboxylation reaction unlike reaction 3 is very similar to the oxidative decarboxylation of pyruvate. It is catalysed by *2-oxoglutarate dehydrogenase* which is a multienzyme complex and requires the same cofactors as does the pyruvate dehydrogenase complex (page 232). The products of the reaction are succinyl-CoA, which is analogous to acetyl-CoA, and NADH.

$$
\begin{array}{ccc}
\underset{|}{\text{COO}^-} & & \underset{|}{\text{COO}^-} \\
\underset{|}{\text{CH}_2} & \text{2-Oxoglutarate} & \underset{|}{\text{CH}_2} \\
\underset{|}{\text{CH}_2} + \text{NAD}^+ \overset{\text{dehydrogenase}}{\underset{+ \text{cofactors}}{\longrightarrow}} & & \underset{|}{\text{CH}_2} + \text{NADH} + \text{H}^+ + \text{CO}_2 \\
\underset{|}{\text{CO}} \quad + \text{CoASH} & & \underset{||}{\text{C}\sim\text{SCoA}} \\
\text{COO}^- & & \text{O}
\end{array}
$$

2-Oxoglutarate	Succinyl-CoA

The activity of 2-oxoglutarate dehydrogenase is inhibited by high ratios of $NADH/NAD^+$ and ATP/ADP. Ca^{2+} ions activate 2-oxoglutarate dehydrogenase in a similar way to that described above for isocitrate dehydrogenase. The concentration of 2-oxoglutarate required for half-maximal velocity in the absence of Ca^{2+} is approximately 1.7 mM; in the presence of 30μM Ca^{2+} half-maximal activity is obtained at 0.095 mM oxoglutarate (Figure 17.7).

Thus an increase in intramitochondrial Ca^{2+} concentration in the range $0-10 \mu$M causes the coordinate activation of the three Ca^{2+}-sensitive enzymes, pyruvate dehydrogenase, isocitrate dehydrogenase and oxoglutarate dehydrogenase with a consequent activation of the citrate cycle.

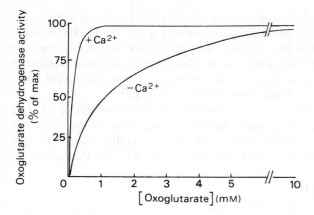

Figure 17.7 Effect of Ca^{2+} on the K_m of oxoglutarate dehydrogenase for oxoglutarate. (After McCormack and Denton (1979) *Biochemical Journal,* **180**, 533)

Reaction 5: The conversion of succinyl-CoA to succinate

Succinyl-CoA is a high-energy thiol ester compound with a $\Delta G^{0'}$ for hydrolysis of about $-33 \cdot 5\,kJ\,(-8\,kcal)\,mol^{-1}$, i.e. of the same order as that required for the synthesis of ATP from ADP. In the course of the cycle, cleavage of the thioester bond is coupled with the phosphorylation of guanosine diphosphate (GDP) and the $\Delta G^{0'}$ of the overall reaction, which is reversible and is catalysed by *succinyl-CoA synthase*, is close to zero.

$$
\begin{array}{c}
COO^- \\
| \\
CH_2 \\
| \\
CH_2 \\
| \\
CO\text{\textasciitilde}SCoA \\
\text{Succinyl-CoA}
\end{array}
\;+\;GDP\;+\;P_i
\;\;\underset{\text{synthase}}{\overset{\text{Succinyl-CoA}}{\rightleftharpoons}}\;\;
\begin{array}{c}
COO^- \\
| \\
CH_2 \\
| \\
CH_2 \\
| \\
COO^- \\
\text{Succinate}
\end{array}
\;+\;GTP\;+\;CoASH
$$

The GTP formed in the reaction transfers its phosphate to ADP in a reaction catalysed by *nucleoside diphosphokinase:*

$$GTP + ADP \rightleftharpoons GDP + ATP$$

The conversion of succinyl-CoA to succinate yields the only high-energy phosphate bond to be formed directly in the course of the cycle. This reaction is an example of a substrate level phosphorylation (page 228).

Reaction 6: The oxidation of succinate to fumarate

The next three reactions follow a pattern that is met with on a number of occasions notably in the oxidation of fatty acids. To introduce an oxygen atom into a compound two hydrogen atoms are first removed to desaturate it, a molecule of water is added and a further pair of hydrogens is removed. Thus

$$[-CH_2-CH_2-] \xrightarrow{\;-2H\;} [-CH{=}CH-] \xrightarrow{\;+H_2O\;} [-CHOH-CH_2-]$$

$$\xrightarrow{\;-2H\;} [-CO-CH_2-]$$

In the first of these three reactions two hydrogen atoms are removed from succinate and fumarate is formed. In this dehydrogenation the hydrogen acceptor is not NAD^+ but a flavo-protein (FP). The flavoprotein is in fact the enzyme *succinate dehydrogenase* which contains *flavin adenine dinucleotide (FAD)* as a covalently bound prosthetic group and also non-haem iron. It differs from other enzymes of the citrate cycle in being an integral constituent of the inner mitochondrial membrane and directly linked to the electron-transport chain.

Both flavin adenine dinucleotide and the closely related *flavin mononucleotide (FMN)* contain riboflavin (page 163) as an essential component. Riboflavin, a member of the vitamin B complex, is a derivative of isoalloxazine to which is attached ribitol, a pentahydroxy alcohol related to ribose. FMN consists of riboflavin esterified with phosphate on C-5 of the ribitol.

Flavin mononucleotide
(FMN)

Strictly speaking, FMN is not a nucleotide because it contains ribitol instead of ribose. However, the general structural similarity of the molecule to a nucleotide is evident and the name has been retained.

In FAD, adenosine monophosphate and riboflavin phosphate are joined together by a pyrophosphate bond.

Flavin adenine dinucleotide
(FAD)

The functional part of both FMN and FAD is shown below in its oxidized and reduced states.

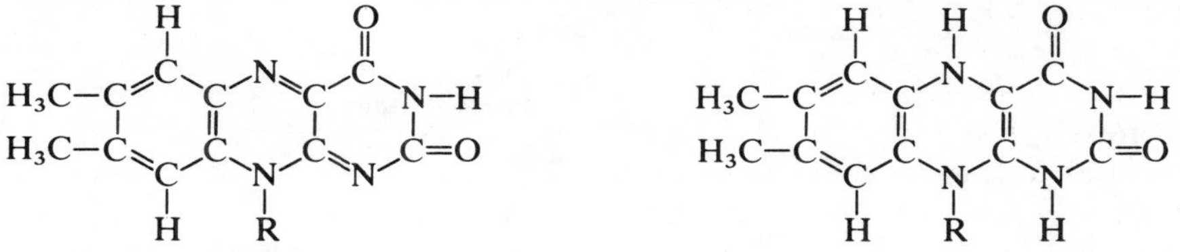

Oxidized form   Reduced form

There is no change in the valency of the nitrogen atoms and two hydrogen atoms are taken up. The reaction is therefore correctly represented as $FP + 2H \rightleftharpoons FPH_2$.

The free energy change in the oxidation of succinate to fumarate is about -150 kJ (-36 kcal) mol^{-1}. This is considerably less than the energy required to reduce NAD^+ to NADH (-220 kJ($-52{\cdot}6$ kcal) mol^{-1}), but it is adequate for the reduction of FAD. This explains why NAD^+ is not used as the hydrogen acceptor in this reaction. In general, reactions that involve the introduction of a double bond into a saturated chain require the participation of a flavoprotein.

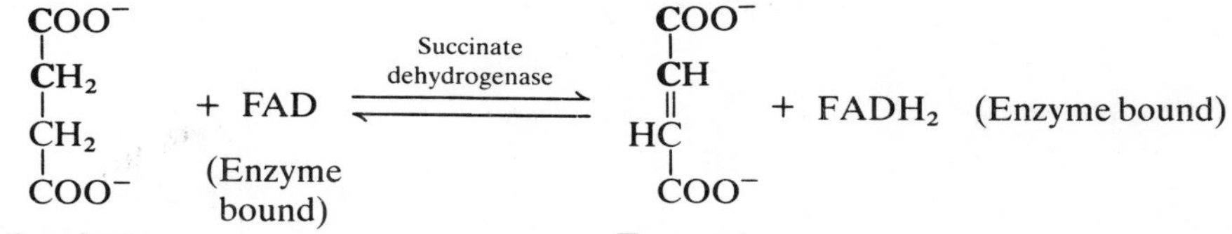

Succinate   Fumarate

Reaction 7: The hydration of fumarate to malate

This is the second preparative reaction, the product being used in the subsequent and final oxidation of the cycle. It is catalysed by *fumarase*.

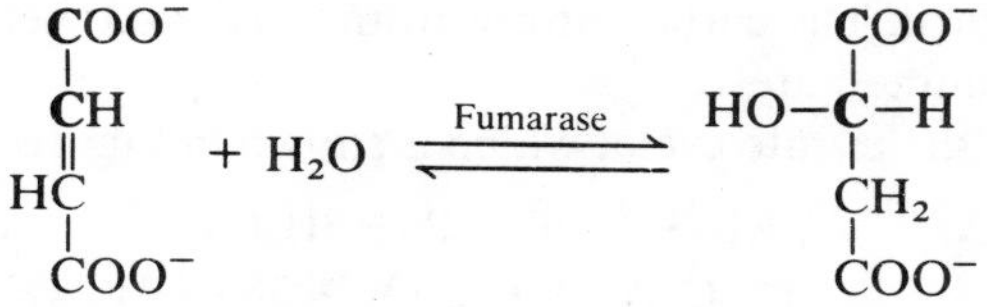

Fumarate   Malate

The free energy change is very small so that small alterations in concentration permit the reaction to proceed in either direction.

Reaction 8: The oxidation of malate to oxaloacetate

The final reaction of this oxidative sequence proceeds with a large negative free energy change which is used to reduce NAD^+ to NADH.

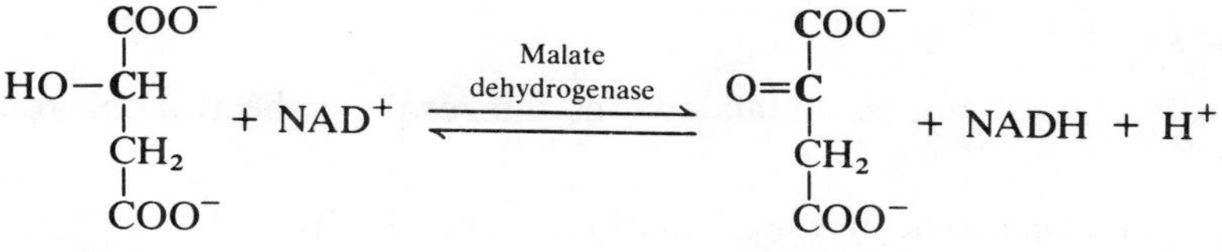

Malate   Oxaloacetate

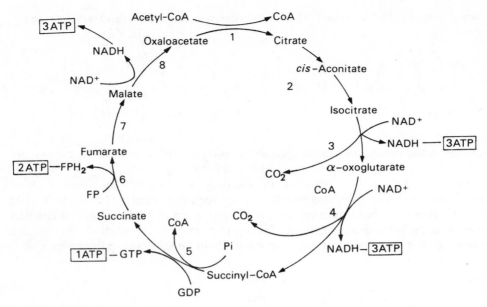

Figure 17.8 Kreb's citrate cycle

With the formation of oxaloacetate the cycle is complete. Condensation of oxaloacetate with a further acetyl fragment from acetyl-CoA sets the stage for the oxidation of another two-carbon fragment. The two-carbon fragment which has just joined with oxaloacetate to form citrate is not the one that is oxidized in the immediately ensuing steps of the cycle, but instead two carbon atoms from the oxaloacetate are oxidized. The oxaloacetate remaining after one turn of the cycle thus contains carbon atoms (shown in heavy type) from the acetyl fragment which was added at the start of that turn. The carbon atoms from the added acetyl fragment are oxidized in the citrate cycle, but not immediately.

The overall reaction of the citrate cycle, which is shown in Figure 17.8, is:

$$CH_3COSCoA + 3NAD^+ + FAD + GDP + P_i + 3H_2O \rightarrow$$
$$CoASH + 2CO_2 + 3NADH + 3H^+ + FADH_2 + GTP$$

ATP production from glucose

Having considered the details of the citrate cycle and respiratory chain, it is now possible to draw up a 'balance sheet' for the production of ATP from glucose when it is oxidized to CO_2 and H_2O.

Stage I: glycolysis

During the first stage of glucose breakdown as the result of the two substrate level phosphorylations:

$$1,3\text{-Diphosphoglycerate} + ADP \rightarrow 3\text{-phosphoglycerate} + ATP$$
$$Phosphoenolpyruvate + ADP \rightarrow pyruvate + ATP$$

and the fact that these occur twice for every molecule of glucose degraded, four molecules of ATP are produced. However, one molecule of ATP is used up in each of the following reactions:

the conversion of glucose $\rightarrow$ glucose 6-phosphate

the phosphofructokinase reaction in which fructose 6-phosphate is converted to
fructose 1,6-bisphosphate

Under anaerobic conditions, therefore, when one molecule of glucose is converted to lactate, the result is the *net* synthesis of two molecules of ATP.

Under aerobic conditions, instead of being used to convert pyruvate to lactate, the two molecules of NADH produced in the reaction

$$2 \times \text{glyceraldehyde 3-P} + 2NAD^+ + 2P_1 \rightarrow 2 \times \text{1,3-diphosphoglycerate} + 2NADH + H^+$$

are oxidized via the respiratory chain. However, since they are produced in the cytoplasm and have to be transported into the mitochondrial by the glycerophosphate shuttle system (page 230) the oxidation of each pair of H atoms is accompanied by the synthesis of only two instead of three molecules of ATP, giving a total production of six molecules of ATP.

Stage II: oxidation of pyruvate

The pyruvate produced in stage I under aerobic conditions passes into the mitochondria where it is oxidatively decarboxylated and gives rise to two molecules of acetyl-CoA and two molecules of NADH. Oxidation of each NADH produces three molecules of ATP giving a net production of six.

Stage III: citrate cycle and respiratory chain

The two molecules of acetyl-CoA produced in Stage II when fed into the citrate cycle each give rise to twelve molecules of ATP since

$$\begin{array}{llr} \text{3 molecules of NADH} & \rightarrow & \text{9 ATP} \\ \text{1 molecule of FPH}_2 & \rightarrow & \text{2 ATP} \\ \text{1 molecule of succinyl-CoA} & \rightarrow & \text{1 ATP} \end{array}$$

Summary

Conversion of glucose to 2 pyruvate	6
Conversion of 2 pyruvate to 2 acetyl-CoA	6
Oxidation of 2 acetyl-CoA to CO_2 and H_2O	24
	36

The free energy of oxidation of 1 mol of glucose

$$= -2872 \text{ kJ } (-686 \text{ kcal})$$

and the synthesis of ATP from ADP requires 31 kJ (7·3 kcal) per mol so that the percentage of the energy conserved as ATP

$$= \frac{36 \times 31}{2872} \times 100 = 39\%$$

The synthetic function of citrate cycle intermediates

The main function of the citrate cycle is undoubtedly that of oxidizing intermediary metabolites so that a large part of their energy is conserved. It is nevertheless an amphibolic pathway and may furnish precursors for synthetic reactions. Succinyl-CoA is a building block for the porphyrins and hence for the haem which is required for the synthesis of haemoglobin and other haem-containing proteins. Oxaloacetate and 2-oxoglutarate serve as precursors for the synthesis of various amino acids, e.g. aspartic acid, alanine, glutamic acid, proline. If there is a constant draining away of citrate cycle intermediates for synthetic purposes, there must also be constant replacement if the efficiency of the cycle is to be maintained. Special reactions known as *anaplerotic reactions* exist by which the cycle intermediates may be replenished. One of the most important of these is the *pyruvate carboxylase* reaction. In this reaction the biotin-containing enzyme catalyses the carboxylation of pyruvate by CO_2 to form oxaloacetate at the expense of ATP.

$$
\begin{array}{c}
COO^- \\
| \\
C{=}O \\
| \\
CH_3
\end{array}
\ +\ CO_2\ +\ ATP
\ \underset{}{\overset{\text{Pyruvate carboxylase}}{\rightleftharpoons}}\
\begin{array}{c}
COO^- \\
| \\
C{=}O \\
| \\
CH_2 \\
| \\
COO^-
\end{array}
\ +\ ADP\ +\ P_i
$$

Pyruvate   Oxaloacetate

Another reaction of lesser importance is the reductive carboxylation of pyruvate to malate. This is catalysed by the *malic enzyme* and the reducing power is supplied by NADPH.

$$
\begin{array}{c}
COO^- \\
| \\
CO \\
| \\
CH_3
\end{array}
\ +\ CO_2\ +\ NADPH\ +\ H^+
\ \underset{}{\overset{\text{Malic enzyme}}{\rightleftharpoons}}\
\begin{array}{c}
COO^- \\
| \\
HCOH \\
| \\
CH_2 \\
| \\
COO^-
\end{array}
\ +\ NADP^+
$$

Pyruvate   Malate

Chapter 18
Lipid metabolism

The digestion and absorption of fats pose considerable problems because of their insolubility in water. The fat splitting enzymes or *lipases* are water-soluble and consequently can only operate at the interface between lipid droplets and the aqueous phase. For this reason the degree of dispersion or emulsification is very important in ensuring that fat is adequately digested and absorbed.

Lipases are secreted both in the stomach and in the pancreatic juice. The value of *gastric lipase* is doubtful since its optimum pH is 8·0 whereas the pH of the normal adult stomach is 1·0–2·0. It may be more effective in infants, where the pH of the stomach contents is much higher and where the fat is mainly milk fat which is already highly emulsified.

The process of emulsification of other fats is probably initiated by the churning motion of the stomach and is greatly facilitated when the chyme passes into the duodenum and is mixed with the bile and pancreatic juice. These secretions, which are both alkaline, neutralize the acid from the stomach so that conditions become suitable for the action of *pancreatic lipase*. Bile contains no enzymes but owes its effects to the presence of the *bile salts*, *sodium glycocholate* and *sodium taurocholate*, which are powerful detergents. The bile salts are derived from *cholic acid*, a sterol, which is joined by a peptide linkage either to glycine or to taurine.

$$CH_2 \cdot NH_2$$
$$|$$
$$COOH \qquad \text{Glycine}$$

$$CH_2 \cdot NH_2$$
$$|$$
$$CH_2 \cdot SO_3H \qquad \text{Taurine}$$

Cholic acid

Lipase is relatively unspecific in its action since it is little affected by either the degree of saturation or the chain length of the fatty acids present in the glyceride. It acts preferentially to remove the fatty acid present in the α-position, so that the first product is an α,β-diglyceride. The fatty acid in the second α-position is then removed to give a β-monoglyceride. Hydrolysis of the monoglyceride probably only occurs after isomerization, involving transfer of the remaining acyl group to one of the α-positions (Figure 18.1). The first, second and third fatty acids are

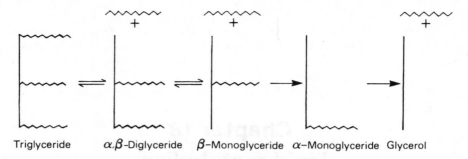

Triglyceride α,β-Diglyceride β-Monoglyceride α-Monoglyceride   Glycerol

Figure 18.1 The hydrolysis of triglycerides

removed with increasing difficulty, so that monoglycerides are a major product of fat digestion and small amounts of diglyceride also remain. It appears that only about 30–40% of the triglycerides are completely hydrolysed to glycerol and fatty acids.

Lipase is activated by bile salts and Ca^{2+} ions. The latter probably act by precipitating the fatty acids which are produced as insoluble calcium soaps.

Absorption of fat

Although fatty acids, glycerol and monoglycerides are the main products of fat digestion, none of these substances appears in the bloodstream in appreciable amounts. Glycerol is water-soluble and readily absorbed by the intestinal epithelial cells. The long chain fatty acids and their monoglycerides, on the other hand, are only sparingly soluble in water and are not readily absorbed. Their absorption is facilitated by the presence of the bile salts with which they form molecular aggregates or *micelles*. It is in such micellar dispersions that the fatty acids and monoglycerides appear to enter the mucosal cells, although how they do so is not clear. Once inside the mucosal cells the fatty acid–bile salt complex dissociates and the bile salts pass into the portal circulation and are returned to the liver. The role of the bile salts in absorption seems to be even more important than in digestion, since if bile is totally excluded from the gut large amounts of fatty acids are found in the faeces.

The fatty acids and monoglycerides released from micelles are resynthesized into triglycerides within the epithelial cells, the mechanism of resynthesis being similar to that for triglyceride synthesis in adipose tissue (page 258). It should be noted that triglycerides that accumulate in the intestinal mucosal cells during fat absorption are different from those originally present in the food, both with respect to the arrangement of their fatty acids and the origin of the glycerol part of the molecule. Glycerol in totally resynthesized fat is derived from intermediates of glycolysis and not from the original glyceride.

From the mucosal cells, the droplets of resynthesized triglyceride pass into the central lacteals of the intestinal villi. They then move into the lymphatics where they appear as small droplets known as *chylomicrons* which are coated with a stabilizing layer of protein, phospholipid and cholesterol. From the lymphatics they pass into the systemic blood via the thoracic duct giving the plasma a milky appearance. This lipaemia is, however, only temporary since the chylomicrons are readily attacked by *lipoprotein lipase* which is produced in a number of tissues and released into the capillaries. This enables the tissues to take up fatty acids from the blood and use them for immediate energy production or for energy storage. The lipoprotein lipase activity of the extrahepatic tissues varies according to the nutritional state. After a meal adipose tissue has a high activity while that of muscle is low; consequently a large proportion of the ingested fatty acids is stored. On the other hand during starvation, exercise or exposure to cold, the lipoprotein lipase activity of muscle is high and that of adipose tissue low so that fatty acids are used mainly for energy production. This adaptation to the changing needs of the organism is probably achieved by hormonal control.

Most of the long chain fatty acids are absorbed into the lymphatic system but the small proportion of fatty acids that contain less than ten carbon atoms do not become re-esterified in the mucosal cells and find their way directly into the portal blood where they circulate as *non-esterified fatty acids* bound to serum albumin. On reaching the tissues these fatty acids are usually oxidized straight away rather than stored.

Body fats

Body fats may be broadly divided into two types, namely the *constant* and *variable elements*. The constant element, which, as the name suggests, is not subject to appreciable variations in amount, is composed mainly of phospholipids and other compound lipids. It represents those lipids present in all regions of the body that fulfil a mainly structural role. The variable element is composed almost entirely of triglycerides and constitutes the main energy reserve. This depot fat is found as a layer under the skin and also surrounding the viscera. It shows wide variations in amount according to the nutritional state. In addition, small amounts of lipid material are present in transport forms in the blood. The plasma of a normal post-absorptive subject contains about 500 mg of total lipid per 100 ml. Free fatty acids are present only in small amounts. Except in the immediate post-absorptive period, the plasma is clear and limpid, since the water-insoluble triglycerides and free fatty acids are associated with various plasma protein fractions to give soluble lipoprotein complexes. It is now clear that adipose tissue fat undergoes rapid and continuous turnover even when the body weight is constant or falling. In line with this is the finding that the small amounts of unesterified or *free fatty acids* (FFA) in the plasma have a high turnover rate. When ample amounts of energy-producing materials are available more are added to than released from the tissue stores and the plasma concentration tends to fall. When extra energy is required, more FFA are released from the tissues and the plasma concentration rises. These two opposing functions of adipose tissue, the accumulation and mobilization of fat, are delicately balanced. However, at certain times, and under certain conditions, one or other process will predominate. Survival of many animal species depends on their ability to store sufficient fat in times of plenty to tide them over lean periods. The amount laid down must not, however, be so great that their mobility is impaired.

Triglycerides are peculiarly well suited to their role as the main food reserve since:

1. On oxidation they produce more than twice the amount of energy released during the oxidation of an equivalent weight of carbohydrate or protein (page 122).
2. Unlike protein and glycogen, fat can be laid down without any concomitant storage of water so that fat depots are compact highly concentrated energy stores.
3. The metabolism of fat produces more water than either protein or carbohydrate

$$1 \text{ g fat} \equiv 1\cdot07 \text{ g water}$$
$$1 \text{ g starch} \equiv 0\cdot55 \text{ g water}$$
$$1 \text{ g protein} \equiv 0\cdot41 \text{ g water}$$
$$(1 \text{ g alcohol} \equiv 1\cdot17 \text{ g water})$$

Although under normal circumstances this may not be an important consideration, when water supplies are restricted it is clearly advantageous that a large proportion of the energy requirement should be derived from fat or better still from alcohol! On the other hand, protein consumption should be kept low since the urea produced from its metabolism requires water for its elimination via the kidneys. The camel's hump is, of course, mainly composed of fat.

The oxidation of fat

In fasting conditions Man and other mammals use fat as the main source of energy and it has been estimated that, even in normally fed animals, the oxidation of fatty acids provides at least half of the energy used by the liver, kidneys, heart and resting skeletal muscle. Brain, however, normally derives little or no energy from this source and is dependent upon the blood glucose.

The oxidation of fatty acids takes place in the mitochondria and involves a series of reactions by which fragments containing two carbon atoms are released one at a time in the form of acetyl-CoA. The reactions are repeated until the entire fatty acid chain has been converted into acetyl-CoA which enters the citrate cycle. Significant amounts of ATP are generated in the oxidative reactions which lead to the formation of acetyl-CoA, but even more is derived from the oxidation of the acetyl-CoA itself.

Oxidation of triglycerides must be preceded by *lipolysis*. Breakdown into their constituent fatty acids and glycerol occurs in the tissues under the influence of lipases. A special *adrenaline-sensitive lipase* in adipose tissue releases FFA and glycerol into the blood when extra energy is required. Glycerol, which represents only a minor fraction of the triglyceride (about 10% in tristearin), is activated by conversion to glycerol 3-phosphate under the influence of the enzyme, *glycerol kinase*. This is present in liver and kidney and various other tissues but is virtually absent from adipose tissue, skeletal and heart muscle. The glycerol 3-phosphate is then dehydrogenated to dihydroxyacetone phosphate which is a normal intermediate of carbohydrate metabolism involved in both glycolytic and gluconeogenetic pathways.

$$
\begin{array}{ccc}
\underset{\text{Glycerol}}{\begin{array}{l}\text{CH}_2\text{OH}\\|\\\text{CHOH}\\|\\\text{CH}_2\text{OH}\end{array}} &
\xrightarrow[\text{Glycerol kinase}]{\text{ATP}\quad\text{ADP}} &
\underset{\text{Glycerol 3-phosphate}}{\begin{array}{l}\text{CH}_2\text{OH}\\|\\\text{CHOH}\\|\\\text{CH}_2\text{O}-\text{P}\end{array}} &
\xrightarrow[\text{dehydrogenase}]{\text{NAD}^+\quad\text{NADH}+\text{H}^+}_{\text{Glycerol 3-phosphate}} &
\underset{\substack{\text{Dihydroxyacetone}\\\text{phosphate}}}{\begin{array}{l}\text{CH}_2\text{OH}\\|\\\text{C}=\text{O}\\|\\\text{CH}_2\text{O}-\text{P}\end{array}}
\end{array}
$$

Similarly the fatty acids must be activated by conversion to their CoA derivatives before they can be metabolized. Formation of the fatty acyl-CoA derivatives is catalysed by various *fatty acid thiokinases* (fatty acid : CoA ligases) whose activity is linked with the breakdown of ATP to AMP and pyrophosphate, the liberated energy being used in the formation of the thiol ester bond:

$$
\text{R}\cdot\text{COO}^- \; \text{CoASH} + \text{ATP} \xrightarrow{\text{Fatty acid thiokinase}} \text{R}\cdot\text{CO}\sim\text{SCoA} + \text{AMP} + \text{PP}_i
$$

Since the reaction is essentially irreversible, fatty acids may be activated and metabolized even when present in low concentration. Furthermore, the reaction will proceed when the ATP concentration is low. The expenditure of the ATP is well worth while in view of the much greater amounts produced during the oxidation of the fatty acids.

Although conversion of FFA to their CoA esters may occur in either the cytoplasm or the mitochondria, their oxidation occurs only within the mitochondria and, since the inner mitochondrial membrane is impermeable to acyl-CoA compounds, a special carrier is needed to take the acyl groups across. The carrier is the compound *carnitine*, to which the acyl group is transferred from acyl-CoA by a *carnitine-CoA acyl transferase* which is associated with the mitochondrial membrane.

$$\underset{\underset{CH_3}{|}}{\overset{\overset{CH_3}{|}}{H_3C-N^{\pm}}}CH_2-CHOH-CH_2-COOH \qquad \text{Carnitine}$$

Once inside the mitochondrion the acyl group is tranferred back to CoA. Thus the extra- and intra-mitochondrial supplies of CoA are kept separate (see Figure 18.5).

Oxidation of fatty acyl-CoA compounds occurs by a well-recognized pattern of reactions similar to those occurring at the four-carbon stages of the citrate cycle. Thus oxidation of the β-carbon atom as shown in Figure 18.2 occurs by: (1) removal of 2H to give an unsaturated derivative; (2) addition of H_2O to give a β-hydroxy derivative; (3) removal of 2H to give a β-keto derivative.

The first reaction of the sequence is catalysed by a *fatty acyl:CoA dehydrogenase*. The reaction requires a stronger oxidizing agent than NAD^+ and the enzymes are flavoproteins containing FAD as the prosthetic group. Before the two hydrogen atoms which have been removed are passed along the carriers in the later stages of the electron-transport chain, they are transferred to a second flavoprotein, known as the *electron-transport flavoprotein*. It is not clear why an extra intermediate is required here but the by-passing of NAD^+ means that only two molecules of ADP are converted to ATP in the course of this particular oxidation.

In the next reaction catalysed by *enoyl hydrase*, water is added at the double bond giving the corresponding β-hydroxyacyl-CoA. This is followed by the second dehydrogenation under the influence of *β-hydroxyacyl-CoA dehydrogenase*, which uses NAD^+ as the electron acceptor. In the presence of a further molecule of CoA the resulting β-ketoacyl-CoA is split by *β-ketothiolase*. This reaction, which is known as *thiolysis*, produces one molecule of acetyl-CoA and one molecule of acyl-CoA in which the acyl group is two carbons shorter than the original. The reaction is highly exergonic and virtually irreversible.

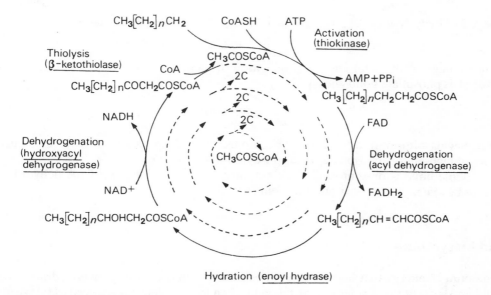

Figure 18.2 The fatty acid oxidation spiral

The shortened fatty acyl-CoA is now drawn back into the oxidative sequence while the acetyl-CoA enters the citrate cycle.

Points worth noting are: (1) All the reactants are acyl derivatives of CoA. (2) All the enzymes are localized within the mitochondria with those of the citrate cycle and electron-transport chain. This ensures efficient utilization of the acetyl-CoA released by the fatty acid oxidation. (3) Only one activation step is necessary, regardless of the length of the fatty acid chain. This uses two high-energy bonds, since ATP is broken down to AMP and pyrophosphate during the thiokinase reaction.

The pathway represents a remarkably efficient and economical method of processing a great variety of fatty acids. It can be used for all those containing an even number of C atoms regardless of the chain length, and also for the unsaturated fatty acids found abundantly in foodstuffs. As a result of the combined action of two addition enzymes, unsaturated fatty acids are converted into standard intermediates for the β-oxidative pathway.

The energy yield from fatty acid oxidation

During the oxidation of palmitate by the pathway described, 8 molecules of acetyl-CoA are produced. Each of these, on oxidation via the citrate cycle, provides for the conversion of 12 molecules of ADP to ATP so that a total of 96 molecules of ATP will be formed. In addition, during each of the seven β-oxidations required to produce the 8 molecules of acetyl-CoA, 1 molecule of reduced flavoprotein and 1 of NADH are formed. In the course of the oxidation of the reduced flavoprotein, 2 molecules of ATP are produced while the oxidation of each molecule of NADH gives rise to 3. Thus every β-oxidation results in the synthesis of 5 molecules of ATP giving a total of 35 (7×5). The balance sheet for the production of ATP is as follows:

7 β-oxidations each producing 5 molecules of ATP	$+35$
Oxidation of 8 molecules of acetyl-CoA each producing 12 molecules of ATP	$+96$
Less 2 ATP equivalents expended during the initial fatty acid activation and conversion of ATP to AMP	-2
	Net gain 129

If the ΔG of hydrolysis of ATP is taken as -31 kJ ($-7\cdot3$ kcal) then the energy conserved

$$= -129 \times 31\,(-7\cdot3) = -4000 \text{ kJ } (-942 \text{ kcal}) \text{ mol}^{-1}$$

The percentage of the total energy of oxidation of palmitate (9800 kJ or 2340 kcal) which is recovered as phosphate bond energy

$$= \frac{4000}{9800} \times 100 = 41\%$$

For fatty acids with more or less than 16 C atoms, every 2 C unit will increase or reduce the number of high-energy phosphate bonds produced by $5 + 12$, i.e. 17.

If a double bond is present in the original fatty acid, one of the acyl-CoA dehydrogenase reactions becomes unnecessary and the yield is decreased by 2.

Lipid biosynthesis

The amount of energy that higher vertebrates can store in the form of carbohydrate is strictly limited and most of the surplus energy taken in when food is plentiful is stored as fat. Although fatty acids cannot give rise to carbohydrate in the body, all types of energy-producing materials may be converted into depot fat and carbohydrate appears to be a major source. In spite of the fact that the carbon residues of the amino acids are readily transformed into pyruvate or citrate cycle intermediates, which may in turn be converted into fat, significant amounts are unlikely to be derived from dietary protein in normal circumstances.

Lipid biosynthesis occurs in two stages: (1) fatty acid synthesis, and (2) incorporation of fatty acids into triglycerides or compound lipids.

Fatty acid synthesis

The long chain fatty acids are built up from units containing two C atoms derived from acetyl-CoA. The process is essentially reductive since, after condensation of the units, a $-CO-$ group must be converted to a $-CH_2$ group. In some respects the synthesis of the acyl residue resembles the oxidative process in reverse, but there are a number of important differences. In the first instance, whereas fatty acids are oxidized within the mitochondria, their synthesis is essentially a cytoplasmic process. Moreover, while the muscles are the principal site of fatty acid oxidation, fatty acid synthesis occurs mainly in the liver and adipose tissue.

During the conversion of carbohydrate to fatty acids the carbohydrate is first oxidized to pyruvate which enters the mitochondria and is oxidatively decarboxylated by pyruvate dehydrogenase to acetyl-CoA and CO_2. Some of the acetyl-CoA will be drawn directly into the citrate cycle to replenish the stocks of ATP. If these are already high, a large proportion of the acetyl-CoA will be used for fatty acid synthesis. However, this is a cytoplasmic process and the mitochondrial wall is not readily permeable to acyl-CoA compounds. The problem is overcome by uniting the acetyl groups with oxaloacetate to form citrate which is able to pass between the extra- and intra-mitochondrial compartments. Thus when citrate is present in high concentration, due to a surplus of substrates for the final stages of oxidative metabolism, it diffuses from the mitochondria into the cytosol. Once in the cytosol, the citrate is subject to the action of the citrate cleavage enzyme *ATP citrate lyase*, which, in the presence of ATP, breaks it down into oxaloacetate and acetyl-CoA once again. In this way, oxaloacetate acts as a carrier of acetyl groups from the mitochondria into the cytoplasm. The acetyl groups are then used for fatty acid synthesis and oxaloacetate is converted to pyruvate by a two-stage process:

$$
\begin{array}{c}
\text{COOH} \\
| \\
\text{CO} \\
| \\
\text{CH}_2 \\
| \\
\text{COOH}
\end{array}
\quad
\underset{\substack{\text{Malate}\\\text{dehydrogenase}}}{\overset{\text{NADH} + \text{H}^+ \quad \text{NAD}^+}{\rightleftharpoons}}
\quad
\begin{array}{c}
\text{COOH} \\
| \\
\text{CHOH} \\
| \\
\text{CH}_2 \\
| \\
\text{COOH}
\end{array}
\quad
\underset{\text{'Malic enzyme'}}{\overset{\text{NADP}^+ \quad \text{NADPH} + \text{H}^+}{\rightleftharpoons}}
\quad
\begin{array}{c}
\text{CH}_3 \\
| \\
\text{CO} \quad + \text{CO}_2 \\
| \\
\text{COOH}
\end{array}
$$

Oxaloacetate   Malate   Pyruvate

As a result of these reactions when energy supplies are plentiful, reducing power (NADH), obtained during the conversion of glucose to pyruvate by the glycolytic pathway, instead of being used for further energy production can be transferred to $NADP^+$ and used for fat synthesis and energy storage. One NADPH is generated for every acetyl unit that passes into the cytosol from the mitochondria but the synthesis of 1 mol of palmitate requires 14 mol of NADPH (see below) and the remaining 6 are obtained from the pentose phosphate pathway. The pyruvate passes back into the mitochondria and is used either for regeneration of oxaloacetate or for conversion to acetyl-CoA (Figure 18.5).

In the first reaction of fatty acid synthesis acetyl-CoA is converted to *malonyl-CoA* by the very important enzyme, *acetyl-CoA carboxylase* which contains biotin (page 166) as its prosthetic group. ATP is needed to provide energy for the carboxylation and magnesium ions are also required:

$$CH_3 \cdot CO \sim SCoA \xrightarrow[\substack{\text{Acetyl-CoA carboxylase} \\ \text{biotin} + Mg^{2+}}]{\substack{ATP \qquad ADP \\ CO_2}} COOH \cdot CH_2 \cdot CO \sim SCoA$$

Acetyl-CoA   Malonyl-CoA

Acetyl-CoA carboxylase is an allosteric enzyme and the reaction is the primary regulating step in fatty acid synthesis (page 341). It is also regulated through phosphorylation/ dephosphorylation reactions which modify specific serine residues on the protein (page 344).

The subsequent series of reactions that lead eventually to the formation of palmitate in mammals are carried out by a multienzyme complex known as *fatty acid synthase*. The initial two carbons, which eventually form C-15 and C-16 of palmitate, are supplied in the form of acetyl-CoA which acts as a primer for the subsequent condensation of malonyl-CoA units which lose CO_2 in the process. The hydrogens required for the reductive reactions are all supplied by NADPH and the overall process may be represented as follows:

1 acetyl-CoA + 7 malonyl-CoA + 14NADPH + 14H$^+$ →

1 palmitate + 7CO$_2$ + 8CoASH + 14NADP$^+$ + 6H$_2$O

As in gluconeogenesis, alternate carboxylation and decarboxylation reactions are involved.

The fatty acid synthase system of mammals, birds and yeast is a complex of six enzymes and an *acyl carrier protein* that cannot be dissociated without loss of activity. The acyl intermediates are linked to the low molecular weight acyl carrier protein which plays a role in the synthesis of fatty acids comparable with that played by coenzyme A in their degradation. It contains two types of reactive –SH group. One of these belongs to *phosphopantetheine* (PhPT) which is also a constituent of coenzyme A. This –SH group occurring at the end of the long chain-like phosphopantetheinyl group is responsible for binding acyl groups to the complex by a thioester linkage. The second –SH group affords temporary accommodation for the growing acyl chain.

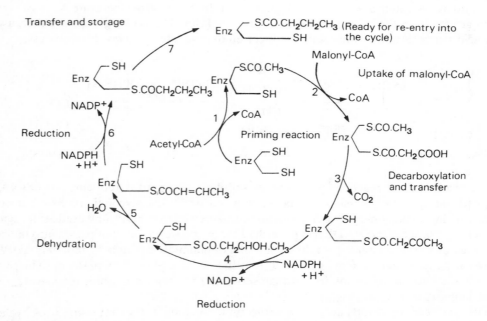

Figure 18.3 Fatty acid synthesis

The long PhPT group appears to be mobile so that it can swing round and carry the growing C chain through wide arcs, bringing it in contact with the active sites of the enzymes responsible for the successive reduction, dehydration and second reduction needed to produce the saturated fatty acyl group. The saturated group is then transferred to the other –SH group while a new malonyl group is attached to the swinging chain phosphopantetheinyl group. The sequence of reactions, which is summarized in Figure 18.3, is as follows:

Reaction 1

This is the priming reaction in which the acetyl group of acetyl-CoA reacts with the storage –SH group and free CoA is released.

Reaction 2

A malonyl group from malonyl-CoA is transferred to the long chain PhPT group.

Reaction 3

The acetyl group reacts with the malonyl group releasing CO_2 and condensing with the remainder to give an acetoacetyl group. Because of the loss of CO_2 this reaction is irreversible; the use of a malonyl rather than an acetyl group for the condensation gives the reaction a greater 'thermodynamic pull' and shifts the overall equilibrium in the direction of synthesis.

Reactions 4, 5 and 6

The acetoacetyl group is now reduced by NADPH to a β-hydroxybutyryl group which is then dehydrated to the corresponding unsaturated acyl–enzyme complex. In this case, it is the crotonyl–enzyme complex that is formed and subsequently reduced to the butyryl derivative, once again using NADPH as the reducing agent.

Reaction 7

Once the saturated fatty acyl radical has been formed it is transferred from the long arm of the PhPT group to the storage –SH group and a new malonyl group attaches to the long arm

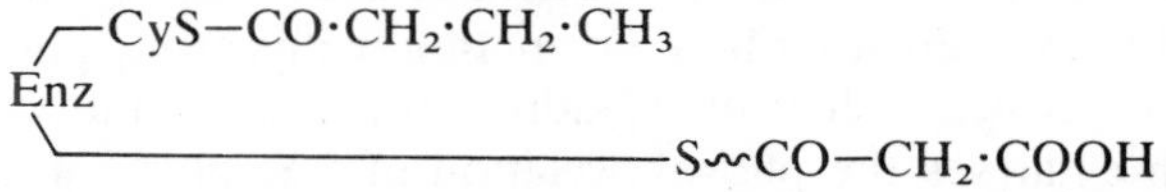

$$\text{Enz}\begin{cases} -\text{CyS}-\text{CO}\cdot\text{CH}_2\cdot\text{CH}_2\cdot\text{CH}_3 \\ \\ -\text{S}\sim\text{CO}-\text{CH}_2\cdot\text{COOH} \end{cases}$$

The butyryl group reacts with the malonyl group displacing CO_2 and forming a β-ketoacyl group containing six carbon atoms which is subjected to the same sequence of reactions as before. The whole process continues until the C_{16} palmitoyl group is formed. At this point, for some reason which is not clear, the palmitate is released from the enzyme and must be converted to palmitoyl-CoA before it can be metabolized further. Usually it will be esterified to form triglyceride.

The main differences between the synthesis and oxidation of fatty acids are shown in Table 18.1.

Although the *de novo* synthesis of fatty acids is essentially a cytoplasmic process, pre-existing fatty acid chains may be lengthened by two different enzyme systems, one occurring in the mitochondria and the other in the endoplasmic reticulum. Both show significant differences from the pathway described above but both have a requirement for reduced NADP. Between

Table 18.1 Differences between the processes of fatty acid oxidation and synthesis

	Oxidation	Synthesis
Most active tissues	Heart, skeletal muscle	Liver, adipose tissue
Site of activity	Mitochondrial matrix	Cytosol
Enzymes	Various separate enzymes	Multienzyme complex
Hydrogen carriers	NAD^+, FAD	NADPH
Form in which 2-C units are added or removed	Acetyl-CoA	Malonyl-CoA (+1 acetyl-CoA as primer)

them these systems are believed to be responsible for extending the palmitoyl chain to provide those fatty acids which contain more than 16 carbon atoms.

Pre-existing fatty acids may be modified not only by lengthening and shortening of the chain by two carbon atoms at a time, but also, to a limited extent, by the introduction of double bonds. Oleic acid (18 : 1) is the most abundant fatty acid in human depot fat and it can be formed quite readily in the body. An enzyme system capable of oxidizing stearoyl-CoA at the central bond is present in the endoplasmic reticulum; it uses molecular oxygen and NADPH in the process.

$$\text{Stearoyl-CoA} + \text{NADPH} + \text{H}^+ + \text{O}_2 \rightarrow \text{oleolyl-CoA} + \text{NADP}^+ + 2\text{H}_2\text{O}$$

Although mammalian systems are able to desaturate fatty acids in this way, and also at the β-carbon atom in the course of their oxidation, no mechanism exists by which double bonds can be introduced between C-9 and the CH_3-terminus of the chain. This explains why the polyunsaturated (polyenoic) fatty acids, linoleic (18 : 2) and arachidonic (20 : 4), must be supplied in the diet (page 123).

Triglyceride synthesis

Fatty acids do not occur free in the body to any appreciable extent. In fact, in high concentration they are toxic and, when being transported in the plasma, are found in combination with protein.

Normally, after synthesis or modification, fatty acids are combined with glycerol to form triglycerides or compound lipids such as phospholipids and glycolipids. For the combination of fatty acids and glycerol both must be present in activated forms as acyl-CoA derivatives and glycerol 3-phosphate respectively. The mechanism of activation of the fatty acids by the thio-kinase reaction has already been described. Formation of glycerol 3-phosphate can occur in two different ways. Certain tissues such as liver, kidney and intestinal mucosa contain the enzyme *glycerol kinase* which catalyses the phosphorylation of free glycerol at the expense of ATP, a reaction comparable to the activation of glucose by hexokinase. Only tissues that possess glycerokinase can utilize free glycerol for triglyceride formation:

$$\begin{array}{ccc}
\text{CH}_2\text{OH} & & \text{CH}_2\text{OH} \\
| & \text{ATP} \quad \text{ADP} & | \\
\text{CHOH} & \xrightarrow{\text{Glycerol kinase}} & \text{CHOH} \\
| & & | \\
\text{CH}_2\text{OH} & & \text{CH}_2\text{O}-\text{\textcircled{P}} \\
\text{Glycerol} & & \text{Glycerol 3-phosphate}
\end{array}$$

At first sight it may be surprising that adipose tissue should lack this enzyme and, consequently, be unable to retrieve any of the glycerol released during triglyceride breakdown. Fat cells must obtain the glycerol 3-phosphate required for triglyceride synthesis from dihydroxyacetone phosphate produced in the course of glycolysis. This, by a simple hydrogenation, can readily be converted to glycerol 3-phosphate and all the glycerol present in stored fat must be derived from carbohydrate in this way

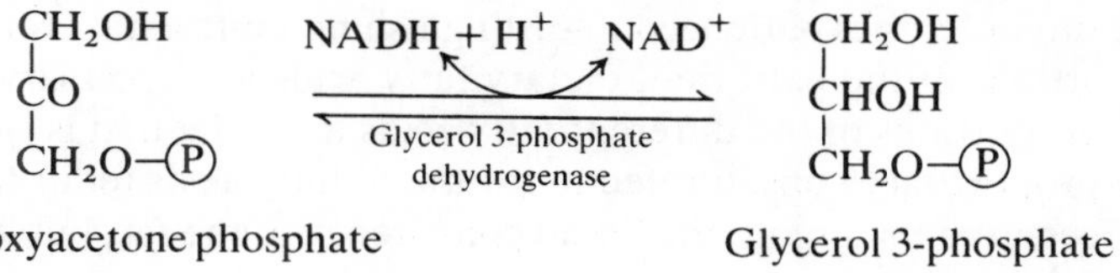

$$
\begin{array}{ccc}
\text{CH}_2\text{OH} & & \text{CH}_2\text{OH} \\
| & \text{NADH} + \text{H}^+ \quad \text{NAD}^+ & | \\
\text{CO} & \xrightleftharpoons[\substack{\text{Glycerol 3-phosphate} \\ \text{dehydrogenase}}]{} & \text{CHOH} \\
| & & | \\
\text{CH}_2\text{O}-\text{(P)} & & \text{CH}_2\text{O}-\text{(P)}
\end{array}
$$

Dihydroxyacetone phosphate   Glycerol 3-phosphate

When both fatty acyl-CoA and glycerol 3-phosphate are available, triglyceride synthesis occurs in the manner shown in Figure 18.4. The free hydroxyl groups of the glycerol 3-phosphate are each esterified by combination with a fatty acyl group transferred from the corresponding CoA derivatives, and *phosphatidic acid* (α,β-diglyceride phosphate) is produced. The phosphate is then released from phosphatidic acid under the influence of a phosphatase and the resulting diglyceride is esterified with a third molecule of fatty acyl-CoA. The enzymes responsible for this series of reactions are, for the most part, found in association with the endoplasmic reticulum.

Both the α,β-diglyceride and the phosphatidic acid may be used for the synthesis of phospholipids. The choline and ethanolamine required respectively for the synthesis of lecithins and cephalins must be available in an active form as their cytidine diphosphate derivatives.

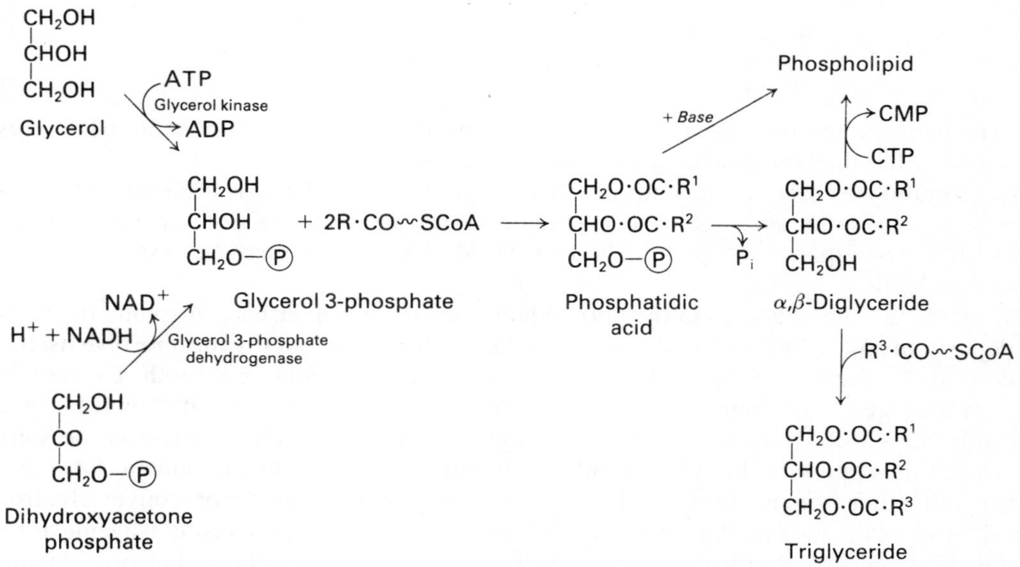

Figure 18.4 The synthesis of triglycerides

Adipose tissue

Two types of adipose tissue are now recognized, namely ordinary white adipose tissue and brown adipose tissue, which is found in hibernating animals and newborn infants but is very poorly defined in adult humans. Ordinary white adipose tissue acts as an energy reserve and a heat insulator, while brown adipose tissue is specialized for the production of heat instead of ATP.

White adipose tissue

In any particular species, the pattern of fatty acids present in stored fat is quite consistent. For example, little difficulty is experienced in distinguishing mutton fat from the much softer beef fat. Major distortions of the pattern of dietary fatty acids are necessary to induce appreciable changes in the proportions of the different fatty acids in the fat that is stored. Nevertheless, an increase in the proportion of unsaturated to saturated fatty acids tends to occur on exposure to cold. This is necessary to maintain the liquid consistency of the fat, but it is not known how this adaptation occurs.

The conversion of the dietary pattern of fatty acids into the characteristic pattern for the species depends on several features of metabolism.

1. Any short chain fatty acids that are absorbed into the bloodstream are usually rapidly oxidized as they pass through the liver.
2. Long chain fatty acids may be elongated or shortened and may also undergo limited desaturation.
3. A considerable proportion of the fatty acids deposited is derived, not from those of the food, but from carbohydrate. Such fatty acids are commonly saturated so that the fattening of animals on high-carbohydrate–low-fat diets tends to produce a hard fat with a high melting point.

The approximate percentage composition of human depot fat is as follows:

Myristic (14 : 0)	2	Palmitoleic (16 : 1)	4
Palmitic (16 : 0)	27	Oleic (18 : 1)	53
Stearic (18 : 0)	7	Linoleic (18 : 2)	7

It can be seen that the ratio of saturated to unsaturated fatty acids is about 36 : 64. Traces of fatty acids other than those listed above may be present.

The amount of stored fat depends on the point at which a balance is achieved between the rates of its deposition and mobilization. In normal people adipose tissue represents between one-fifth and one-quarter of the total body mass, although it may increase in some subjects to more than half!

When there is a breakdown in the normal homoeostatic mechanisms controlling the rates of fat deposition and mobilization, obesity may result. Ultimately, obesity must resolve itself into a question of too great a food intake or too low an energy expenditure or both. Except where there is damage to the appetite or satiety centres in the hypothalamus, it should be readily controllable. In fact, it is a question of great complexity and it is still not clear why one person can eat a great deal and stay slim while another eats comparatively little and remains fat. Obesity must result either from a failure to adapt metabolism to the food intake or, conversely, from a failure to adapt the food intake to a change in metabolism occurring as a result of ageing or some pathological process. Storage of depot fat occurs in any subject whose diet provides more calories than he expends. The source of the calories, be it fat, carbohydrate, or even, in exceptional circumstances, protein, is immaterial. The fact that carbohydrate can be converted into body fat was demonstrated by Lawes and Gilbert in 1860, long before anything was known about the relevant metabolic pathways. These workers fed young pigs on a diet containing a high proportion of carbohydrate and very little fat. Subsequent analysis of their carcasses showed that a large proportion of the fat, which had been laid down during the experimental feeding period, could only have been derived from carbohydrate.

Although carbohydrate readily supplies the carbon atoms for both the glycerol and fatty acid elements of triglycerides, net conversion of fatty acids into glucose or glycogen does not occur.

A summary of fat metabolism is given in Figure 18.5.

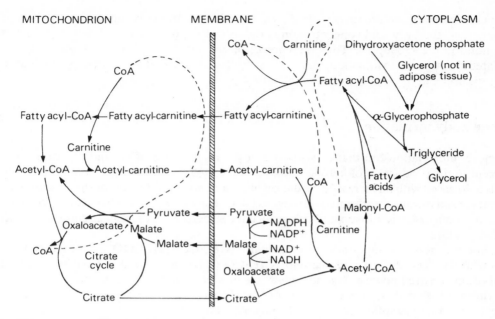

Figure 18.5 Summary of fat metabolism

Brown adipose tissue

This is a specialized form of adipose tissue which is found in newborn children and hibernating animals but, until relatively recently, was not thought to occur in adults. It now appears, however, that it may be present in adult humans and that it is more abundant than normal in subjects exposed to cold. It is found at multiple sites but mainly in the interscapular and cervical regions.

Brown adipose tissue owes its name to the fact that it has a high content of mitochondria and cytochromes which give it its characteristic colour; also it is highly vascularized. The mitochondria are different from those of other tissues. The inner mitochondrial membrane contains a special protein of molecular weight 32 000 which has been termed *thermogenin*. This constitutes about 10% of the protein of the inner mitochondrial membrane and is present in increased amounts in cold-adapted animals. Thermogenin acts as a *proton channel* which allows protons to cross the membrane. Brown fat mitochondria, as isolated, are uncoupled since the pH gradient and membrane potential produced by the respiratory chain are dissipated by the inward movement of the protons through the thermogenin proton channel. This uncoupling is reversible, however, since the mitochondria can be recoupled by the addition of low concentrations of purine nucleotides which bind to the proton channel on the outer surface of the membrane and effectively close it. In the presence of purine nucleotides, isolated brown fat mitochondria behave like mitochondria from other tissues and maintain a pH gradient and membrane potential which are used for ATP synthesis.

In unstimulated brown adipose tissue, the mitochondria are coupled, since purine nucleotides are present in the cytosol and the proton channel is closed. When the tissue is stimulated by noradrenaline, the adenylate cyclase in the cell membrane is stimulated to produce cyclic AMP which, in turn, stimulates triglyceride breakdown and the release of fatty acids. It is believed that fatty acids at low concentration displace nucleotides from the proton channel and cause it to open, thus uncoupling the mitochondria. The tissue is then able to generate heat from the energy supplied by fatty acid oxidation. When the stimulation of the tissue ceases, the fatty acid concentration is reduced, the proton channel closes again and the mitochondria are recoupled. Thus the control of enzyme activity in brown adipose tissue is mediated through the sympathetic nervous system, and its activity as an energy dissipator and heat producer can be turned on and off at very short notice.

Ketone body formation

The close interrelationship that exists between the metabolism of fat and of carbohydrate is apparent in the production of ketone bodies and the abnormal metabolic condition of *ketosis*. This is associated with an increased oxidation of fat and decreased metabolism of carbohydrate. It occurs in starvation after the glycogen stores have been depleted, or when a diet rich in fat and low in carbohydrate is consumed. It also occurs in certain pathological conditions such as diabetes mellitus.

In ketosis, three compounds, acetoacetate ($CH_3 \cdot CO \cdot CH_2 \cdot COO^-$), β-hydroxybutyrate ($CH_3 \cdot CHOH \cdot CH_2 \cdot COO^-$) and acetone ($CH_3 \cdot CO \cdot CH_3$), which are normal products of fat metabolism and are known as *ketone bodies*, are produced in much greater amounts than usual with the result that their concentrations in both blood and urine are greatly increased. The subject is then said to suffer from *ketonaemia* and *ketonuria*.

Acetoacetate is the primary metabolic product but a substantial proportion of it is reduced to β-hydroxybutyrate under the influence of *β-hydroxybutyrate dehydrogenase* and NADH. Acetoacetate also undergoes a slow spontaneous decarboxylation to acetone which appears in the urine and, since it is volatile, is also lost from the lungs and may be smelt in the breath.

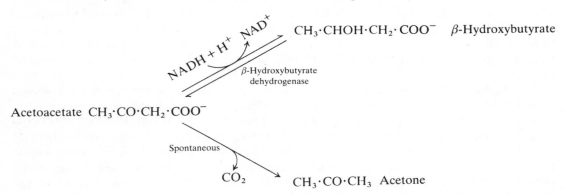

Acetoacetic and β-hydroxybutyric acids are moderately strong acids and their ionization tends to release protons into the plasma which react with the plasma bicarbonate. As a result of this, there is a depletion of buffer cations and the subject suffers from secondary *acidosis*.

In non-ruminant animals, including Man, the liver is the only organ that adds ketone bodies to the blood since its enzymes are active in ketone body production but inactive in ketone body utilization. This is exactly the reverse of the condition in muscle and other extrahepatic tissues which oxidize ketone bodies but do not produce them.

In ketosis, for one reason or another, there is a reduction in the amount of carbohydrate which can be oxidized so that the demands of the body for high-energy phosphates have to be met by an increase in the oxidation of fat. The tendency for the blood glucose to fall results in an increased rate of lipolysis in adipose tissue. The rate at which fatty acids are released exceeds the rate at which they can be re-esterified since, because of the reduced carbohydrate metabolism, little glycerol 3-phosphate is available. As a result, large amounts of free fatty acid are released into the circulation and pass to the liver where two possible fates await them. Either they can be re-esterified or they can be caught up into the β-oxidation process and converted to acetyl-CoA. However, in the liver as in adipose tissue, the glycerophosphate required for the esterification process is in short supply. It is certainly not available in the quantities required to esterify the greatly increased amounts of FFA arriving from the depots. As a result, a large proportion of the FFA are drawn into the oxidative pathway and converted to acetyl-CoA. Some of this is fully oxidized to CO_2 and H_2O by the reactions of the citrate cycle and respiratory chain, but the very large amounts of acetyl-CoA produced cause reversal of the thiolase (acetyl-CoA acetyltransferase) reaction leading to synthesis of acetoacetyl-CoA.

$$2CH_3CO—SCoA \xrightleftharpoons{\text{Thiolase}} CH_3 \cdot CO \cdot CH_2 \cdot CO—SCoA + CoA—SH$$

Present in the liver, but not in other tissues, are enzymes which convert the acetoacetyl-CoA into acetoacetate which the liver is unable to metabolize further.

The acetoacetyl-CoA is converted into acetoacetate in two stages.

1. A molecule of acetoacetyl-CoA condenses with a further molecule of acetyl-CoA to give β-hydroxymethylglutaryl-CoA (HMG-CoA), a reaction reminiscent of the formation of citrate from oxaloacetate and acetyl-CoA.
2. The β-hydroxymethylglutaryl-CoA is then cleaved into acetoacetate and one molecule of acetyl-CoA is regenerated:

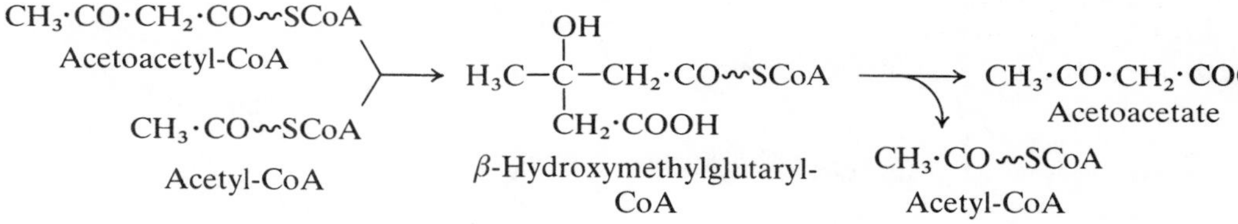

Since the activity of *HMG-CoA synthase* and *HMG-CoA cleavage enzyme* in liver is high, under conditions of carbohydrate shortage, large amounts of acetoacetate and β-hydroxybutyrate are added to the blood.

The formation of ketone bodies is useful in allowing the liver to dispose of large quantities of potentially toxic fatty acids without increasing its overall energy production. Thus in experiments with isolated perfused livers it was found that (1) the greater the quantity of fatty acids supplied, the greater the ketone body production; (2) the proportions of acetyl-CoA that were used for oxidation and for ketone body production were adjusted so that the total ATP production from the fatty acids was kept constant.

In the non-ketotic animal the ketone bodies produced by the liver pass to the muscles and other extrahepatic tissues where acetoacetate can be converted into acetoacetyl-CoA by one of two methods.

The first reaction involves the transfer of CoA from succinyl-CoA produced in the citrate cycle to acetoacetate under the influence of *succinyl-CoA : acetoacetate CoA-transferase*.

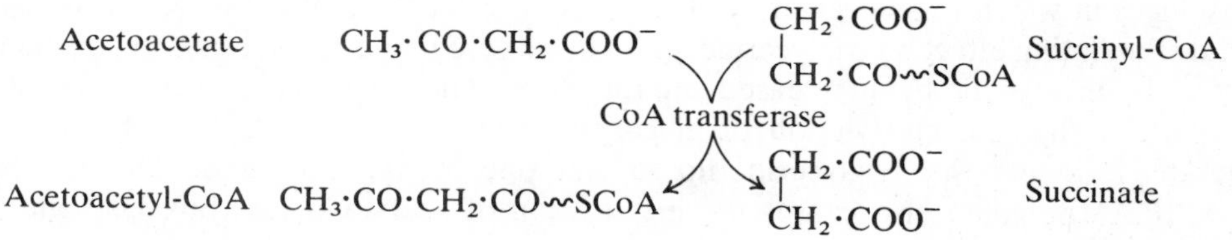

The second is a thiokinase reaction during which ATP is split into AMP and pyrophosphate:

$$CH_3 \cdot CO \cdot CH_2 \cdot COO^- + ATP + CoA\text{-}SH \xrightarrow{\text{Thiokinase}} CH_3 \cdot CO \cdot CH_2 \cdot CO \sim SCoA + AMP + PP_i -$$

Once acetoacetate has been activated by conversion into acetoacetyl-CoA it can be cleaved by thiolase in the usual way, the resulting two molecules of acetyl-CoA being fed into the citrate cycle.

The capacity of the extrahepatic tissues to oxidize ketone bodies is more than adequate to deal with the amounts reaching them under normal conditions. However, when the liver is forced to metabolize large quantities of fat it releases excessive quantities of acetoacetate and β-hydroxybutyrate into the blood. Under these circumstances the extrahepatic tissues are unable to cope with them and there is a progressive accumulation leading to both ketonaemia and ketonuria. Although the capacity of the extrahepatic tissues to oxidize ketone bodies is limited, it has been found that ketone bodies may be metabolized in preference to glucose and fatty acids.

The possible fates of acetyl-CoA are summarized in Figure 18.6.

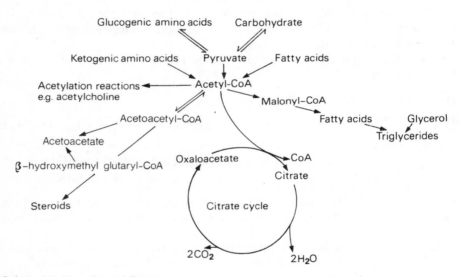

Figure 18.6 Possible fates of acetyl-CoA

Hormonal control of fat metabolism

Throughout this chapter reference has been made to a variety of factors that play a part in controlling fat metabolism within the cells of various tissues. The balancing of the metabolic activities of these tissues and overall control of fat metabolism is achieved largely as a result of the activity of the hormones adrenaline and insulin. Adrenaline, which is secreted in circumstances in which it is necessary to have plenty of fuel available for oxidation, exerts a powerful stimulating effect on triglyceride lipase in adipose tissue. This results in large amounts of fatty acids and glycerol being released into the blood. The reaction may be considered as the counterpart of the phosphorylation of glycogen in the process of glycolysis and there is considerable evidence that triglyceride lipase, like phosphorylase, is under the influence of cyclic AMP. Adrenaline also causes the inactivation of acetyl-CoA carboxylase and this is equally important as it reduces fatty acid biosynthesis. Thus a futile cycle of fatty acid synthesis and oxidation is avoided.

Insulin, on the other hand, is secreted when the blood glucose level is raised and the fuel supply exceeds demands. It not only antagonizes the effect of adrenaline on adipose tissue lipase, but also promotes carbohydrate metabolism and the process of lipogenesis by increasing the uptake of glucose into adipose tissue. The hormone also increases the disposal of glucose once it has entered the cell. The increased metabolism of glucose ensures the availability of both NADPH for fatty acid biosynthesis and glycerol 3-phosphate for esterification of the fatty acyl-CoA compounds. Efficient storage as carbohydrate and lipid is facilitated by an increase in the activity of glycogen synthase, pyruvate dehydrogenase and acetyl-CoA carboxylase through changes in the phosphorylation state of these key enzymes. These topics are dealt with more fully in Chapter 23.

Phospholipid metabolism

The most obvious function of phospholipids is structural and based on their ability to interact with both hydrophilic and hydrophobic compounds. They are essential cell constituents but are unevenly distributed in living tissues. They are present only in small amounts in depot fat but are found in appreciable amounts in liver, plasma and myelin, as well as in egg yolk and in the seeds of legumes. Their role in metabolism has not been clearly established but certain fractions undergo rapid turnover. The half-life of liver lecithin is less than 24 hours, although that of brain cephalin is over 200 days. The importance of liver lecithin is indicated by the finding that if choline, or the methyl groups required for its synthesis, are lacking from the diet, large amounts of fat accumulate in the liver cells.

Recently the metabolism of one of the more highly labile phospholipid fractions, the *phosphatidylinositides*, has been shown to be closely associated with intracellular calcium metabolism. The phosphatidylinositides are esters of the cyclic hexahydric alcohol, *inositol*.

Inositol

Cholesterol metabolism

The naturally occurring steroids include the bile salts and various hormones. Steroids are also present as membrane constituents. They are derived from cholesterol, which is present in appreciable amounts in normal diets.

A large fraction of the cholesterol present in lymph and blood plasma is found in the chylomicrons and about two-thirds of the plasma cholesterol is esterified with fatty acids giving *cholesteryl esters*. Cholesterol and its esters constitute a large fraction of the lipid present in the atheromatous plaques which are deposited in the intima of arteries in the condition of atherosclerosis (page 267). Cholesterol, which is insoluble in aqueous media, is also a major constituent of most gallstones.

Dietary cholesterol appears, on average, to contribute only about 10% to the total serum cholesterol and cholesterol synthesis presents no difficulty. All the C atoms of the steroid

Table 18.2 Cholesterol content of commonly used foods (mg 100^{-1} edible portion)

Food and description	Cholesterol content	Food and description	Cholesterol content
Beef, lean, cooked, total edible	91	Herring, flesh only	85
Brains, raw	>2000	Ice cream, 10% fat	40
Butter	250	Ice milk	20
Buttermilk, from skim milk	2	Lamb, cooked, total edible	98
Cake, chocolate	48	Lard	95
Cheese		Liver	
American, pasterurized processed	90	Beef, calf, hog, lamb, cooked	438
Cheddar, natural	99	Chicken, cooked	746
Cottage, creamed 4% fat	19	Margarine	
Cottage, uncreamed	7	All vegetable fat	0
Cream	111	$^2/_3$ animal fat–$^1/_3$ vegetable fat	50
Parmesan, grated	113	Mayonnaise, commercial	70
Swiss, pasteurized processed	93	Milk	
Chicken		Dry non-fat	22
Breast, cooked, total edible	80	Low fat, 1% fat	6
Drumstick, cooked, total edible	91	Whole fluid	14
Chicken fat	65	Pork, cooked, total edible	89
Clams	50	Salmon, raw, canned	35
Crab meat	101	Sausage, all meat, cooked	62
Cream		Shrimp, raw, flesh only	150
Light	66	Sweetbreads, cooked	466
Sour	66	Tuna, drained solids	65
Eggs		Turkey, cooked	
Whole	504	Light meat, no skin	77
White	0	Dark meat, no skin	101
Yolk	1480	Veal, cooked, total edible	101
Frankfurter, all meat, cooked	62	Yogurt	
Flounder, flesh only	50	Plain or vanilla	8
Haddock, flesh only	60	Fruit, all kinds	7
Halibut, flesh only	50		

Data from R. M. Feeley *et al.* (1972). Cholesterol content of foods. *Journal of the American Dietitians Association*, **61**, 134–149

nucleus are derived from acetyl-CoA, three molecules of which condense to form β-hydroxy-methylglutaryl-CoA (HMG-CoA) as described above. HMG-CoA is the immediate precursor of *mevalonic acid* ($CH_2OH \cdot CH_2 \cdot C(OH)CH_3 \cdot CH_2 \cdot COOH$), an intermediate in the synthesis of steroids and of coenzyme Q. The reduction of HMG-CoA to mevalonate is catalysed by *HMG-CoA reductase*. This reaction is rate-limiting and irreversible and is the first committed step in steroid synthesis.

The amount of cholesterol synthesized in the body is partly regulated by the dietary intake. The cholesterol content of some commonly used foods is given in Table 18.2. In the West the average daily intake is 500–800 mg, of which about 300–400 mg are absorbed in spite of its insolubility in water. One of the effects of dietary cholesterol is to inhibit HMG-CoA reductase. The absorbed cholesterol not only reduces the activity of the enzyme already present but also suppresses the synthesis of additional enzyme. Increases in plasma cholesterol have another important effect on cholesterol metabolism. Cells other than those of the liver and intestine obtain most of their cholesterol from the plasma and the cholesterol is carried to these tissues in the form of *low-density lipoproteins* (LDL). These complexes have *apoprotein B* as their main shell protein and this reacts with high-affinity receptors in the plasma membrane of non-hepatic cells. The complex enters the cell by endocytosis and the resulting vesicles fuse with lysosomes which release cholesterol which may then be used for membrane synthesis. Alternatively the cholesterol may be re-esterified and stored within the cell. The *LDL receptor proteins* are very labile and are rapidly broken down and resynthesized. This process of degradation and resynthesis is subject to feedback control. When there is plenty of cholesterol within the cell no new LDL receptors are formed and the uptake of further cholesterol is prevented. Conversely when the cell cholesterol content starts to fall, new LDL receptors are synthesized and uptake is renewed. There is a genetic disorder known as *familial hypercholesterolaemia* in which the plasma cholesterol level is abnormally high. This is due to the absence or deficiency of LDL receptors and is caused by a single autosomal mutation. In the homozygous condition the plasma cholesterol level may rise to about 700 mg dl^{-1} instead of the normal fasting value of 120–240 mg dl^{-1} and, because of this, cholesterol is deposited in various tissues including arterial walls. This produces the condition of *atherosclerosis* and normally leads to death in childhood. The heterozygous condition is less severe since, whereas homozygotes have almost no LDL receptors, heterozygotes have half the normal number. With plasma cholesterol levels of about 300 mg dl^{-1}, heterozygotes are still at grave risk from atherosclerosis and coronary heart disease at a relatively early age.

Dietary fat and coronary heart disease

Coronary heart disease results from a failure of the coronary arteries to maintain an adequate blood supply to the heart muscle. It is usually associated with the condition of *atherosclerosis* in which there is 'hardening of the arteries', i.e. patchy thickening of the intima and media of the arterial walls. The plaque-like thickenings consist of proliferating muscle cells, connective tissue components, fibrin and calcium as well as lipids, mainly in the form of cholesteryl esters. This deposition causes a narrowing of the blood vessels and notably of the coronary, cerebral and femoral arteries causing, respectively, heart attacks, strokes and intermittent claudication. A connection between diet and coronary heart disease (CHD) was suggested by the observation that, in Europe, during World War II, the number of deaths from arteriosclerotic disease declined significantly, and that, as diets improved, mortality from this condition returned to its former level. Many epidemiological studies have since been carried out and it has emerged that in countries such as Asia and Africa where diets are very restricted the incidence of CHD is low; thus it seems clear that atherosclerosis and the diseases which result from it are associated with a high standard of living. This is supported by the finding that the incidence of CHD in Japanese living in California is ten times that of those living in Japan where the diet has a relatively low fat content. Coronary heart disease and cerebrovascular disease account for 40% of deaths in men and 38% of deaths in women in the UK. The chief difficulty in relating unequivocally the risk of atherosclerotic conditions with diet is that smoking, alcohol consumption, physical fitness and stress are all recognized as being contributory factors.

The cholesterol question

The presence of cholesterol in atherosclerotic plaques and the fact that atherosclerotic-type lesions can be produced in animals by manipulating the diet so as to cause a significant rise in the serum cholesterol level led to the suspicion that a high cholesterol intake might have deleterious effects. There is fairly clear evidence in humans of a correlation between serum cholesterol levels greater than 220 mg dl^{-1} (5·7 mmol l^{-1}) and the incidence of CHD but, within the same culture, no correlation could be found between total serum cholesterol levels and the dietary intake of either cholesterol or of saturated fatty acids. Genetic rather than dietary factors seem to be the main determinants of serum total cholesterol and LDL levels. They may also be responsible for raised *high-density lipoprotein* (HDL) levels which appear to protect against atherosclerosis. That innate factors are more important than dietary ones in determining the concentration of cholesterol in the blood is borne out by the difficulty experienced in lowering the concentration by restricting the cholesterol intake. Dietary cholesterol, on average, only contributes about 10% to the serum cholesterol and, in normal subjects, as cholesterol intake increases, cholesterol absorption and cholesterol synthesis both decrease. Thus the association between dietary cholesterol and blood cholesterol levels is weak and it now appears that it is only those people who are known to be at risk of CHD who need to restrict their cholesterol intake. This does not mean that the evidence supporting a relationship between diet and CHD is at fault but the association is now believed to be with the total amount of fat and with the ratio of saturated (SFA) to polyunsaturated (PUFA) fatty acids in the diet rather than with the cholesterol content. An increase in the intake of saturated fatty acids causes an increase in plasma cholesterol, while an increased intake of polyunsaturated fatty acids lowers it. The recent (1984) report of the Committee on Medical Aspects of Food Policy (COMA) recommends that the PUFA/SFA ratio should be increased to approximately 0·45.

The SFA probably act by an adverse effect on the balance between the accumulation and clearance of cholesteryl esters from the arterial wall while the effect of increasing the PUFA intake may, at least in part, be due to the corresponding reduction in SFA consumption. The PUFAs also act as precursors for the synthesis of *prostacyclin* (page 364) which prevents thrombus formation in animals and disperses circulating platelet aggregates in Man.

Two extensive clinical trials using diets enriched with PUFA showed that it was possible to reduce serum cholesterol by 10–15% and that there was concomitant reduction in the incidence of cardiovascular disease. However, mortality from non-cardiovascular conditions was increased and it is suggested that gradual depletion of membrane cholesterol over many years may have an adverse effect on cell function.

The majority of the COMA panel believed, on the basis of current evidence, that the incidence of CHD would be reduced or its onset delayed by decreasing the consumption of saturated fatty acids and total fat. They recommended that (i) the percentage of food energy consumed in the form of fat should not exceed 35%, (ii) that the energy derived from SFA should not exceed 15% and (iii) that the PUFA/SFA ratio should be increased to about 0·45. They made no specific recommendations for cholesterol intake and considered that the average intake of 350–450 mg day^{-1} for adults is not excessive.

Energy balance and obesity

Obesity is the most common nutritional disorder in Britain today and leads to increased susceptibility to many diseases as well as to shorter life expectancy. For insurance and similar purposes the definition of obesity is usually based on actuarial analyses which give an acceptable range of body weights for each sex and height. Persons who weigh 110–119% of the acceptable average are classed as overweight, while those who weigh 120% or more of the average value are classified as obese.

In general, at all ages women tend to have a greater proportion of adipose tissue than men. At 25 years the average male contains about 14% of body fat compared with 26% in the female, while at 55 these figures have increased to 25% and 28% respectively. In Britain from the age of 50 and upwards roughly half the population is overweight if not obese. Since it has been found that with increasing weight there is an increasing risk of diabetes, hypertension, ischaemic heart disease, gall-bladder disease, arthritis and even of cancer, this is a matter which concerns both personal and community health.

Obesity in children is relatively uncommon but is even more detrimental than in adults. It was once thought that the overfeeding of infants caused a permanent increase in the number of adipocytes and that this led to obesity in the adult but later studies have failed to confirm this. Nevertheless, there is little doubt that, for both genetic and environmental reasons, children of overweight parents are more likely to become overweight adults than children of average weight parents. A fact observed, but not explained, is that in affluent societies it is the children and adults from the lower income groups who are more frequently overweight.

The amount of stored fat depends on the level at which a balance is achieved between the rates of its deposition and mobilization and it has been suggested that each person has a physiologically determined 'set point' at which energy intake and energy output are balanced. This is open to question but nevertheless it is necessary to consider the factors which control food intake, energy expenditure and the means by which they are balanced.

Food intake

Whereas hunger has been defined as the sum of sensations aroused by the physical need for food, appetite is a psychic or emotional desire to eat which may or may not be associated with the need for food. Appetite is largely dependent on pleasurable past experience and is therefore acquired, while hunger and satiety are innate sensations which depend on physiological factors. From studies of lesions of the hypothalamus, evidence has been obtained for the presence of 'feeding' and 'satiety' centres but gastrointestinal and metabolic mechanisms are also involved in appetite control. The effects of gastrointestinal stimuli, e.g. degree of filling of the stomach, help to determine the amount of food consumed, while metabolic factors, e.g. the levels of glucose, insulin and other substances circulating in the blood, may influence the choice of food. Superimposed on these are a variety of social and psychological factors which, although of considerable interest, cannot be considered here.

Energy expenditure

The energy expended by the body can be divided into three categories:

1. Basal metabolism
2. Muscular activity
3. The thermic response to cold or food

Basal metabolic rate (BMR)

In sedentary subjects the BMR accounts for a major fraction of the total energy output. Individuals at rest, however, show wide differences in their BMRs but it has not been possible to show that the BMR of obese subjects is appreciably and consistently lower than that of normal weight subjects. On the contrary there is some evidence that it may be slightly greater in obese subjects.

Physical activity

Since it is clear that fat people often eat less than thin people it has been suggested that fat people may be fat because they are more leisurely than thin people. This again does not necessarily appear to be the case. An accurate measurement of the amount of every day physical activity is difficult to obtain. Not only does it include the degree of muscular tone but also small fidgeting movements which vary markedly between individuals. As a result of increasing mechanization both at work and in the home, the amount of physical work carried out by people in the West has undergone a progressive decline, so that recognizable physical activity may account for only 12–15% of the total energy expenditure.

Exercise is the most important means of increasing energy expenditure, but, in relation to total energy turnover each day, the effect is small. For example a brisk 2 hour walk will increase energy expenditure only by about 1505 J (360 kcal) which represents about 15% of the daily energy expenditure, although obese subjects expend more energy than lean ones for the same amount of exercise owing to the greater weight they have to move. It should be remembered that the exercise may stimulate the appetite and, if extra food is taken, there will be little object in the exercise. It is claimed, but not proved however, that exercise taken soon after a meal increases the thermogenic effect of food (see below). If this is so, walking off a large meal may have a beneficial effect for those tending to obesity.

The thermogenic effect of food – dietary-induced thermogenesis

Since obesity seems to occur in individuals whose food intake and energy output in terms of BMR and obvious physical activity appear to be little different from those of normal weight, the question arises as to whether normal and obese subjects show significant differences in their response to food. There are two different types of *thermic response*.

1. A short-term response which immediately follows the taking of food and lasts for a few hours. Its duration is related to the size and composition of the meal, and on normal diets it accounts for a 5–10% increase in the metabolic rate taken over 24 hours. This corresponds to what was previously known as the 'specific dynamic action' of food and is greater for a diet rich in carbohydrate than for one rich in fat.
2. An adaptive effect which depends on long-term changes in feeding patterns, i.e. chronic over- or under-nutrition. Fasting or underfeeding induces a progressive reduction in the metabolic rate which may amount to 20% or so after 20 days. This can be attributed to a lower expenditure of ATP since, during fasting, essential energy is mobilized from endogenous sources and little or no ATP is required for storage reactions. Protein synthesis is also reduced. The reduction in metabolism in fasting and underfeeding enhances the chances of survival in adverse conditions.

Some years ago it was found that rats which were chronically restricted in their energy intake, lived longer than those allowed to feed *ad libitum*. A recent revival of interest in this finding has occurred but there are obvious difficulties in discovering whether it is true for humans. There seems little doubt that overfeeding and obesity are risk factors for many degenerative diseases but whether dietary restriction has a positive effect in determining health and longevity in humans has not been conclusively established.

If, on the other hand, an individual is continuously overfed, initially he will show a steady gain in weight but this results in increased metabolism which will eventually reach a point at which the energy expenditure once again equals the energy of the food including the excess. In this way energy balance is established at a new and higher level. This was clearly shown in an experiment carried out on volunteer inmates of a Vermont prison. It was found that, when they were subjected to overfeeding with a high fat diet for several months, lean men had a remarkable ability to buffer major increases in food intake, i.e. there seemed to be some way in which they could dissipate some of the extra energy they were consuming.

Mechanisms of dietary-induced thermogenesis

It has been suggested that changes in thyroid hormone production and in the activity of the sympathetic nervous system may act together to adjust the metabolic rate to the energy intake. However, this still does not explain the biochemical mechanisms by which excess energy may be dissipated. Various suggestions have been made but the one of greatest current interest involves brown adipose tissue.

Brown adipose tissue

The activity of brown adipose tissue (BAT see page 261) as a heat producer was first demonstrated in connection with 'non-shivering thermogenesis' in the body's response to cold. Subsequently it was suggested that it might also play a part in dietary-induced thermogenesis and it was shown that rats given a varied and highly palatable diet could be induced to overfeed and put on weight although their weight increase was by no means as great as might have been expected from the extra amount of food they consumed. It was also found that there was an adaptive increase in their brown adipose tissue. It is uncertain, however, how fully changes in brown adipose tissue metabolism can account for the increased (or reduced) energy expenditure which occurs when men or animals are over- or under-fed. It is an interesting fact that a genetically obese strain of rats (*ob/ob*) has been found to have a deficient mechanism for non-shivering thermogenesis; furthermore, obese women and women who had been obese but had managed to reduce to a normal weight showed a rise of only 9·6% in their O_2 consumption after an infusion of noradrenaline, whereas a control group of thin women showed a rise of 21·2%. A connection between a tendency to obesity and a reduced ability to dissipate energy by thermogenesis associated with brown fat remains to be proved.

Other possible mechanisms of thermogenesis

Substrate cycles

Many reactions and metabolic conversions that take place in the body are either directly or indirectly reversible. The breakdown and synthesis of triglyceride in adipose tissue is, of course, a major example. Furthermore, glycogen is interconvertible with glucose, glucose with pyruvate, and fatty acids with the acetyl group of acetyl-CoA. In each case, however, the synthetic pathway, i.e. synthesis of triglycerides, glycogen, glucose or fatty acids utilizes appreciably more energy than when a corresponding amount of the material is broken down. Hence, if there is a continuous cycle of breakdown and synthesis of such compounds the net outcome is merely an expenditure of energy. Even more restricted cycles may occur in the body, for example

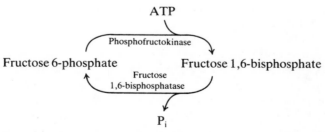

(This particular cycle could only occur in liver and kidney but is a good illustration of the principle.) Usually one or other reaction is predominant, the direction of the conversion being

appropriate to the prevailing conditions but it is suggested, when the energy intake is excessive and the body overloaded with substrates, it may be functionally appropriate to waste energy so that futile cycling occurs resulting in its dissipation. It is not, however, generally believed that substrate cycling makes a major contribution to dietary-induced thermogenesis.

Protein turnover

As explained in Chapter 19 the body proteins are being continuously synthesized and broken down. This is turnover of functional protein and not of storage compounds. The energy cost of protein turnover which involves the synthesis of large numbers of peptide bonds is high and the rate of turnover is increased by overfeeding. This being so, protein turnover must make a contribution to the increased energy output which occurs under such conditions but it has not yet been possible to determine its extent and there is no evidence that protein turnover is abnormal in obese subjects.

The sodium pump

It has been suggested that alterations in cellular sodium pumping (page 198) may be involved in the regulation of energy balance but it has not been clearly demonstrated that there is a lower rate of pumping in obese subjects.

In conclusion it may be said that there is evidence to show that the body can dissipate energy when it is overfed and a number of cellular mechanisms have been suggested to account for this. Their relative importance and how far they contribute to the control of body weight has yet to be established.

The treatment of obesity

Many attempts have been made to promote weight loss by modifying the diet, reducing the appetite or increasing the energy expenditure, but the only way that body fat can be reduced is to create an energy deficit, i.e. to adjust the energy intake so that it is lower than the energy output. Owing to the great adaptability of the body, short of prolonged starvation, this may not be easy. However, by both reducing the food intake and increasing the energy expenditure this can sooner or later be achieved. The question is ultimately whether or not the subject considers the effort and self-control required for the maintenance of such a rigorous regime worthwhile. For health reasons, especially if the obesity is due to excessive energy intake rather than being of genetic origin, there is good reason to think that it should be, but serious dieting should be undertaken with caution and be properly supervised.

Chapter 19
The metabolism of proteins and amino acids

Proteins play an essential part in every biological activity, and since they are built up from about twenty different amino acids, their metabolism, like their structure, is complex. The present chapter is planned to give only a general picture of protein and amino acid metabolism. Examination of the individual metabolic pathways of the various amino acids is beyond the scope of this book. Protein biosynthesis, which is dependent on the nucleic acids, is dealt with in Chapter 20.

Nitrogen balance

Normal adults of any mammalian species are in a state of *nitrogen balance* in which the total amount of nitrogen lost from the body, most of which is derived from protein, exactly balances the amount of nitrogen that is consumed in the diet. There are, of course, hour-to-hour and day-to-day fluctuations in intake and output, but, taken over long periods the statement is, in general, true. It is another illustration of the necessity of steady state conditions for long-term survival. In the short term, if the nitrogen intake is increased or diminished the nitrogen output will also be increased or diminished but, after a short period of adjustment, provided the change is not too drastic, balance will be achieved at a slightly higher or lower level than before.

During growth, pregnancy and recovery from injury or wasting disease, the nitrogen intake is likely to exceed the nitrogen output since new tissue is being formed. When there is retention of nitrogen in this way the subject is said to be in *positive nitrogen balance*. Conversely negative balance and a net loss of nitrogen from the body occur when the protein intake is reduced, during a wasting disease and almost imperceptibly in ageing.

The body is made up of a variety of tissues or compartments within which it is possible for material to be redistributed. Thus a particular organ or tissue may grow or be repaired even though the body is in overall *negative nitrogen balance*. This occurs in pregnancy and lactation if the mother's protein intake is inadequate in which case her tissues will be raided in order to supply the needs of her offspring. Evidently it is not primarily the dietary supply of amino acids which determines the rate of protein synthesis but rather some local anabolic quality which ensures that, when amino acids are in short supply, certain tissues have priority. This is borne out by the redistribution of material that occurs in starvation. Even though no food is being consumed energy must still be expended if the body is to remain alive. Initially the energy is obtained mainly at the expense of body fat, although some tissue breakdown also occurs. The protein of some tissues appears to be more labile than in others. The losses, which are losses of functional protein, are greatest and occur most rapidly from the liver, the pancreas and the intestinal mucosa all of which normally synthesize large amounts of protein. Substantial losses of plasma proteins also occur, and may result in waterlogging of the tissues and oedema. Organs such as kidneys and muscles lose protein more slowly although, because of their mass, the muscles account for a large proportion of the total protein loss. The organ which retains its protein most avidly is the brain.

Protein digestion

Protein molecules are too large to be transported through the gut wall to the bloodstream by the normal absorptive processes and, even if this were possible, it would be dangerous because foreign proteins cause toxic reactions in the body. Consequently the first step in the metabolism of food proteins is their hydrolysis to amino acids by the proteolytic enzymes of the gastrointestinal tract. The proteolytic enzymes break peptide bonds and may thus be regarded as *C–N hydrolases*. Since the equilibrium of hydrolysis favours breakdown there is no need for coupling to an energy-producing system. On the other hand, since peptide bonds only release about 2·1 kJ (0·5 kcal) mol^{-1}, their free energy of hydrolysis cannot be used for ATP synthesis and is lost as heat.

As the food proteins pass along the gastrointestinal tract they undergo a systematic attack, being first subjected to three *endopeptidases* (pepsin, trypsin and chymotrypsin) which act on proteins and large polypeptides, splitting them at definite points along the chain. The peptides so produced are then subjected to the action of several types of *exopeptidase* which break off terminal amino acids. A list of the proteolytic enzymes of the gastrointestinal tract is given in Table 19.1.

The proteases and particularly the endopeptidases are potentially very dangerous to the organism and must be kept in an inactive state until they have reached the place where they are required at the time that they are required. The endopeptidases and carboxypeptidases, which like trypsin and chymotrypsin are produced in the pancreas, are secreted in precursor or *zymogen* form which only becomes active after a masking peptide or peptides have been removed.

Although all the peptide bonds between the amino acids in a polypeptide chain are identical they are not all equally susceptible to attack by proteolytic enzymes. These show a distinct preference for certain bonds depending on the nature of the amino acids that participate in the formation of the bonds and, in the case of the exopeptidases, of free amino and/or free carboxyl groupings attached to the α-C atom. Peptides containing proline are particularly resistant to enzymic cleavage and there appear to be specific enzymes for splitting such peptides. Denaturation of proteins by the acid of the stomach, by heating or, as in the case of egg white, by mechanical agitation, causes the highly organized protein molecules to uncoil and expose a larger surface to enzyme attack. However, excessive or prolonged cooking may cause extra linkages to be formed so that the protein becomes less, instead of more, digestible.

Protein digestion starts in the stomach where the acid secreted by the oxyntic cells both assists the denaturation of the proteins and activates the *pepsinogen* secreted by the peptic cells by removing about 20% of the molecule. Activation is autocatalytic; exposure to the very low pH of the stomach contents also provides optimum conditions for the activity of the enzyme. *Pepsin* is not very specific but is most active with respect to bonds in which an aromatic amino acid

Table 19.1 The main proteolytic enzymes of the digestive tract

Enzyme		Source	Mode of activation	Linkages preferentially attacked	Optimum pH
Zymogen form	*Active form*				
Endopeptidases					
Pepsinogen	Pepsin	Gastric mucosa	Hydrochloric acid and autocatalysis	Those in which Phe, Tyr or Trp contribute the –NH– group	1·5–2·0
Trypsinogen	Trypsin	Pancreas	Enterokinase and auto-catalysis	Those in which Lys or Arg provide the –CO– group	7·0–9·0
Chymo-trypsinogen	Chymo-trypsin	Pancreas	Trypsin	Those in which Phe, Tyr, Trp and, to a lesser extent, Leu and Met contribute the –CO– group	7·5–9·0
Exopeptidases					
Procarboxy-peptidase	Carboxy-peptidase	Pancreas	Trypsin	The bond linking the C-terminal amino acid to the rest of the chain	7·2
—	Amino-peptidase	Intestinal epithelium	—	The bond linking the N-terminal amino acid to the rest of the chain	7·4
—	Dipeptidase	Intestinal epithelium	—	The bond joining two amino acids to form a dipeptide	

provides the –NH– group. Usually about 10% of the bonds in food proteins are cleaved by pepsin and this produces peptides of molecular weight 600–2000, which are the 'peptones' used in preparing bacteriological media.

On passing into the duodenum the chyme from the stomach is mixed with the pancreatic juice which contains *trypsin, chymotrypsin* and *carboxypeptidase* in their zymogen forms. Trypsinogen is converted into trypsin either by *enterokinase*, an enzyme secreted by the duodenal mucosa, or autocatalytically by trypsin itself. In the conversion a hexapeptide Val-(Asp)$_4$-Lys is split off, exposing the active centre of the enzyme which consists of the hydroxyl group of serine in close proximity to two histidine residues. Trypsin is highly specific in its action and only breaks bonds which involve the carbonyl groups of either lysine or arginine.

Chymotrypsinogen, which consists of a single chain containing 246 residues and five disulphide bonds, is activated in several stages. Activation is initiated by trypsin and completed by chymotrypsin itself, the final form consisting of three residual chains held together by disulphide bonds. Chymotrypsin attacks bonds involving the carbonyl groups of the aromatic amino acids, phenylalanine, tyrosine and tryptophan.

Procarboxypeptidase is the inactive precursor of the pancreatic exopeptidase which hydrolyses the peptide bonds joining the amino acid in the C-terminal position to the rest of the chain.

Trypsin is unique among pancreatic enzymes in that it is capable of activating all the pancreatic proenzymes including itself. The pancreas of all mammals contains a potent tryptic inhibitor which protects the gland against autodigestion by small amounts of active trypsin formed within it but which does not prevent proteolysis of food by the fully activated juice.

The oligopeptides formed by the action of the endopeptidases are broken down into their constituent amino acids by the action of the exopeptidases. The carboxypeptidase of the pancreas splits amino acids one by one from the *C*-terminus so that, by the time they reach the absorbing cells of the small intestine, the dietary proteins have been converted into a mixture of amino acids and small peptides. The mucosal cells which contain both *aminopeptidases* and *dipeptidase* take up the small peptides which are then hydrolysed either within the brush border or in the layer immediately beneath it. Thus the final stages of protein digestion, like those of carbohydrates, are intracellular. Under normal circumstances no peptides pass across the mucosa to enter the bloodstream.

Amino acid absorption

Amino acids are rapidly absorbed in the intestine. The intestinal wall is lined with specialized absorptive cells whose primary function is the transport of nutrients from the lumen of the gut into the portal circulation. These cells contain active transport systems for both sugars and amino acids in the brush border membrane.

The transport of most amino acids in the intestine is linked to the transport of Na^+ ions in the same direction (symport). The Na^+ ions are carried down a concentration gradient on the same carrier as the amino acids which are carried against a concentration gradient. The inward Na^+ gradient is maintained by the action of a Na^+/K^+-ATPase which pumps the Na^+ ions out of the cell in exchange for K^+ ions.

Thus the energy for the active transport of amino acids is derived indirectly from the hydrolysis of ATP (Figure 19.1). After uptake into the absorptive cells by this method, the amino acids pass into the portal circulation by a passive transport process. The brush border membrane contains a number of different transport systems for amino acids, which have overlapping specificity. It is probable that similar systems are responsible for the uptake of amino acids into other tissues such as kidney and liver. As a result of the operation of such transport systems, the total free amino acid concentration in the plasma is kept at between 2 and 4 mM but in the tissues it is between 15 and 30 mM. Amino acids derived exogenously from the food are mixed with amino acids derived endogenously from the tissues to form a metabolic

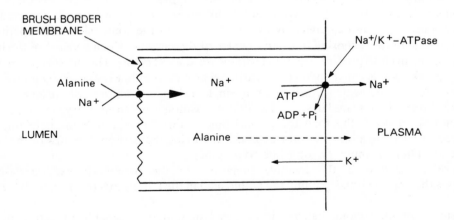

Figure 19.1 Na^+ -linked transport of alanine in the intestine

pool. The essential amino acids (see below) are taken up by the tissues with great avidity and the non-essential amino acids, notably glycine, alanine, glutamic acid and glutamine, account for 80% of the total free amino acid nitrogen.

The absorption of intact protein

Occasionally large polypeptides and even complete proteins are absorbed. These cannot be used for protein synthesis and may lead to immunological sensitization and allergic reactions. Absorption of native protein is, however, a normal process in certain newborn animals. In Man passive immunity is conferred on the newborn infant by placental transfer of maternal antibodies. In some other species including the cow, horse, goat, sheep and pig this does not occur and, instead, antibodies are supplied in the colostrum, the secretion of the mammary glands which is produced prior to the start of lactation proper. The colostrum proteins are protected against digestion by the presence in colostrum of a trypsin inhibitor and also by the failure of the neonate to secrete hydrochloric acid. In the first few hours the proteins are absorbed in large quantities by pinocytosis but after about 36 hours the intestine loses its ability to absorb intact protein.

Essential amino acids

Although plants and many microorganisms are able to synthesize all the amino acids they require from simple carbon compounds and non-specific sources of nitrogen such as ammonia, higher animals are unable to do this and must obtain some of the amino acids from the protein in the diet. An essential amino acid is one that an animal is either unable to synthesize for itself or which it cannot synthesize at a sufficient rate to meet the needs for metabolism and growth. Different species vary to some extent in their essential amino acids. Humans require at least eight and probably ten. They are valine, leucine, isoleucine, lysine, methionine, phenylalanine, threonine and tryptophan with arginine and histidine having a doubtful status.* The latter are 'relatively indispensable' in that they can be synthesized in the body but their rate of synthesis may be too slow fully to supply the needs of the growing child. On a similar basis glycine is an essential amino acid for rapid growth of feathers in young birds such as the chick. Young rats require the same ten amino acids as are needed by children.

  The quantities of the various essential amino acids required daily in the diets of individual humans were determined by Rose who fed young adult volunteers on diets containing adequate amounts of purified carbohydrate, fats, minerals and vitamins but provided mixtures of amino acids in the place of protein. The mixtures contained all the amino acids except the one under investigation which was given separately and, by slight alterations in the level of intake, the subject could be made to go reproducibly from positive to negative balance and back again. This indicated the daily requirement of the individual for this amino acid. The experiment was repeated for each essential amino acid in turn thus giving a picture of the overall needs of that person. Particular individuals were found to have well-defined requirements although there was considerable variation from one person to another. Average results for men, women and infants are given in Table 19.2. As mentioned in Chapter 10 the 'safe' level of a given amino acid is taken as being considerably higher than the minimum requirement.

* A useful mnemonic for remembering these runs as follows: These (Thr) Ten (tyr) Valuable (Val) Amino acids (Arg) Have (His) Long (Leu) Preserved (Phe) Life (Lys) In (Ile) Man (Met)).

Table 19.2 Estimated daily requirements for the essential amino acids

Amino acid	Minimum requirement		
	Infants (mg kg^{-1})	Men (g)	Women (g)
Arginine	*	0	0
Histidine	34	0	0
Isoleucine	126	0·7	0·55
Leucine	150	1·1	0·73
Lysine	103	0·8	0·54
Methionine (in the presence of cysteine)	45	1·1	0·70
Phenylalanine (in the presence of tyrosine)	90	1·1	0·70
Threonine	87	0·5	0·37
Tryptophan	22	0·25	0·17
Valine	105	0·8	0·62

* No figure given

The requirements for the essential amino acids are further complicated by the finding that two non-essential amino acids can only be synthesized in the body if two of the essential amino acids are present in sufficient amounts. Tyrosine is formed directly from phenylalanine so that the requirement for phenylalanine is less when tyrosine is present than when it is absent from the diet. Similarly the sulphur that is required for the synthesis of cysteine can only be obtained from methionine so that the dietary requirements for the sulphur-containing amino acids should be considered together. If cysteine is present in ample amounts the requirement for methionine will be minimal, but if cysteine is in short supply more methionine is needed.

It should perhaps be pointed out that the 'non-essential' amino acids are just as important in metabolism as the 'essential' amino acids, the distinction being the need for an external supply of the latter. If protein is to be synthesized, all its constituents must be simultaneously available and experiments have shown that if a missing essential amino acid is fed an hour or so after the others it is inefficiently utilized.

In most instances it is the α-oxo acid corresponding to the essential amino acid that the body is unable to synthesize and, if this oxo acid is supplied it can be quite readily converted into the corresponding amino acid. Exceptions to this rule are lysine and threonine which have to be supplied in the amino acid form.

Amino acid metabolism

A summary of amino acid metabolism is given in Figure 19.2. Amino acids are used for protein synthesis and as N and C donors for the synthesis of other types of macromolecule, e.g. the nucleic acids as well as numerous small molecular compounds. After *deamination*, i.e. removal of the amino group, the carbon skeleton may be used for the formation of glucose or even fats or it may be oxidized to CO_2 and water with the production of metabolic energy. *Decarboxylation*, i.e. removal of the carboxyl group of certain of the amino acids, leads to the production of *biogenic amines* such as histamine, serotonin and γ-aminobutyrate.

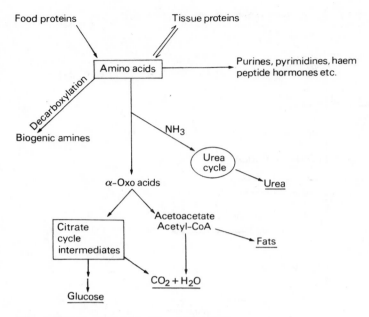

Figure 19.2 Summary of amino acid metabolism

Tissue interrelationships in amino acid metabolism

While dietary carbohydrate in excess of immediate requirements may be stored in the form of glycogen, and lipid may be stored as triglyceride, there is no analogous short-term storage of amino acids. Amino acids in excess of requirements are immediately degraded. In fact, it has been shown that after eating a balanced meal, degradation of excess amino acids precedes the metabolism of carbohydrates and fats.

The breakdown of amino acids involves the liberation of the α-amino group in the form of ammonia. Ammonia is extremely toxic, especially, for reasons which are still not fully understood, to the brain and one of the major functions of the mammalian liver is to detoxify ammonia by converting it to *urea* ($CO(NH_2)_2$); this is non-toxic, highly water-soluble and readily excreted via the kidneys. Different mechanisms of *ammonia* detoxification occur in fish where ammonia is excreted directly via the gills, and in birds and reptiles where ammonia is converted to *uric acid*. Uric acid is insoluble in water and is thus suitable for excretion under conditions where the water supply may be limited.

The metabolism of amino acids proceeds by pathways which are common to most tissues, but the pathway for the conversion of ammonia to urea occurs only in the liver. During the degradation of amino acids in peripheral tissues such as skeletal muscle, the ammonia formed is not released directly into the bloodstream. Instead it is used to form the amino acids alanine and glutamine from pyruvate and glutamate which are readily available, and it is these amino acids that are then released. The alanine produced by the tissues is taken up by the liver and converted to urea and glucose. Although some glutamine is metabolized by the liver, the major site of glutamine metabolism is the intestine where it is used as a major respiratory fuel. The ammonia produced by glutamine metabolism in the gut returns immediately via the portal circulation to the liver, where it is detoxified. These tissue interrelationships in amino acid degradation are illustrated in Figure 19.3.

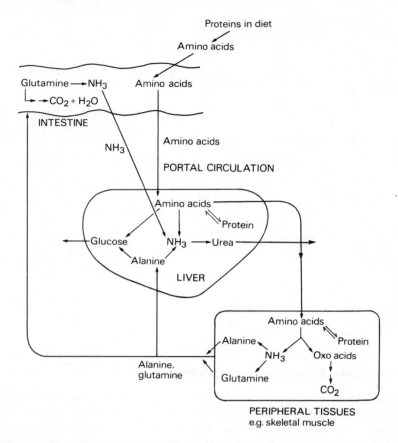

Figure 19.3 Schematic diagram of interrelationships between liver, intestine and peripheral tissues in nitrogen metabolism in mammals

Pathways of amino acid catabolism

Transamination and deamination

The initial step in the degradation of many amino acids is a transamination reaction whereby the α-amino group of the amino acid is transferred to α-oxoglutarate with the formation of glutamate and the α-oxo acid corresponding to the amino acid in question. Transamination reactions are catalysed by a group of enzymes called *transaminases* or *aminotransferases*. The most important of these are *glutamate–oxaloacetate transaminase* (GOT) and *glutamate–pyruvate transaminase* (GPT); the reactions catalysed by these enzymes are shown below.

$$
\begin{array}{ccc}
\text{COO}^- & & \text{COO}^- \\
| & & | \\
\text{CH}_2 & \text{COO}^- & \text{CH}_2 & \text{COO}^- \\
| & | & | & | \\
\text{CH}_2 & + & \text{CH}_2 & \xrightarrow[\text{pyridoxal phosphate}]{\text{GOT}} & \text{CH}_2 & + & \text{CH}_2 \\
| & \text{CO} & | & \text{CHNH}_3^+ \\
\text{CHNH}_3^+ & | & \text{CO} & | \\
| & \text{COO}^- & | & \text{COO}^- \\
\text{COO}^- & & \text{COO}^-
\end{array}
$$

Glutamate Oxaloacetate   2-Oxoglutarate Aspartate

$$
\begin{array}{ccc}
\begin{array}{c} COO^- \\ | \\ CH_2 \\ | \\ CH_2 \\ | \\ CHNH_3^+ \\ | \\ COO^- \end{array}
&+&
\begin{array}{c} CH_3 \\ | \\ CO \\ | \\ COO^- \end{array}
\quad\underset{\substack{\text{pyridoxal}\\\text{phosphate}}}{\overset{\text{GPT}}{\rightleftharpoons}}\quad
\begin{array}{c} COO^- \\ | \\ CH_2 \\ | \\ CH_2 \\ | \\ CO \\ | \\ COO^- \end{array}
&+&
\begin{array}{c} CH_3 \\ | \\ CHNH_3^+ \\ | \\ COO^- \end{array}
\end{array}
$$

| Glutamate | Pyruvate | 2-Oxoglutarate | Alanine |

Transaminase reactions are freely reversible so that they function in both the synthesis and breakdown of amino acids. All transaminases require pyridoxal phosphate, a derivative of vitamin B_6 (page 165), as a cofactor which transfers the α-amino group from an amino acid to a keto acid. In general, transaminases have a high K_m value for the appropriate amino acid but a much lower K_m for 2-oxoglutarate.

The glutamate formed by the transamination of amino acids with 2-oxoglutarate then undergoes oxidative deamination via the *glutamate dehydrogenase* reaction:

$$
\begin{array}{c} CH_2 \cdot COO^- \\ | \\ CH_2 \\ | \\ H_3\overset{+}{N}-CH-COO^- \end{array}
\; + \; NAD(P)^+ \quad\underset{-H_2O}{\overset{+H_2O}{\rightleftharpoons}}\quad
\begin{array}{c} CH_2 \cdot COO^- \\ | \\ CH_2 \\ | \\ O=C-COO^- \end{array}
\; + \; NAD(P)H + H^+ + NH_4^+
$$

| Glutamate | 2-Oxoglutarate |

Glutamate dehydrogenase is a mitochondrial enzyme which can use either NAD^+ or $NADP^+$ as the hydrogen acceptor.

Although the equilibrium of this reaction is very much in favour of glutamate formation, in the cell the rapid removal of the 2-oxoglutarate and NAD(P)H allows the enzyme to function efficiently in the direction of glutamate deamination. Liver glutamate dehydrogenase is a very active enzyme, and the reaction is not rate-limiting for amino acid deamination.

Glutamate dehydrogenase is responsible not only for the deamination of glutamate itself but also indirectly for the deamination of many other amino acids. For example, when alanine is transaminated with 2-oxoglutarate, pyruvate and glutamate are produced. The glutamate is then deaminated via the glutamate dehydrogenase reaction and 2-oxoglutarate is regenerated and is available to transaminate with another molecule of amino acid. The net result of the two reactions is the deamination of one molecule of the amino acid with the production of one molecule of its corresponding α-oxo acid and one molecule of ammonia and the reduction of one molecule of $NAD(P)^+$.

$$
\begin{array}{ccc}
\text{Amino acid} \searrow \quad \nearrow \text{2-Oxoglutarate} & \leftarrow & NAD(P)H + H^+ + NH_4^+ \\
\textit{Transaminase} & \textit{Glutamate} & \\
& \textit{dehydrogenase} & \\
\alpha\text{-Oxo acid} \nearrow \quad \searrow \text{Glutamate} & & NAD(P)^+
\end{array}
$$

Not all amino acids are deaminated in this way. The amino groups of glutamine and asparagine are directly hydrolysed by the enzymes *glutaminase* and *asparaginase* with the production of ammonia. The hydroxyamino acids serine and threonine are acted upon by the enzymes *serine dehydratase* and *threonine dehydratase* respectively, again with the direct production of ammonia, while proline, arginine and histidine are metabolized to form glutamate and the amino group is then removed by glutamate dehydrogenase.

The fate of the carbon skeleton

In general, the deaminated residues of the various amino acids are converted into intermediates of the citrate cycle, acetyl-CoA or acetoacetyl-CoA. The pathways involved are long and complex and will not be considered in detail. An outline of the metabolic fate of the various amino acids is given in Figure 19.4. The amino acids which produce pyruvate, 2-oxoglutarate, succinyl-CoA, oxaloacetate or fumarate are said to be *glucogenic*, since, in the liver, these intermediates can be converted to phosphoenolpyruvate and hence to glucose by the gluconeogenic pathway (page 237). The acetyl-CoA and acetoacetyl-CoA formed from amino acids can be converted to ketone bodies in the liver, and amino acids that are metabolized to these compounds are termed *ketogenic*. Some amino acids such as tyrosine, phenylalanine and isoleucine are both glucogenic and ketogenic since their breakdown produces both acetyl-CoA (or acetoacetyl-CoA) and citrate cycle intermediates. Leucine is, in fact, the only amino acid which is ketogenic but not glucogenic. Alternatively citrate cycle intermediates generated by amino acid degradation may be oxidized to produce energy or they may be used in various synthetic pathways.

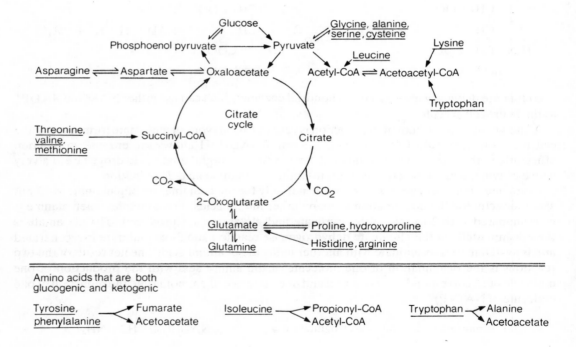

Figure 19.4 An outline of the fates of the various amino acids

The urea cycle

In mammalian organisms, the ammonia produced by amino acid degradation is detoxified by conversion to urea in the liver. The metabolic pathway by which this occurs was elucidated by Krebs in 1935. Each molecule of urea contains the equivalent of two molecules of ammonia, one of which is derived from carbamoyl phosphate and one from aspartate. The urea cycle which is energetically fairly expensive is depicted in Figure 19.5.

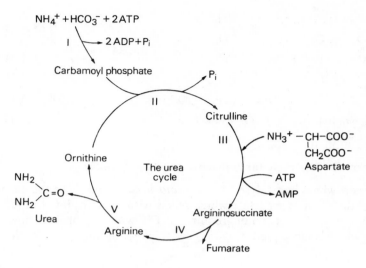

Figure 19.5 The urea cycle

Individual reactions of the urea cycle

1. This reaction, while not strictly part of the urea cycle as such, converts one NH_4^+ ion and one HCO_3^- ion into *carbamoyl phosphate* which has a high phosphate transfer potential because of its anhydride bond

$$NH_4^+ + HCO_3^- + 2ATP \xrightarrow{Mg^{2+}} NH_2-\overset{O}{\overset{\|}{C}}-O-\overset{O}{\overset{\|}{\underset{\underset{O^-}{|}}{P}}}-O^- + 2ADP + P_i$$

The reaction is catalysed by *carbamoyl phosphate synthase* which is Mg^{2+}-dependent and has an absolute requirement for *N-acetylglutamate* as a cofactor. Carbamoyl phosphate synthase is a mitochondrial enzyme and comprises approximately 15% of the matrix protein in liver mitochondria. As a consequence of the hydrolysis of two molecules of ATP, the formation of carbamoyl phosphate is effectively irreversible, so that any ammonia undergoing this reaction is committed to excretion.

N-Acetylglutamate is itself synthesized in the mitochondria by the reaction of glutamate with acetyl-CoA that is catalysed by *N-acetylglutamate synthase* (acetyl-CoA:glutamate *N*-acetyltransferase):

$$\underset{\text{Glutamate}}{\overset{\overset{\displaystyle CH_2-COO^-}{|}}{\underset{H_3^+N-CH-COO^-}{\overset{\displaystyle CH_2}{|}}}} + \underset{\text{Acetyl-CoA}}{CH_3\overset{O}{\overset{\|}{C}}SCoA} \underset{\text{synthase}}{\overset{\text{Acetylglutamate}}{\rightleftharpoons}} \underset{N\text{-Acetylglutamate}}{CH_3-\overset{O}{\overset{\|}{C}}-NH-\underset{\overset{\displaystyle CH_2}{\underset{\overset{\displaystyle CH_2-COO^-}{|}}{|}}}{CH}-COO^-} + CoA$$

2. The carbamoyl group of carbamoyl phosphate is transferred to the amino acid *ornithine* to form *citrulline* under the influence of the mitochondrial enzyme *ornithine transcarbamylase* (ornithine carbamoyltransferase). Ornithine and citrulline are α-amino acids which do not occur in proteins (page 36). The ornithine transcarbamylase reaction is also effectively irreversible.

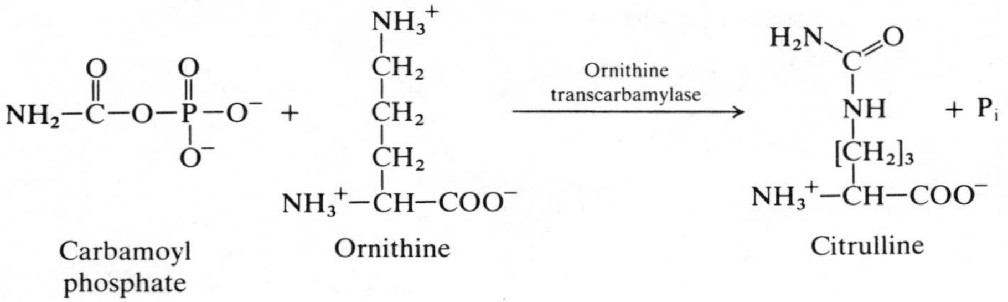

$$NH_2-\overset{\overset{\displaystyle O}{\|}}{C}-O-\overset{\overset{\displaystyle O}{\|}}{\underset{\underset{\displaystyle O^-}{|}}{P}}-O^- \quad + \quad \underset{\underset{\displaystyle NH_3^+-CH-COO^-}{|}}{\overset{\overset{\displaystyle NH_3^+}{|}}{\underset{\underset{}{}}{CH_2}-CH_2-CH_2}} \quad \xrightarrow{\text{Ornithine transcarbamylase}} \quad \underset{\underset{\displaystyle NH_3^+-CH-COO^-}{|}}{\overset{\overset{\displaystyle H_2N}{}}{C}=O,\ NH,\ [CH_2]_3} \quad + P_i$$

Carbamoyl   Ornithine   Citrulline
phosphate

The remainder of the urea cycle takes place in the liver cytosol.

3. In this reaction which is catalysed by *argininosuccinate synthase* the second amino group is introduced in the form of aspartate which reacts with the citrulline formed in Reaction 2 to give *argininosuccinate*. The reaction requires ATP, which is broken down into AMP and pyrophosphate which is subsequently hydrolysed to inorganic phosphate so that this reaction too is irreversible.

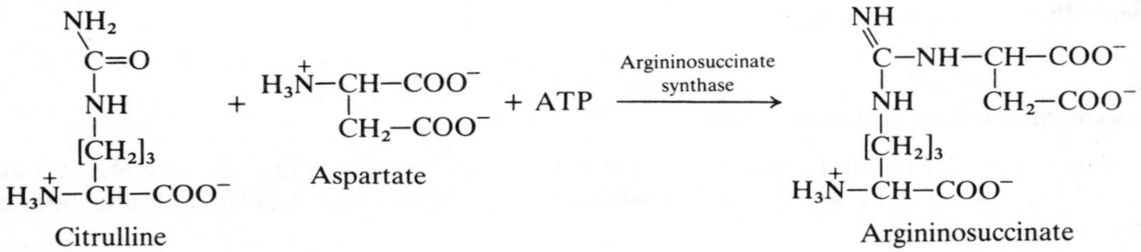

$$\underset{\text{Citrulline}}{\overset{\overset{\displaystyle NH_2}{|}}{\underset{\underset{\displaystyle H_3\overset{+}{N}-CH-COO^-}{|}}{C=O,\ NH,\ [CH_2]_3}}} \quad + \quad \underset{\text{Aspartate}}{\overset{\overset{\displaystyle +}{}}{\underset{\underset{\displaystyle CH_2-COO^-}{|}}{H_3N-CH-COO^-}}} \quad + ATP \quad \xrightarrow[\text{synthase}]{\text{Argininosuccinate}} \quad \underset{\text{Argininosuccinate}}{\overset{\overset{\displaystyle NH}{\|}}{\underset{\underset{\displaystyle H_3\overset{+}{N}-CH-COO^-}{|}}{C-NH-CH-COO^-,\ NH,\ CH_2-COO^-,\ [CH_2]_3}}}$$

4. In the next reaction the argininosuccinate is hydrolysed by the enzyme *argininosuccinase* into arginine and fumarate.

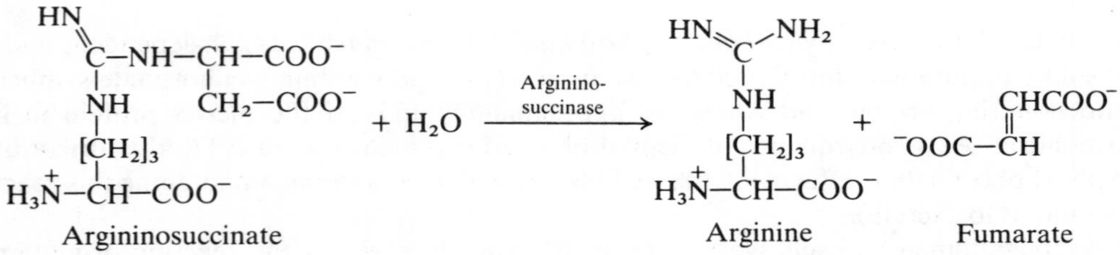

$$\underset{\text{Argininosuccinate}}{\overset{\overset{\displaystyle HN}{\|}}{\underset{\underset{\displaystyle H_3\overset{+}{N}-CH-COO^-}{|}}{C-NH-CH-COO^-,\ NH,\ CH_2-COO^-,\ [CH_2]_3}}} \quad + H_2O \quad \xrightarrow[\text{succinase}]{\text{Arginino-}} \quad \underset{\text{Arginine}}{\overset{\overset{\displaystyle HN,\ NH_2}{\diagdown\ \diagup}}{\underset{\underset{\displaystyle H_3\overset{+}{N}-CH-COO^-}{|}}{\underset{\displaystyle [CH_2]_3}{NH}}}} \quad + \quad \underset{\text{Fumarate}}{\overset{\overset{\displaystyle CHCOO^-}{\|}}{^-OOC-CH}}$$

5. The final reaction, like the previous one, is a simple hydrolysis. In this case *arginase* hydrolyses arginine to form urea plus ornithine. The ornithine formed is then available to react with more carbamoyl phosphate in the next turn of the cycle. Arginase is very active in mammalian liver.

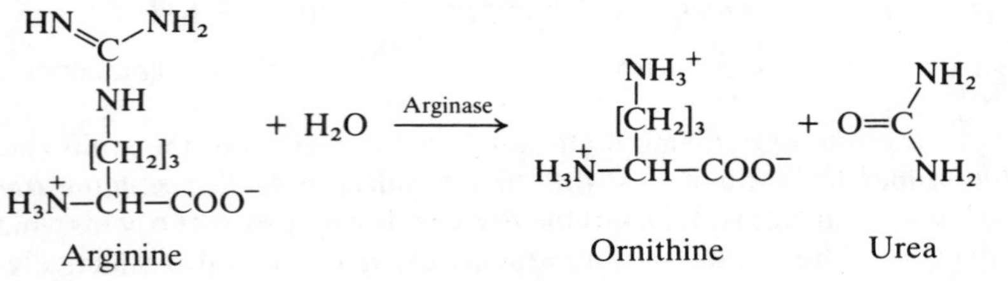

$$\underset{\text{Arginine}}{\overset{\overset{\displaystyle HN,\ NH_2}{\diagdown\ \diagup}}{\underset{\underset{\displaystyle H_3\overset{+}{N}-CH-COO^-}{|}}{\underset{\displaystyle [CH_2]_3}{NH}}}} \quad + H_2O \quad \xrightarrow{\text{Arginase}} \quad \underset{\text{Ornithine}}{\overset{\overset{\displaystyle NH_3^+}{|}}{\underset{\underset{\displaystyle H_3\overset{+}{N}-CH-COO^-}{|}}{[CH_2]_3}}} \quad + \quad \underset{\text{Urea}}{\overset{\overset{\displaystyle NH_2}{\diagup}}{\underset{\underset{\displaystyle NH_2}{}}{O=C}}}$$

The overall reaction of the urea cycle is thus:

$$NH_4^+ + HCO_3^- + aspartate + 3ATP \rightarrow urea + fumarate + AMP + 2ADP + 2P_i + PP_i$$

Two ATP molecules are used in the carbamoyl phosphate synthase reaction and one in argininosuccinate synthesis. Thus urea synthesis may be regarded as an energetically expensive process, although ATP is synthesized during the mitochondrial oxidation of the NADH produced by the oxidative deamination of the amino acids.

Both the ammonia and the aspartate required for argininosuccinate synthesis are derived from glutamate. The ammonia is formed by the glutamate dehydrogenase reaction while aspartate is formed by the transamination of glutamate with oxaloacetate via the glutamate–oxaloacetate transaminase (GOT) reaction.

$$\underset{\text{Glutamate}}{\overset{\displaystyle CH_2{-}COO^-}{\underset{\displaystyle H_3\overset{+}{N}{-}CH_2{-}COO^-}{\overset{\displaystyle |}{\underset{\displaystyle |}{CH_2}}}}} + \underset{\text{Oxaloacetate}}{\overset{\displaystyle CH_2{-}COO^-}{\underset{\displaystyle O{=}C{-}COO^-}{|}}} \underset{\text{transaminase}}{\overset{\text{Glutamate–oxaloacetate}}{\rightleftharpoons}} \underset{\text{2-Oxoglutarate}}{\overset{\displaystyle CH_2{-}COO^-}{\underset{\displaystyle O{=}C{-}COO^-}{\overset{\displaystyle |}{\underset{\displaystyle |}{CH_2}}}}} + \underset{\text{Aspartate}}{\overset{\displaystyle CH_2{-}COO^-}{\underset{\displaystyle H_3\overset{+}{N}{-}CH{-}COO^-}{|}}}$$

The fumarate formed in the urea cycle is converted to malate and then to oxaloacetate by enzymes of the citrate cycle and is available for the production of more aspartate by transamination.

$$\underset{\text{Fumarate}}{\overset{\displaystyle CHCOO^-}{\underset{\displaystyle {}^-OOCCH}{\|}}} + H_2O \underset{\text{Fumarase}}{\rightleftharpoons} \underset{\text{Malate}}{\overset{\displaystyle CH_2COO^-}{\underset{\displaystyle HOCHCOO^-}{|}}} + NAD^+ \underset{\text{dehydrogenase}}{\overset{\text{Malate}}{\rightleftharpoons}} \underset{\text{Oxaloacetate}}{\overset{\displaystyle CH_2COO^-}{\underset{\displaystyle O{=}CCOO^-}{|}}} + NADH + H^+$$

It is of interest that many of the key enzymes in urea synthesis are located in the mitochondria. The mitochondrial enzymes include several transaminases, especially glutamate–oxaloacetate transaminase, as well as glutamate dehydrogenase, carbamoyl phosphate synthase, ornithine transcarbamylase and *N*-acetylglutamate synthase.

Regulation of urea synthesis

Under many conditions the rate-limiting step in urea synthesis is the carbamoyl phosphate synthase reaction. Isolated liver mitochondria will synthesize citrulline from added ammonia under appropriate conditions. The rate of citrulline synthesis can be shown to depend on the intramitochondrial content of acetylglutamate, and both the mitochondrial acetylglutamate content and the rate of citrulline synthesis increase on adding glutamate to the mitochondria.

If rats are injected with a mixture of amino acids, there is a rapid increase in the liver content of glutamate. This is followed by an increase in acetylglutamate, a consequent increase in carbamoyl phosphate synthase activity and an increase in urea production. If excess amino acids are injected, the liver carbamoyl phosphate synthase becomes saturated with acetylglutamate and ammonia appears in the circulation. Thus regulation of carbamoyl phosphate synthase by *N*-acetylglutamate appears to be an important factor in the control of nitrogen disposal by the liver.

The importance of glutamine

Glutamine occurs in the plasma at higher concentrations than those of any other amino acid. In addition to its involvement in protein synthesis glutamine undergoes a number of other important reactions.

Glutamine is formed by the enzyme *glutamine synthase*, which catalyses the reaction:

$$\text{Glutamate}^- + \text{ATP} + \text{NH}_4^+ \rightleftharpoons \text{Glutamine} + \text{ADP} + \text{P}_i$$

As already discussed, this enzyme is primarily involved in ammonia detoxification in extrahepatic tissues, although it also occurs with high activity in liver. Little is known of the regulation of this enzyme in mammalian tissues.

Glutamine acts as a nitrogen donor for the synthesis of a number of complex molecules. In particular two nitrogen atoms of the purine ring and one of the pyrimidine ring are derived from glutamine. Glutamine is also involved in the synthesis of amino sugars.

Glutamine is hydrolysed by the enzyme *glutaminase* with the production of glutamate and ammonium ions:

$$\text{Glutamine} + \text{H}_2\text{O} \rightarrow \text{Glutamate} + \text{NH}_4^+$$

In the kidney, this reaction is of importance in the regulation of acid/base balance, since ammonium salts are excreted and the glutamate formed is converted to glucose with the net uptake of acid. In the intestine, glutamine is used in preference to glucose as a major energy source. Glutamine is also required as an energy source for a number of cells which turn over rapidly such as lymphocytes, thymocytes and retinal cells. Importantly, tumour cells have an absolute requirement for glutamine for growth. The glutamine analogue *Acivin* competes with glutamine for synthetic reactions and has been found to be effective clinically in the treatment of certain tumours.

Acivin

Other nitrogenous compounds

The body contains a great variety of nitrogenous compounds which are derived from amino acids. These include the purine and pyrimidine bases, haem, various hormones and a number of biogenic amines which are formed by amino acid decarboxylation. Some of these compounds are depicted in Table 19.3.

Protein turnover

Apart from the turnover of material caused by cell death and replacement and the loss of proteins by secretion, intracellular proteins are continuously being hydrolysed to their constituent amino acids and replaced by newly synthesized proteins. The breakdown of particular polypeptide chains within a species appears to be a random event since proteins, unlike whole cells, are not believed to 'age' and newly formed proteins are as likely as older ones to be broken down. Different proteins are degraded at very different rates. For example, the total proteins of rat liver have been found to have a *half-life* (the time required for half of the material in question to disappear) of 3·5 days but the half-lives of specific liver enzymes range from 11 minutes to 19 days.

Table 19.3 Some nitrogenous substances derived from amino acids

Substance	Amino acids from which derived	Function
Pyrimidines (cytosine, thymine and uracil)	Gln and Asp	Constituents of nucleotides and nucleic acids
Purines (adenine and guanine)	Gly, Gln and Asp	Constituents of nucleotides and nucleic acids
Haem	Gly	Prosthetic group of Hb, Mb and various enzymes
Choline	Ser and Met	Constituent of acetylcholine and phospholipids
Carnitine	Glu and Met	Mitochondrial fatty acid transport
Creatine	Gly, Arg, Met	Precursor of phosphocreatine of muscle
Glutathione	Glu, CySH, Gly	Maintenance of –SH groups
Thyroxine	Tyr	Active principle of thyroid gland
Adrenaline	Tyr	Numerous effects
Noradrenaline	Tyr	Transmission of nerve impulses
Melanin	Tyr	Pigment of hair and skin
Histamine	His	Vasodilator
Serotonin	Trp	Neurohumoral agent and vasoconstrictor
Nicotinic acid	Trp	Constituent of NAD^+ and $NADP^+$
γ-Aminobutyrate	Glu	Regulator of neuronal activity
Tyramine	Tyr ⎫	
Putrescine	Orn ⎬	Noxious amines produced by bacterial action
Cadaverine	Lys ⎪	
Agmatine	Arg ⎭	

Peptide and protein hormones

Vasopressin	Gastrin
Oxytocin	Secretin
Calcitonin	ACTH (adrenocorticotropic hormone)
Parathormone	TSH (thyrotropic hormone)
Glucagon	Growth hormone
Insulin	Gonadotropic hormone

In terms of their life-span it seems possible to divide proteins into three categories.

1. *Long-lived proteins*. Evidence suggests that most of the cytosolic and membrane-bound proteins fall in this group. They have a compact structure and are fairly resistant to proteolytic attack. At the same time they appear to be continuously, if slowly, sequestered by the lysosomes, i.e. by autophagy. Thus the lysosomal system is believed to function as a general pathway for the breakdown of most enzymes and structural proteins to free amino acids.

2. *Short-lived proteins*. Certain cellular proteins seem to be subject to fairly rapid turnover. Many of the proteins in this group are enzymes that catalyse rate-limiting reactions and whose rates of synthesis are regulated according to environmental conditions. By combining a fairly high rate of degradation with a variable rate of synthesis the most efficient use of the metabolic pathway is ensured.

3. *Very-short-lived proteins*. The body seems to be able to recognize defective and abnormal proteins and to get rid of them very rapidly. Such proteins are usually less compact than the normal form and more susceptible to proteolytic attack which may help to explain the speed of their disposal.

Breakdown of the long-lived proteins appears to be more or less non-selective but it is affected by such factors as nutritional deprivation, hormones and inhibitors of protein synthesis and is effected by the various proteases present in the lysosomes.

The breakdown of the short-lived and abnormal proteins, unlike that of the long-lived ones, appears to be ATP-dependent and may occur by more than one pathway. One of the routes involves a recently discovered heat-stable polypeptide containing 70–80 amino acid residues. This has been found in all species studied and has consequently been named *ubiquitin*. Ubiquitin forms a conjugate with the protein in question and in this way marks it for rapid degradation. Formation of the ubiquitin–protein conjugate requires ATP and at least three proteins. The ubiquitin is bonded to the protein by an isopeptide bond in which the ε-group of lysine is joined to the C-terminal glycine residue of ubiquitin. The conjugation appears to be the recognition signal for protein breakdown and to lead to endoproteolytic cleavage. The resulting fragments are then hydrolysed to their constituent amino acids by normal non-ATP-dependent proteases, the ubiquitin being released during the process.

The amount of protein synthesized by a 70 kg man and therefore, if he is in nitrogen balance, of protein broken down is estimated to be about 200 g day^{-1}. In terms of energy expenditure it is therefore quite an expensive process but it is obviously of great physiological significance since it plays an indispensable role in tissue growth and remodelling. More specifically protein turnover:

1. Increases the organism's ability to adapt to changes in its environment. If a protein is broken down rapidly its concentration can also change rapidly in response to a change in conditions. The rate of catabolism of proteins varies under different physiological conditions such as the supply of nutrients, the degree of activity, hormonal influences and denervation. Moreover, the rates of catabolism of individual proteins show changes that are appropriate to the new conditions. Thus, starvation retards the breakdown of certain enzymes such as arginase and the gluconeogenic enzymes that are responsible for amino acid breakdown, and accelerates the catabolism of acetyl-CoA carboxylase and other proteins, e.g. ribosomal proteins, which play a part in anabolic processes. In this way protein turnover allows the characteristics of a population of protein molecules to evolve, just as the physical characteristics of a human population are able to evolve only as a result of the death and replacement of individuals.
2. Enables the organism to mobilize protein and use it for the provision of energy when the energy intake is decreased. The labile proteins of the tissues mentioned earlier provide amino acids that can either be oxidized directly or converted into glucose.
3. Is responsible for the removal of abnormal proteins, which for one reason or another, are liable to occur in the body from time to time.

Lysomal protein degradation is without doubt subject to physiological regulation. The current list of regulatory substances seems almost endless and includes: amino acids, insulin, various growth factors, glucagon, catecholamines, serotonin (5-hydroxytryptamine), cAMP, Ca^{2+}, prostaglandins and glucocorticoids. The picture is still further complicated by the fact that a given agent may stimulate the process, or inhibit it, or have no effect at all according to the cell type. Regulation seems to be tailored to the needs of the individual tissue. For example, comparatively small decreases in the concentration of particular amino acids in the liver seem to signal deprivation and impending starvation and they initiate a large degradative response with the result that the liver may lose as much as 40% of its protein in 24 hours. In this way it provides free amino acids which may be taken up by other tissues and used for their maintenance and for gluconeogenesis. The skeletal muscles respond much more slowly although, because of their bulk, if starvation is prolonged, they lose more protein overall. On the other hand the brain retains its protein more or less intact. It is, however, affected in more subtle ways since starvation victims show noticeable psychological changes. A great deal remains to be learnt about intracellular proteolysis and protein turnover which is clearly a most important process.

Chapter 20
DNA replication and gene expression

DNA – the genetic material

The year 1944 was a landmark in nucleic acid biochemistry. Prior to that time it was generally believed that chromosomal proteins carried the genetic information in cells. This was hardly surprising since the limited chemistry which had been carried out on DNA and RNA suggested that they were composed of four nucleotides in no particular order and it was felt that such a simple structure could not possibly encode the complex genetic information. Instead it was believed that the DNAs of all species were similar and probably played a structural role.

However, research which ultimately led to the discovery that DNA is the genetic material began as early as 1928, and came from experiments with the *Pneumococcus* bacterium. This organism possesses a slimy polysaccharide capsule which is required for pathogenicity in animals, and enables it to form 'smooth' colonies on agar plates. Mutants exist which cannot synthesize this capsule; they are therefore non-pathogenic and form 'rough' colonies on agar. In 1928, Griffith found that if a mixture of live 'rough' (non-pathogenic) pneumococci and heat-killed 'smooth' (pathogenic) pneumococci were injected simultaneously into mice, they died from pneumonia (Figure 20.1). Consequently a factor from the killed smooth cells was being transferred to the mutant rough cells, thereby making them pathogenic. This change or *transformation* was permanent and resulted in the appearance of live smooth pneumococci in the blood of the animal. Work then began on identifying the 'transforming activity' and in 1944 Avery and others finally showed that purified DNA extracted from killed smooth cells was able to transform unencapsulated rough pneumococci into encapsulated smooth cells *in vitro*, thereby establishing DNA as the transforming factor or genetic material.

Further support for the genetic nature of DNA came 8 years later from studies with a virus, bacteriophage T2, which infects the bacterium *Escherichia coli*. Phage T2 is composed of a central DNA core surrounded by a protein coat. By differential labelling of the phage DNA with the radioactive isotope ^{32}P, and the phage protein coat with ^{35}S, Hershey and Chase were able to show that when T2 infects a bacterial cell the phage DNA enters the host and is able to induce viral replication, whereas the phage protein coat remains outside the bacterial cell. Hence it was concluded that the phage's genetic information must reside within its DNA.

It is now firmly established that DNA, present in a double-stranded helical form, is the genetic material in all prokaryotic and eukaryotic cells although this is not always the case for viruses

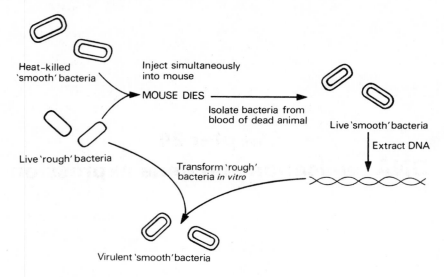

Figure 20.1 Bacterial transformation by DNA

which may use single-stranded DNA, or even RNA, as their genetic material. An example of the latter is *tobacco mosaic virus* (TMV) which infects the leaves of tobacco plants. TMV consists of a single spiral RNA molecule surrounded by a rod-like protein coat composed of over 2000 identical subunits. The RNA alone may be extracted from the virus and shown to cause infection of tobacco plants.

The structure of genes

For any molecule to be recognized as the material responsible for transmitting genetic information, it must fulfil certain requirements dictated by our knowledge of the continuity of species and the process of evolutionary change. (1) It must contain biologically useful information in a stable form. This information is contained in the form of a linear array of *genes*, i.e. specific stretches of DNA, most of which code for a single protein. An average gene is perhaps 1000–2000 base pairs in length. (2) The genetic material must be capable of being accurately replicated, and transmitted faithfully from generation to generation. (3) The genetic material must be able to express itself in such a way as to direct the synthesis of all the different proteins characteristic of the organism, cell type or developmental stage. The amino acid sequence of each individual protein is determined by the nucleotide sequence of its corresponding gene(s). However, it will be seen later that proteins are not synthesized on the genes directly. Instead, an RNA intermediary, called *messenger RNA* (mRNA), is first synthesized (transcribed) using the DNA as a template. This mRNA then directs the synthesis of a specific polypeptide, the amino acid sequence being determined by the order of nucleotides in the mRNA which in turn reflects the DNA sequence from which it was transcribed. Gene expression therefore represents the flow of information from DNA to RNA to protein (page 202). (4) Finally, although in general the genetic information should be stable, it must nevertheless be capable of some variation or *mutation*, even if only very infrequently, to explain the observed characteristics of evolutionary change.

The bacterial chromosome

The whole of the genetic information contained within a single bacterial cell or eukaryotic nucleus is called the *genome*. In eukaryotes this is distributed between a number of different chromosomes, the number being characteristic of the species. Each eukaryotic chromosome is a highly condensed structure composed of both DNA and nuclear proteins, organized in a very specific manner (page 311), while the bacterial genome is present as a single chromosome (i.e. a single DNA duplex), with very little associated protein. The *E. coli* chromosome contains about 4 million base pairs in its DNA and is circular, although *in vivo* this circle must be folded very compactly since the contour length of the DNA is about 1000 times the diameter of the bacterial cell. A property of circular DNA molecules which contributes to this tight packing is supercoiling: the twisting of the double-helical axis itself to form a higher order of twisting, known as a *superhelix* or *supercoil*.

Not all simple DNA molecules are circular. Some viral DNAs are linear, whereas others may interconvert between a linear form in the virus particle and a circular form in the bacterial host cell.

DNA replication

The Meselson–Stahl experiment

It is essential that DNA should be able to replicate since, after cell division, both daughter cells must each contain the genetic information. Watson and Crick suggested that this was possible with a double-stranded helix since the two strands could separate and each could then direct the synthesis of its complement by means of specific base-pairing (Figure 20.2). Such a mechanism

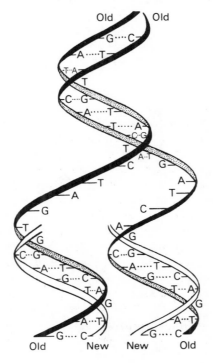

Figure 20.2 Semi-conservative replication of DNA

would be described as *semi-conservative* since each daughter double helix would contain one parental DNA strand and one newly synthesized strand. Semi-conservative DNA replication was actually shown to occur by Meselson and Stahl. For this they labelled *E. coli* DNA with a 'heavy' isotope of nitrogen, ^{15}N, by growing the bacteria for many generations in ^{15}N-labelled ammonium chloride as the sole nitrogen source. Some of the bacteria were removed for analysis immediately and the remainder were transferred to a medium containing normal ^{14}N ammonium chloride. Cells were removed from this medium at intervals and their DNA extracted, and analysed by isopycnic or *equilibrium density gradient centrifugation*. This technique involves placing a tube of concentrated caesium chloride (CsCl) solution in an analytical ultracentrifuge. The CsCl, because it is denser than water, tends to sediment to the bottom of the tube when centrifuged at high speed. However, the tendency to sediment is opposed by diffusion and after a number of hours an equilibrium is reached with the CsCl forming a continuous stable density gradient. If a mixture of macromolecules is dissolved in the original CsCl solution they will come to equilibrium at a position in the gradient where the density of the CsCl solution exactly matches their own, causing them to separate into bands, the positions of which can be located by optical means. This technique is sufficiently sensitive to allow the separation of 'heavy' DNA (containing ^{15}N) from normal 'light' DNA (containing ^{14}N). Their results are summarized in Figure 20.3, which shows that after one bacterial generation, centrifugation of purified DNA produced a single band with a buoyant density intermediate between that of the original ^{15}N-labelled 'heavy' DNA and 'light' DNA from cells grown only on non-isotopic medium. After two cell generations, two DNA bands of equal intensity were obtained; one of hybrid density, and one of 'light' (^{14}N) density. These were exactly the results predicted for semi-conservative replication.

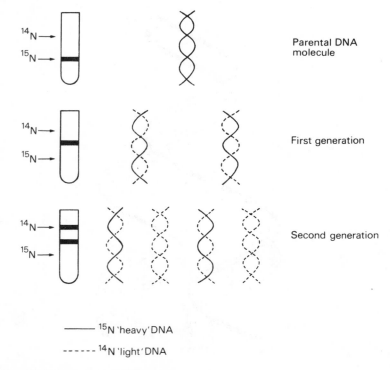

Figure 20.3 Results of the Meselson and Stahl experiment

The mechanism of DNA synthesis

The first DNA-synthesizing enzyme to be discovered was isolated from *E. coli* in 1956 by Kornberg and became known as *DNA polymerase I* or the *Kornberg enzyme*. For DNA synthesis *in vitro*, DNA polymerase requires (a) all four *deoxynucleoside triphosphates* (dATP, dGTP, dCTP and TTP) – these are the immediate precursors of DNA – (b) Mg^{2+}, (c) a small amount of DNA or RNA *primer* – this is necessary because DNA polymerase I can only add deoxyribonucleotides to the 3′-OH terminus of a pre-existing DNA or RNA molecule, it cannot initiate DNA synthesis *de novo* – and (d) a DNA *template*. During DNA synthesis, DNA polymerase I synthesizes a complementary copy of the template, from which it follows that the primer must be able to base pair with the template.

DNA synthesis proceeds by a nucleophilic attack by the 3′-OH group of the primer on the α-phosphorus atom of the incoming deoxynucleoside triphosphate, to form a phosphodiester bond (Figure 20.4). Pyrophosphate is released and is hydrolysed by *pyrophosphatase*, thereby driving the polymerization reaction in the forward direction. Synthesis therefore occurs in a

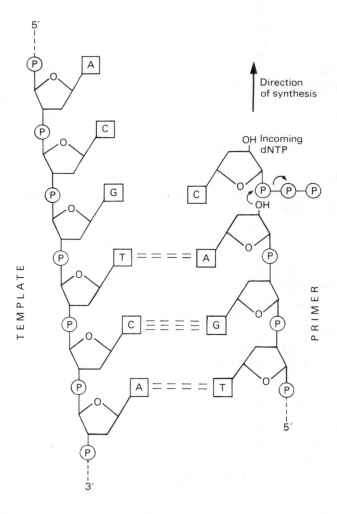

Figure 20.4 Phosphodiester bond formation during DNA synthesis

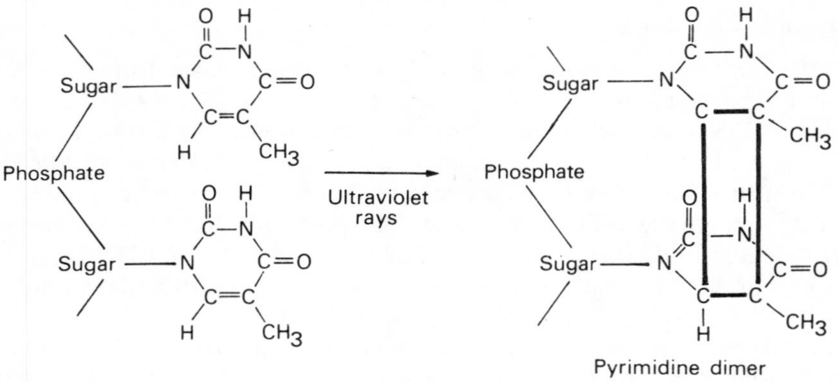

Figure 20.5 The formation of pyrimidine dimers under the influence of ultraviolet light

5′ to 3′ direction; the enzyme remains attached to the DNA throughout and is not released after each nucleotide addition.

As stated above, DNA polymerase I requires a template. The probability of making a covalent phosphodiester bond is very low unless the incoming deoxynucleotide is the correct one to base pair with the corresponding one on the template. Nevertheless, since the possibility exists, DNA polymerase must possess a 'proof-reading' mechanism to correct the occasional mistakes which might otherwise lead to a mutated gene and be detrimental to the organism. Proof-reading is achieved by a $3′ \rightarrow 5′$ *exonuclease* activity associated with the DNA polymerase, which is able to recognize an incorrectly incorporated nucleotide and hydrolyse the corresponding bond, thereby ensuring extremely accurate DNA replication.

DNA polymerase I also has another exonuclease activity, but in this case hydrolysis occurs in a $5′ \rightarrow 3′$ direction and appears to serve two functions *in vivo*; (i) it is involved in removing RNA primers during DNA replication (see later) and (ii) it plays a role in DNA repair processes. That this is an important function is illustrated by experiments in which *E. coli* was exposed to ultraviolet light, which in large doses can cause adjacent pyrimidine residues situated in the same polynucleotide strand to become covalently cross-linked (Figure 20.5). Whereas normal *E. coli* cells are able to excise these pyrimidine dimers and repair their DNA, a mutant form which lacked DNA polymerase I was unable to do so and was therefore more readily killed by ultraviolet light. In humans, as in *E. coli*, exposure to ultraviolet light causes the production of stable pyrimidine dimers but, as shown in studies on skin fibroblasts, these are rapidly excised from the DNA of normal subjects. Sufferers from the rare inherited condition of *xeroderma pigmentosa*, however, appear to lack the enzyme responsible for nicking the DNA backbone in the vicinity of the pyrimidine dimers and skin cancer is a frequent result.

DNA replication in bacterial cells

DNA replication in *E. coli* (Figure 20.6) has the following properties. (a) Replication starts at a unique site on the circular bacterial genome, called the *origin of replication*. (b) Replication proceeds simultaneously in both directions around the genome, that is, it is *bidirectional*. In other words, there are two *replication forks*, one travelling clockwise and one anticlockwise, at about the same rate. (c) Replication is terminated at a point diametrically opposite the origin of replication.

Such an overall mechanism poses a number of problems at the molecular level. First, at a

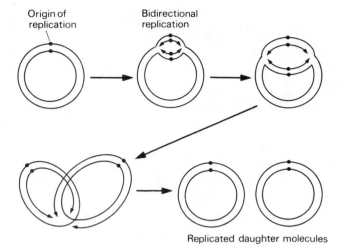

Figure 20.6 Replication of the circular *E. coli* chromosome

replication fork, both strands of the double helix must be replicated, but since they are antiparallel this would suggest $5' \rightarrow 3'$ synthesis on one strand and $3' \rightarrow 5'$ on the other; yet DNA polymerase can only synthesize in the $5' \rightarrow 3'$ direction. This dilemma was resolved by Okazaki who found that one DNA strand is synthesized continuously in the expected $5' \rightarrow 3'$ direction, whereas the opposite strand is synthesized discontinuously as short pieces of DNA known as *Okazaki fragments* (Figure 20.7). Each of these fragments is synthesized in the expected $5' \rightarrow 3'$ direction and adjacent pieces are rapidly joined together by another enzyme called *DNA ligase* giving the appearance that overall growth is in the $3' \rightarrow 5'$ direction.

The second problem is that the initiation of DNA synthesis requires a primer, base paired to the template, and each Okazaki fragment requires its own primer. In fact there is a specific RNA polymerase, called *primase*, which can synthesize short RNA primers of about ten nucleotides. RNA synthesis, unlike DNA synthesis, does not require a primer for initiation (page 000). These short RNA molecules then act as primers for DNA polymerase (Figure 20.8). It is now known that DNA polymerase I is not the major replicating enzyme in *E. coli*. Instead another enzyme, *DNA polymerase III*, carries out most of the replication *in vivo*, whereas DNA polymerase I is responsible for degrading the RNA primers after DNA synthesis by means of its

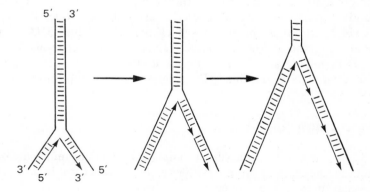

Figure 20.7 Discontinuous DNA replication

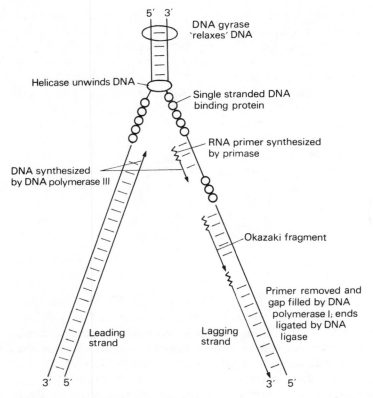

Figure 20.8 Proteins involved in DNA replication

$5' \rightarrow 3'$ exonuclease activity and replacing it with DNA using its polymerase and $3' \rightarrow 5'$ proof-reading activities.

The final problem in DNA replication is the unwinding of the double helix that is necessary for replication to occur, and the subsequent rewinding of the daughter molecules. The whole molecule does not unwind. Instead a small region of the helix around the replication fork is unwound with the aid of a number of specific proteins (Figure 20.8) including a *helicase*, which carries out the actual unwinding, and *single-stranded DNA binding protein*, which stabilizes the single strands and prevents them from base pairing. Finally, when the DNA helix of a circular genome is unwound this puts a tortional strain on the rest of the molecule. This strain is relieved by *DNA gyrase* which acts as a 'molecular swivel' and allows the DNA to relax. Having successfully unwound a region of double-stranded DNA, primase can then bind and synthesize an RNA primer, DNA polymerase III can bring about DNA synthesis, DNA polymerase I can replace RNA primer with DNA, and finally DNA ligase can join adjacent Okazaki fragments.

Gene expression – transcription

As already stated DNA is not itself the direct template which determines the order of amino acids during protein synthesis, since protein synthesis can be carried out *in vitro* in the absence of DNA. Furthermore, protein synthesis in eukaryotic cells occurs in the cytoplasm whereas DNA is confined to the nucleus (and mitochondria; page 201). Instead, a particular class of RNA molecule, the *messenger RNAs* (mRNA), act as templates for protein synthesis. Each mRNA has a nucleotide sequence which is complementary to that of the gene from which it is transcribed. Hence the mRNA is capable of transmitting the genetic information contained within that gene. The existence of mRNA was first shown during experiments carried out on *E. coli* cells infected with bacteriophage T2. Following infection, nearly all the proteins synthesized by the host cell are phage-specific not host-specific proteins, i.e. they are genetically determined by the phage DNA. A minor RNA fraction, with a very short half-life, was found to appear soon after infection. This RNA had a base composition which was complementary to that of one of the phage DNA strands but was unlike that of *E. coli* DNA, and it was found to be associated with pre-existing host ribosomes which were synthesizing new phage proteins. It was therefore concluded that this unstable mRNA fraction carried the genetic information necessary to direct the synthesis of phage proteins. Further investigations showed that this new RNA could be made to associate or *hybridize* with DNA isolated from the same type of phage to form a *hybrid* molecule which contained one strand of RNA and one of DNA. Since it could not be made to hybridize with any other form of DNA the experiment showed that the nucleotide sequence of the newly synthesized RNA was complementary to that of the phage DNA.

Two other classes of RNA molecules are also involved in protein synthesis. These are *ribosomal RNA* (rRNA), a major component of the ribosomes, the organelles responsible for protein synthesis; and *transfer RNA* (tRNA), which plays a key role in the mechanism of protein synthesis. Unlike mRNA, rRNA and tRNA are much more stable and account for about 80% and 15% respectively of the total RNA in a bacterial cell.

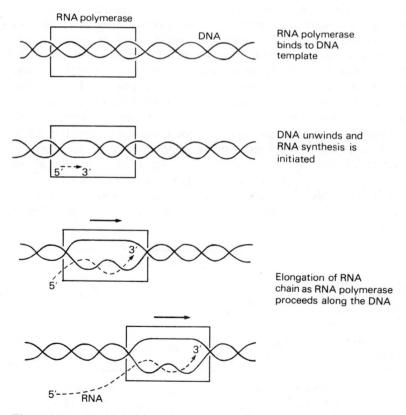

RNA polymerase binds to DNA template

DNA unwinds and RNA synthesis is initiated

Elongation of RNA chain as RNA polymerase proceeds along the DNA

Figure 20.9 Transcription by RNA polymerase

RNA synthesis

All RNA molecules are synthesized on a DNA template by the process known as *transcription*. The enzymes involved, *DNA-dependent RNA polymerases*, catalyse a reaction very similar to that involved in DNA synthesis. In both reactions the immediate precursors are nucleoside triphosphates although in the case of RNA synthesis ribo- and not deoxyribo-nucleotides are utilized. Polymerization involves the formation of a phosphodiester bond between the 3'-OH group of the growing RNA chain and the 5'-α-phosphate of the incoming base-paired nucleoside triphosphate. Pyrophosphate is released and hydrolysed, making the overall reaction essentially irreversible. For each gene only one DNA strand acts as a template for RNA synthesis (Figure 20.9); the complementary strand is not transcribed. However, different genes may be transcribed from different strands of the same DNA molecule. Synthesis of RNA, like that of DNA, always proceeds in a 5' → 3' direction. RNA polymerases do not possess proof-reading activities, and consequently RNA synthesis is less accurate than DNA synthesis. However, since RNA is not self-replicating, occasional mistakes in its synthesis do not become genetically inherited and are therefore not appreciably detrimental to the organism.

The mechanism of transcription in bacterial cells

The RNA polymerase of *E. coli* has been the most extensively studied and its properties seem to be typical of those of many other bacterial systems. It is composed of five different types of subunits (α, β, β', ω and σ) in the ratio $2:1:1:1:1$. The whole complex is known as the *holoenzyme* and can be readily dissociated into the *core enzyme* ($\alpha, \beta, \beta', \omega$) and the *sigma factor* (σ). The sigma factor itself has no catalytic activity but enables the holoenzyme to bind to specific sites on the DNA. These sites, which are located at the beginning of genes, are called *promoters*, and possess certain general features (Figure 20.10). Firstly, the sequence –TTGACA– (or a close derivative of it) is usually found about 35 nucleotides upstream from the point at which RNA synthesis is initiated. This sequence is initially recognized by the RNA polymerase, which then binds more strongly to a second region (further downstream) with the general sequence –TATAAT–. Initiation of RNA synthesis then occurs about ten nucleotides still further downstream. Following initiation, the sigma factor dissociates from the RNA polymerase and the core enzyme continues transcription until a *termination signal* is reached. In some cases this is simply a particular DNA sequence, while in others a protein factor, such as the *rho factor* (ϱ), is required for termination. Bacterial messenger RNAs are not usually modified after transcription. Transfer RNAs and ribosomal RNAs on the other hand are generated by the cleavage of larger precursors and in addition are often chemically modified; for example, several of the bases in tRNA are methylated.

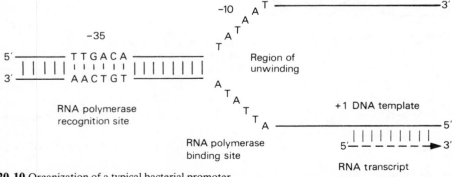

Figure 20.10 Organization of a typical bacterial promoter

Viral RNA synthesis

While all bacteria and eukaryotes contain DNA as their genetic material and synthesize RNA by the process of transcription, many viruses do not contain any DNA, but instead possess an RNA genome. Some are able to replicate this RNA using an *RNA replicase*, while others, such as the *retroviruses*, e.g. Rous sarcoma virus, use quite a different method. In 1964 Temin observed that infection by such viruses is blocked by inhibitors of DNA synthesis, from which he concluded that DNA synthesis is necessary for their replication. This finding led to the discovery of a DNA polymerase which uses RNA as its template. This RNA-directed DNA polymerase is known as *reverse transcriptase*. The immediate product of reverse transcriptase is an RNA–DNA hybrid molecule in which the DNA strand is complementary to that of the viral RNA. This single-stranded DNA copy may then be converted into double-stranded DNA, which can then be normally transcribed in the host to give RNA-containing viral progeny.

At first the discovery of reverse transcriptase appeared to disprove Crick's 'central dogma' (page 202). However, Crick himself pointed out that the dogma merely excluded transfer of information from protein to protein, or protein to nucleic acid, and that with minor modification the original statement was still valid:

$$\text{DNA} \rightleftharpoons \text{RNA} \longrightarrow \text{protein}$$

Protein synthesis – translation

As already stated DNA itself is not directly involved in protein synthesis. Instead it is the mRNAs which define the amino acid sequence during protein synthesis. This assembly of amino acids on an mRNA template, to form a polypeptide, is an extremely complex process and is known as *translation*. It requires many factors including the amino acids, mRNA, ribosomes, a whole series of different tRNAs, many enzymes, protein factors, ATP, GTP and Mg^{2+}.

Amino acid activation

The formation of a peptide bond between two amino acids is thermodynamically unfavourable. This is overcome by activating the carboxyl group of the amino acids in the form of amino acid esters, by linkage to the 2' or 3' OH group of the ribose unit at the 3' end of a tRNA molecule. This reaction, which requires ATP, is carried out by a class of enzymes called the *aminoacyl-tRNA synthases*; there is a separate enzyme for each different amino acid. In addition, there is at least one specific tRNA for each amino acid and it is the synthase which recognize a particular tRNA and its specific amino acid. To a large extent the accuracy of protein synthesis relies on the specificity of these synthases and many of them possess a 'proof-reading' activity to distinguish between similar amino acids.

All tRNAs have a similar overall structure (Figure 20.11). They contain about 75 nucleotides, several of which are modified, e.g. by methylation; and they possess extensive regions of internal base pairing. The 3' end, to which the amino acid is attached during activation, has the sequence –CCA, while the 5' end is usually G. The single-stranded loop opposite the 3' end contains a sequence of three bases known as the *anticodon* which is able to base pair with a complementary sequence of three bases, known as a *codon*, in the mRNA. Transfer RNAs, therefore, have two important functions; they activate amino acids in the form of esters, and they align the resulting aminoacyl-tRNAs on the mRNA in a specific manner by means of *anticodon–codon base pairing*. Consequently, if each different amino acid binds to a different

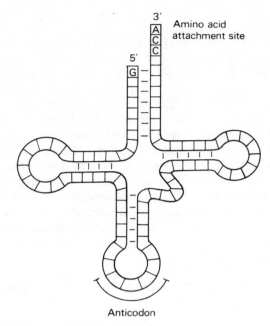

Figure 20.11 Generalized structure of transfer RNA molecules

tRNA, which in turn has a different anticodon, the sequence of a protein can be directed by the nucleotide sequence of the mRNA and hence of the gene (Figure 20.12). The tRNAs therefore act as adaptor molecules to align the amino acids, one at a time, into the correct position. This relationship between the sequence of bases in the mRNA and the sequence of amino acids in proteins is known as the *genetic code*.

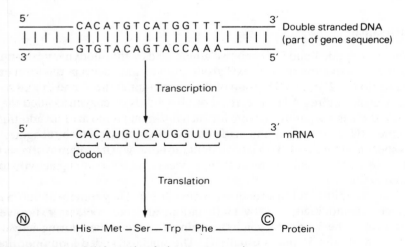

Figure 20.12 Transfer of genetic information during gene expression

The genetic code

It should be possible, with the aid of a triplet (three base) code, to encode 64 different tRNAs and hence 64 amino acids. However, there are only 20 different amino acids but some amino acids have more than one tRNA and hence more than one *coding triplet*; for example, both UUU and UUC code for phenylalanine, while serine has six different coding triplets. Because of this redundancy the genetic code is said to be *degenerate*.

The complete genetic code is shown in Table 20.1. From this it can be seen that degenerate codons specifying the same amino acid are grouped together, usually differing only in the third base position. All possible triplets are utilized; 61 code for amino acids and the remaining three are *termination codons* which signal the end of a polypeptide chain.

Table 20.1 The genetic code

First position (5' end)	Second position				Third position (3' end)
	U	C	A	G	
U	Phe	Ser	Tyr	Cys	U
	Phe	Ser	Tyr	Cys	C
	Leu	Ser	Stop	Stop	A
	Leu	Ser	Stop	Trp	G
C	Leu	Pro	His	Arg	U
	Leu	Pro	His	Arg	C
	Leu	Pro	Gln	Arg	A
	Leu	Pro	Gln	Arg	G
A	Ile	Thr	Asn	Ser	U
	Ile	Thr	Asn	Ser	C
	Ile	Thr	Lys	Arg	A
	Met	Thr	Lys	Arg	G
G	Val	Ala	Asp	Gly	U
	Val	Ala	Asp	Gly	C
	Val	Ala	Glu	Gly	A
	Val	Ala	Glu	Gly	G

On this basis a cell might be expected to contain at least 20 different aminoacyl-tRNA synthases (one for each amino acid) and 61 different tRNAs (one for each amino acid codon). In fact this is not the case; there are less than 61 different tRNAs, and instead some can recognize more than one codon. However, the first two bases in the codon always pair with the expected bases in the anticodon, whereas the third base is allowed a certain degree of 'wobble'; it can often pair with more than one base, for example U can pair with A or G. This produces a second level of degeneracy in the genetic code and explains why many of the degenerate codons specifying the same amino acid are grouped together, differing in only the third base position. If they were not grouped in this way, 'wobble' would allow a tRNA to recognize codons for more than one amino acid.

Apart from mitochondria, the genetic code appears to be *universal*; a particular codon specifies the same amino acid in all species. It is also *non-overlapping*; triplets are read sequentially along the mRNA in a 5' → 3' direction, starting at a specific point known as the *initiation codon*.

The mechanism of protein synthesis

Once charged with the appropriate amino acid, the aminoacyl-tRNAs diffuse to the ribosomes where the peptide bonds are formed. The main function of the ribosomes is to orientate the

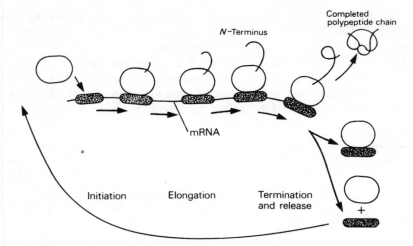

Figure 20.13 The synthesis of polypeptide chains by a polyribosomal complex

aminoacyl-tRNAs correctly on the mRNA template. Ribosomes are complex particles containing both ribosomal RNA and a large number of proteins. Bacterial and mitochondrial ribosomes have a sedimentation coefficient of 70S and are composed of two subunits: a large subunit of 50S and a smaller one of 30S. Most of the components appear to play a structural rather than an active role. During protein synthesis many ribosomes can attach to a single mRNA molecule to form a *polyribosome* or *polysome* (Figure 20.13). Within the polysome, the ribosomes travel progressively along the mRNA, in a 5' → 3' direction, 'translating' the mRNA sequence into a protein chain. Hence a cell can synthesize a relatively large amount of protein using only a small amount of mRNA, since each ribosome in a polysome is synthesizing an identical protein molecule.

Polypeptide chains are synthesized by the stepwise addition of amino acids, starting with the *N*-terminus and terminating with the *C*-terminus. Protein synthesis or translation can be divided into three processes, *initiation*, *elongation* and *termination*.

Initiation

The first amino acid in the synthesis of all bacterial polypeptides is *N-formylmethionine* (fMet), i.e. a modified methionine residue with a formyl group attached to its amino group. Two types of methionyl-tRNA exist; one binds formylmethionine and the other, normal methionine. Both have the same anticodon and recognize the AUG codon characteristic of methionine. However, only formylmethionyl-tRNA binds at the initiating AUG codon while normal methionyl-tRNA is bound at all internal AUG codons.

Initiation in bacteria starts with the formation of a complex between the small 30S ribosomal subunit, the mRNA and fMet-tRNA (Figure 20.14), the latter binding to the initiating AUG (or occasionally GUG) codon near the 5' end of the mRNA. A 50S large ribosomal subunit then attaches to form a functional initiation complex. A number of initiation factors and GTP are also required.

Elongation

Each ribosome has two cavities into which tRNA molecules can fit. The initiating fMet-tRNA binds to the *P (peptidyl) site* and the next aminoacyl-tRNA dictated by the codon following the

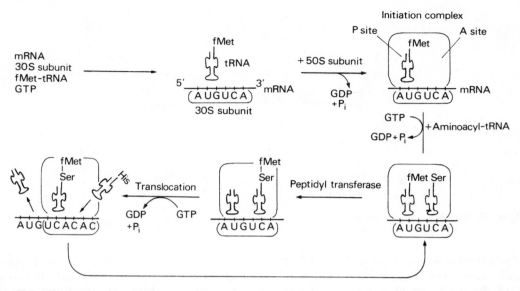

Figure 20.14 Mechanism of protein synthesis

initiating AUG, binds to the *A (aminoacyl) site* (Figure 20.14). A covalent peptide bond is then formed between the two adjacent amino acid residues, by the enzyme *peptidyltransferase*, an integral protein of the 50S ribosomal subunit. Peptide bond formation involves the transfer of the formylmethionine residue to the aminoacyl-tRNA bound at the A site. The uncharged tRNA now leaves the P site, the dipeptidyl-tRNA is *translocated* from the A site to the P site, and the mRNA moves along three nucleotides (one codon). As a result the third codon is now located in the A site, the appropriate aminoacyl-tRNA can bind, and peptidyltransferase activity will produce a tripeptide. This cycle continues until the whole polypeptide has been synthesized. As in the case of initiation, various protein factors and GTP are required for the elongation phase of protein synthesis.

Termination

Chain termination is signalled by one of the three codons UAA, UGA or UAG which do not code for any amino acid and for which there are no tRNAs. Consequently, protein synthesis halts at any of these termination codons. The codon is then recognized by a *protein release factor* which hydrolyses the nascent polypeptide chain from the peptidyl-tRNA bound at the A site.

Many bacterial mRNAs are *polycistronic* (Figure 20.15), i.e. a single mRNA molecule may code for several polypeptides. Each coding region has its own initiation codon (AUG) and termination codon, the translated regions being separated by non-coding regions of RNA. In addition, each mRNA molecule has a 5' non-coding region and a 3' non-coding region. Usually polycistronic mRNAs code for proteins involved in the same metabolic pathway.

Post-translational protein modification

In many cases proteins are modified during or after translation. (i) The *N*-terminal formyl group of bacterial proteins is usually removed by a *deformylase* and one or more *N*-terminal residues may be removed by *aminopeptidases*. (ii) *Disulphide bonds* may be formed by the oxidation of

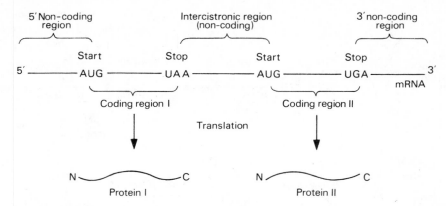

Figure 20.15 Organization of polycistronic mRNA

two cysteine residues in the same or different chains. (iii) Certain amino acid side chains may be modified by *hydroxylation*, *phosphorylation*, *glycosylation* or the addition of *prosthetic groups*. (iv) Polypeptide chains may be specifically cleaved to convert a precursor form into a mature active form.

Control of bacterial gene expression

Bacterial cells have quite sophisticated control mechanisms to ensure that many of their enzymes are synthesized only when required, according to their changing environment. This increases their efficiency and allows them to achieve maximal rates of proliferation under many conditions. External food substances often regulate the levels of enzymes involved in their metabolism by controlling the rates of synthesis and hence levels of their corresponding mRNAs. In other words, transcriptional control plays a major part in regulating bacterial gene expression. Such enzymes, which are expressed only when required, are called *inducible enzymes*, in contrast to *constitutive enzymes*, which are present in approximately constant amounts, regardless of the growth conditions.

Precise details of their control mechanisms are only known for a few bacterial proteins. One of the best studied examples is the *E. coli* enzyme *β-galactosidase* which splits the sugar lactose into its glucose and galactose moieties. *β*-Galactosidase is an important enzyme since lactose cannot be utilized as either a carbon or an energy source until it has been broken down into its monosaccharide components. *E. coli* cells growing in the presence of lactose as their sole carbon source contain about 3000 molecules of *β*-galactosidase; yet in the absence of lactose there are less than three enzyme molecules per cell. In fact, two other proteins are synthesized in parallel with *β*-galactosidase, namely *galactoside permease* and *thiogalactoside transacetylase*. The observation that the levels of the three enzymes was always coordinately controlled led Jacob and Monod to propose the *operon model* for the regulation of bacterial protein synthesis. An *operon* is composed of an *operator region* and one or more associated *structural genes*. In the case of the lactose or *lac operon* the operator region (O) is followed by the *β*-galactosidase (*z*), the permease (*y*) and the transacetylase (*a*) genes, in that order (Figure 20.16). All three structural genes are transcribed as a single polycistronic mRNA molecule, thereby explaining the coordinate synthesis of these three enzymes.

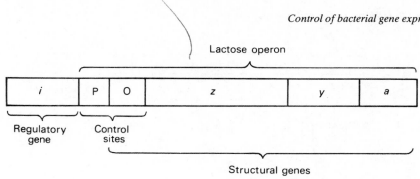

Figure 20.16 The lactose operon and its regulatory gene

A special group of proteins called *repressors* control the expression of operons. Repressors are the products of *regulatory genes*, and the *lac repressor*, which is the product of the *i* gene, is particularly well understood. It readily aggregates to form tetramers which appear to be the active form. There are usually about 10–20 *lac* repressor tetramers per bacterial cell.

Repressors act by binding to the operator region on the corresponding operon, thereby blocking the initiation of mRNA transcription. In fact the *lac* operator region overlaps the first 20 bases that are transcribed into *lac* mRNA. Consequently, in the absence of lactose, *lac* repressor molecules bind to the *lac* operator region and prevent transcription by physically blocking the path which the polymerase must take (Figure 20.17a). As a result synthesis of the β-galactosidase and associated enzymes is repressed. However, this inhibition must be reversed in the presence of lactose. To achieve this, *allolactose* (a lactose metabolite), which acts as the *inducer*, binds to the *lac* repressor and inactivates it by preventing it from binding to the *lac* operator region (Figure 20.17b). *Lac* mRNA transcription and subsequent β-galactosidase

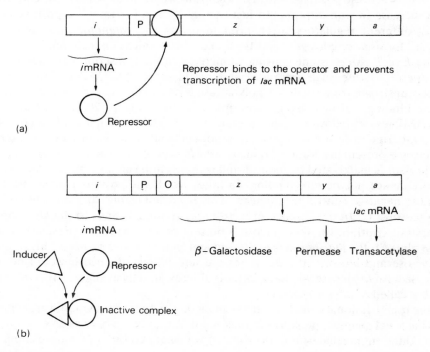

Figure 20.17 Control of the *lac* operon

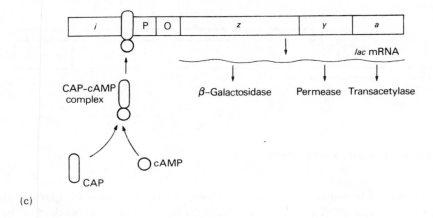

(c)

Figure 20.17 (*cont.*)

synthesis can then occur. Consequently addition of lactose to the medium of growing cells permits *lac* mRNA synthesis by decreasing the concentration of active *lac* repressor. The binding of the inducer to the repressor is non-covalent and readily reversed upon depletion of lactose from the medium.

The action of repressors in preventing transcription is an example of *negative control* since an increase in the controlling factor (*lac* repressor in this case) causes a decrease in mRNA synthesis. There are also positive control mechanisms where an increase in the controlling factor causes an increase in transcription. In fact the *lac* operon is subject to positive control by a completely different regulatory mechanism involving the *catabolite gene activator protein* (CAP). CAP forms a complex with cAMP (cyclic AMP) which can then bind to several specific sites on the *E. coli* chromosome causing an increase in the transcription of adjacent operons. The *lac* operon is one such example, and in this case the CAP–cAMP complex binds immediately upstream from the RNA polymerase binding site, thereby in some way enhancing polymerase binding and increasing transcription 50-fold (Figure 20.17c). In the presence of glucose, cAMP levels are lowered, the amount of CAP–cAMP complex will be correspondingly low, and transcription of the *lac* operon (and other CAP-sensitive operons) is therefore low. Even if lactose is present in addition to glucose, the *lac* operon remains repressed since, although the *lac* repressor is inactivated by inducer and transcription can take place, CAP–cAMP is not present to enhance polymerase binding. In other words the positive control mechanism can over-ride the negative control mechanism. This is advantageous to the bacterial cell for the following reasons. (i) In the absence of lactose, *lac* repressor binds to the *lac* operon thereby preventing transcription, whether glucose is present or not. (ii) In the presence of lactose, but absence of glucose, the *lac* operon is expressed and lactose is metabolized. (iii) In the presence of both lactose and glucose, the *lac* genes are not expressed since it would be wasteful to metabolize lactose to glucose when the latter is already directly available. This inhibitory effect by glucose is called *catabolite repression*.

While the transcriptional control mechanisms acting on the lactose operon are typical of those for many bacterial genes, it must be emphasized that they serve only as an example and many other quite different mechanisms exist, some of which are considerably more complex and are only just beginning to be understood.

Inhibitors of nucleic acid and protein synthesis

A wide range of substances interfere with nucleic acid and protein synthesis; many of them form invaluable research tools while others are used as antibiotics and antitumour agents. As in all chemotherapy the usefulness of a drug depends on its selectivity and ability to destroy bacteria, viruses or malignant cells without causing damage to normal cells and tissues. Anticancer agents exert their effects primarily on malignant cells but many have an overlapping toxicity on normal cells and cause unpleasant side effects.

Anticancer drugs

1. Alkylating agents

Mechloroethamine, chlorambucil and various *nitrosoureas* are able to transfer their alkyl groups to various cell constituents. They cause impairment of DNA function and inhibition of both nucleic acid and protein synthesis. Such drugs have a palliative effect on malignancies of many tissues that have a rapid rate of cell proliferation, but do not cure them.

2. Antimetabolites

Cell proliferation may be decreased by using various structural analogues to inhibit nucleic acid synthesis. *Amethopterin* (*methotrexate*) closely resembles folic acid (page 165) in structure and prevents the formation of the purine precursors of DNA, RNA and ATP. *6-Mercaptopurine* is a purine analogue which interferes with the pathway in which the phosphoribosyl precursors of the purine nucleotides are formed. *5-Fluorouracil* is a competitive inhibitor of the conversion of uridylic acid (dUMP) into thymidylic acid (dTMP).

Antibiotics

1. Inhibitors of transcription

Rifampicin and other members of the rifamycin group bind to the β subunit of bacterial RNA polymerase and block the formation of the first phosphodiester bond. They therefore inhibit initiation, with little effect on elongation or termination of previously initiated chains. *Actinomycin D* binds tightly to double-stranded DNA and prevents it from acting as a template for transcription. It binds between adjacent base pairs, particularly in G-rich regions, by a process known as *intercalation*. At low concentration, RNA synthesis is effectively inhibited with little effect on DNA or protein synthesis.

2. Inhibitors of protein synthesis

Streptomycin binds to the small 30S subunit of bacterial ribosomes and inhibits initiation. It can also cause misreading of the genetic code, resulting in the synthesis of functionally deficient proteins. *Tetracycline* also inhibits the initiation of prokaryotic protein synthesis, but in this case by preventing the binding of aminoacyl-tRNAs. Tetracycline is taken up by calcifying teeth and, if taken during pregnancy or early childhood, may cause permanent staining of the teeth. *Chloramphenicol, sparsomycin* and *lincomycin* all inhibit the peptidyltransferase activity of bacterial ribosomes and therefore block the elongation phase. Finally, *puromycin* has a structure which mimics the 3′ end of aminoacyl-tRNA and is consequently able to bind to the A site of the ribosome. There it acts as a substrate for the peptidyltransferase which transfers the growing polypeptide chain to the puromycin. These prematurely terminated chains are then released without further elongation.

Genetic manipulation

Genetic manipulation involves the introduction of DNA isolated from one organism into a different species in such a way that it is capable of continued propagation. This process of *gene cloning* provides a means of obtaining large amounts of a particular gene or DNA sequence. This is particularly important since individual genes, unlike proteins, are not readily purified by conventional biochemical means since they are present in very small amounts and are physically linked to other genes within chromosomes.

Cloning techniques

Ever since the classical experiments of Avery and others (page 289) it has been apparent that some bacterial species can take up exogenous DNA and undergo the process of *transformation*. In fact most transformable strains cannot discriminate between the uptake of DNA from a similar species and that from a completely different organism. This is the basis of gene cloning in bacteria. Unfortunately, if it does not impose a selective advantage on the organism, such acquired DNA is usually lost. However, this problem may be overcome by inserting the 'foreign' DNA into either a bacteriophage or a *plasmid*, prior to transformation. Such carriers of foreign DNA are usually called *vectors*. Plasmids are small circular extrachromosomal double-stranded DNA molecules that are found naturally in bacteria. They are capable of autonomous replication, and frequently carry drug resistance genes, thereby conferring a selective advantage on their bacterial hosts. Foreign DNA can be inserted into either plasmid or viral vectors and, after subsequent transformation of a suitable bacterial host, is stably maintained.

Such recombinant plasmids may be constructed with the aid of a number of enzymes. Perhaps the most important are a class of nucleases known as *restriction enzymes* which cleave double-stranded DNA at specific base sequences, different restriction enzymes recognizing different

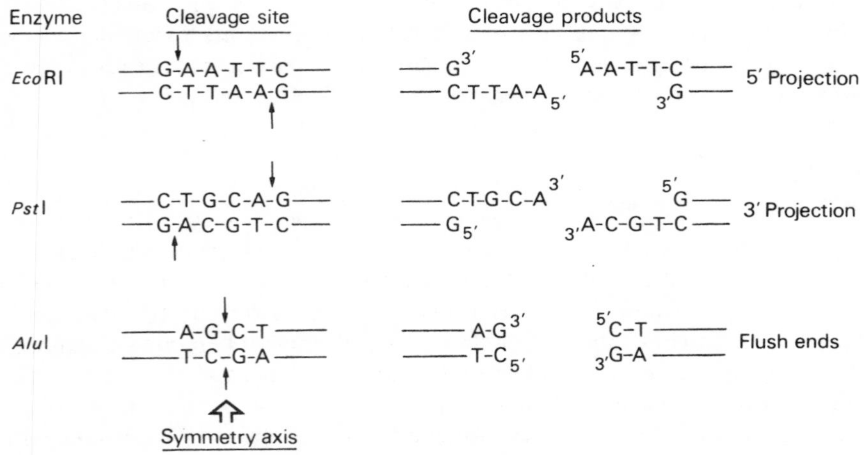

Figure 20.18 Cleavage sites of some common restriction enzymes

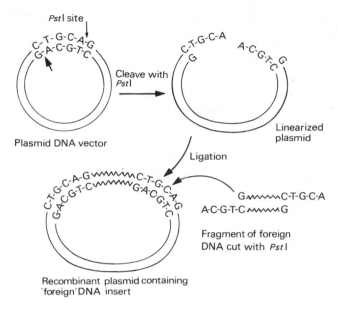

Figure 20.19 Construction of a recombinant plasmid

sequences. Most of these sequences, or restriction sites, possess a twofold axis of symmetry, and many are cleaved in such a way that they leave single-stranded projections or 'sticky ends' (Figure 20.18). Because of the symmetry, the sticky ends of two different DNA molecules cut with the same restriction enzyme will be complementary and can associate by base pairing. If then treated with the enzyme *DNA ligase*, these two molecules will be covalently joined. It can therefore be seen how a circular plasmid molecule may be linearized by treatment with a restriction enzyme which cleaves the molecule only once, and then a piece of foreign DNA, cut with the same enzyme to produce complementary ends, inserted into the plasmid (Figure 20.19). Such *recombinant plasmids* may then be used to transform bacterial cells in which they become stably maintained. In practice it is usual to generate a 'gene library', where the foreign DNA is cut up randomly with the restriction enzyme, such that different plasmids will then each contain a different foreign DNA fragment. After transformation, it is then necessary to use a suitable *probe* to select the bacterial clone containing the particular gene of interest for subsequent analysis. The most widely used methods for clone selection make use of *nucleic acid hybridization techniques*. Such radioactively labelled DNA or RNA probes need to be complementary to the cloned sequence of interest for hybridization to occur. The type of probe used will depend on the specific application (details of which are beyond the scope of this book), but may be a purified mRNA, a DNA copy of an mRNA synthesized *in vitro* using reverse transcriptase, or a short chemically synthesized oligonucleotide whose base sequence may be predicted if part of the amino acid sequence of the cloned gene's product is known. Alternatively, genes may be cloned in such a way that they become expressed as proteins in the transformed bacterial cells, and clones of interest can then be identified using specific antibodies raised against these known gene products.

Similar techniques can be used to insert foreign DNA into *bacteriophage* (instead of plasmid) *vectors*, which are then used to infect bacterial host cells; or to insert DNA into *animal virus vectors* for transformation into mammalian tissue culture cells.

Applications of recombinant DNA technology

Recombinant DNA technology has opened up many fields of biological research, as well as having important medical applications. With regard to biological research it has made it possible to study:

1. the structure and organization of individual genes and their controlling elements;
2. the manner in which genes are expressed, both with respect to different cell types and under varying physiological conditions;
3. gene abnormalities;
4. protein modifications by applying *site-directed mutagenesis*.

With this powerful new application it is now possible to engineer specific changes into a protein molecule (ranging from altering a single amino acid residue to building new hybrid proteins) by changing the corresponding bases in its gene. In this way it should be possible to produce new proteins with novel properties, such as altered substrate specificity, kinetic parameters or enhanced thermal stability.

In medicine, recombinant DNA techniques can be used for:

1. the diagnosis of diseases and investigation of their pathogenesis;
2. the detection of carriers of genetic diseases;
3. the large-scale synthesis of medically important peptides which would otherwise be in short supply, such as human insulin, growth hormone and interferon;
4. in addition, DNA technology may ultimately be of value in *gene therapy* (page 326) in cases where a disorder is attributable to a defective gene.

Chapter 21
Gene organization and expression in eukaryotes

Genes and chromosomes

There are a number of fundamental differences between the way genes are arranged, expressed and controlled in eukaryotic cells, when compared with bacteria.

1. Eukaryotes, because of their greater complexity, must possess much more genetic information. For example, a human cell contains about 1000 times more DNA than an *E. coli* cell. As a result the DNA may have an overall length of several centimetres which must be packed into a few micrometres. Hence the DNA of eukaryotic cells is very highly condensed and this is aided by the presence of a class of basic proteins called *histones*. Bacterial DNA is not associated with histones.
2. Eukaryotic chromosomes are located within a nucleus bounded by a nuclear membrane and, since proteins are synthesized in the cytoplasm, the sites of transcription and translation are physically separated. Consequently these two processes are not as closely coupled as they are in bacteria.
3. Primary RNA transcripts in eukaryotic cells are extensively modified, cleaved and spliced in the nucleus before being transported to the cytoplasm in the form of mRNA.
4. The control of gene expression is much more complex and diverse in eukaryotes, with many levels of regulation. In addition to transcriptional control, post-transcriptional mechanisms also play a major role. Furthermore, the primary translation products may in turn be subjected to post-translational modification.

Eukaryotic chromosome structure

It was not known for many years whether each eukaryotic chromosome contained a single linear DNA duplex molecule. Very large DNA molecules are readily broken down during isolation and handling, due to the shearing forces involved when working with molecules several millimetres or more in length. Eventually this problem was overcome by using a sophisicated *viscoelastic technique* which involved stretching the DNA molecules out in a flow of liquid, and then allowing them to recoil to their normal state. A measure of the rate of recoiling provides a measure of the molecular weight of the largest molecules in the preparation. When cells from fruit flies were lysed and subjected to this technique the mass of the largest DNA molecule was found to be 41×10^9 daltons; a value which agreed well with that for the DNA content of the largest fruit fly chromosome. Subsequent autoradiographic studies of radioactively labelled DNA confirmed the existence of very long DNA molecules and showed them to be linear and unbranched.

As mentioned above, the DNA in eukaryotic chromosomes is tightly bound to a group of small basic proteins called *histones*. The protein:DNA ratio is about 1:1 and the complex is known as *chromatin*. Histones can be fractionated into five types called H1, H2A, H2B, H3 and H4. They are all extremely basic, about one-quarter of their residues being either lysine or arginine. Each type of histone can be found in a variety of forms due to varying levels of post-translational modification of some of the amino acid side chains. These include acetylation, methylation and phosphorylation, and may be important in regulating DNA replication and transcription although this has yet to be firmly established. Histones H3 and H4 are highly conserved between species. In fact calf and pea H4 histones only differ by two conservative changes in their amino acid sequence, indicating that these histones play a crucial role in chromatin structure that was established early in the evolution of eukaryotes and has hardly diverged since.

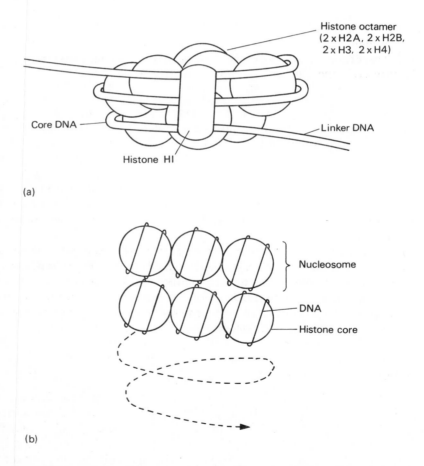

Figure 21.1 Structure of a single nucleosome (a) and proposed solenoid model of packing of the nucleosomes (b)

Nucleosomes

In 1974, Roger Kornberg proposed that chromatin is composed of regularly repeating units which he called *nucleosomes*. When observed in the electron microscope adjacent nucleosomes were joined together giving the appearance of beads on a string.

Several lines of evidence have shown that each nucleosome is composed of a *core particle* containing 140 base pairs of DNA (Figure 21.1), irrespective of the species or cell type. This DNA is wound in the form of 1·75 turns of a left-handed *superhelix*, round a histone octamer composed of two molecules each of H2A, H2B, H3 and H4. Adjacent nucleosomes are then joined by a short stretch of DNA, called *linker DNA*, thereby maintaining the integrity of the chromosome. Consequently a typical mammalian gene of 10 000 base pairs will contain about 40 nucleosomes. Histone H1, which is present at only one molecule per nucleosome and is absent from the core particle, may be associated with the linker DNA and serve as a bridge between adjacent nucleosomes.

If stretched out a 200 base pair piece of DNA (140 base pairs in a nucleosome core plus about 60 base pairs of linker DNA) would have a length of 680 Å (68 nm). This is packed within a 100 Å (10 nm) diameter nucleosome by winding round the outside. Hence the packing ratio of a nucleosome is about 7. However, the overall packing ratio of DNA in interphase nuclei is about 100–1000 and this is further increased to 10 000 during metaphase. Consequently the formation of nucleosomes must be only the first step in DNA packing. At the moment it is not certain what other higher levels of chromatin packing exist. However, one popular model is the *solenoid model*. This proposes that chromatin forms a solenoid with six nucleosomes to the turn of the helix (Figure 21.1) giving an overall structure with a diameter of about 360 Å (36 nm) and a packing ratio of 40. Further folding of the solenoid into loops would then result in an even more condensed structure with a packing ratio approaching that found in interphase chromosomes. A class of nuclear proteins called the *non-histone proteins* may play an important part in stabilizing such postulated higher levels of chromatin structure.

Repetitive DNA

Unlike bacteria, all eukaryotic cells, except perhaps yeast, contain DNA sequences that are repeated many times. In most cases the eukaryotic genome can be divided into three classes of DNA; namely, highly repetitive, moderately repetitive and single-copy DNA. The proportion of each of these classes may vary considerably between different species. In the mouse, the *highly repetitive DNA* fraction, which represents about 10% of the genome, is composed of approximately one million copies of a repeating sequence of about 300 base pairs. Although its function is unknown (it does not appear to be transcribed into RNA), the fact that it is confined to the centromeric regions of chromosomes might suggest a role in chromosome alignment during mitosis and meiosis. The *moderately repetitive* DNA fraction accounts for about 20% of the mouse genome, being composed of several thousand different sequences, each reiterated several hundred times. In this case the sequences appear to be distributed throughout the whole genome, interspersed between the single-copy DNA, although again their function is unknown.

The remaining 70% of the mouse genome constitutes the *single-copy DNA* fraction, i.e. those sequences present at only one (or very few) copies per haploid genome. This fraction contains most of the *structural genes*, i.e. those sequences which are transcribed into mRNA, and then translated into protein. Even the genes encoding many of the more abundant proteins (e.g. globin, ovalbumin, silk fibroin, milk proteins), which must be capable of very high levels of expression at times, are present at only one (or just a few) copies per genome. However, there are exceptions, and the histone genes, for example, are each reiterated about 10–50 times in mammals and up to 1000 times in sea-urchins. In the latter case it has been shown that the genes for each of the five histone types are clustered into a group and these groups are then tandemly repeated many times. Finally, the genes coding for ribosomal RNA are also tandemly repeated at least 100 times in eukaryotic cells, and the transfer RNA genes are even more highly reiterated.

Eukaryotic DNA replication

DNA replication in eukaryotic cells is fundamentally the same as that in bacteria. Replication is semi-conservative, occurs in a $5' \rightarrow 3'$ direction, and requires a template, a primer and deoxy-ribonucleoside triphosphates for synthesis to occur. Replication also proceeds bidirectionally, but in view of the large size of eukaryotic chromosomes, synthesis is initiated simultaneously at many origins; otherwise chromosome replication would take many days. Eukaryotic cells contain three types of DNA polymerase, α, β and γ. The first two are found in the nucleus and are involved in replication and repair respectively; the latter is mitochondrial and replicates the DNA of this organelle. These polymerases all lack a proof-reading activity. This function is probably performed by a separate enzyme.

Since the amount of DNA is duplicated during chromosome replication, more histone molecules are required. Unlike the DNA strands, the existing histones segregate conservatively, becoming associated exclusively with the continuously replicating DNA strand, whereas the new histone molecules become associated with the discontinuously replicating strand. This is probably because histones bind much more strongly to double-stranded DNA than to single-stranded DNA and hence would tend to stay with the continuously replicating DNA strand which does not contain the single-stranded regions characteristic of the discontinuous strand.

Eukaryotic gene structure

In prokaryotes, mRNAs are exactly complementary to the genes from which they are transcribed. Consequently the linear arrangement of codons found within the mRNA, which is used to direct protein synthesis, is also reflected in the gene itself. For many years it was assumed that a similar situation would exist with regard to eukaryotic genes. However, in 1977 this was shown not to be the case. Instead most eukaryotic genes contain additional *intervening sequences* which are not found in their mature mRNA transcripts. Those regions which are common to both the genes and their mRNA transcripts are known as *exons* and the intervening sequences are called *introns*. Thus, for example, the β-globin gene is split into three exons by two introns (Figure 21.2). The globin-coding capacity is restricted to the exon regions of the gene since these are the only regions which appear in the mature mRNA.

The β-globin gene is a relatively simple gene with only two introns. Most genes have many more introns; for example, ovalbumin has seven introns and conalbumin has 17. The combined lengths of the introns is usually much greater than the combined lengths of the exons. The sequences of introns tend to change more rapidly than those of exons during evolution. Although their function is as yet unclear, in some cases the positions of introns appear to break the protein up into *functional domains*, suggesting that the exons may represent the building blocks from which large complex proteins with intricate regulatory mechanisms have evolved. However, in other cases the positions of introns within protein-coding regions appear to be random.

How can an mRNA lacking introns be transcribed from a gene containing them? In fact, the *primary RNA transcript* (that is, the initial transcript) is much larger than the mature mRNA which it eventually becomes (Figure 21.2). This short-lived primary transcript is a

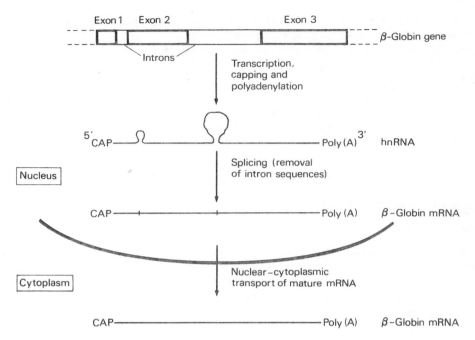

Figure 21.2 Transcription and processing of β-globin mRNA

complementary copy of the whole gene (exons plus introns), is confined to the nucleus and is called *heterogeneous nuclear RNA* or hnRNA. Those regions which are complementary to the introns and do not appear in the mature mRNA are excised and the regions corresponding to the exons are spliced together by specific processing enzymes in the nucleus. The whole process which is known as *RNA splicing* takes place before the mRNA is transported into the cytoplasm.

Transcription in eukaryotic cells

Although the mechanism of RNA synthesis in higher organisms is similar to that in bacterial cells, the overall process of transcription is much more complex, particularly with respect to mRNA synthesis. Eukaryotic cells contain three different RNA polymerases, each responsible for the synthesis of a different class of RNA (mRNA, rRNA and tRNA). Here again, RNA polymerase binds to specific regions of the DNA at the start of genes, called *promoters*, but the sequence and spacing between conserved regions in these promoters are different from those found in bacterial cells. Most eukaryotic structural genes have two conserved sequences within the promoter region; one situated about 19–26 nucleotides upstream from the start of transcription, with the sequence –TATAAA–, and the other about 70–80 nucleotides from the start site, with the sequence –CAAT–.

The most important difference between RNA synthesis in eukaryotic and prokaryotic cells is, however, at the level of the primary transcript, particularly in the case of hnRNA which must undergo three types of post-transcriptional modification (Figure 21.2) before it is transported to the cytoplasm as a fully mature mRNA molecule. These processes are as follows. (i) Modification of the 5′ end of the RNA to form a *cap structure*. This entails the enzyme addition of a guanosine residue via a 5′–5′ triphosphate linkage to the 5′ end, as well as varying degrees of methylation of the first two or three nucleotides. (ii) In most eukaryotic mRNAs the addition of a long tract of adenosine residues to produce a poly(A) tail at the 3′ end. (iii) Removal of the intervening sequences by nuclear splicing enzymes.

Having undergone capping, polyadenylation and splicing, the mature mRNA may now be transported to the cytoplasm where it is able to direct protein synthesis. Unlike prokaryotic mRNAs, all eukaryotic mRNAs are monocistronic and only code for a single polypeptide. This primary translation product may in some cases, however, be proteolytically cleaved to produce two or more peptide products. To summarize, a eukaryotic mRNA contains a single coding region enclosed by two non-coding regions and possesses a cap structure at the 5′ end and a poly(A) tail at the 3′ end.

Cytoplasmic processes

Eukaryotic protein synthesis

The mechanism of protein synthesis in eukaryotic cells is also essentially the same as in bacteria. However, since eukaryotic protein synthesis occurs in the cytoplasm, the processes of transcription and translation are not as closely coupled as they are in bacteria. In eukaryotes the initiating methionine is not formylated, but is attached to a different form of tRNA from that involved in incorporating internal methionine residues.

Post-translational modification

Many of the post-translational modifications observed in bacterial cells also occur to eukaryotic proteins. These include disulphide bond formation, hydroxylation, glycosylation, phosphorylation and cleavage of precursor forms to mature proteins.

Signal sequences and protein secretion

In eukaryotic cells some polysomes (polyribosomes) are free in the cytoplasm while others are bound to the membranes of the endoplasmic reticulum, forming the rough endoplasmic reticulum (page 192) and there is a functional difference between these two classes of polysome. Membrane-bound polysomes synthesize secretory and membrane proteins, whereas those free in the cytoplasm synthesize internal or 'housekeeping' proteins. There is no difference between the ribosomes themselves in these two populations, just in the proteins they synthesize. To enable the cell to distinguish between secretory (or membrane) and housekeeping proteins, before they have been completely synthesized, nearly all secretory proteins have a *signal sequence* at their *N*-terminus. This signal sequence is a stretch of about 15–30 residues, a high proportion of which are hydrophobic and do not appear in the final mature protein. In fact, all protein synthesis is initiated on free polysomes in the cytoplasm, but those with a signal peptide attach to the endoplasmic reticulum by means of this signal sequence (Figure 21.3), soon after its synthesis. The signal peptide then passes through the membranes of the endoplasmic reticulum into the lumen, and is followed by the rest of the protein chain as it is synthesized. During this process the signal peptide is cleaved off by a *signal peptidase* located on the inner surface of the endoplasmic reticulum. Almost all proteins synthesized on membrane-bound polysomes are glycosylated after translation and this occurs in the endoplasmic reticulum. The secretory proteins then pass through the Golgi complex where they may be further glycosylated and in some cases may also be phosphorylated, before being secreted via secretory vesicles.

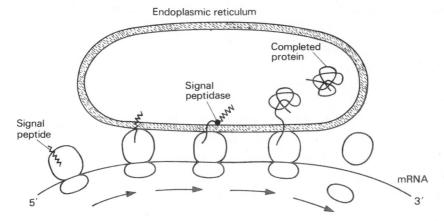

Figure 21.3 The signal hypothesis

Control of gene expression in eukaryotes

Eukaryotic organisms contain many different cell types, each with a distinctive pattern of proteins or *phenotype*. Since every somatic cell has the same genetic constitution, differentiation clearly depends on the selective expression of certain genes. The fact that, for example, liver cells do not synthesize haemoglobin and kidney cells do not synthesize insulin suggests that differentiated cells must contain a great deal of genetic information that is never expressed as protein. However, although there clearly are some proteins which are completely tissue-specific, the majority of differences in gene expression between different cell types are quantitative rather than qualitative. Broadly speaking, therefore, the control of gene expression in higher organisms falls into two categories: (i) the selective expression of certain tissue-specific genes which occurs when a cell differentiates, and (ii) the regulation of gene expression within differentiated cells in response to physiological, nutritional or pharmacological stimuli.

Owing to the complexity of higher organisms, the ways in which the expression of eukaryotic genes is regulated are only just beginning to be understood. Much of the work depends on recombinant DNA techniques, which have made it possible to obtain large amounts of pure gene sequences for analysis and for use as probes. In bacterial cells, transcriptional control was seen to be the predominant form of gene regulation. In eukaryotes this is also clearly important, but in addition there are many other levels at which control can, and does, operate (Figure 21.4).

Control at the level of the gene

When isolated chromatin is partially digested with deoxyribonuclease I, actively transcribed genes are often degraded much more readily than those which are not being expressed. For example, the globin genes are preferentially degraded in chick red blood cells whereas the ovalbumin genes are not. On the other hand, in the oviduct the ovalbumin genes are degraded in preference to the globin genes. Two non-histone proteins, HMG14 and HMG17, appear to be involved, and have therefore been implicated with actively transcribed genes.

In addition, about 2–7% of the cytidine residues in animal cell DNA are methylated, and there is some evidence of a correlation between the extent of methylation at particular sites and the level of transcription.

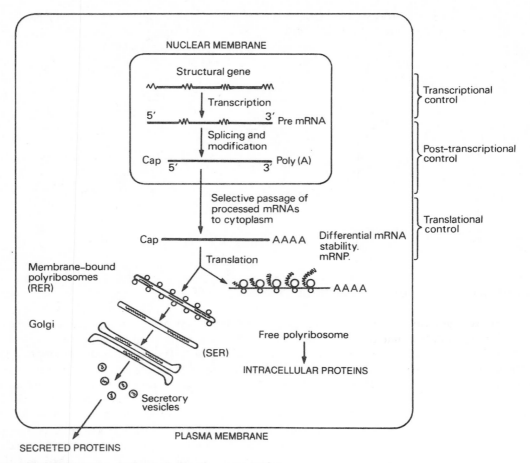

Figure 21.4 Multiple steps in the regulation of gene expression

Transcriptional control

Typically less than 5% of the eukaryotic genome is transcribed into hnRNA in any given tissue or cell type and consequently most genes would appear to be 'switched off'. In the case of certain genes which are controlled by steroid hormones (page 349) it has been established that the hormone binds to a specific receptor in the cytoplasm and the resulting hormone–receptor complex is translocated to the nucleus where it binds in close proximity to the promoter regions of hormone-responsive genes, thereby in some way enhancing their transcription. This is a rather specialized case and for the vast majority of eukaryotic genes we know virtually nothing about the mechanisms which operate to bring about their transcriptional control.

Post-transcriptional regulation

Again very little is known about the mechanisms involved in regulating hnRNA processing and the transport of the resulting mature mRNAs to the cytoplasm. However, it is clear that such regulatory mechanisms are extremely important in eukaryotes since in most cell types as many as 80% of the different transcribed hnRNA sequences are completely degraded in the nucleus and are not detectable in a processed form in the cytoplasm. Clearly mechanisms exist which are able to identify those hnRNAs which need to be processed and transported in that particular cell type, and those which are not required. Furthermore, in some specific cases, the hnRNA transcript is spliced in different ways to produce different mRNAs in different tissues, e.g. the mouse α-amylase gene.

Control of mRNA stability

Different eukaryotic mRNAs may have widely differing half-lives and the more stable the mRNA, the more protein that can be translated from it. Various factors may affect the stability of specific mRNAs. For example, in the presence of the peptide hormone prolactin, casein mRNAs are specifically stabilized during lactation, thereby increasing the level of expression of these milk proteins.

Translational control

Large amounts of some mRNAs may be stored within the cytoplasm, complexed with protein, in the form of ribonucleoprotein (RNP) particles. In this form they are inactive and are not translated into protein, but they may become active at a later stage of development or differentiation. The translational efficiency of specific mRNAs may be modulated under certain conditions, e.g. extracts of reticulocytes synthesize globin subunits efficiently only when there is an adequate supply of haem.

Overall it can be seen that the control of eukaryotic gene expression is highly complex and it will probably be some time before precise details of the mechanisms have been worked out even for a few well-characterized genes.

Chapter 22
Mutations, evolution and inherited disease

Mutations and mutagens

Genetic differences within a species arise as a result of random mutations which, as well as being the basis of individuality, provide new characteristics which can either be maintained or eliminated as a result of natural selection. Mutations are changes in the nucleotide sequence of DNA and fall into three classes: (1) *Substitutions* involve the replacement of a base pair by a different one. They are sometimes referred to as *point mutations*. (2) *Deletions* involve the loss of one or more base pairs. (3) *Insertions* involve the acquisition of one or more base pairs. The substitution of one base pair for another is the most common type of mutation. Causes of mutation in DNA include rare tautomerization of bases to form base pairs other than A-T and G-C, imprecise replication and proof-reading by DNA polymerase, natural background radiation, damage by strong ultraviolet light and exposure to chemical mutagens. Among the chemical mutagens are: (1) base analogues such as 5-bromouracil and 2-aminopurine which become incorporated into DNA in place of the normal bases and lead to errors in base pairing; (2) acridine dyes such as proflavin and Acridine Orange which intercalate or bind between adjacent base pairs, thereby distorting the DNA helix and leading to the insertion or deletion of one or more base pairs; (3) alkylating agents such as the nitrogen mustards, and other compounds such as hydroxylamine and nitrous acid which chemically modify specific bases.

Mutations in protein-coding sequences

Point mutations (base substitutions)

Mutations of this type within the protein-coding regions of genes can have a variety of effects on the resulting protein (Figure 22.1).

(i) Since the genetic code is degenerate and there are alternative codons for most of the amino acids, a base substitution can occur without having any effect on the structure of the protein synthesized. For example, UUU and UUC are both codons for phenylalanine, so a mutation which converts one to the other is known as a *silent mutation*.

(ii) If, on the other hand, the codon UUU is converted to either UUA or UUG, there will be an amino acid replacement since UUA and UUG code for leucine instead of phenylalanine, and

a. *Wild type – original message*
   THE MAN AND THE DOG HID BUT SAW THE RAT NIP THE FOX WHO RAN OFF.

b. *Point mutation – amino acid substitution*
   THE MAN AND THE DOG HID BUT SAW THE ⒸAT NIP THE FOX WHO RAN OFF.

c. *Phase shift – deletion*
   THE MAN AND THE *OGH IDB UTS AWT HER ATN IPT HEF OXW HOR ANO FF*
                    —

d. *Phase shift mutation – insertion*
   THE MAN AND THE DOG HID *BUT TSA WTH ERA TNI PTH EFO XWH ORA NOF F*
                            +

e. *Double mutant – suppression*
   THE MAN AND THE DOG *IDB UTS* SAW THE RAT NIP THE FOX WHO RAN OFF
                        —   +

f. *Triple mutant – Crick and Benzer's experiment*
   THE MAN *NAN DTH EDD OGH* HID BUT SAW THE RAT NIP THE FOX WHO RAN OFF.
            +   +   +

Figure 22.1 An illustration of the effects of different types of mutation

at this one position in the protein chain the mutant will differ from the normal or wild type. In many instances single amino acid replacements, particularly if the substitutions occur between similar types of amino acid, e.g. both neutral or both acidic, may have little or no effect on the functional efficiency of the protein (Figure 22·1b). Occasionally, however, even a single amino acid replacement may have a profound effect, especially if it involves an active site residue or if it causes a gross change in protein tertiary structure, as for example in sickle cell haemoglobin, HbS.

(iii) If the mutation causes the codon for a particular amino acid, e.g. UCA (serine), to be replaced by a chain termination codon (UAA or UGA), then a truncated protein will be produced. Mutations of this type, unless they occur very close to the *C*-terminus of the protein, will usually result in complete or severe loss of protein function.

(iv) Conversely, if a chain termination codon is converted into one coding for an amino acid, e.g. UGA to AGA, a larger protein will be synthesized, its length being determined by the distance to the next in-phase termination codon.

From what is known of the degeneracy of the code it can be calculated that of all possible point mutations 20–25% would be silent, about 3% would result in chain termination to produce truncated proteins, and the remaining 70–75% would lead to an amino acid substitution.

Phase-shift mutations (insertions and deletions)

Phase-shift or frame-shift mutations arise from the insertion or deletion of one or more base pairs into the protein-coding region of a gene. If, for example, as a result of a deletion within a gene, an mRNA molecule lacks a base at some point, the reading of all subsequent triplet codons will be out of phase and hence very different; the addition of a single base will have a similar effect (Figure 22·1c and d). Thus, while point mutations may cause only a slight, but possibly significant, alteration in the sequence of a protein, insertions and deletions are likely to result in products with long stretches of completely different amino acid sequence. However, the deleterious effect of a single base addition may be partly overcome or suppressed by a second mutation involving the deletion of a single base close to the site of the first mutation; only the region between the two mutations will now differ from the wild-type protein sequence. A highly significant finding was that if the phage carried either 3(+) or 3(−) mutations in close proximity it hardly differed from the wild type (Figure 22.1f). In these cases the equivalent of a whole new codon had been added to or subtracted from the DNA so that one amino acid was either introduced into, or eliminated from, the protein. Only in the short stretch of DNA separating the first and third mutation was the message garbled. This work gave proof to the suggestion, which was originally based on theoretical considerations, that the genetic code is a triplet code.

Mutations in non-coding regions

Mutations which occur in non-coding regions of the genome may also have adverse effects. For example, mutations within promoter regions may result in a loss of transcription or tissue-specific regulation. Mutations close to exon–intron boundaries, or even within introns themselves, may prevent correct splicing of the hnRNA transcript. Even changes in the 5' or 3' non-coding regions of mature mRNAs may affect their secondary structure and hence stability, thereby affecting their translational efficiency.

Sequence divergence

Most major changes in protein structure occur by the gradual accumulation of small mutations. Many of the mutations that result in amino acid changes are deleterious and will rapidly be eliminated by natural selection. On rare occasions, however, a mutation may have a beneficial effect and may be retained and spread throughout the population, eventually to replace the former sequence. The rate at which mutational changes accumulate will vary from protein to protein, depending on the particular constraints. For example, the histones apparently can tolerate only very minor changes and are therefore extremely highly conserved, whereas other less structurally constrained proteins show much higher rates of mutation.

The presence within a population of two or more variants of a protein is called a *polymorphism*. This can be either a stable situation in which neither form is advantageous or disadvantageous, or it can be a transient stage during which one variant is replacing the other. When we compare corresponding proteins from two different species of organism, we see the differences which have accumulated since the divergence of those species. While the histones are highly conserved between species, other proteins, e.g. the haemoglobins, show greater divergence.

One way of facilitating sequence divergence is by means of *gene duplication*. This falls into three types. (i) If two identical copies of a gene exist, then one can mutate at a higher rate without depriving the organism of a functional protein as supplied by the other gene copy. In this way the faster mutating copy may eventually diverge to encode a new function. The separation of functions between embryonic and adult globin genes (page 371) probably arose by this type of mechanism. (ii) In other cases duplicated genes have retained the same function with selective pressure being maintained on both copies. For example, there are two human α-globin genes which code for proteins with identical sequence. The reason for maintaining two identical copies in such cases is unknown. (iii) Finally, one of the duplicated gene copies may mutate in such a way that it can no longer be expressed to produce a functional protein, for example as a result of a mutation in a promoter region, at a splice site, or within an essential part of the coding region. Such non-functional copies are called *pseudogenes*. They often contain several deleterious mutations, presumably because once they have become inactive selective pressures will become relaxed and additional changes will then accumulate at a faster rate. Pseudogenes are generally regarded as being dead ends of evolution.

Inherited disease

When one considers the huge amount of DNA present in a eukaryotic cell and the rate of spontaneous mutation, it is easy to explain why no two individuals are alike. Instead each person possesses a number of traits which distinguishes that individual from the population as a whole, although in most cases these differences are concealed, either due to their unobtrusive nature, or because of the remarkable efficiency of the body's homoeostatic mechanisms. However, deleterious mutations do sometimes occur and such genetic defects may lead to inherited diseases. In fact there are some 2500 genetic defects known to occur in Man, although many are extremely rare and their genetic lesion is often unknown. Within Northern Europe, recognizable genetically inherited diseases may affect 1% of all live births.

Sickle cell anaemia

The human haemoglobins have been extensively studied for many years and many examples of genetically determined defects have been identified. These defects, which are collectively known as the *haemoglobinopathies*, fall into two groups: (i) the *structural variants*, haemoglobins with altered polypeptide chains caused by amino acid substitutions, and (ii) the *thalassaemias*, caused by the absence of reduced synthesis of globin α or β chains, resulting in a relative excess of the other chain.

A large number of structural variants have been identified. Although some of these are almost indistinguishable from normal haemoblobin A (HbA) in their properties, many of the others cause anaemia of varying degrees of severity. One of the most notorious is *sickle cell haemoglobin* (HbS) whose molecular properties are so profoundly affected that persons who are homozygous with respect to the mutant gene usually die before reaching maturity. The disease for which it is responsible, *sickle cell anaemia*, is common in Central Africa and is seen in Negro populations living in other parts of the world. A milder form known as *sickle cell trait* is found in patients heterozygous for the mutant gene. The cause of the anaemia is the fragility of the red blood cells which, although normal in shape when the blood is oxygenated, become elongated, sickle-shaped and readily destroyed at low oxygen tension. In 1949 Pauling and his associates showed that the haemoglobin (HbS) isolated from sickle cell anaemic patients behaved differently from that from normal patients (HbA) when subjected to electrophoresis. Moreover it was found that the blood of sickle cell trait individuals contained both HbS and HbA. Subsequent studies of the abnormal HbS involving the *'fingerprinting' technique* showed that, although the α-globin chain was identical to that of normal HbA, the β chain was different (Figure 22.2). In fact the difference is due solely to the substitution of valine for glutamate at position 6 in the β-globin chain, brought about by a single base change in the corresponding gene. This single amino acid change markedly reduces the solubility of deoxygenated HbS but has little effect on the oxygenated form, ultimately accounting for the clinical characteristics of sickle cell anaemia.

An interesting feature of the disease is that heterozygotes suffering from sickle cell trait are less severely affected by malaria than normal individuals, so that in malarial districts natural selection has favoured this condition since it confers a specific advantage in this particular environment.

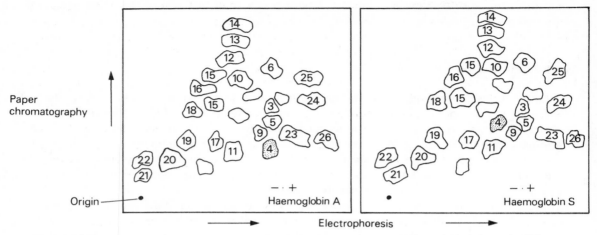

Figure 22.2 'Fingerprints' of tryptic digests of the β chain of haemoglobin A and haemoglobin S. Note the different positions of peptide 4.

Inborn errors of metabolism

Sickle cell anaemia results from the congenital abnormality of a transport protein but similar abnormalities may occur in any of the proteins found in the body whether they be structural, enzymic or regulatory in function. The realization that inherited diseases might result from deficiency of a specific enzyme came from the work of Garrod (1909) and was derived largely from his studies on the condition of *alkaptonuria*. In this rare disorder large amounts of *homogentisic acid* are excreted in the urine which becomes black on standing as a result of the oxidation of this abnormal constituent. Garrod noticed that the condition appeared to be inherited. He found that the homogentisic acid was derived from phenylalanine and tyrosine and that its secretion resulted from an inability to degrade the benzene ring. If homogentisic acid was given to normal subjects it was readily metabolized. Garrod then searched for, and found, various other genetically determined peculiarities which he designated *inborn errors of metabolism* and suggested that in such conditions the body was unable to perform some particular metabolic step due to lack of the necessary enzyme.

If one considers such a condition and takes a sequence of reactions:

$$A \rightarrow B \rightarrow C \nrightarrow D \rightarrow E$$
$$w \qquad x \qquad y \qquad z$$

in which enzyme y is lacking, it can be seen that compound C will tend to accumulate and that, if the preceding reactions are reversible, compounds A and B may also be present in increased amounts. On the other hand, there will be a deficiency of compound D, as well as of E and any other metabolites originating from them, unless there are alternative routes of production that can be correspondingly increased. Thus excess of compound C or lack of compound D can result in secondary metabolic disturbances.

A great variety of disorders can now be explained in these terms including *phenylketonuria*, *galactosaemia*, *fructosuria*, *hypophosphatasia* and *acatalasia*, but, although it has been possible to demonstrate their association with the deficiency of a specific enzyme, only in a few cases is the exact genetic nature of the defect known. The deficiency may be due to either the synthesis of an abnormal protein or to the synthesis of reduced amounts of normal protein, depending on whether the genetic lesion is in the structural gene or a regulatory region respectively. Moreover, a change in the structure of a protein might result in changes in its catalytic or substrate-binding properties, or in its stability and rate of degradation. Hence the deficiency of a particular enzyme activity may arise in a number of different ways, thereby resulting in wide variability in the clinical expression and severity of a particular inherited disease.

Some inherited metabolic disorders are extremely damaging while the effects of others are so mild that they can hardly be called diseases. For example, alkaptonurics are usually quite healthy although in later life they are prone to a particular form of arthritis. Similarly the conditions of fructosuria and pentosuria, in which fructose and pentose sugars respectively appear in the urine, have no pathological consequences. At the other end of the scale is phenylketonuria in which the enzyme *phenylalanine hydroxylase*, which is responsible for converting phenylalanine to tyrosine, is lacking. In this condition phenylpyruvic acid and other intermediate products of phenylalanine metabolism accumulate in the blood and tissues and are so injurious to the central nervous system that, although physical development is essentially normal, there is severe mental retardation.

Any function performed by protein in the body is subject to inherited abnormality as a result of a mutation. *Haemophilia*, a sex-linked hereditary defect of the blood-clotting mechanism, is caused by deficiency of *antihaemophilic globulin (Factor VIII)* (page 389) in the plasma and is only detectable as a result of trauma. It is exceedingly serious since a major haemorrhage may result from quite trivial damage, e.g. tooth extraction. If bleeding should occur into a joint it is excruciatingly painful, and subsequent organization of the blood clot can cause deformity with limitation of movement.

Apart from this, congenital diseases are known which result from defects in the matrix of connective tissue; others, such as *cystinuria* in which cystine and the basic amino acids are continuously excreted in the urine, seem to be caused by disorders of active transport, presumably as a result of alterations in the carrier proteins.

Rare congenital enzyme deficiencies which have effects that are of particular interest to the dental profession include *hypophosphatasia*, *acatalasia* and the *Lesch–Nyhan* syndrome. Furthermore, some drug idiosyncracies are known to result from inherited defects in an enzyme which, in normal subjects, is concerned with the metabolism of the drug. For example, certain subjects who are deficient in serum cholinesterase show an abnormally prolonged respiratory paralysis after administration of suxamethonium given to produce muscular relaxation. Other subjects develop an acute haemolysis when given the antimalarial drug primaquine or certain sulphonamides.

Mutant genes may be dominant, co-dominant or recessive. If the mutant gene is dominant the corresponding abnormality will be apparent even in heterozygotes who inherit a normal gene from one parent and the abnormal gene from the other. This is the case in the dental defect *dentinogenesis imperfecta*. More commonly, however, biochemical defects are inherited as recessive characteristics so that the defect is only apparent in homozygotes, although sometimes the normal and abnormal genes are co-dominant and, as in the case of heterozygotes carrying the sickle cell trait, both are expressed. In such instances it is possible to detect persons who are carriers of the defect and to provide genetic counselling for individuals in whose families they are known to exist.

It has been estimated that the average healthy individual is a heterozygous carrier of at least three harmful mutations which, in the homozygous state, would produce genetic disorders; this being so the undesirability of consanguinous marriages becomes obvious.

Early diagnosis and treatment of genetic disorders

At one time it seemed that little could be done to treat congenital abnormalities, but advances are continually being made. As both pre- and post-natal care improve, so that the survival rate of sufferers is increased, it is clear that genetic disorders are causing an increasing burden on the medical services. Although most genetic disorders cannot, as yet, be 'cured', in some cases palliative treatment is possible. Methods used or suggested include.

1. Supplying a missing protein or metabolite if its production is blocked, e.g. injections of antihaemophilic globulin to haemophiliacs, thyroxine administration to goitrous cretins, blood transfusion for thalassaemic patients.
2. Limiting the intake of a substance that cannot be metabolized and leads to the accumulation of toxic material. Considerable success has been achieved in the treatment of infants suffering from galactosaemia by replacing the lactose of milk with another sugar. Similarly, phenylketonuric infants may be fed a low-phenylalanine diet which provides just enough phenylalanine for protein synthesis but not enough to allow its intermediate metabolites to accumulate.
3. Treatment with metabolic inhibitors. For example allopurinol which inhibits *xanthine oxidase*, an enzyme responsible for the oxidation of purines, has been used to regulate uric acid production in gout.

Although such methods may alleviate the condition they will not cure it. To achieve the latter one must either correct the genetic mutation causing the disorder, or introduce a normal copy of the mutated gene. With the recent advances in *recombinant DNA technology*, it is now possible to microinject purified genes into early embryos, which, following reimplantation give rise to offspring which express the introduced gene. Such experiments, with *transgenic animals*, suggest that successful *gene replacement therapy* may one day be a practical reality, although clearly much more research has first to be done. In the meantime much effort has been directed towards developing or improving the antenatal diagnosis of genetic disorders (to enable the option of abortion to be offered within the legal time limits) and again recombinant DNA techniques have played a major role. This can be illustrated by taking the haemoglobinopathies as an example. There are two current approaches to the problem. First, it is possible to take a fetal blood sample at about 16 weeks gestation and look for both α- and β-globin variants using routine procedures. However, fetal blood sampling and analysis requires expensive equipment and a high level of expertise. In addition, the antenatal diagnosis of β-thalassaemia by this method has a fetal death rate of about 10%. Fortunately the alternative more modern approach overcomes most of these problems. This involves *amniocentesis*, the extraction of a small amount of amniotic fluid surrounding a 16–18-week fetus, which contains fetally derived fibroblasts. These fibroblasts may then be used either directly, or after culture *in vitro*, for the preparation of fetal DNA and subsequent globin gene analysis using rapid recombinant DNA techniques. In this case it is only necessary to establish whether the fetus has inherited a single normal globin gene since all of the haemoglobinopathies have clinically mild carrier (heterozygous) states. At the moment the reliability of this approach is variable but improvements are continually being made. However, its main advantage over fetal blood analysis is in the lower risk associated with amniocentesis. In fact the fetal death rate associated with this procedure is only 3%, the same as the spontaneous abortion rate during the second trimester of normal pregnancies. In some of the other genetic diseases where a suitable biochemical assay is not available, the DNA approach may be the only solution at the moment.

Oncogenes and cancer

A growing number of vertebrate genes appear to be involved in tumorigenesis. In their normal form, such genes are known as *proto-oncogenes*. However, abnormal forms of these proto-oncogenes, known as *oncogenes*, are found in tumours as well as in a number of turmour-producing retroviruses. Consequently the retroviruses, which can cause virtually every major form of neoplasia known, have been the subject of much study. Both the retroviruses and the DNA tumour viruses transform normal cells (page 289) by inserting viral genetic material into the host chromosomal DNA. In this way the viral genes become part of the genome of the host and are replicated along with the hosts own DNA. It is the protein products of the viral oncogenes which cause the tumorigenesis by attacking crucial cellular processes. Hence, when the oncogene of Rous sarcoma virus (page 299) was deleted, the virus was still capable of replication, but its carcinogenic potential was lost. The deleted gene was found to code for an *oncogenic protein* (molecular weight 60 000) that could transform normal chicken cells in culture. The product of the Rous sarcoma oncogene, known as the *src* gene, has been identified as a protein kinase that catalyses the phosphorylation of specific tyrosine –OH groups in specific proteins. This is then thought to trigger cell proliferation.

However, not all retroviruses contain oncogenes, yet they may still cause tumour growth. In these cases, integration of viral genetic material into the host chromosome, which occurs more or less at random sites, will sometimes occur in the proximity of a cellular proto-oncogene, converting it into an oncogene, and resulting in tumorigenesis.

Recently active oncogenes have been identified in some human and animal tumours in which there appears to be no viral involvement. Furthermore, the DNA of such tumour cells has been found to be carcinogenic when introduced into normal cells in culture. In their normal form such genes are known as proto-oncogenes and it is abnormal forms of these genes which are found in tumours and which appear to have been the origin of the oncogenes present in the retroviruses.

Two suggestions have been made as to the means by which oncogenes may induce tumorigenesis.

1. Malignancy results from overexpression of a normal control gene. An amplification of a proto-oncogene, or an increase in its expression, results in an overproduction of a normal gene product associated with the control of cell division, leading to excessive cell proliferation. For example, amplification and increased expression of the *N-myc* proto-oncogene may be one factor involved in the progression of human neuroblastomas and small cell carcinoma of the lung to advanced malignancy.

2. In other instances it is thought that translocation of segments of DNA in the proximity of a normal cellular proto-oncogene may cause an alteration in its expression, converting it into an oncogene. Many tumours contain chromosomal translocations and in some cases proto-oncogenes have been identified at, or close to, the breakpoints. For example, the trans-locations associated with *Burkitt's lymphoma* and *chronic myelogenous leukaemia* both affect a known proto-oncogene. Although there is no direct evidence to implicate such translocations with the cancerous state, it is easy to envisage how such translocations might affect the expression of the proto-oncogene or its protein product, thereby resulting in tumorigenesis.

About 20 different oncogenes have been identified, each causing a different type of neoplasia. The proteins coded for by different oncogenes and proto-oncogenes are very diverse in their properties, with sites of action which include the nucleus, the cytoplasm and the plasma membrane. Some act by phosphorylating proteins or phosphoinositides. As with the *src* gene, the product may itself be the kinase, or it may be some other factor involved in phosphorylation, e.g. the subunit of *platelet-derived growth factor* (page 366) which is coded by the *sis* oncogene. Several oncogene products represent abnormal growth factor receptors. Yet other oncogene and proto-oncogene products may act by regulating adenylate cyclase, transcription or DNA replication.

Section 5

Control processes

Chapter 23
The integration and control of metabolism

The main pathways of carbohydrate, fat and protein metabolism, that is of the major sources of energy, were described earlier in terms of the enzymes responsible for them. However, the bodies of vertebrates contain about a hundred different types of cell each with a distinctive enzyme pattern. Some of the differences involve tissue-specific enzymes but many are differences in the amounts and sensitivity of particular enzymes within the metabolic pathways. Not every tissue can burn all types of fuel (glucose, fatty acids, ketone bodies, amino acids and lactate). Tissues which depend on glucose as a major energy source include red and white blood corpuscles, brain, retina, renal medulla, intestinal mucosa, and skeletal muscle in severe exercise. Liver, kidney cortex, heart muscle and skeletal muscle, except in severe exercise, can obtain most of their energy from the oxidation of fatty acids, while the brain and renal cortex, as well as both heart and skeletal muscle, can utilize ketone bodies. Not only are there fundamental differences of this sort in the metabolism of different tissues but, furthermore, the pathways which predominate in the various tissues can alter significantly in response to external factors such as dietary variation. The necessary control and integration of energy and other types of metabolism within and between the tissues is brought about by the action of hormones which, in conjunction with the nervous system, ensure that the cells of the body exist in a controlled environment of more or less constant composition.

The major pathways of carbohydrate and lipid metabolism and the enzymes that are mainly responsible for their control are as follows:

1. Glycolysis – *phosphofructokinase*
2. Glycogenolysis – *phosphorylase*
3. Conversion of pyruvate to acetyl-CoA – *pyruvate dehydrogenase*
4. Lipolysis – *adipose tissue lipase*
5. Citrate cycle – *citrate synthase*
6. Glycogenesis – *glycogen synthase*
7. Gluconeogenesis – *pyruvate carboxylase*
8. Fatty acid synthesis – *acetyl-CoA carboxylase*

The metabolic characteristics of some individual tissues

The liver

The liver is generally recognized as the organ which serves the metabolic needs of the body as a whole, and specialized as well as general metabolic pathways are found within it. The liver derives most of its blood supply from the portal vein which drains the intestinal tract, and materials absorbed from the intestine must pass through the liver before entering the general circulation. Consequently the liver is exposed to widely varying concentrations of incoming metabolites as well as to certain potentially toxic substances so that it requires considerable metabolic versatility. The liver contains the enzymes necessary for the pathways of glycogen synthesis and breakdown and for glycolysis and gluconeogenesis. In particular, it contains the enzyme glucose 6-phosphatase which converts glucose 6-phosphate obtained from glyco-genolysis or gluconeogenesis into glucose which can then be released into the plasma.

Unlike most other tissues the liver contains two enzymes, *hexokinase* and *glucokinase*, which catalyse the phosphorylation of glucose:

$$\text{Glucose} + \text{ATP} \rightarrow \text{glucose 6-phosphate} + \text{ADP}$$

Liver hexokinase is similar to the hexokinases in other tissues and has a low K_m for glucose (0·01–0·1 mM) but glucokinase which catalyses the same reaction has a much higher K_m for glucose ($\simeq 10$ mM). The concentration of glucose in the blood is normally of the order of 3–7 mM, and glucose equilibrates rapidly across the liver cell membrane. Hexokinase is there-fore normally operating at its maximum rate which is relatively low in liver. The presence of glucokinase with its high K_m allows the liver cell to respond to an increased concentration of blood glucose by increasing the rate of glucose phosphorylation (Figure 23.1) and hence of overall glucose metabolism.

The liver also contains pathways for both the synthesis and the oxidation of fatty acids as well as the urea cycle enzymes and many enzymes involved in amino acid catabolism and amino acid synthesis. Other important overall reactions catalysed by the liver are the formation of ketone bodies, cholesterol and bile acid synthesis, the synthesis and breakdown of triglycerides,

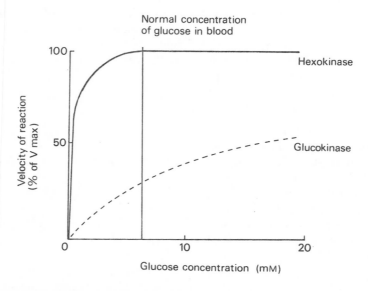

Figure 23.1 Substrate concentration curves for hexokinase and glucokinase

phospholipid synthesis and the detoxification of foreign compounds such as drugs. It is clear that control mechanisms must exist to prevent the simultaneous operation of the many opposing pathways such as glycogen synthesis and glycogenolysis which would lead to the futile cycling of metabolites and net loss of cell ATP.

Adipose tissue

Adipose tissue is required to store fuel in the form of triglycerides in times of plenty and to release fatty acids and glycerol into the blood for use by other tissues when glucose is in short supply. Thus the major metabolic pathways in this tissue are those for lipogenesis and lipolysis. Adipose tissue takes up glucose readily and contains an active glycolytic pathway, which generates both acetyl units for fatty acid synthesis and dihydroxyacetone phosphate for production of the glycerophosphate needed for triglyceride synthesis. The enzymes pyruvate dehydrogenase, ATP citrate lyase, acetyl-CoA carboxylase and fatty acid synthase are present with relatively high activity, as are the enzymes of the pentose phosphate pathway which is responsible for the generation of some of the NADPH required for fatty acid synthesis. It also contains an adrenaline-sensitive lipase which releases fatty acids and glycerol into the blood when extra energy is required. Adipose tissue does not catalyse gluconeogenesis or the metabolism of glycogen to any extent and the pathways of amino acid metabolism and fatty acid oxidation are of little quantitative significance in this tissue. Since adipose tissue is capable of both the synthesis and the breakdown of triglycerides, the key enzymes in these pathways are subjected to coordinated metabolic control so that both pathways are not active simultaneously.

Muscle

Skeletal muscles are specialized for the production of large quantities of ATP and the conversion of its chemical energy into mechanical energy for the contraction process. They are required to vary their activity, and hence their energy production, to a far greater degree than any other tissue. When resting they must prepare themselves for bursts of intense activity during which, in spite of a tremendous increase in blood supply, there may be a shortage of oxygen which necessitates anaerobic functioning for limited periods.

A particular feature of muscle is the presence of *phosphocreatine* which acts as a second source of readily available high-energy phosphate. Creatine is a substituted guanidine compound, methylguanidine acetic acid, which is synthesized in the body from glycine, arginine and methionine.

$$\text{From arginine} \quad
\begin{array}{l}
\quad\quad NH_2 \\
HN=C \\
\quad\quad N\cdot CH_2\cdot COOH \quad \text{From glycine} \\
\quad\quad CH_3
\end{array}$$

From methionine

Creatine is readily phosphorylated by ATP in a reversible reaction catalysed by *creatine kinase*. The standard free energy of hydrolysis of phosphocreatine is $-43\,kJ$ ($-10\cdot3$ kcal) so the equilibrium favours ATP formation.

In resting muscle phosphocreatine is present at at least five times the molar concentration of total adenine nucleotides and during contraction the creatine kinase reaction helps to maintain the intracellular concentration of ATP.

$$\begin{array}{c} NH_2 \\ | \\ HN{=}C \\ \backslash \\ N{\cdot}CH_2{\cdot}COOH \\ | \\ CH_3 \end{array} \quad + \quad ATP \quad \underset{\substack{Creatine \\ kinase}}{\rightleftharpoons} \quad \begin{array}{c} NH{\sim}\textcircled{P} \\ | \\ HN{=}C \\ \backslash \\ N{\cdot}CH_2{\cdot}COOH \\ | \\ CH_3 \end{array} \quad + \quad ADP$$

Creatine   Phosphocreatine

A further feature of muscles is the presence of appreciable amounts of *myoglobin* which acts as an auxiliary source of oxygen (page 373). The muscles of diving mammals such as seals, whales and dolphins and the flight muscles of birds owe their deep red colour to myoglobin, which in Man is present in significant amounts only in heart muscle.

Heart muscle, like skeletal muscle, is essentially an energy expender and is required to adapt itself to a tremendously varied work load. The oxygen supply of heart muscle, unlike that of skeletal muscle, is nearly always adequate since, when during contraction the blood supply is cut down, oxygen can be obtained from the store held by the myoglobin.

Skeletal muscle takes up glucose from the circulation and stores it in the form of glycogen. Under resting conditions, muscle uses fatty acids or ketone bodies rather than glucose as a energy source. During contraction, stored glycogen is broken down. Muscle cells do not contain glucose 6-phosphatase, and the glucose 6-phosphate formed is metabolized internally to pyruvate, and oxidized via the citrate cycle. If pyruvate is produced more rapidly than it can be oxidized it is converted to lactate which is released into the bloodstream.

Protein breakdown and amino acid metabolism are also of importance in muscle, and the major nitrogen-containing products are glutamine and alanine, which are released by the tissue. The pathways of gluconeogenesis and fatty acid synthesis do not exist in muscle. Heart muscle differs from skeletal muscle in that at high work loads it can use the lactate released by skeletal muscle as an energy source. Pyruvate produced by glycolysis in the heart is not converted to lactate. Heart lactate dehydrogenase is inhibited by high concentrations of pyruvate while lactate dehydrogenase from skeletal muscle is not (page 230).

The brain

The brain is very active and has a high rate of energy utilization at all times. Although it accounts for only about 1·4% of the total body weight it accounts for nearly 25% of the basal energy expenditure. Thus it uses about 120 g of glucose (= 2000 kJ) per day. It has not been found possible to demonstrate any significant increase in the overall energy consumption of subjects performing tasks requiring intense mental concentration.

Under normal conditions glucose is the only source of energy that is used by the brain which, as a result, is extremely sensitive to alterations in the blood glucose concentration. This is clearly demonstrated by the convulsions which occur in hypoglycaemia and the coma which results from prolonged hyperglycaemia. When the blood sugar is maintained within the normal range, the properties of hexokinase described earlier will ensure that the glucose 6-phosphate will be kept sufficiently high to provide the necessary energy. But when, as a result of prolonged starvation, glucose is in short supply and the only source is gluconeogenesis, the brain develops the ability to oxidize ketone bodies which circulate in appreciable amounts during starvation conditions. Studies on obese subjects undergoing 5–6 weeks of therapeutic starvation showed that the utilization of glucose by the brain was reduced to about 24 g day^{-1} and that nearly 40 g of ketone bodies were oxidized.

Another notable feature of brain metabolism is the high rate of turnover of its proteins. A steady supply of amino acids is therefore essential even if it has to be at the expense of other tissues. These amino acids cannot replace glucose as substrates for energy production even though glutamate and glutamine are present in high concentration and are actively metabolized. Glutamate serves not only as a precursor of *γ-aminobutyrate* (GABA), which plays a role in the regulation of neuronal activity, but also as a 'scavenger' for ammonia which is highly toxic and acts as a convulsive agent.

From this we may conclude that the most active of the common metabolic pathways in the brain are glycolysis, the citrate cycle and protein synthesis and breakdown.

The kidney

The main function of the kidney is to regulate the composition of the body fluids and a pathway of particular importance in this respect is the conversion of glutamine to ammonia and glucose. This conversion is involved in acid/base homeostasis (page 395), and is greatly stimulated in metabolic acidosis. The kidney uses fatty acids as a major energy source and much of the ATP produced from their oxidation is utilized in the active transport of metabolites. The kidney is the only tissue other than the liver which is capable of gluconeogenesis, and, under certain conditions, kidney gluconeogenesis can make a significant contribution to the overall glucose requirements.

From what has been said it is apparent that it is the different enzyme patterns which arise from the tissue-specific expression of genes that mainly account for the varying metabolic capabilities of different tissue. Thus, for example, the enzymes fructose 1,6-bisphosphatase and glucose 6-phosphatase occur only in liver and kidney and these are the only tissues capable of gluconeogenesis. Similarly, carbamoyl phosphate synthase, which is involved in the synthesis of urea and is ammonia dependent, occurs in the mitochondria of liver but not of other tissues. At the same time, the enzymic profile of tissues can vary to some extent in response to external factors such as diet.

The adjustment of tissue metabolism to different physiological states

The metabolic pathways which predominate in various tissues may vary according to the conditions prevailing at the time, notably with respect to (a) substrate availability, i.e. nutritional state and (b) substrate utilization, i.e. muscular activity and, in the longer term, with growth and ageing processes.

Absorptive state

During the period immediately after eating a meal, synthetic and storage processes predominate. Under these conditions, the major pathways operating in the liver are the synthesis of glycogen and fatty acids from glucose and the conversion of the fatty acids into triglycerides (Figure 23.2). The amino acids which are not needed for protein and other synthetic processes cannot be stored and are catabolized. The nitrogen atoms derived from the amino groups are excreted as urea whereas the carbon skeletons are mostly oxidized.

In adipose tissue as in liver, glucose is taken up from the plasma and used as a substrate for the synthesis of fatty acids and triglycerides. Muscle takes up plasma glucose and stores it as glycogen, while the brain uses glucose as its major energy source.

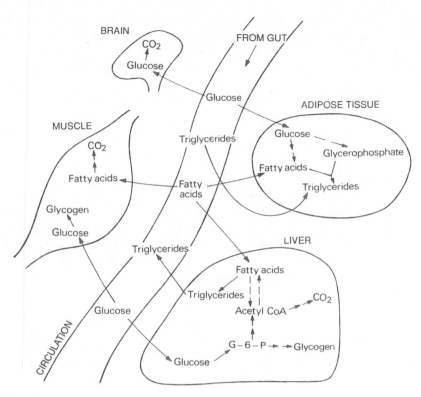

Figure 23.2 Summary of metabolism in the absorptive state

Starvation

The average well-nourished human body contains energy stores which amount to the equivalent of about 7500 kJ (1800 kcal) in the form of glycogen and glucose, 82 000 kJ (19600 kcal) of usable protein and 470 000 kJ (112 000 kcal) of triglyceride. In starvation, the liver glycogen reserves are rapidly depleted and fat and ketone bodies derived from the oxidation of fatty acids are then used as a major source of energy. Eventually, protein breakdown contributes significantly to the requirement for energy and for glucose and the body becomes severely wasted.

In starvation, the metabolic pathways which predominate in the various tissues are different from those which are important immediately after a meal (Figure 23.3). In the liver, glycogen is broken down to glucose 6-phosphate which is then hydrolysed to glucose and released into the blood for use by other tissues. But, in Man, the liver glycogen is exhausted within 48 hours, after which fatty acid oxidation is increased. This results in the extensive formation in the liver of ketone bodies which are released into the plasma. Glucose, which is essential for the brain and certain other tissues, is synthesized from (1) any available lactate, (2) glycerol derived from the breakdown of triglycerides and (3) glucogenic amino acids.

In adipose tissue glucose uptake is diminished and triglyceride breakdown is increased. The fatty acids produced are exported via the plasma and are oxidized by other tissues, while the glycerol is used for gluconeogenesis in the liver. Muscle oxidizes mainly fatty acids and ketone bodies while the brain adapts to use ketone bodies rather than glucose as a major energy source. This ability of the brain to use ketone bodies reduces the requirement for amino acids as a source of glucose, and is a factor of importance in the conservation of body protein.

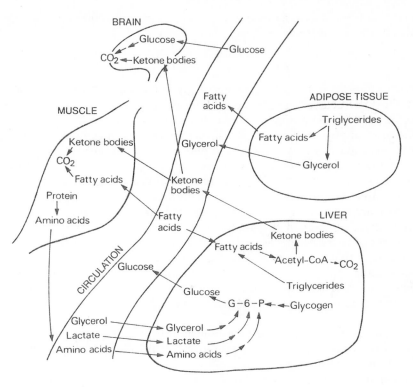

Figure 23.3 Summary of metabolism during starvation

Even though ketone bodies can be used by various extrahepatic tissues, during starvation the liver may produce them in such large quantities that the metabolic capacity of these tissues is exceeded. If this is so, ketone bodies accumulate in the blood with consequent ketosis and metabolic acidosis.

A general feature of starvation is the conservation of glucose and the preferential oxidation of fat. It should be remembered, however, that some cells, e.g. red blood cells have an obligatory requirement for glucose and that there is no pathway for the conversion of fatty acids to glucose in mammals.

High-carbohydrate low-protein diet

In this situation, the liver converts excess glucose to fat, and the pathways of gluconeogenesis and glycogenolysis are depressed. A particular feature of this dietary state is *protein sparing* i.e. the conservation of body nitrogen. Amino acids from protein catabolism are required neither as an energy nor a glucose source and, since they are not available in excess, amino acid breakdown and urea synthesis are greatly reduced. However, if the body's minimum requirement for protein (page 126) is not fulfilled, tissue breakdown will occur and *kwashiorkor* (page 128) may result.

Physical activity

A sudden increase in the activity of skeletal muscles causes a rapid breakdown of ATP and also of phosphocreatine which acts as a reserve supply of energy. An additional source of ATP is the *myokinase reaction* which is freely reversible:

$$2ADP \xrightleftharpoons[]{\text{Myokinase}} ATP + AMP$$

The breakdown of ATP initiates a flare-up of glycolytic activity mainly as a result of the activation of phosphofructosekinase (page 226) for which the AMP produced in the myokinase reaction may be partly responsible. The breakdown and use of muscle glycogen as a source of energy at the onset of physical activity has the advantage that it can occur anaerobically and, moreover, for every glucose unit converted to pyruvate and subsequently to lactate, there is a net synthesis of three molecules of ATP whereas only two molecules would be formed from the breakdown of glucose as such (page 231). There is, however, a price to pay for the provision of extra ATP at the time it is most urgently required because, when glycogen is resynthesized, two molecules of ATP are needed for every glucose unit stored. This resynthesis will, however, only take place when there is plenty of energy available.

Further supplies of energy are provided by the breakdown of liver glycogen to replenish the blood glucose and by the hydrolysis of triglycerides to fatty acids and glycerol in both liver and adipose tissue. In this way there is a general mobilization of the body's energy reserves.

These changes are reversed after exercise when lactate is converted to glucose by the liver, triglycerides are resynthesized and muscle glycogen is replenished from plasma glucose.

The above outline of tissue-specific metabolism illustrates the necessity for the activity of metabolic pathways within any tissue to be rigorously controlled and for the metabolism of the various tissues to be integrated. The biochemical mechanisms by which control of metabolism is achieved in mammalian organisms will nwow be considered.

The regulation of metabolic pathways

The flux through a metabolic pathway is, generally speaking, subject to two types of control.

Long-term control

Long-term control occurs over hours, days or even longer and is brought about by a *change in the amount* of a particular enzyme or enzymes in a tissue.

The amount of an enzyme present in a cell at any given time depends on the balance between the rate of its synthesis and breakdown. Different enzymes have very different half-lives ranging from a few minutes to several days (page 286). Those with short half-lives are inducible and repressible, i.e. their rates of synthesis and/or breakdown, and hence the level in the cell, are readily altered in response to environmental factors. Some enzymes are very sensitive to the nutritional state. Thus, many of those concerned with amino acid breakdown are affected by the supply of amino acids as well as by hormonal factors. The changes are particularly large in the case of the aminotransferases that are responsible for the deamination of the essential amino acids. These enzymes virtually disappear when the protein intake is very low so that the essential amino acids are effectively conserved. The enzymes of the urea cycle are also significantly reduced.

The means by which alterations in enzyme levels are brought about are not well understood but it appears that hormones act by altering the rate of enzyme synthesis rather than of enzyme breakdown. This is accomplished by the specific induction or repression of enzymes. This type of regulation is considered in Chapter 24. It is particularly important in metabolic adaptation to long-term factors such as variation of diet, growth and ageing.

Short-term control

This refers to *changes in activity* of metabolic pathways which occur over periods of minutes rather than hours. Such changes are brought about by influencing the activity of certain key enzymes present in the tissue without affecting the overall amount of these enzymes present. This can occur (a) directly by a change in the intracellular concentration of an activator or inhibitor of the enzyme or (b) indirectly via a hormonal signal originating from another tissue. Hormonal control is superimposed on control mechanisms initiated within the cell. Short-term control is important in metabolic homoeostasis and in adaptation to short-term factors such as fasting or physical stress.

Control of the flux through a metabolic pathway

In any metabolic pathway there are one or two enzymes whose activity is particularly important from the point of view of regulation. Consider a general unbranched pathway represented as follows:

$$A \rightleftharpoons \underset{\text{I}}{B} \rightleftharpoons \underset{\text{II}}{C} \rightleftharpoons \underset{\text{III}}{D} \rightleftharpoons \underset{\text{IV}}{E}$$

Here, the tissue is able to convert the primary substrate A to the eventual product E. B, C and D are intermediates which do not accumulate and the pathway consists of four consecutive enzyme reactions represented by I–IV. The flux through the pathway is the rate of disappearance of A or the rate of appearance of E; in the steady state these will be equal. For each individual enzyme step, the net flux in the forward direction is the difference between the rates of the forward and back reactions for that step.

For many enzymes which have relatively high activity, the net flux through the enzyme will be much less than the rates of the forward and back reactions, i.e. the enzyme will maintain its substrates and products at concentrations near to those determined by the equilibrium constant of the enzyme. However, for every pathway, there will be one or more enzyme steps where net flux through the pathway is nearly equal to the rate of the forward reaction catalysed by the enzyme. In this case, the rate of the back reaction is negligible, the enzyme is working at its maximum capacity and can be regarded as *rate-limiting* for the pathway concerned. Such enzymes are often said to catalyse 'effectively irreversible' reactions.

From the above considerations, it follows that regulation of a metabolic pathway as a whole is achieved by modifying the activity of its rate-limiting enzyme. An increase in the activity of an enzyme which is already active enough to maintain the tissue concentrations of its substrates and products near equilibrium cannot affect the net flux through the pathway.

The identification of rate-limiting reactions

Rate-limiting steps in metabolic pathways can be identified using a combination of approaches.

(i) The kinetic constants of the various enzymes can be determined in cell homogenates or after partial purification. Enzymes with a relatively high V_{max} are unlikely to be regulatory, and potential rate-limiting enzymes generally have V_{max} *values much lower* than those of other enzymes in the particular pathway. This criterion can give no more than a general indication because of the difficulties of relating the behaviour of enzymes as assayed *in vitro* to their likely behaviour under the conditions operating in the intact cell.

(ii) The intracellular concentrations of intermediates in the pathway can be measured, and for each enzyme *the mass action ratio* can be calculated. Where the mass action ratio for a particular enzyme reaction approaches the equilibrium constant of the enzyme, then that reaction cannot be rate-limiting. For potential rate-limiting reactions, the mass action ratio will be much lower than the equilibrium constant. A major problem here is the determination of the concentration of metabolites in different subcellular compartments such as the mitochondrial matrix.

(iii) The *'cross-over' theorem* can be used. In the pathway depicted above, suppose that enzyme II catalysing the interconversion of B to C is rate-limiting. When the pathway is stimulated, e.g. by the addition of a hormone to the tissue, this stimulation must be attributed to an increase in the activity of enzyme II. As a result of this increase in activity, the steady-state level of B will fall while that of the immediate product, C, will increase. In such an experiment as that shown in Figure 23.4, the decrease in B and increase in C during an increase in flux in the pathway identifies enzyme II as the rate-limiting step. In practice, a decrease in the intracellular concentration of a substrate of a particular enzyme accompanied by an increase in flux through that enzyme is sufficient to identify a rate-limiting reaction.

(iv) In some cases, a specific inhibitor of a particular enzyme may be available. The metabolic pathway concerned is then *titrated with the inhibitor*. If the enzyme is rate-limiting, the concentration of inhibitor which inhibits the enzyme to a particular extent must inhibit the overall pathway to the same extent. If, for example, the activity can be reduced by 50% by a certain concentration of inhibitor but the overall pathway is not inhibited at all at this concentration, it follows that the enzyme cannot be rate-limiting.

Having identified a potential rate-limiting enzyme, the effect of various activators and inhibitors can be studied *in vitro*. The intracellular concentrations of such activators and inhibitors must then be determined in the intact tissue or in isolated cells and shown to increase or decrease in the appropriate concentration range when the pathway is stimulated or inhibited.

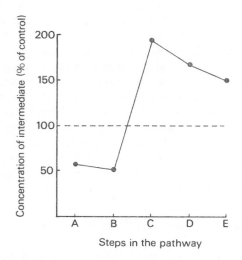

Figure 23.4 Diagrammatic representation of a cross-over plot. The pathway A → E is assumed to be stimulated by a hormone or some other external factor. This stimulation is accompanied by a fall in the concentration of A and B and a rise in the concentrations of the subsequent intermediates, indicating that the enzyme catalysing the reaction B → C is rate-limiting for this pathway.

The importance of this approach is illustrated by the finding that, in several cases, the activation or inhibition of various enzymes by metabolic intermediates observed *in vitro* has been shown to have no importance in the regulation of a metabolic pathway *in vivo*. This may be because these particular activators or inhibitors do not occur at a high enough concentration in the cell, or because their concentrations do not change appropriately when the pathway is stimulated. Alternatively, enzymes which appear to be highly regulated from studies *in vitro* may turn out not to be rate-limiting for the metabolic pathways in which they participate. A notable example is the enzyme glutamate dehydrogenase in liver which is involved in the deamination of amino acids (page 281). This enzyme is inhibited *in vitro* by ATP and GTP and is activated by ADP. However, it is now recognized that the enzyme is active enough to catalyse a near-equilibrium reaction in the hepatocyte and is thus not a rate-limiting enzyme; the control by purine nucleotides observed *in vitro* is therefore not of physiological significance.

The rate-limiting step occurs early in the reaction sequence. If this were not so, there would be a tendency for products occurring earlier in the sequence to accumulate; this would not only be wasteful but might lead to undesirable side reactions. Where a pathway is branched, the rate-limiting reaction usually occurs soon after the branch point at the first committed step, i.e. the first reaction to have no other function than the production of the end product which exerts the *feedback control*.

$$A \xrightarrow{} B \xrightarrow{} C \rightarrow D \rightarrow E \rightarrow F$$
$$W \rightarrow X \rightarrow Y \rightarrow Z$$

The above concept of a single rate-limiting enzyme for any particular pathway, while useful, is in fact an oversimplification. More than one enzyme may contribute to the control of a metabolic pathway and the contribution made by any enzyme can, in principle, be quantified.

Factors affecting the activity of regulatory enzymes in metabolic pathways

Substrate concentration

The activity of an enzyme within a cell depends on a number of factors including the concentration of available substrate. However, in the case of mammalian cells, the composition of the extracellular fluid is kept more or less constant and it is not usual for metabolic pathways to be regulated simply by changes in the concentration of the primary substrate.

This does, however, happen with respect to the non-essential amino acids. When they are taken into the body in excess of the immediate requirements, they cannot be stored and there is a significant rise in their concentration in both the plasma and the tissues. This rise causes an automatic increase in their rate of breakdown because the K_m values of the *aminotransferases* which initiate their degradation are much higher than the concentration of the amino acids in the tissues. Consequently, the rate of breakdown is more or less directly related to their concentration.

Activating ions

As will be discussed in the next chapter control may sometimes be exerted by changes in the concentration of ions resulting from the action of hormones.

Energy charge

This has been discussed in Chapter 16.

Most commonly the activity of key enzymes in the cell is controlled by allosteric regulators or covalent modification, which are discussed below.

Allosteric activation and inhibition

Many regulatory enzymes are allosterically controlled by a product or products of the reaction sequence; that is to say they are subject to *feedback control*. The binding of an effector to the enzyme causes a conformational change which is transmitted to the active site and causes either an increase or a decrease in activity over a range of substrate concentrations. Frequently, in the absence of an activator or in the presence of an inhibitor, the enzyme exhibits sigmoidal kinetics with respect to substrate concentration. Addition of the activator or removal of the inhibitor restores normal saturation kinetics.

Reactions of this type show limited sensitivity to changes in the concentrations of their substrates and it is often found that the flow of material through the reaction increases despite a decrease in substrate concentration and vice versa. This results from the effect of allosteric regulators in altering the affinity of the enzyme for its substrate and sometimes also the maximum velocity of the reaction.

Certain allosteric effectors have reciprocal effects on enzymes that catalyse directly opposite reactions. For example, AMP activates phosphofructokinase and hence promotes glycolysis and the formation of ATP, while at the same time it inhibits liver fructose 1,6-bisphosphatase, thereby suppressing gluconeogenesis and this form of ATP expenditure. This is one means by which futile cycling may be prevented.

Phosphofructokinase (PFK)

Muscle phosphofructokinase is a classical example of an allosteric enzyme. It catalyses the rate-limiting step for glycolysis and is allosterically controlled by ATP and certain other ligands including AMP. Although small amounts of ATP are essential for the phosphofructokinase reaction (page 226), at high concentrations ATP binds to a special inhibitory site and changes the shape of the substrate concentration curve from hyperbolic to sigmoidal (Figure 23.5). As a

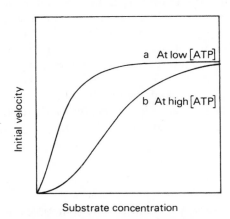

Figure 23.5 The effect of (a) low and (b) high concentrations of ATP on phosphofructokinase

result large changes in activity occur within the limited range of concentrations of fructose 6-phosphate present in muscle. The inhibitory effect of ATP is enhanced by a build-up of citrate which, like that of ATP, signals that plenty of energy is available and that it is not necessary to break down any more glucose. In resting muscles which are oxidizing fatty acids the levels of ATP and of citrate are inhibitory to phosphofructokinase so that glycolysis is reduced and glucose is conserved. Conversely phosphofructokinase is activated by ADP and AMP which serve to indicate that more energy is required. The changes in intracellular ATP and AMP concentrations that occur in anoxia are sufficient to account for the activation of phosphofructokinase and increased rate of glycolysis observed in such conditions. An even more potent allosteric activator of phosphofructokinase has recently been discovered. This is *fructose 2,6-bisphosphate* which also acts as an allosteric inhibitor of fructose 1,6-bisphosphatase the enzyme responsible for directing fructose 1,6-bisphosphate towards glycogenesis. Thus high concentrations of this metabolite inhibit glycogenesis at the same time as they promote glycolysis.

Acetyl-CoA carboxylase

This is an allosteric enzyme which catalyses the primary regulating step in the synthesis of fatty acids (page 256). It can exist in monomeric and polymeric forms, the latter being more active. Citrate activates the enzyme probably by favouring the polymeric configuration. Thus, citrate serves not only to transfer acetyl groups from the mitochondria to the cytoplasm (page 255) but also to activate the initial enzyme on the path of fatty acid biosynthesis which uses the acetyl groups. Acetyl-CoA carboxylase is also regulated through covalent modification (page 344).

2-Oxoglutarate dehydrogenase

This is another important enzyme which, as explained earlier (page 242), has been found to be activated by very low concentrations of Ca^{2+} ions. This activation may play a significant part in the regulation of metabolism in heart and liver by certain hormones.

Regulation of metabolic pathways by changes in the concentration of allosteric activators and inhibitors of regulatory enzymes is an example of short-term control. This sort of regulation is important in the minute-to-minute regulation of tissue function and is involved in the action of certain hormones.

Phosphorylation/dephosphorylation reactions

A considerable number of regulatory enzymes have been shown to undergo phosphorylation by the following type of reaction:

$$\text{Enzyme + ATP} \rightarrow \text{Enzyme-P + ADP}$$

such reactions are catalysed by enzymes known as *protein kinases* some of which are dependent on cyclic AMP and under hormonal control and have a wide substrate specificity. The phosphate group is usually incorporated into a specific serine residue or residues in the protein substrate. Phosphorylation reactions of this type proceed with a large negative standard free energy change and are effectively irreversible. The protein kinase of liver catalyses the incorporation of phosphate from ATP into a number of enzymes with consequential changes in their activity. The protein kinase comprises two pairs of subunits namely two identical catalytic subunits and two

Table 23.1 Some enzymes regulated by covalent modification

Enzyme	Process promoted	Energy relationship	Effect of phosphorylation on activity
Phosphorylase	Glycogen breakdown	Release	Increases
Phosphorylase *b* kinase	Glycogen breakdown	Release	Increases
Triglyceride lipase	Triglyceride breakdown	Release	Increases
Glycogen synthase	Glycogen synthesis	Storage	Decreases
Pyruvate dehydrogenase	Fatty acid synthesis	Storage –conversion of carbohydrate to fat	Decreases
Acetyl-CoA carboxylase	Fatty acid synthesis	Storage	Decreases
Liver pyruvate kinase	Gluconeogenesis		Decreases

identical regulatory subunits. In the absence of cAMP the complex is inactive but when cAMP is present, it binds to the regulatory subunits and causes the complex to dissociate. The catalytic subunits are released from restraint and are then free to act.

The phosphate group which has been added to a protein in this way can be removed by *protein phosphatases* which are present in the cell and which, like the protein kinase, may have wide specificity. Here again the action of the enzymes is effectively irreversible. Phosphorylation of an enzyme in some cases leads to an activation and in other cases to an inhibition. Table 23.1 lists some of the enzymes which are known to be phosphorylated *in vivo*. In general enzymes involved in catalytic pathways are activated by phosphorylation while those involved in synthetic pathways are inhibited. The proportion of an enzyme which, at any one time, is in the phosphorylated form, is dependent on the relative activities of the appropriate kinase and phosphatase. An increase in the activity of the kinase will increase the steady-state phosphorylation of the enzyme and an increase in the activity of the phosphatase will have the opposite effect.

Enzymes that undergo such phosphorylation/dephosphorylation reactions play an important role in the regulation of both carbohydrate and lipid metabolism. Those involved in carbohydrate metabolism include the following.

Pyruvate dehydrogenase (PDH)

This enzyme complex (page 232) which is responsible for the reactions by which pyruvate is irreversibly converted into acetyl-CoA is subject to end product inhibition by raised concentrations of acetyl-CoA and NADH. It is, in addition, subject to phosphorylation/ dephosphorylation.

The PDH complex possesses an intrinsic kinase which is not dependent on cAMP and can catalyse the phosphorylation of up to three unique serine residues on certain of its subunits. The phosphorylation of one particular serine residue inactivates the enzyme. The role of the other two serines that are phosphorylated by the kinase is not clear. The phosphorylated form has a V_{max} of less than 1% of the non-phosphorylated form.

The complexity of the control of PDH activity is increased by the fact that the kinase responsible for the phosphorylation of pyruvate dehydrogenase is itself affected by the NADH/

NAD^+, acetyl-CoA/CoA and ATP/ADP ratios all of which are indicative of the overall energy state. Furthermore the phosphatase responsible for dephosphorylation, and hence for activation of the PDH complex, is stimulated by Mg^{2+} and Ca^{2+} ions. As mentioned in the next Chapter, insulin is thought to stimulate PDH activity by increasing the activity of the phosphatase relative to the kinase so that there is a net dephosphorylation of the complex.

Phosphorylase

The initial reaction of glycogen breakdown, by which terminal glucosyl residues are removed in the form of glucose 1-phosphate is finely controlled. The enzyme phosphorylase, which is responsible for the breakdown, exists in two forms, phosphorylase *a* which is active and phosphorylase *b* which is relatively inactive. Inactive phosphorylase *b* is converted into active phosphorylase *a* by phosphorylation. The enzyme responsible for the conversion is *phosphorylase b kinase* whose full activity is only manifest when Ca^{2+} ions are present (Figure 23.6) and it has itself been phosphorylated by cAMP-dependent protein kinase (page 341).

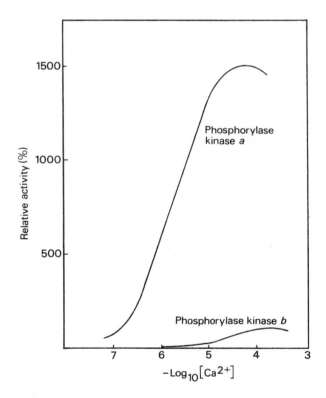

Figure 23.6 Dependence of phosphorylase kinase activity on calcium ions. (After P. Cohen (1983) *Control of Enzyme Activity*, Chapman and Hall, London)

As with PDH, specific serine residues in the phosphorylase are phosphorylated to cause the change in activity. When the need for glycogen breakdown is over a *phosphoprotein phosphatase* causes the dephosphorylation of phosphorylase *a*. The activity of this phosphatase is also under complex control.

Glycogen synthase

This is the enzyme which is responsible for adding glucosyl units to a pre-existing glycogen primer (page 236) and consequently for promoting the storage of glucose when it is freely available. Like phosphorylase it exists in both active and inactive forms which are inter-convertible by a phosphorylation/dephosphorylation process. In this case, however, it is the relatively inactive form that is phosphorylated and, as will be described later, there is a reciprocal relationship between the activities of glycogen synthase and phosphorylase. The relative inactivity of glycogen synthase *b* can be overcome by high concentrations of glucose 6-phosphate which occur when there is a large excess of glucose available for disposal.

The phosphorylation of glycogen synthase which occurs directly under the influence of cAMP-dependent protein kinase (page 341) is more complex than that of phosphorylase as five separate phosphorylation sites, some containing more than one phosphoserine residue, have been demonstrated on the glycogen synthase molecule. Thus a number of hormones acting independently through a variety of different phosphorylation/dephosphorylation reactions may regulate the activity of glycogen synthase in a very subtle manner.

Acetyl-CoA carboxylase

Acetyl-CoA carboxylase promotes the first committed step in fatty acid synthesis, namely the conversion of acetyl-CoA to malonyl-CoA (page 256). Not only is it regulated allosterically as already described but it is also regulated by phosphorylation/dephosphorylation reactions. Specific sites have been shown to be phosphorylated by cAMP-dependent protein kinase and these phosphorylations inactivate the enzyme. Another site which is phosphorylated in response to insulin stimulation of the cell appears to increase the activity of the enzyme and thereby to stimulate fatty acid synthesis.

Chapter 24
Hormones and growth factors

Cells are highly sensitive to a variety of chemical signals and the overall activities of tissues in different metabolic states are to a large extent controlled by hormones. Hormones are involved in both short- and long-term control.

Hormones may be defined as substances that are produced in very small amounts and are carried in the blood from the site of their production to a specific target tissue or tissues where they bring about a response that is appropriate to the functioning of the body as a whole. Hormones are essential for normal development and activity and most of them are produced continuously at a slow rate. Under certain conditions, however, much larger amounts are released and the factors that trigger their release are more or less specific for each endocrine gland.

The effects of hormones are individual and striking. Hormones produced by specialized cells but not by clearly defined endocrine glands include gastrin, secretin, pancreozymin and enterogastrone, which are produced in the alimentary canal, and renin and erythropoietin, which are produced by the kidney.

Several other substances which have hormone-like activity are widely distributed and exert their effects in the area in which they are produced. Histamine, serotonin and various plasma kinins may be considered to be *local hormones*.

The nature of hormones

Chemically speaking there are three types of hormone, steroids, amino acid derivatives and polypeptides. The steroid hormones include the adrenal cortical hormones and the sex hormones. The amino acid derivatives are adrenaline, noradrenaline and thyroxine which are all derived from tyrosine. The remainder, which constitute the largest group, are oligo- and poly-peptides with chain lengths varying from three amino acid residues in thyrotropin-releasing hormone to nearly 200 residues in growth hormone and prolactin. Sometimes a hormone has completely different effects in different species. For example prolactin, which stimulates the development of the mammary glands in pregnant mammals, acts as a general growth stimulant in amphibians and reptiles, and plays a part in the regulation of salt and water balance in certain fishes. On the other hand, human, pig, rabbit and beef insulins show small structurual differences but have similar activities. This is fortunate for diabetics who have been able to lead normal lives with the help of insulin derived from other species. With growth hormone the situation is different since humans only respond to growth hormone from humans or other primates. Consequently only a very few of the people who suffer from lack of growth hormone can be given replacement therapy although recombinant DNA techniques give hope for the future.

Hormone release

The factors that trigger hormonal release are many and varied, their nature depending on the hormone in question; for example, *adrenaline* and *noradrenaline* are secreted in response to stimulation of the sympathetic system. *Insulin* is secreted in response to an increase in the blood sugar level, while *glucagon* is secreted when the level falls. A dual control system also operates with respect to the regulation of the level of Ca^{2+} ions in blood. When this is lowered *parathormone* is secreted, while *calcitonin* is secreted when the level is raised. These systems both appear to operate on a simple negative feedback basis, and when the level of glucose or Ca^{2+} ions in the blood has been restored to normal, the hormone levels are also restored.

In many instances the regulation of hormone output is more complex. The *gonadotropins* and several other hormones are under the control of the anterior pituitary which secretes a whole range of peptide hormones, including *growth hormone*, *adrenocorticotropic hormone* (ACTH), *thyroid-stimulating hormone* (TSH), *follicle-stimulating hormone* (FSH) and *luteinizing hormone* (LH) which exert their effects on other endocrine glands.

Since hormones are needed in particular circumstances, means for their destruction or removal are required. This usually involves enzymic modification which either inactivates the hormone or converts it into a form suitable for excretion in the urine.

The determination of hormone concentrations by radioimmunoassay

Hormones such as insulin occur in the plasma at concentrations in the range 10^{-9}–10^{-10}M, which is a million times lower than the concentration of metabolites in cells. For measurement of the latter very sensitive spectrophotometric techniques are required while the understanding of hormone function has largely depended on the development of the *radioimmunoassay technique* for estimating peptide hormones.

In order to assay insulin by this method, a specific *insulin-binding antibody* must be produced. A sample of insulin is then radioactively labelled by incorporation of ^{125}I into some of its tyrosine residues. When the radiolabelled hormone is mixed with the antibody, a complex is formed which can be separated by centrifugation, and the radioactivity that has been bound measured. The assay is calibrated by mixing a constant amount of radiolabelled insulin with known amounts of a standard solution of unlabelled insulin, adding an exact amount of antibody and measuring the radioactivity bound. Since the antibody will bind native insulin and iodinated insulin with the same affinity, there will be competition between labelled and unlabelled insulin for the available binding sites. The more unlabelled insulin there is present, the less labelled insulin will be bound and *vice versa*. A typical calibration curve for such an assay is shown in Figure 24.1. The concentration of insulin in an unknown solution may then be measured by mixing the solution with radioactive insulin and antibody as before, measuring the radioactivity bound and reading the insulin concentration from the calibration curve.

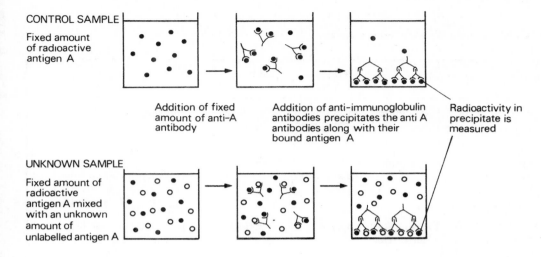

CONTROL SAMPLE

Fixed amount of radioactive antigen A

Addition of fixed amount of anti-A antibody

Addition of anti-immunoglobulin antibodies precipitates the anti A antibodies along with their bound antigen A

Radioactivity in precipitate is measured

UNKNOWN SAMPLE

Fixed amount of radioactive antigen A mixed with an unknown amount of unlabelled antigen A

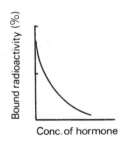

Figure 24.1 Radioimmunoassay

Similar principles may be used for the assay of many other hormones. The radioimmunoassay technique is widely used in research into the mechanism of hormone synthesis and secretion, and is also used to determine the concentration of hormones in plasma in normal and pathogenic conditions.

The mode of action of hormones

The actions of hormones are very diverse. Some, e.g. glucagon, have specific and clearly defined effects on the metabolism of particular tissues. Others such as growth hormone and the sex hormones have more general effects on growth and development while the *tropic hormones* stimulate their target tissues to secrete further hormones. For example the adrenocorticotropic hormone (ACTH), which is produced in the anterior pituitary, promotes the synthesis and release of glucocorticoids by the adrenal cortex. A list of some of the hormones and their effects on metabolism is given in Table 24.1.

Since hormones regulate pre-existing processes within the cell, before they can act they must either enter the cell themselves or they must use a messenger molecule which the hormone causes to enter or to be produced within the target cell. The ability of the target cell to respond

Table 24.1 Hormones and their effects on metabolism

Hormone	Type	Site of production	Target	Effect
Insulin	Polypeptide	β-Cells of pancreatic islets	Most tissues	Regulation of carbo-hydrate, fat and protein metabolism. Lowers blood glucose
Glucagon	Polypeptide	α-Cells of pancreatic islets	Liver	Increase in glycogenolysis. Hyperglycaemia. Increased gluconeo-genesis. Mobilization of fat
Thyroxine (T_4) Tri-iodothyronine (T_3)	Tyrosine derivatives	Thyroid	Most tissues	Increase in metabolic rate. General role in growth and development
Calcitonin	Polypeptide	Thyroid	Bones and kidney	Decrease in blood calcium concentration. Inhibition of calcium release from bones. Increased excretion of calcium and phosphorus
Parathormone	Polypeptide	Parathyroid	Bones and kidney	Elevation of blood calcium concentration. Mobiliz-ation of calcium from bones and decreased excretion by kidney
Adrenaline	Tyrosine derivative	Adrenal medulla	Most cells	Numerous vascular effects. Increased glycolysis and lipolysis. Hyperglycaemia
Cortisol Cortisone etc.	Steroids	Adrenal cortex	Most cells	Hyperglycaemia. Increased gluconeogenesis. Balancing carbohydrate, fat and protein metabolism. Anti-inflammatory effects
Aldosterone	Steroid	Adrenal cortex	Kidney	Promotes reabsorption of Na^+ in the kidney
Growth hormone (somatotropin)	Polypeptide	Anterior pituitary	All tissues	Growth of tissues. Promotes nitrogen retention
Adrenocortico-tropin (ACTH)	Polypeptide	Anterior pituitary	Adrenal cortex	Promotion of synthesis and release of glucocorticoids
Thyrotropin (TSH)	Polypeptide	Anterior pituitary	Thyroid	Promotion of synthesis and release of thyroid hormones
Oxytocin	Polypeptide	Posterior pituitary	Uterus and mammary glands	Contraction of smooth muscle. Milk ejection
Vasopressin	Polypeptide	Posterior pituitary	Kidneys and blood vessels	Reabsorption of water. Contraction of smooth muscle

to any particular extracellular signalling molecule depends on it posssessing a specific *receptor protein* which binds the signalling molecule with high affinity. The receptor protein may either be built into the cell membrane or may be located inside the cell.

Most hormones, as well as other chemical signals, e.g. neurotransmitters, have been found to act in one of three ways. They may

1. Alter the properties of existing proteins.
2. Alter the rate of synthesis of existing proteins or initiate the synthesis of new ones.
3. Alter the permeability of cell membranes (probably using method 1).

Each different type of cell possesses a distinctive set of protein *hormone receptors* which determines the signals to which it will respond but the actual response of the target cells to a particular signal is characteristic of the tissue in question.

Most hormones are water-soluble, the main exceptions being the steroid and thyroid hormones. These are more or less insoluble in water and are carried in the bloodstream bound to special carrier proteins. Being hydrophobic, once they have been released from their carrier, they are able to pass through the plasma membrane and bind to specific receptor proteins inside the cell. Whereas water-soluble hormones are usually removed from the bloodstream or broken down within a few minutes, the steroid hormones may remain in the blood for hours and the thyroid hormones for days, so that their effects are usually of relatively long duration.

Steroid hormones

Not only do steroid hormones persist for a relatively long time in blood but they are also responsible for relatively long-term alterations in the metabolism of their target cells. A typical target cell possesses about 10 000 steroid receptors and the effect of their activation is usually to change the amounts of particular enzymes within the cell. *Cortisol* is a typical steroid hormone which operates in this way but much of the work on the mechanism of action of the steroid hormones has been carried out using the female sex hormone *oestradiol* and it is thought likely that the mechanism of its action may be common to all steroid hormones.

After entering the target cell, each type of steroid hormone binds with high affinity to a specific type of receptor in the cytoplasm. The *hormone–receptor complex* then undergoes some sort of *transformation*, as shown by an increase in its sedimentation rate, after which it migrates to the nucleus and binds to the DNA at specific sites (Figure 24.2). After binding to the chromatin the hormone–receptor complex seems to stimulate the transcripton of specific genes with the production of the corresponding mRNA molecules. The response to a steroid hormone may take place in two stages. In the primary response there is a direct induction of transcription

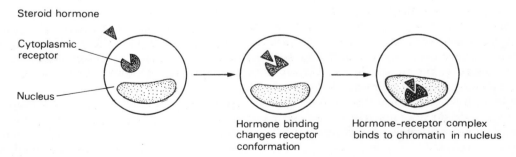

Steroid hormone

Cytoplasmic receptor

Nucleus

Hormone binding changes receptor conformation

Hormone-receptor complex binds to chromatin in nucleus

Figure 24.2 The mode of action of steroid hormones

of certain genes while, in the secondary response, further genes are activated by the products of the primary response. The actual nature of the response is determined by the nature of the target cell. For example, oestradiol causes epithelial development in the uterus and mammary glands while it decreases the resorption of bone.

The water-soluble hormones

Most of the non-steroid hormones are unable to enter their target cells directly and instead they bind to high-affinity receptors on the cell surface. Some of them, e.g. insulin and thyroid-stimulating hormone (TSH), are taken into the cell by *receptor-mediated endocytosis* but it is uncertain whether, once inside the cell, they have a direct effect on cell processes or use an intermediary.

The majority of hormones that bind to cell surface receptors do not enter the cell at all but instead they generate an intracellular signal or *second messenger* and it is this which is responsible for altering the behaviour of the cell. They may do this by changing the activity of an enzyme bound to the plasma membrane or by opening or closing gated ion channels (page 197) within the plasma membrane. The most important membrane-bound enzyme with respect to such hormones is *adenylate cyclase* which catalyses the synthesis of cAMP from ATP in the cytoplasm.

cAMP acts as an intracellular regulator in both eukaryotes and prokaryotes and all its known effects result from the activation of *cAMP-dependent protein kinases* which use ATP to phosphorylate proteins. Other enzymes or *phosphodiesterases* which are present in the cytosol break down cAMP to 5'-AMP.

The two reactions

$$\text{ATP} \xrightarrow{\overset{\text{Adenylate}}{\text{cyclase}}} \text{cAMP} + \text{PP}_i$$

and

$$\text{cAMP} \xrightarrow{\text{Phosphodiesterase}} \text{5'-AMP}$$

result in a continual synthesis and breakdown of cAMP so that at any particular moment the concentration of cAMP depends on the relative activities of the two enzymes. Phosphodiesterase, and hence the breakdown of cAMP, is inhibited by *caffeine* which is present in tea and coffee and by the related drug *theophylline*.

Many hormones have been found to act by stimulating adenylate cyclase and each type of cell responds to an increase in cAMP concentration in a characteristic way. This can be seen from Table 24.2 which shows that a rise in cAMP concentration causes glycogenolysis in liver and muscle and hormone production in the thyroid gland. On the other hand a cell of any one type, e.g. liver cell, will respond to cAMP in the same manner regardless of the nature of the hormone responsible for raising its concentration. Five different hormones, namely glucagon, adrenaline, adrenocorticotropic hormone (ACTH), thyroid-stimulating hormone (TSH) and luteinizing hormone, have been found to stimulate triglyceride breakdown in rat adipose tissue cells by activating adenylate cyclase. While each hormone has a specific receptor it is believed that they share a common set of adenylate cyclase molecules.

Recent work has shown that, at least in liver and probably in other tissues, the hormone–receptor complex does not activate adenylate cyclase directly but requires the intervention of a third membrane protein, the *G protein*, which binds GTP on its cytoplasmic surface and is needed to couple the hormone–receptor complex with the adenylate cyclase. Once formed, the GTP–G protein complex is self-inactivating, since it hydrolyses the GTP to GDP and P_i, and, in

Table 24.2 Hormonal responses that involve cAMP

Hormone	Tissue	Response
Adrenaline	Liver, muscle	Glycogenolysis
	Adipose tissue	Lipolysis
	Heart	Increased force of contraction
Glucagon	Liver	Glycogenolysis
Adrenocorticotropic hormone	Adrenal cortex	Steroid production
Thyroid-stimulating hormone	Thyroid	Thyroid hormone production
Parathyroid hormone	Bone	Calcium resorption
Luteinizing hormone	Corpus luteum	Steroid synthesis
Vasopressin	Renal medulla	Water reabsorption
Melanocyte stimulating	Frog skin	Darkening of skin

this form, has no effect on adenylate cyclase. As a result, the activation of the adenylate cyclase is short-lived and the response to changes in hormonal levels is very sensitive and rapid.

As mentioned earlier cAMP affects a wide range of cellular processes ranging from triglyceride and glycogen breakdown to a reduction in platelet aggregation, darkening of the skin and water resorption in the kidneys. In this latter connection the effect of *cholera toxin* is of interest. The toxin has the effect of altering the G protein in such a way that it no longer hydrolyses the bound GTP. As a result the adenylate cyclase molecules remain indefinitely active and the intracellular cAMP level remains indefinitely raised. This, in the intestinal cells, causes a loss of water and Na^+ ions into the gut with a consequent severe diarrhoea.

Calcium ions as second messengers

Evidence is accumulating that Ca^{2+} ions, like cAMP, may act as a second messenger for certain hormones and other extracellular signals. The concentration of free Ca^{2+} ions in the cytosol is kept at a very low level ($\simeq 10^{-7}$ M). This is because (a) Ca^{2+} ions are actively extruded by ion pumps present in the plasma membrane and (b) Ca^{2+} ions are bound to intracellular proteins and structures, especially the endoplasmic reticulum and sarcoplasmic reticulum of muscle fibres (Figure 24.3). Some cell surface receptors, instead of being coupled with adenylate cyclase molecules, are coupled to Ca^{2+} ion channels in the plasma membrane. Several hormones, including adrenaline and vasopressin and also the neurotransmitter acetylcholine, alter the distribution of Ca^{2+} ions within the cell and cause a transient opening of the channels allowing Ca^{2+} ions to enter the cytoplasm where they act as a second messenger with wide-ranging effects. They cause depolarization of the plasma membrane which changes its permeability to ions including Ca^{2+} ions themselves, and they also have a direct effect on the activity of various enzymes. The effects are transient because the extra Ca^{2+} ions are rapidly pumped out of the cell or taken up by Ca^{2+} ion-binding molecules. It is now believed that an early event by which the hormone-activated receptor induces the uptake of Ca^{2+} ions by the cell involves the hydrolysis of a specific phospholipid namely *phosphatidylinositide*.

Calcium ions have been found to be used as a secondary messenger in secretory cells which are stimulated by extracellular ligands. The increase in the concentration of free Ca^{2+} ions initiates exocytosis causing the secretory vesicles to fuse with the plasma membrane and release their contents to the exterior. It appears that ATP is required for exocytosis as well as the Ca^{2+} ion flux and it is also likely that a Ca^{2+}ion-binding protein such as the recently discovered *calmodulin* is required. Calmodulin is clearly a very important protein since it has been found in every plant and animal cell so far examined and has been highly conserved in the course of

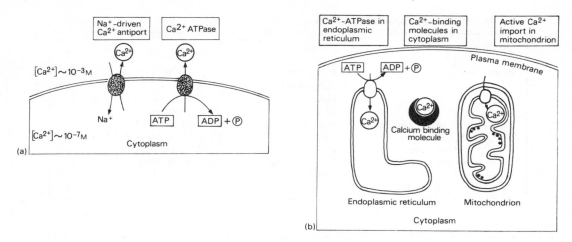

Figure 24.3 The maintenance of a low concentration of Ca^{2+} in the cytoplasm. Ca^{2+} is actively pumped out of the cytosol to the cell exterior (a) as well as into the intracellular membrane-enclosed organelles such as the endoplasmic reticulum and mitochondria (b). In addition, various molecules in the cell bind free Ca^{2+} tightly

evolution. It consists of a single polypeptide chain made up of 148 amino acid residues and it has four Ca^{2+} ion-binding sites. When it binds Ca^{2+} ions it undergoes major conformational changes and it seems to play a part in most Ca^{2+} ion-regulated processes.

Calmodulin has been found to be a constituent of muscle phosphorylase kinase, the enzyme responsible for the activation of the phosphorylase which breaks down glycogen (page 234). Muscle phosphorylase kinase is made up of four subunits one of which is catalytic the other three being regulatory and enabling the enzyme to be activated by both cAMP and Ca^{2+} ions. The calmodulin subunit is responsible for the fact that the catalytic subunit can be activated by protein kinase only when Ca^{2+} is bound.

Although calmodulin appears as a regulatory subunit in the phosphorylase kinase molecule, in most instances the binding of Ca^{2+} ions by calmodulin allows it to bind to and regulate certain target proteins inside the cell, e.g. adenylate cyclase, cAMP phosphodiesterase and some membrane-bound ATPases. Thus there is an overlap between the regulatory effects of cAMP and Ca^{2+} ions.

Hormones and energy metabolism

The hormones chiefly responsible for coordinating the energy metabolism of the various tissues are glucagon, adrenaline and insulin; noradrenaline and ACTH also play a part. All of them, except insulin, have the effect of raising the blood sugar level.

Glucagon

Glucagon is a polypeptide hormone which is secreted by the α cells of the pancreatic islets in response to a low blood glucose concentration. It acts mainly on the liver and increases the concentration of blood glucose by stimulating glycogenolysis and gluconeogenesis; it also increases triglyceride breakdown and the mobilization of fat. Glucagon achieves these effects by increasing the activity of adenylate cyclase and hence the production of cAMP and active protein kinase as described earlier. The series of reactions needed to activate phosphorylase which are shown in Figure 24.4 have a major *amplification effect* (page 388) so that, for every molecule of glucagon bound to a cell surface receptor, many thousands of molecules of phosphorylase are activated. Triglyceride breakdown is increased by the phosphorylation and activation of cAMP-dependent lipase. Glycogen synthase and acetyl-CoA carboxylase are also phosphorylated but this inhibits their activity so that the synthesis of glycogen and of fatty acids is inhibited. A further enzyme phosphorylation, namely of pyruvate kinase, is indirectly responsible for the increased rate of gluconeogenesis which results from glucagon secretion. Phosphorylation inhibits pyruvate kinase and reduces the cycling which occurs between phosphoenolpyruvate and pyruvate under the influence of pyruvate kinase, pyruvate carboxylase and phosphoenol-pyruvate phosphokinase (page 238). In this way the net flux from pyruvate to phosphopyruvate is increased. Interestingly in muscle where gluconeogenesis does not occur, the pyruvate kinase is not phosphorylated by protein kinase. The effect of glucagon on liver enzymes is summarized in Figure 24.5.

The metabolic response to glucagon can be seen to be a coordinated series of phosphorylations of key enzymes brought about by protein kinase. The result is the activation of

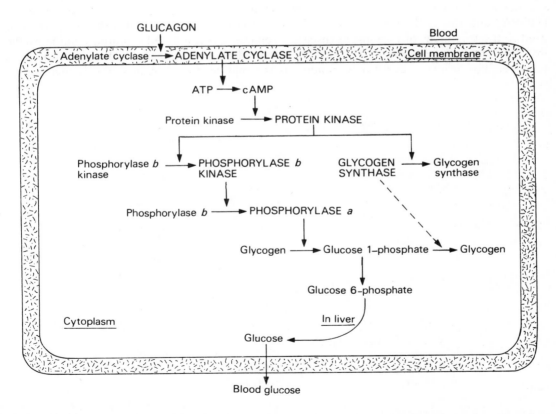

Figure 24.4 The action of glucagon in promoting the breakdown of glycogen and inhibiting its synthesis. The active forms of the enzymes are shown in capital letters

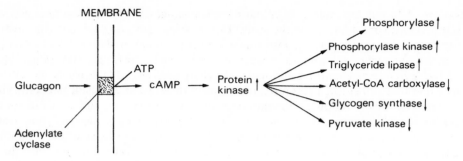

Figure 24.5 Effect of glucagon on liver metabolism

the pathways of glycogen breakdown, triglyceride breakdown and gluconeogenesis and the inhibition of glycogen and fatty acid synthesis.

Adrenaline

Adrenaline is a derivative of tyrosine, and its synthesis and that of noradrenaline is shown in Figure 24.6. Adrenaline and noradrenaline are both amines which, as shown in Figure 24.6, are derived from tyrosine. Tyrosine is first hydroxylated to give dihydroxyphenylalanine (DOPA) and this is then decarboxylated to form dopamine, a natural metabolite which is used in the treatment of Parkinsons disease. Dopamine is converted to noradrenaline by the insertion of a hydroxyl group in the side chain and adrenaline is formed by the methylation of noradrenaline using *S*-adenosylmethionine as the methyl donor. Adrenaline is secreted by

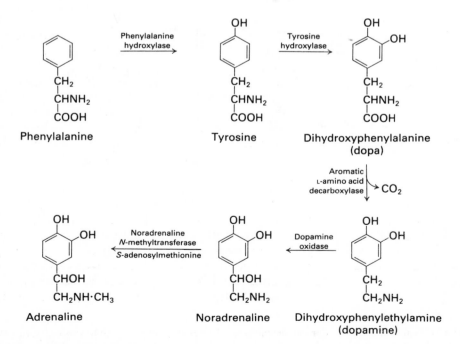

Figure 24.6 The synthesis of catecholamines

the adrenal medulla in response to stress. It has wide-ranging physiological and biochemical effects. Thus it causes the mobilization of food stores by stimulating glycogen breakdown in muscle and liver, and triglyceride breakdown in liver and adipose tissue.

There are two types of cell membrane receptor (α and β) for adrenaline. *β-Receptors* which are inhibited by *β-blockers* such as propanolol are the main type of receptor in muscle, heart, adipose tissue and many other tissues. They interact with and activate adenylate cyclase in the cell membrane so that the effect of adrenaline on muscle or adipose tissue is to increase the concentration of cAMP in the cell and thus to activate protein kinase. Stimulation of glycogen breakdown by adrenaline in muscle is then mediated by a *cascade mechanism* similar to that involved in the stimulation of glycogenolysis in liver by glucagon (page 353). Breakdown of triglycerides in adipose tissue, as in liver, occurs as a result of activation of triglyceride lipase by phosphorylation.

In rat liver, β-blockers do not completely abolish the response to adrenaline due to the presence of the second type of adrenaline receptor, the *α-receptor*. α-Receptors are characterized by their sensitivity to phenoxybenzamine. The binding of adrenaline to α-receptors does not increase the cAMP concentration, but nevertheless it stimulates glycogen breakdown by causing an increase in the cytosolic concentration of free Ca^{2+} ions. This calcium is initially released from the endoplasmic reticulum. The non-phosphorylated form of phosphorylase kinase is activated by calcium ions so that an increase in cytoplasmic calcium concentration increases the activity of phosphorylase kinase, and hence glycogen breakdown, independently of a change in cAMP. Thus Ca^{2+} ions act as a second messenger for the α-receptor-mediated effects of adrenaline. In most tissues there are more β than α receptors but the ratio varies with both the tissue and the species of animal and also with age. The significance of such variation is not understood.

Another catecholamine, *noradrenaline*, is produced mainly at the nerve endings of the sympathetic system and also in small amounts in the adrenal medulla. Secretion from this gland appears to be under nervous control and occurs rapidly as an appropriate response to stressful situations.

The hormones are stored in special granules which are present in the sympathetic nerve endings and medullary cells and the net hormonal output depends on the rates of both the synthesis and release. Any catecholamine that diffuses from the synapse into the remainder of the neuron is destroyed by a *monoamine oxidase*. Sympathomimetic drugs such as ephedrine and the amphetamines act by inhibiting monoamine oxidase and slowing the removal of catecholamines and 5-hydroxytryptamine (serotonin) from within neurons. In this way they increase the sensitivity of the neuron to stimulation and act as antidepressants. Any catecholamines that are released into the bloodstream are rapidly removed and inactivated by the liver.

Insulin

Insulin is the only hormone known to reduce the blood sugar level. It is secreted by the β-cells of the islets of Langerhans in the pancreas in response to an elevated level of blood glucose. The overall action of insulin is to promote storage pathways. More specifically it stimulates the transport of glucose across the plasma membrane of certain cells, especially of muscle and adipose tissue, but not of liver. In this way it promotes the synthesis of glycogen in the liver and fatty acids in both liver and adipose tissue. Insulin also stimulates protein synthesis.

Insulin binds to special receptors in cell membranes, but the sequence of events after this has occurred is still not clear.

1. Under some conditions insulin reduces the cell concentration of cAMP or opposes the rise induced by other hormones.

2. It causes the dephosphorylation and hence the activation of pyruvate dehydrogenase in adipose tissue mitochondria. Pyruvate dehydrogenase in adipose tissue may be regarded as a regulatory enzyme in the synthesis of fatty acids from glucose. Insulin operates by stimulating the phosphatase for this enzyme but how it causes this change inside the mitochondria is unknown.

3. On stimulation of adipocytes with insulin, some of the specific glucose-transport proteins that have been found to be present, both in the cell membrane and in the endoplasmic reticulum of these cells, migrate from the endoplasmic reticulum into the plasma membrane. This increases the uptake of glucose into the cells but, here again, it is not known how insulin causes this effect.

4. Insulin has recently been found to cause the phosphorylation of certain proteins in adipose tissue, e.g. acetyl-CoA carboxylase (page 256), via a protein kinase that is independent of cAMP.

Final elucidation of the mechanism of action of insulin is still a major subject of research.

The synthesis and secretion of insulin

Some features of the synthesis and secretion of hormones can be illustrated by consideration of the mechanisms involved in the secretion of insulin from pancreatic β-cells.

Insulin consists of two peptide chains linked together by two –S–S– bridges but it is synthesized on the ribosomes of β-cells of the pancreatic islets as a precursor, *pre-proinsulin*, which is a single polypeptide chain (Figure 24.7). A sequence of 16 amino acids at the *N*-terminus represents the *signal peptide* (page 316) which is removed in the endoplasmic reticulum after directing the remainder of the p.o.ein to the Golgi apparatus. Here the *proinsulin* is packaged into granules and hydrolysed to active insulin by the cleavage of two peptide bonds. This results in the removal of a *connecting peptide* containing 33 amino acid residues leaving the A and B chains held together by the disulphide bonds.

Insulin is stored as such in granules in the cytoplasm of the β-cells. When the cells receive the stimulus for secretion, the granules fuse with the cell membrane and insulin is released by exocytosis. This storage mechanism enables the cells to respond rapidly to a requirement for increased insulin in the blood without the immediate necessity for *de novo* synthesis. The fusion of granules with the cell membrane is known to be preceded by an increase in the intracellular calcium concentration.

The major physiological stimulus for insulin secretion is an elevated concentration of blood glucose. The pancreatic β-cells, like liver cells, contain a glucokinase with a high K_m for glucose. It has been suggested that, owing to the presence of this enzyme, the cell responds to an increased extracellular glucose concentration by increasing the rate of glucose metabolism. The link between glucose metabolism and an increase in cell calcium, however, is still obscure. A current hypothesis is that some direct or indirect metabolite of glucose is responsible for the opening of calcium channels in the cell membrane and/or the release of calcium from intracellular stores. The nature of this putative metabolic signal is still under investigation. Progress is difficult because of the very small amount of material which can be obtained for investigation.

Regulation of blood glucose concentration

The regulation of blood glucose concentration serves as a useful example of the control and integration of metabolism. The level of glucose in the portal circulation may vary widely as a

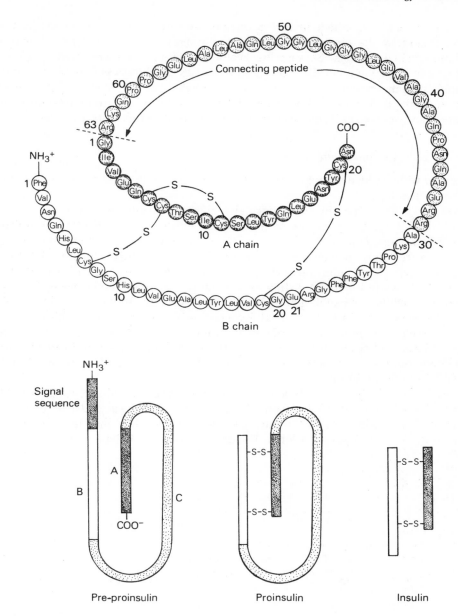

Figure 24.7 Pre-proinsulin and its conversion to insulin

consequence of fasting or carbohydrate feeding but, under normal conditions, the plasma concentration of glucose in the systemic circulation is kept within the range 3·3–7 mM. A balance is maintained between the utilization of glucose via glycolysis, glycogen synthesis and fatty acid synthesis and glucose production via glycogenolysis and gluconeogenesis all of which are subject to hormonal control.

In the absorptive period when the portal glucose concentration is high, there is a rise in the concentration of glucose in the systemic circulation. The β-cells of the pancreas respond to this by secreting insulin, which increases the rate of glucose metabolism in the liver and peripheral tissues by the mechanisms considered above, thus lowering the plasma glucose concentration. When this falls below a critical value insulin secretion is reduced, and glucagon is secreted by the pancreatic α-cells. Glucagon increases the blood glucose concentration by stimulating glycogenolysis in the liver and by increasing the synthesis of glucose from lactate and amino acids, as discussed earlier. The hormonal responses involved in the regulation of blood glucose are finely balanced and the insulin/glucagon concentration ratio is critical.

Diabetes as a failure of metabolic control

Many diseases result from a failure of control mechanisms and this is particularly well illustrated in the case of diabetes.

Diabetes is characterized by an abnormally high blood glucose concentration, and an intolerance to ingested glucose. The preliminary diagnosis of diabetes relies on a procedure known as the *glucose tolerance test*. The patient fasts overnight and his blood and urine glucose concentrations are determined before and after oral ingestion of 50 g of glucose. Blood and urine glucose concentrations are determined at 30 min intervals for the next 3 h. Typical results of this procedure are shown in Figure 24.8. In a normal subject there is an increase in blood glucose concentration reaching a maximum after 30 min but this returns to the fasting level within 2 h. No glucose appears in the urine. Diabetics have a fasting blood glucose level which is higher than normal and develop a *hyperglycaemia* of long duration. At the same time glucose is excreted in the urine (*glycosuria*) because the normal renal threshold (approximately 10 mM) is exceeded. The degree and duration of hyperglycaemia observed in the glucose tolerance test is indicative of the severity of the condition.

Other symptoms of diabetes include dehydration and excessive thirst, excessive output of urine, an excess of ketone bodies in the blood with associated acidosis, and loss of body protein. The brain is very sensitive to the plasma glucose concentration and, in prolonged hyperglycaemia, the subject may go into a coma. The underlying basis of diabetes is usually a failure of

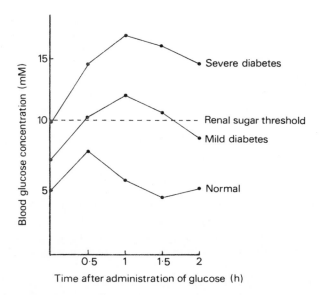

Figure 24.8 Glucose tolerance curves

the subject to produce enough insulin to allow the delicately balanced metabolic control mechanisms discussed above to operate properly. Occasionally diabetes results from a failure of the patient to respond to insulin in the normal way.

Some of the symptoms of diabetes can be understood in the context of the actions of insulin already considered. In the absence of adequate insulin levels, glucose will not be taken up by the tissues and the blood glucose level will remain high. Excess water is excreted with the glucose leading to dehydration and salt loss. In the absence of the antilipolytic effect of insulin, fat breakdown and fatty acid oxidation increase and lead to excess ketone body production in the liver and consequent acidosis. Protein breakdown similarly increases. In the liver, amino acids produced from proteolysis, and glycerol produced from fat breakdown, are converted to glucose. This glucose cannot be used by the tissues and is to a large extent excreted.

Mild diabetes can be controlled by strict regulation of the diet, but the more severe forms require the administration of regular doses of insulin by injection. This administration must be carefully controlled since an excess of insulin may cause a sudden drop in blood glucose which is too large to be overcome by the glucagon-dependent compensatory mechanisms. Severe *hypoglycaemia* may lead to a rapid loss of consciousness, convulsions and even death. Diabetes can produce serious long-term complications such as blindness and gangrene of the extremities, which are not directly related to the increased blood glucose concentration or to ketoacidosis.

The adrenal cortex

Two types of steroid hormone are secreted by the adrenal cortex: the *glucocorticoids*, so called because they function in the regulation of carbohydrate metabolism, and the *mineralocorticoids* of which the most important is *aldosterone*, which regulates salt loss via the kidneys.

The main glucocorticoid is *hydrocortisone* and only relatively small amounts of the other glucocorticoids, including corticosterone, are secreted in Man. Hydrocortisone is responsible for the induction of enzymes that promote gluconeogenesis and lipolysis. In this way it has the effect of raising the blood sugar level and mobilizing stored adipose tissue fat; it also increases

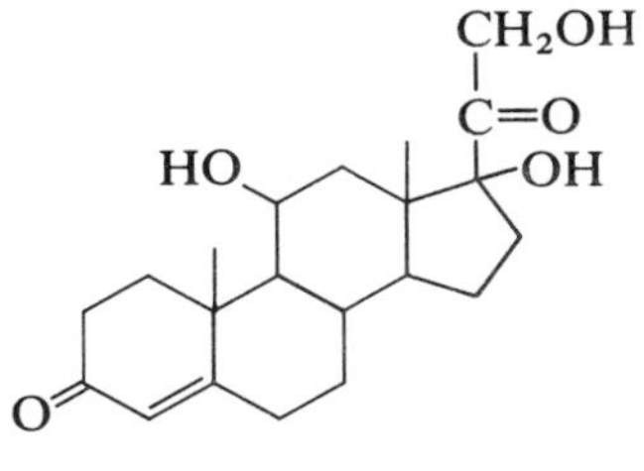

Cortisol (hydrocortisone)

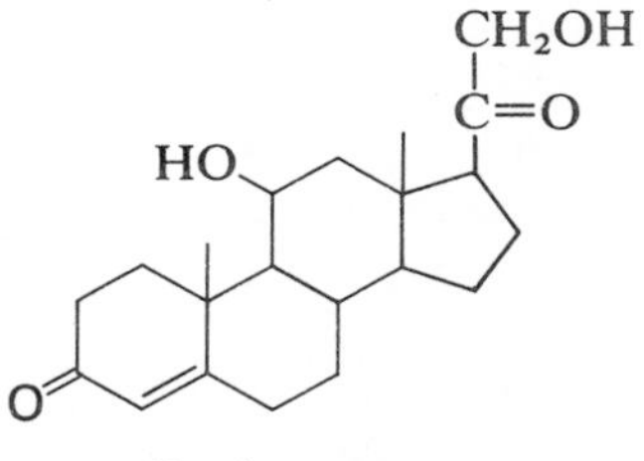

Corticosterone

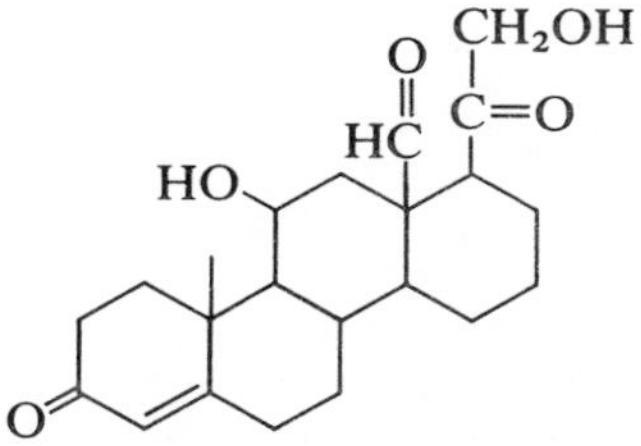

Aldosterone

fatty acid oxidation in the liver. The function of hydrocortisone is to help ensure that, when glucose is in short supply, the blood glucose level is maintained so that glucose is available for those tissues, notably the brain, that need it most, while at the same time an alternative energy supply is made available for the other tissues.

When administered in large amounts hydrocortisone has an anti-inflammatory action; it inhibits vasodilatation, the proliferation of fibroblasts and the deposition of collagen in connective tissue. These effects may result from stabilization of the lysosomes and evidence has been obtained that hydrocortisone may actually be incorporated into the lysosomal membrane.

In addition to their anti-inflammatory effects large doses of hydrocortisone have been found to increase the excretion of calcium. Since calcium absorption from the gut may be simultaneously decreased, if care is not taken, hydrocortisone treatment may cause a dangerous loss of calcium from the body, resulting in osteoporosis.

The thyroid gland

The thyroid gland not only plays a role in growth and development but also has profound effects on energy metabolism and protein synthesis. Lack of the thyroid hormones causes *cretinism* in children and *myxoedema* in adults. Cretins are both physically and mentally retarded, while in myxoedematous subjects there is a general slowing down of metabolism and an accumulation of proteoglycans under the skin, which coarsens the features and gives the subject a puffy appearance.

The thyroid hormones and their mode of synthesis are shown in Figure 24.9. Both the iodenation and the coupling of the tyrosine residues appear to occur within the thyroglobulin molecule and it is in this form that the hormones are stored in the colloid-containing vesicles of the gland. The thyroid hormones, like the steroid hormones, bind to intracellular receptors in their target cells but these receptors are present within the nucleus even before the hormone is bound, and how the thyroid hormones exert their effects is still a mystery. It has been known

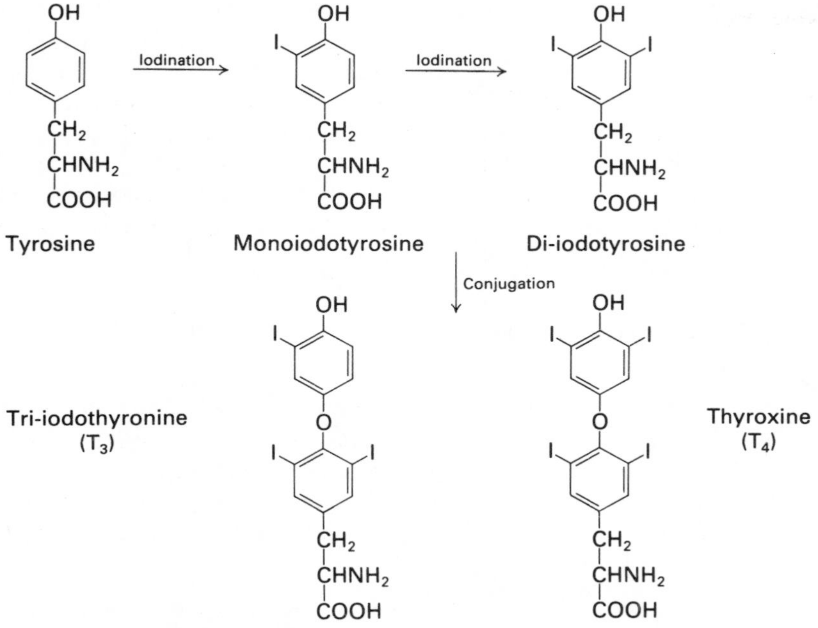

Figure 24.9 The synthesis of thyroid hormones

since the end of the last century that thyroxine increases oxygen consumption and the metabolic rate. Thyroxine also causes changes in the mitochondria, but its effects vary from tissue to tissue and no clear pattern has emerged. The hormones increase protein synthesis in certain tissues and protein breakdown in most, so that they have the effect of increasing the turnover of protein as well as of many other body constituents.

The formation of thyroglobulin and the release of *thyroxine* (T_4) and *tri-iodothyronine* (T_3) is controlled by the *thyroid-stimulating hormone* (TSH or *thyrotropin*) of the anterior pituitary, which is secreted on a feedback basis when the level of circulating T_4 and T_3 falls, or as a result of neural stimulation of the hypothalamus.

The pituitary gland

Hormones produced in the anterior pituitary are *corticotropin* (ACTH), *somatotropin* (growth hormone), *follicle-stimulating hormone* (FSH), *luteinizing hormone* (LH), *prolactin* and *β-lipotropin*.

Growth hormone

Normal growth and development depends on the production and secretion of adequate amounts of many hormones, notably the pituitary hormones, adrenal cortical hormones, thyroxine and the sex hormones.

Growth hormone or somatotropin is of special importance in the development of normal stature. Deficiency of growth hormone leads to *dwarfism* while overproduction results in the condition of *gigantism* in the immature subject and *acromegaly* in adults. In the latter condition, since epipysial fusion has already occurred, abnormal bone growth results in thickening of all bones and overgrowth of the extremities.

Human growth hormone is a single-chain protein containing about 190 amino acid residues. As mentioned earlier, it is species-specific and cannot be replaced by growth hormone derived from other species.

The effects of growth hormone are numerous and complex. When injected it causes retention of nitrogen (positive N balance) and of many electrolytes. The nitrogen retention appears to result from increased protein synthesis rather than decreased breakdown. The hormone not only increases the uptake of amino acids by the tissues from the blood but also promotes the incorporation of amino acids into protein, apparently by increasing the activity of RNA polymerase and the speed of transcription. Growth hormone is only fully active in the presence of insulin. If large doses of growth hormone are injected into animals, e.g. rats and dogs, over a long period it causes a form of diabetes.

The neurohypophyseal system

The nervous and endocrine systems are linked by the hypothalamus which contains *neuro-secretory cells*. These, on stimulation by electrical impulses, secrete relatively short chain highly active peptides which pass in special blood vessels directly to the pituitary gland. The hypothalamic hormones include *somatostatin*, which inhibits growth hormone release, and various hormones that stimulate the release of those anterior pituitary hormones that control the secretion of hormones in various other endocrine glands. For example the secretion of thyroid hormone requires

1. stimulation of the neurosecretory cells of the hypothalamus leading to secretion of *thyrotropin-releasing hormones* (TRH);

2. the passage of TRH along the special vessels of the pituitary stalk to the anterior lobe of the pituitary gland where it causes the release of *thyrotropin* (thyroid-stimulating hormone – TSH);
3. carriage of the TSH in the blood stream to the thyroid gland where it stimulates the synthesis and secretion of *thyroid hormone* (TH).

   The posterior lobe of the pituitary is responsible for the production of the hormones *vasopressin* and *oxytocin* each of which contains nine amino acid residues and is derived from a larger precursor molecule. These are stored in intracellular vesicles and processed by proteolytic cleavage to the peptide hormone and a large protein called *neurophysin*. The secretion of vasopressin and oxytocin, like that of the other pituitary hormones, is controlled by the hypothalamus. The intracellular vesicles containing vasopressin and oxytocin travel down the neurohypophyseal tract bound to neurophysins.

   Oxytocin causes contraction of the smooth muscle of the uterus and mammary glands and the ejection of milk. Vasopressin, as the name suggests, causes a rise in blood pressure by

Table 24.3 Some mammalian peptides (all these may be classified as *neuropeptides* since they have been found within the mammalian central nervous system)

	Number of residues
Pituitary hormones	
Corticotropin (ACTH)	39
β-Endorphin	32
Lipotropin	91
α-Melanocyte-stimulating hormone (α-MSH)	13
β-Melanocyte-stimulating hormone (β-MSH)	22
Oxytocin	9
Vasopressin	9
Hypothalamic releasing hormones	
Thyrotropin-releasing hormone (TRH)	3
Corticotropin-releasing hormone (CRH)	—
Gonadotropin-releasing hormone (GnRH)	10
Growth hormone-releasing hormone (GHRH)	43
Somatostatin	14
Nervous tissue	
Met-enkephalin	5
Leu-enkephalin	5
Pancreas	
Insulin	51
Glucagon	29
Heart	
Cardionatrin	—
Gut	
Gastrin	17
Secretin	27
Cholecystokinin	33
Parathyroid	
Parathormone	84
Calcitonin	32

constricting small blood vessels. It also increases water resorption in the kidney tubules. Its effects on the kidney are mediated by the activation of adenylate cyclase and the production of cAMP but liver vasopressin receptors resemble the α-receptors for adrenaline in that their activation causes an increase in the cytosolic Ca^{2+} ion concentration without affecting the tissue cAMP levels. This increase in Ca^{2+} ion concentration stimulates phosphorylase kinase, as described above. The action of vasopressin on the liver, while of uncertain physiological significance, provides a very useful experimental system to study Ca^{2+}-dependent effects of hormones on metabolism.

A list of pituitary and other hormones which have been found in the mammalian central nervous system is given in Table 24.3.

Endogenous opiates and other neuropeptides

In the middle 1970s two pentapeptides with pain-suppressing effects similar to, but even more powerful than, those of morphine were isolated from the brains of pigs. These endogenous opiate-like substances were found to have the structure

$$^+H_3N\text{-Tyr-Gly-Gly-Phe-Met-COO}^-$$
$$^+H_3N\text{-Tyr-Gly-Gly-Phe-Leu-COO}^-$$

and are known as *Met-enkephalin* and *Leu-enkephalin* respectively. Subsequently some larger peptides known as *endorphins* with similar effects were isolated from mammalian pituitary glands. The best known of these, *β-endorphin*, contains 32 amino acid residues and the structure of its *N*-terminal region is identical with that of Leu-enkephalin.

It was found that the effects of these opiate-like substances could be rapidly reversed by administration of the morphine antagonist *naloxone* and this and other findings led to the conclusion that the enkephalins and endorphins bind to the same receptors in the central nervous system, of which there appear to be at least three types, as morphine itself. Evidence was also obtained that the natural opiates may play a part in normal emotional responses as well as in the control of pain perception. The natural opiates differ from morphine and its derivatives in that they do not accumulate and lead to the tolerance which occurs with morphine. It has been suggested that the effects of acupuncture may result from the release of natural opiates.

Altogether about 18 opioid peptides have now been isolated all of which have an *N*-terminal sequence corresponding to one or other of the enkephalins. They appear to be derived from three precursor proteins, namely *proopiocortin* (pituitary), *proenkephalin* (adrenal medulla) and *prodynorphin* (hypothalamus). The peptides are released from the precursors by proteolytic fragmentation, the cleavage sites usually being marked by pairs of basic amino acids (lysine and/or arginine), as is also the case with proinsulin (page 356) and proparathormone. The facts that (a) processing is not uniform among all tissues and the products vary in their potency and receptor selectivity, (b) the various *neuropeptides* frequently co-exist with each other or with a monoamine transmitter and (c) the various target neurons differ in the numbers and types of their receptors, mean that provision exists for a precise and complex chemical communication system which is independent of any anatomical connections.

Proopiocortin

As recorded above, the enkephalins have been found to be derived from larger precursors. β-Endorphin is derived from the pituitary hormone *β-lipotropin* which contains 91 amino acid residues and stimulates the release of fatty acids from adipose tissues. β-Lipotropin is, in turn, derived from the even larger precursor *proopiocortin* which contains 265 residues.

From proopiocortin are derived two lipotropins, corticotropin, three endorphins and two melanocyte-stimulating hormones! All these peptides are derived from the *C*-terminal half of the proopiocortin molecule and the fate of the *N*-terminal half is unknown. It is quite possible that it gives rise to a completely different set of biologically active peptides, from which it is apparent that there may be many other biologically active peptides yet to be discovered!

Chemical messengers other than hormones

It should not be thought that hormones are the only type of chemical messenger or signalling molecule to be found in living organisms since it is now clear that a wide variety of substances transmit information and instructions within the bodies of animals. Indeed, in a sense, all molecules are chemical messengers and distinctions are based merely on the manner in which the information is passed and the distance between the origin of the message and its destination. Gene repressors, neurotransmitters and embryonic inducing agents are all types of chemical messenger, as are the growth factors, chalones and pheromones.

Prostaglandins

These are a complex group of unsaturated fatty acids containing 20 carbon atoms and a five-membered ring structure. They are synthesized *in vivo* from arachidonic acid (page 103). The prostaglandins (PG), which include *thromboxane A* and *prostacyclin*, are among the most potent biological substances known. They were first discovered about 50 years ago as vasoactive principles derived from the prostate gland and hence the name. Since then they have been found in a variety of tissues. In many respects they resemble hormones but they act locally exerting their effects on the cells that produce them. Since they are not stored in the producing cells and are rapidly destroyed, their actions depend on continuous biosynthesis.

Variations in the structure of the five-membered ring allow them to be divided into groups designated the A, B, E, F, G, H and I series, the two major groups being PGE and PGF. The PGs are very difficult to study because of their evanescent nature and their minute concentrations. Nevertheless they have been found to influence a great many systems and events in the body. The picture is further complicated in that different PGs often have opposing influences in cell processes (Table 24.4). In general they have two types of action, namely effects on the contractile state of smooth muscle and a modulating influence on a number of hormonal responses.

Table 24.4 Some antagonistic effects of PGE and PGF

	PGE	*PGF*
Muscle (smooth)		
General	—	Contraction
Vascular	Relaxation	—
Gut	Contraction	—
Uterus	—	Contraction
Bronchi	Relaxation	Contraction
Blood pressure	Reduces	Increases
Adrenergic responses in general	Opposed	Accentuated
Cellular cyclic nucleotide level	cAMP increased	cGMP increased

Two of the prostaglandins have been found to be implicated in blood clotting and the development of thrombosis.

Thromboxane (TXA2)

This compound has an aggregating effect on platelets (page 385). It suppresses the level of cAMP within the thrombocytes and also acts as a vasoconstrictor for the neighbouring blood vessels. Shortly after the discovery of thromboxane another compound was found with effects which are essentially the opposite of those of thromboxane. This is *prostacyclin* (PGI_2) which is a powerful inhibitor of platelet aggregation and an active vasodilator. However, whereas thromboxane is produced within the platelets, prostacyclin is formed in blood vessel walls. The two compounds together provide a finely balanced control system (Table 24.5).

Table 24.5 Opposing effects of thromboxanes and prostacyclins on the cardiovascular system

	Thromboxane (platelets)	Prostacyclins (vascular wall)
Platelets	Aggregates	Inhibits aggregation
Platelet cAMP level	Raises	Lowers
Blood vessels	Constricts	Dilates
Blood pressure	Increases	Decreases

Synthesis of prostaglandins

The enzyme primarily responsible for the synthesis of prostaglandins is *cyclooxygenase* which converts arachidonic acid into endoperoxide intermediates (PGG and PGH) which are the

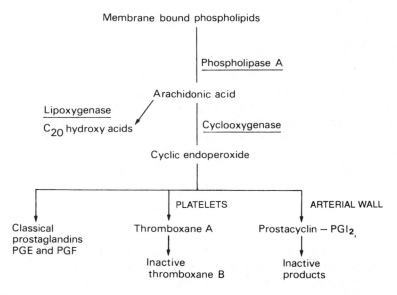

Figure 24.10 The synthesis of prostaglandins

immediate precursors not only of prostaglandins PGE and PGF but also of thromboxane and prostacyclin (Figure 24.10). Presumably the nature of the end product is determined by the enzyme system present in the tissue in question.

The rate of PG production seems to be determined by the concentration of free essential fatty acids (page 123), chiefly arachidonic acid. This, in turn, depends on the relese of the essential fatty acids from position 2 of cellular phospholipids. The enzyme responsible for this release is *phospholipase A* which is activated when the cell is injured. PG synthesis is inhibited by anti-inflammatory agents such as aspirin, indomethacin and acetaminophen which inhibit cyclooxygenase.

Prostaglandins have, potentially, very important applications in a wide range of clinical conditions, e.g. in the treatment of hypertension and thrombosis, as well as for contraception, the induction of abortions and the relief of asthma and peptic ulcers. However, much more work needs to be done before they can be put to routine use.

Tissue growth factors

An important and relatively recently discovered group of proteins and protein derivatives are the tissue growth factors. These are synthesized in a number of widely distributed cells and tissues but, because they are active in tiny amounts and are not produced in a discrete gland, their isolation and characterization, like that of prostaglandins, is very difficult. The first to be discovered was *nerve growth factor* (molecular weight 13 000) which for some undisclosed reason is highly concentrated in the submaxillary gland of the male mouse. Nerve growth factor is needed for the development, survival and functioning of sympathetic and some peripheral sensory neurons. Other recognized tissue growth factors are the *somatomedins, epidermal growth factor* and the *platelet-derived growth factors*.

When growth hormone, which is produced in the anterior pituitary, binds to receptors in its target tissues it stimulates the production of *somatomedins*. These local growth factors are polypeptides (molecular weight about 7500) which resemble insulin both in their structure and effects so that they are sometimes referred to as *insulin-like growth factors* (IGF I and IGF II). On the basis of their structural similarities, it has been suggested that proinsulin, the somatomedins and nerve growth factor may well have shared a common ancestral gene. *Epidermal growth factor* is also a polypeptide, similar in size to the somatomedins, which induces proliferative changes in epithelial and other tissues. Like the somatomedins and platelet-derived growth factors, epidermal growth factor promotes cell division.

These growth factors react with receptors on the surface of their target cells and, in the process, activate a cascade system (page 388) which results in mitogenesis. Thus the growth factors may play a critical role in the control of both normal and abnormal cell proliferation. They are currently arousing considerable interest because there is evidence that the genes which encode proteins that render cells responsive to growth factors may be potential oncogenes (page 326), i.e. may be responsible for neoplastic transformations by which the cells are altered in such a way as to predispose them to cancer.

Chalones

Chalones are tissue-specific substances that are responsible for the inhibition of mitosis in tissues such as skin and liver which retain the potential for cell division. The rate of division is related to the need for replacement; for example, liver cells normally divide slowly at a rate that is just sufficient for the replacement of worn-out and damaged cells so that the organ size remains constant. If part of the liver is removed the remaining cells divide at a greatly increased rate until, within a relatively short time, the missing tissue is replaced and the organ is restored to almost exactly its original size.

A chalone extracted from the skin inhibits epidermal mitosis; it is tissue-specific in that it inhibits cell division in the epidermis but not in other tissues, but it is not species specific.

It is suggested that the intracellular concentration of chalone is responsible for controlling the rate of cell division within a tissue; after injury to the skin, chalone is lost from the epidermal cells in the region of the wound and the mitotic machinery becomes activated until the wound is sealed and intracellular chalone levels have been restored. Such substances that cause specific inhibition of tissue growth could be of great significance in the treatment of cancer.

Pheromones

Pheromones may be defined as substances produced by one member of a species which alter the behaviour pattern of other members of the species. Pheromones are found in most animal phyla and are used to assemble individuals, as sex attractants and aphrodisiacs, in marking territories, in group recognition and also to produce social and alarm associations.

In mice the smell of other mice causes their adrenals to increase in size and produce more corticosteroids. This brings about a decrease in fertility and population limitation. As a result of studies on many species it has been suggested that stress, resulting from overcrowding, may explain the fluctuations of population that occur in natural conditions even when plenty of food is available.

The question of how far animals and men are masters of their fate or subjects of their body chemistry is worth considering, but is beyond the scope of this book.

Section 6

Soft tissues

Chapter 25
The body fluids

The human body may in a sense be regarded as a colloidal solution of great complexity since there is a continuous aqueous phase throughout. The obvious differences in composition which occur from one region to another are maintained by physiological barriers which take the form of membranes and intercellular macromolecules.

Except in the case of oxygen, entry of material into the body occurs by absorption across the intestinal epithelium which is subjected to a constantly changing chemical environment. Apart from the great variety of natural food constituents it may also be exposed to a tremendous range of synthetic compounds devised by food scientists and pharmaceutical chemists. It is not surprising, therefore, to find that the life of an intestinal epithelial cell is extremely short and that the whole of the intestinal lining is replaced in rather less than 2 days.

Although energy-requiring transport mechanisms ensure that valuable materials such as sugars and amino acids are actively absorbed into the bloodstream, useless and even harmful substances may pass across the intestinal barrier if their physicochemical characteristics are such as to allow them to traverse it by passive means. Once water and other materials have been absorbed they are distributed among the various fluid compartments.

Of the 40 litres of water contained in the body of a man weighing 65 kg about 2·5 litres are exchanged with the environment every 24 hours. This is made up as follows:

Gain	(ml)	Loss	(ml)
Drinks	1000	Urine	1500
Solid and semi-solid food	1200	Expired air	350
Metabolic water	300	Through the skin	500
		In faeces	150
	2500		2500

It will be noticed that about 12% of the water gained by the body is produced in the course of metabolism.

Intracellular fluid

It is very difficult to obtain information about the composition of intracellular fluid under physiological conditions. Not only does it vary from one type of cell to another but also from cell compartment to cell compartment. Nevertheless certain generalizations may be made, such as that the concentration of Na^+ and Ca^{2+} in intracellular fluids is low. This is also true for Cl^-, except in the case of red blood corpuscles and the HCl-secreting gastric glands. The chief cellular cations are K^+ and Mg^{2+} and the anions phosphate, sulphate and protein, the bulk of the phosphate being covalently bound to organic material. Data about intracellular pH values are scant but it appears to vary from 4·5 in the cells of the prostate gland to about 8·5 in osteoblasts. Most cells are believed to be slightly more acid than the plasma.

Extracellular fluids

In order to integrate the needs of the various tissues of the body and to maintain the constant conditions required for the survival of the delicate organization of their cells, higher organisms have evolved circulatory systems. In Man the relatively small volume of rapidly circulating blood (about 5 litres) is backed up by 12–15 litres of interstitial or tissue fluid. This continuously exchanges material with the cellular elements both of the blood and tissues. The extracellular fluids are the chief agents through which the homoeostatic mechanisms of the body operate to maintain the necessary balance of water, ions, respiratory gases and metabolites. The precise steady state conditions within which an organism is maintained are characteristic for the species and, whereas the body temperature of Man is held at 37–38°C, that of birds is about 41°C. Similarly while the fasting blood glucose concentration for Man is 4–5 mM that for sheep is 1·7–2·8 mM. It is not known how the various control mechanisms are set to the appropriate value.

The extracellular fluids are essentially solutions of sodium chloride and sodium bicarbonate but they also contain small amounts of calcium, magnesium and potassium, and of phosphate, sulphate and organic ions. Their pH is maintained in the range 7·35–7·45. Organic constituents include glucose, amino acids, urea and a multitude of other compounds in very small amounts. The main difference in composition of the various extracellular fluids lies in their protein contents which range from 7% in plasma down to 0·1% in subcutaneous interstitial fluid.

The composition of the interstitial fluid also differs from that of plasma with respect to other substances which are either inherently indiffusible or rendered indiffusible by combination with the plasma proteins, e.g. lipid, bilirubin and Ca^{2+} ions.

The blood

The main function of the blood is to act as a rapid transport system for oxygen, carbon dioxide, absorbed nutrients, intermediary metabolites, waste products and hormones. It also plays a role in acid–base regulation, water balance and the distribution of body heat and provides defence against infection and intrusion by foreign substances.

Blood consists of about 55% plasma and 45% of formed elements, chiefly red corpuscles but also white corpuscles and platelets. The red corpuscles are mainly concerned with O_2 and CO_2 transport, the white corpuscles with body defence mechanisms and the platelets with the clotting process.

Although many of the constituents of blood are present in simple solution, others exist in combination with one or other of the blood proteins. For example, almost all the oxygen is combined with the haemoglobin present in the red corpuscles at a concentration of $14–18\,g\,dl^{-1}$ in men and $12–16\,g\,dl^{-1}$ in women. Carriage of oxygen is the most important commitment of blood and the evolution of blood pigments of one sort or another was essential for the development of large specialized organisms.

Three closely related forms of haemoglobin are found in Man. They are present in different proportions according to the stage of development. The α chain is common to all three forms and their subunit constitution is as follows:

$$\left.\begin{array}{l} \text{HbA}\ \alpha_2\beta_2 \\ \text{HbA}_2\ \alpha_2\delta_2 \end{array}\right\} \text{ adult haemoglobin} \quad \left\{\begin{array}{l} \text{major component (97·5\%)} \\ \text{minor component (2·5\%)} \end{array}\right.$$

$$\text{HbF}\ \alpha_2\gamma_2 \qquad \text{fetal haemoglobin}$$

Fetal haemoglobin, the properties of which enable it to take up oxygen from the maternal blood while the fetus is *in utero*, is gradually replaced by the adult forms. This shows that bone marrow cells possess some form of temporal specificity with respect to the proteins that they synthesize. The α, β, γ and δ polypeptide chains, of which the various forms of haemoglobin are composed, are coded for by different genes, which are believed to have arisen from a common ancestral gene shared with myoglobin.

The structure and metabolism of haem

Haemoglobin is interesting from many points of view and it has probably been studied more extensively than any other protein. Its shape and general characteristics and its relationship to myoglobin have already been described (page 65) but little has been said about the haem group. Myoglobin, which consists of a single polypeptide chain, has one haem group while haemoglobin, which has four globin subunits, correspondingly has four haem groups, each of which can combine with one molecule of oxygen. Globin itself is colourless and contains a greater proportion of basic amino acids than any of the other blood proteins. Although the haemoglobins of all mammals are similar in shape and structure, they show appreciable differences in their amino acid composition, affinity for O_2 and other gases, and in their crystalline form. All these differences are attributable to the globin since the haem group is the same in all species. Haem is an *iron–porphyrin* compound.

The *porphyrin ring* is a planar structure formed from four pyrrole rings which are joined into a larger ring by methine (–CH=) bridges. Four methyl (M), two vinyl (V) and two propionate (P) groups are attached to the ring. The highly polar propionate side chains of the haem are situated on the surface of the molecule and are ionized at physiological pH values. The centrally

Pyrrole

Haem

placed iron atom is bound to the four N atoms of the pyrrole rings leaving two of the six coordination valencies on the iron atom free. In both myoglobin and haemoglobin the iron atom of the haem is directly bonded to a histidine residue. This is known as the *proximal histidine*. Oxygen binding occurs at the sixth coordination position near which the second important or *distal histidine* is situated. In deoxyhaemoglobin this position is empty.

$$
\begin{array}{ccc}
COO^- & & COO^- \\
| & NH_2 & | \\
CH_2 & | & CH_2 \\
| & CH_2 & | \\
CH_2 & + & CH_2 \quad \longrightarrow \quad CH_2 \quad + CO_2 + CoASH \\
| & COOH & | \\
C{\sim}S{-}CoA & & C{-}CH_2{-}NH_2 \\
\| & Glycine & \| \\
O & & O \\
\end{array}
$$

Succinyl–CoA   δ-Aminolaevulinate

Synthesis of haem is readily accomplished from simple precursors. In the first step of porphyrin synthesis succinyl-CoA, which is produced in the citrate cycle and during the metabolism of various amino acids, is condensed with glycine to give *δ-aminolaevulinic acid*, and it is this reaction which is rate-controlling. Subsequently two molecules of δ-aminolaevulinic acid condense to form *porphobilinogen* and four molecules of porphobilinogen undergo a series of reactions to produce *protoporphyrin* which combines with ferrous ions to form haem.

$$
2 \quad
\begin{array}{c}
COO^- \\
| \\
CH_2 \\
| \\
CH_2 \\
| \\
O{=}C \\
| \\
CH_2 \\
| \\
NH_2 \\
\end{array}
\quad \longrightarrow \quad
\begin{array}{c}
HOOC \quad CH_2 \\
H_2C \quad CH_2 \\
C{-}C \\
C \quad \| \quad CH \\
H_2C \quad NH \\
H_2N \\
\end{array}
\quad + 2H_2O
$$

δ-Aminolaevulinate   Porphobilinogen

Bile pigments

When, at the end of their life span, for unknown reasons the red cells rupture, the haemoglobin is released. It first combines with *haptoglobins* (page 379) present in the plasma which have a special affinity for Hb and, while combined in this way, the iron is oxidized to the ferric form. Either before or after combination with haptoglobins the haemoglobin is taken up by cells of the reticuloendothelial system, mainly in the liver, spleen and bone marrow. Here it is split into its constituent parts which are independently processed. The globin is broken down to amino acids which pass into the metabolic pool while one of the methine bridges of the porphyrin ring is oxidized, the iron is released and a chain-like *tetrapyrrole compound* is produced. The first bile pigment to be formed is *biliverdin* which is green. This is readily reduced to *bilirubin* which is golden brown and the chief pigment of human bile. The bilirubin is transported from the reticuloendothelial cells to the liver in combination with serum albumin. In the liver it is conjugated with glucuronic acid and the conjugated bilirubin, which is water-soluble, is excreted in bile into the intestine.

Bilirubin is not itself usually found in the faeces. It is subjected to the reductive action of bacteria in the lower reaches of the intestine and converted to *stercobilinogen* (urobilinogen)

Haem

$$O_2 + NADPH + H^+$$
$$\rightarrow H_2O + NADP^+$$
$$\rightarrow Fe^{3+}$$

Biliverdin

$$NADPH + H^+$$
$$\rightarrow NADP^+$$

M = methyl group
V = vinyl group
P = propionate group

Bilirubin

which is colourless, but this is subsequently oxidized to orange–yellow *stercobilin* (urobilin) which contributes to the normal colour of the faeces.

The functions of haemoglobin and myoglobin

In the haemoglobin molecule, although the four haem groups are separated by appreciable distances, the state of one haem is influenced by that of the other three and these *haem–haem interactions* are of considerable physiological importance. This can be judged by comparing the properties of haemoglobin and myoglobin. As can be seen from Figure 25.1, the O_2 dissociation curve of myoglobin is a simple rectangular hyperbola while that of haemoglobin is sigmoid. The

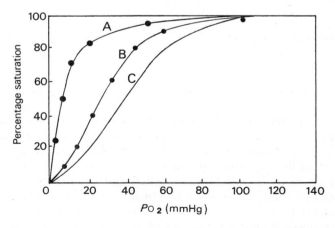

Figure 25.1 Oxygen dissociation curves for myoglobin (A) and haemoglobin at P_{CO_2} values of 40 mmHg(B) and 80 mmHg (C)

two pigments are well suited for their respective physiological roles. Thus myoglobin acts as a store of O_2 in muscles that may be deprived of O_2 for relatively long periods. For this purpose it is important that it should take up O_2 when it is readily available and release it only when it cannot be obtained from the atmosphere. From the curve it can be seen that at an O_2 pressure of 20 mmHg myoglobin is 80% saturated with O_2 and only releases significant amounts at O_2 pressures below this. Haemoglobin on the other hand, although it also has storage capacity for O_2, is essentially a carrier and is required alternately to pick up and release O_2 with changes of O_2 pressure operating at a higher range.

The difference in properties between the two proteins, whose tertiary structures are very similar (page 67), is due to the superimposed quaternary structure of haemoglobin and the fact that the ease with which any haem group binds O_2 is determined by the state of the other three. Starting with deoxyhaemoglobin the first O_2 molecule is taken up very slowly, the second and third are taken up more and more readily and the fourth is taken up several hundred times more rapidly than the first; hence the sigmoid shape of the curve.

Changes in haemoglobin in response to the environment

When deoxyhaemoglobin is converted into oxyhaemoglobin or *vice versa* subtle changes occur in the tertiary structure of the subunits which cause relatively large changes in the quaternary structure.

In deoxyhaemoglobin the iron atom lies about 0.6 Å (0.06 nm) out of the plane of the ring but, on oxygenation, it moves into the plane of the ring and is able to form a strong bond with oxygen (Figure 25.2). This tiny structural change within the subunits is translated into a shift in the relationship between them. One pair of $\alpha\beta$ subunits rotates relatively to the other pair causing the β chains to move closer together and the α chains to move slightly away from one another. This change in the quaternary structure on oxygenation and deoxygenation may be regarded as a 'breathing movement' at the molecular level.

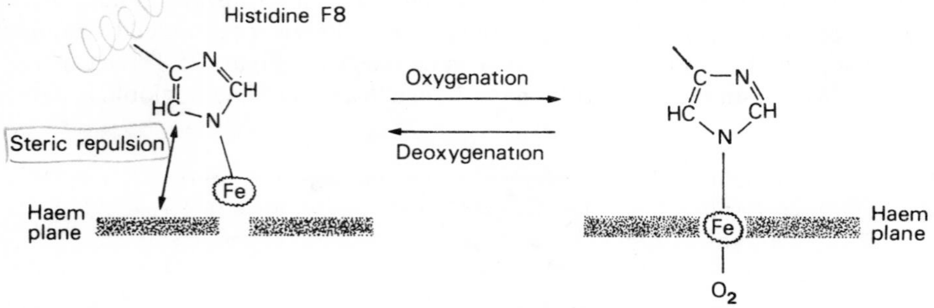

Figure 25.2 Movement of the Fe^{2+} atom into the plane of the haem group on oxygenation

Not only does haemoglobin have multiple binding sites for oxygen which, as described above, show positive cooperativity, it also combines at different sites with CO_2 and H^+ ions and also with the substance *2,3-diphosphoglycerate*, and a complex relationship exists between the binding of these various ligands. This is physiologically highly advantageous and has the result that when oxygenated blood from the lungs reaches the tissues where H^+ and CO_2 are being produced, the combined effects of the lower O_2 tension and higher H^+ and CO_2 concentrations ensure that O_2 is released in appropriate amounts while, at the same time, CO_2 is taken up. The promotion of O_2 dissociation by an increase in CO_2 tension and therefore of acidity is known as the *Bohr Effect* and is illustrated in Figure 25.1.

The effect of 2,3-diphosphoglycerate

The concentration of 2,3-diphosphoglycerate which is derived from the glycolytic intermediate 1,3-diphosphoglycerate is higher in red corpuscles than in other cells. 2,3-Diphosphoglycerate binds specifically to deoxyhaemoglobin and reduces its O_2 affinity so that binding of O_2 and 2,3-diphosphoglycerate are mutually exclusive. The 2,3-diphosphoglycerate binds to the central cavity of the haemoglobin molecule which is lined by numerous positively charged groups and crosslinks the two β subunits. But, when the haemoglobin is oxygenated, the central cavity is reduced in size and the 2,3-diphosphoglycerate is extruded.

The effect of the 2,3-diphosphoglycerate is to regulate the O_2 binding affinity of haemoglobin in relation to the partial pressure in the lungs. This is of special importance in circumstances when the O_2 tension is low, as for example at high altitudes or in patients suffering from hypoxia, i.e. when either the lungs or the circulatory system are not operating efficiently. In such cases the 2,3-diphosphoglycerate concentration in the blood increases and this allows the haemoglobin to release its O_2 more readily.

The uptake of O_2 by the fetus from the maternal blood is made possible by the fact that fetal haemoglobin (HbF page 371) binds 2,3-diphosphoglycerate less strongly than the maternal haemoglobin (HbA) and consequently has a higher affinity for oxygen.

The modifying effects of O_2, CO_2, H^+ and 2,3-diphosphoglycerate on the properties of haemoglobin provide a good illustration of the extra functional dimension conferred by the evolution of the quaternary level of protein structure.

The role of haemoglobin in carbon dioxide transport

As already stated when oxygenated blood from the lungs reaches the tissues where acid metabolites are being produced, oxyhaemoglobin tends to lose O_2 and the combined effects of the lower O_2 and higher CO_2 tensions ensure that O_2 is released in appropriate amounts.

Haemoglobin plays a part in the carriage of CO_2 from the tissues to the lungs in two ways:

1. It combines directly with the CO_2 which reacts with free amino groups to form *carbamino compounds*.

$$R-NH_2 + CO_2 \rightleftharpoons R-NH-COOH$$
Carbamino compound

This reaction is not peculiar to haemoglobin and all proteins with free amino groups will react in this way. The important point about haemoglobin is that the degree to which the reaction takes place depends almost entirely on its state of oxygenation and hardly at all on the CO_2 tension. Thus deoxyhaemoglobin readily forms carbamino compounds but when it is converted to oxyhaemoglobin most of the CO_2 is released. Although only about 5% of the total CO_2 in venous blood is present in the form of *carbaminohaemoglobin* it represents a very labile form of CO_2 and may account for as much as 30% of the CO_2 that is taken up in the tissues and released in the lungs.

2. It has a buffering effect. When haemoglobin, which is notably rich in histidine, is oxygenated the resulting conformational changes increase the tendency for specific protonated histidine residues to lose H^+, i.e. their pK value in oxyhaemoglobin is 7·16 compared with 7·3 in deoxyhaemoglobin. Thus, in the lungs, the proportion of HbO_2 is increased and that of HHb is reduced. Conversely, in the tissues, deoxyhaemoglobin binds H^+; at the same time the plasma bicarbonate is increased (see the next paragraph). In this way a large proportion of the acid produced in the course of the tissue metabolism is carried as H^+ by haemoglobin in the corpuscles and as bicarbonate in the plasma.

Formation of carbonic acid from H_2O and CO_2 is a relatively slow process, but within the corpuscles it is speeded up by the presence of the enzyme *carbonic anhydrase*. As a result the concentration of bicarbonate ions rises more rapidly in the corpuscles than in the plasma and some of them leave the corpuscles in exchange for chloride ions. This chloride–bicarbonate exchange ensures that a large fraction of the acidic CO_2 produced in the tissues is carried as plasma bicarbonate. Consequently there is very little increase in the acidity of venous blood.

It can be calculated that, if the respiratory quotient is 0·7 (i.e. 1 volume of O_2 is utilized for every 0·7 volume of CO_2 produced), all the H^+ resulting from the conversion of $CO_2 + H_2O \rightarrow H_2CO_3 \rightarrow H^+ + HCO_3^-$ can be buffered by haemoglobin without any alteration in pH. However, since the respiratory quotient is usually greater than 0·7, other blood buffer systems, notably the Na_2HPO_4/NaH_2PO_4 system, also operate to keep the pH change within narrow limits.

The overall process of CO_2 uptake and O_2 release can be represented as follows:

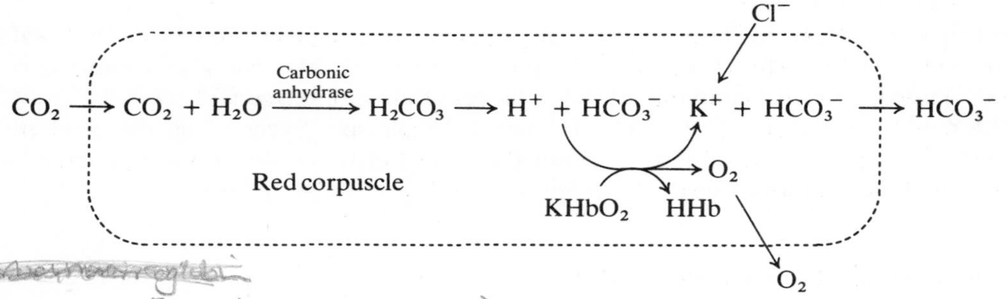

The role of the plasma bicarbonate in acid–base regulation

In addition to the 13 mol or so of CO_2 produced each day most of which is buffered by haemoglobin, small amounts of certain non-volatile acids are produced. These usually account for rather less than 0·1 mol of H^+ per day and, since they cannot be eliminated through the lungs, they must be excreted via the kidneys. The non-volatile acids include sulphuric acid, formed by oxidation of the sulphur present in cysteine and methionine, phosphoric acid from phospholipids and phosphoproteins, and lactic acid produced during severe exercise. Appreciable amounts of acetoacetic acid and β-hydroxybutyric acid are released into the blood in ketosis. All these acids are buffered by the plasma bicarbonate according to the following reaction:

$$HA + NaHCO_3 \longrightarrow NaA + H_2CO_3$$
$$\downarrow$$
$$H_2O + CO_2 \longrightarrow Lungs$$

The carbonic acid which is produced causes a fall in the $NaHCO_3/H_2CO_3$ ratio and a slight drop in the pH of the blood. The overall effect is to stimulate the respiratory centre of the brain causing an increase in pulmonary ventilation so that the extra CO_2 is lost from the lungs and the normal $NaHCO_3/H_2CO_3$ ratio is restored. However, in the course of the reaction some of the plasma bicarbonate has been used up so that, although the $NaHCO_3/H_2CO_3$ ratio and pH are normal, the plasma bicarbonate is reduced. The responsibility for regulating the absolute amount of bicarbonate in the plasma belongs to the kidney (page 395).

Disturbances of acid–base balance

In spite of the variety and efficiency of the body's mechanisms for maintaining a constant pH, disturbances of acid–base balance can and do occur. They may result from gross dietary imbalance, and also from respiratory, metabolic or renal disorders in which there is either too great a production or a failure of elimination of acid or base.

Acidosis is a fairly common condition in which the total concentration of buffer base (chiefly HCO_3^-) is less than normal; *alkalosis* in which the total concentration of buffer base is greater than normal (i.e. HCO_3^-/H_2CO_3 is increased) is far less common. It may occur when diets containing large amounts of vegetables are consumed, as a result of hyperventilation or of continuous vomiting, and after taking alkalizing salts such as potassium citrate and sodium lactate. In these circumstances the increased alkalinity of the blood reaching the brain causes respiration to be depressed so that less CO_2 is lost from the lungs. This causes a build-up in P_{CO_2}, and the plasma H_2CO_3 rises until the normal HCO_3^-/H_2CO_3 ratio is restored but there is still an increase in total concentration of buffer base. This is reduced to normal by excretion of $NaHCO_3$ by the kidney. Owing to the interplay of the various regulatory mechanisms such conditions are complicated and may be confused by ambiguous terminology.

In prolonged acidosis in which there is a reduction in the pH of the blood, calcium may be drawn from the bones and some of the Na^+ of the urine replaced by Ca^{2+}. Although this use of calcium phosphate to neutralize acid is extremely efficient in preventing excessive depletion of the plasma bicarbonate, demineralization of the hard tissues does not do them any good!

Haemoglobin derivatives

A large number of haemoglobin derivatives are known, some of which occur naturally. The following are among the most important.

Methaemoglobin

In order that haemoglobin may combine reversibly with O_2, its iron must be present in the ferrous (Fe^{2+}) state. If the haem is oxidized to the corresponding ferric derivative *haematin*, a new pigment known as *methaemoglobin* is produced. Methaemoglobin is brown in colour and, although it contains O_2, it is unable to release it in the tissues. Methaemoglobin is not normally found in the blood in appreciable amounts since blood contains the enzyme *methaemoglobin reductase* which reduces it to haemoglobin. *Methaemoglobinaemia* may result from exposure to agents which oxidize Fe^{2+} to Fe^{3+} including amyl nitrite, nitrates, nitrobenzene and drugs such as salicylates, phenacetin and the sulphonamides.

Carboxyhaemoglobin

Haemoglobin has an affinity for carbon monoxide which is 200 or more times that for oxygen. This means that if blood is exposed to a mixture of 1 part of CO and 200 parts of O_2 approximately equal amounts of *carboxyhaemoglobin* and oxyhaemoglobin will be formed. Because of the great stability of carboxyhaemoglobin, the blood is deprived of its O_2-carrying power and, when 60–80% of the haemoglobin has been converted into this form, death occurs due to O_2 lack. Carboxyhaemoglobin has a bright cherry-red colour which is quite different from the orange–red of oxyhaemoglobin and the purple-red of deoxyhaemoglobin. The pink and healthy-looking colour of victims of carbon monoxide poisoning is very distinctive and is a useful diagnostic feature.

Cyan-methaemoglobin and sulph-methaemoglobin

The toxic effects of cyanide and sulphide are chiefly due to combination of these substances with the Fe^{3+} of cytochrome oxidase so that the final reaction of the respiratory chain is blocked. Cyanide and sulphide, however, also have the effect of converting haemoglobin into *cyan-methaemoglobin* and *sulph-methaemoglobin* respectively. Both are stable compounds and once formed can only be removed by complete degradation. Cyan-methaemoglobin is used as a stable and reproducible standard in haemoglobin estimations.

Plasma proteins

Normal human plasma contains a very complex mixture of proteins amounting to about 7·0–7·5 g/100 ml. Structural and physicochemical data are available on 22 distinct human plasma proteins. A host of others are known to be present in low concentrations and to have important biological functions, but they have not yet been isolated.

For clinical investigations of the plasma proteins serum is commonly used instead of plasma since fibrinogen and fibrin tend to interfere with some of the tests. The serum proteins are usually separated on a variety of materials when five distinct fractions are produced. These are albumin and the α_1, α_2, β and γ globulin fractions. Typical electrophoretic patterns for normal serum are shown in Figure 25.3 and the percentage composition of the total plasma proteins in Table 25.1.

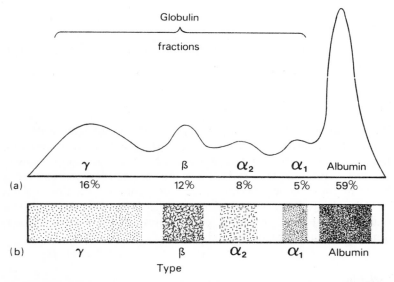

Figure 25.3 Electrophoresis patterns for normal human serum. (a) Stained strip; (b) densitometric scan of strip

The plasma proteins function generally:

1. In the maintenance of normal osmotic relationships between the blood and interstitial fluid.
2. As buffers.
3. As a reservoir of body protein maintaining equilibrium with the tissue proteins.
4. In the transport of substances that are not otherwise soluble in plasma.

Some of the proteins have specialized functions, for example in immunological reactions and blood clotting.

Table 25.1 Plasma protein fractions (approximate values)

		g/100 ml		% of total
Albumin		4·0		55·8
Globulins				
α_1	0·35		4·9	
α_2	0·60	2·9	8·4	40·0
β	0·78		10·4	
γ	1·17		16·3	
Fibrinogen		0·3		4·2
Total		7·2		100·0

Most of the plasma proteins are glycoproteins and, except for the γ-globulins that are synthesized in lymphoid tissue and the widely distributed cells of the reticuloendothelial system, they are synthesized in the liver. They exist in equilibrium with the tissue proteins and are subject to continuous catabolism and replacement. Nevertheless, homologous plasma proteins (i.e. plasma proteins derived from the same species) appear able to pass into the tissue cells without prior degradation. No particular organ has been shown to be the sole site of catabolism of any one plasma protein.

Albumin

Although 20 or so variants have been described, the major form of albumin in the plasma is a single-chain protein containing 610 amino acid residues which has a molecular weight of 69 000 and is present in plasma at a concentration of between 3·4 and 4·5 g/100 ml. It accounts for rather more than 50% of the total plasma protein and, because of its high concentration and low molecular weight, is largely responsible for the colloid osmotic pressure.

Albumin has a great avidity for anions and transports a wide variety of substances including fatty acids, bile acids, uric acid and bilirubin as well as Cu^{2+}, Ca^{2+} and Zn^{2+}. It also combines with a number of drugs including aspirin, barbiturates, penicillin and sulphonamides and mops up excess vitamin A and C as well as histamine and various steroids.

The globulins

The globulin fraction comprises a very complex mixture of hundreds of proteins some of which are listed in Table 25.1. Most of the plasma fat is found as lipoprotein in the α and β fractions. The protein component provides a vehicle for the transport of the water-insoluble material.

Two well-recognized metal-binding proteins are found among the globulins. The first of these is *transferrin* (page 144) which is the principal β-globulin of plasma and the second is the blue–green copper-containing α_2-globulin known as *ceruloplasmin*.

The *haptoglobins* are a heterogeneous group of α_2-globulins which readily combine with haemoglobin. Their function may be to remove haemoglobin from sites of tissue damage and hence to prevent the loss of valuable iron from the body and possible renal damage.

Immunoglobulins

The immune system is concerned with the 'self-identity' of the body and in Man consists of about 10^{12} lymphocytes which secrete proteins called *antibodies*. At an early stage in development the haemopoietic stem cells differentiate and produce two distinct types of lymphocyte. The production of *T-lymphocytes* is dependent on the thymus and these lymphocytes mediate the cellular type of immunity which is responsible for tissue incompatability and the rejection of tissue grafts. By contrast, the *B-lymphocytes* are independent of the thymus and are the precursors of the plasma cells which produce the antibodies. B-lymphocytes and their antibodies circulate in the bloodstream, enter the tissues through the capillary walls and return to the blood by the lymphatic vessels. The antibodies belong to a group of structurally related proteins called *immuno-* or *gamma-globulins*.

The immune response

During the immune response a specific antibody is synthesized as a result of the presence in the body of a foreign macromolecule which acts as an *antigen* or *immunogen*. Innumerable types of large molecule, both natural and synthetic, behave as antigens and cause the production of specific antibodies. The body is also able to form antibodies to small molecules provided that they are attached to a protein carrier of high molecular weight. The small molecule is known as a *hapten* and quite minor changes in its structure can upset the recognition process. The antibody and antigen molecules bind together to form a precipitate which is subsequently removed by phagocytosis so that the immune response provides resistance to infection. The nature of the antigen–antibody reaction has not yet been fully determined but, since size is an important factor, it seems probable that a large number of contacts between the antigen and antibody molecules is required.

The normal human body contains an immense variety of circulating antibodies each able to react with one specific antigen. The immunoglobulins can be divided into five structurally related groups, IgA, IgD, IgE, IgG and IgM; of these, immunoglobulins of the IgG type are present in by far the greatest amount (Table 25.2).

Table 25.2 Types of immunoglobulin

Immunoglobulin	Concentration in serum (mg ml^{-1})	Function
IgG	9–17	Main antibody in serum (80% of total) and gingival fluid
IgA	1·2–1·4	Main antibody in saliva, tears and mucus
IgM	0·5–2·0	Early antibody in serum
IgD	0·03–0·4	Not known
IgE	0·001	Involved in allergic reactions

Immunoglobulins of the IgG type have a molecular weight of about 160 000 and are composed of two light (i.e. short) chains containing 214 amino acid residues and two heavy (i.e. long) chains containing 446 residues. The chains are joined by –S–S– bonds as shown in Figure 25.4. They also possess a large number of intrachain –S–S–bonds. The *C*-terminal portions of both L (light) and H (heavy) chains have constant regions representing about half of the L chain (residues 109–214) and about three-quarters of the H chain, while the remaining *N*-terminal portions show major variations in their constituent amino acids (Figure 25.5). The specificity of antibodies is inherent in the variable parts of the L and H chains both of which are involved in the recognition and binding of the antigen.

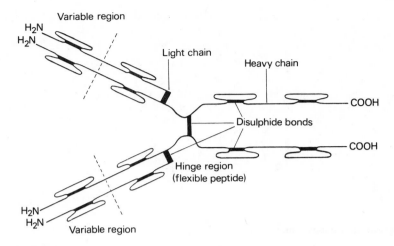

Figure 25.4 Schematic representation of an immunoglobulin (IgG) molecule

The immunoglobulin molecules which have a Y-shape and two identical binding sites are able to link molecules of antigen together to form an unreactive aggregate as shown in Figure 25.6. The Y-shape of the molecules gives a 'hinge' effect so that the distance between the two binding sites may be varied, thus increasing the efficiency of interaction with foreign substances of different shapes and sizes.

When the antigen is a foreign cell, the binding of antibody by antigenic sites on the cell surface is followed by the binding of one of a group of plasma proteins collectively known as *complement*

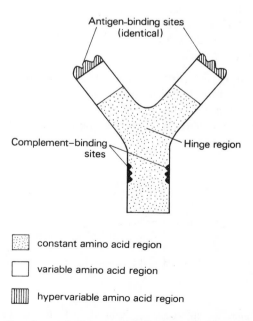

Figure 25.5 The location of binding sites on the immunoglobulin molecule (shown on Figure)

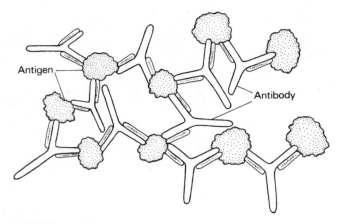

Figure 25.6 An antigen–antibody complex

(Figure 25.7). This triggers a cascade of reactions that causes cell lysis and phagocytosis (Figure 25.8). The sequence involves the activation of enzyme precursors by proteolysis and peptide release. Many of the peptides released in this process possess pharmacological activity attracting phagocytes by chemotaxis, while the C5c peptide promotes histamine release and increased vascular permeability.

Antibody molecules are all alike except for differences in the amino acids in the variable regions of their chains. These regions contain the antigen-binding sites and it is an almost endless variation in their amino acid composition that provides the very large number of antibodies needed to recognize so many different antigens.

Any one lymphocyte contains four antibody genes coding for:

1. The variable region of the short chain
2. The variable region of the long chain
3. The constant region of the short chain
4. The constant region of the long chain.

Different lymphocytes contain different variable region genes which are thought to have been produced by a large number of random mutations and recombinations, which continually occur during multiplication of the lymphocytes.

The high degree of antigen specificity as well as the memory and power of self-recognition

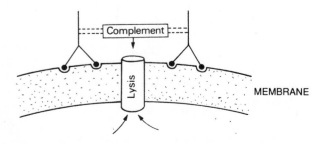

Figure 25.7 The binding of complement to two adjacent antibody molecules on a bacterial surface leading to the loss of cytoplasmic constituents by phospholipase activity

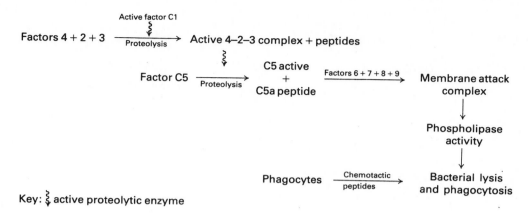

Figure 25.8 Cascade of reactions causing cell lysis and phagocytosis

which characterize the humoral immune response have led to the *clonal selection theory of antibody production*, which states the following.

1. Most lymphocytes are immature, i.e. in a resting state, and do not secrete antibody.
2. Each immature lymphocyte contains a unique set of genes that code for one antibody. Thus any one cell produces only one type of antibody and the information for the synthesis of this antibody is present before the cell encounters the antigen.
3. Each B-lymphocyte, as it matures, produces small amounts of antibody bound to the cell surface. These are known as labelled lymphocytes and their surface antibodies act as antigen receptors. If and when they encounter the appropriate antigen, usually brought to them by macrophages, the lymphocytes are stimulated to grow, change in structure and divide.
4. Stimulated lymphocytes are called *plasma cells* and the identical descendants of any one cell are called a *clone*. A clone of plasma cells produces large amounts of one type of antibody against the antigen which initiated the division of the parent lymphocyte.
5. A few clone cells persist after the disappearance of the antigen. These cells can still be stimulated by the antigen if it ever reappears, and represent an immunological 'memory' which lasts for the lifetime of the individual. Such a renewed stimulation leads to a *secondary response*, i.e. the rapid production of large amounts of the original antibody, the individual being *immune* to that particular antigen (Figure 25.9).
6. Lymphocytes do not produce antibodies against the body's own macromolecules and can, therefore, distinguish between self and non-self. This distinction appears to have been 'learned' in the embryo by the destruction in the thymus of all lymphocytes that have produced self-recognizing antibodies.

The clonal selection theory implies that the B-lymphocytes do not use antigenic information to construct antibodies but that the amino acid sequences of the antigen-binding sites are inherent in the genome. The production of genes that can code for millions of different antibodies, only a few of which are ever used, seems an extremely wasteful process. However, the random generation of different patterns or variations, only some of which are selected, is the basis of Darwin's theory of evolution, and antibody production by a clone descended from one stimulated lymphocyte is an example of the 'survival of the fittest'.

The invaluable protection provided by the immune system against a great variety of hazards may be judged by the devastating effects of AIDS (acquired immune deficiency syndrome). This

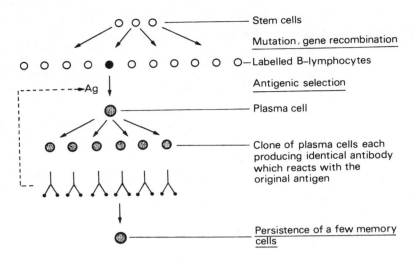

Figure 25.9 The progress of the humoral immune response illustrating antigenic selectivity, clone formation and memory

is caused by a retroviral infection which infects and destroys specific lymphocytes, causing permanent damage to the immune system and making the patient highly susceptible to opportunist bacterial infections.

Immunoglobulins of the IgG type are found in external secretions such as saliva and the lachrymal, nasal, bronchial and intestinal secretions. They may be important in creating an immune barrier against microorganisms at exposed surfaces. The role of salivary IgG and crevicular fluid IgG in protection against dental diseases is discussed in Chapter 36.

The other family of lymphocytes, the T-lymphocytes, which are dependent on the thymus gland, do not secrete appreciable amounts of free antibody but are involved in *cell-mediated immunity* and lead to the production of differentiated cells. These are active against foreign cells, usually bacteria and transplanted tissues; they produce soluble *lymphokines* which attract other lymphocytes, macrophages and polymorphonuclear leucocytes to the site of infection or introduction. The foreign cells which become coated with antibody are destroyed by complement and removed by phagocytosis, a process known as *opsonization*. In addition, there are memory T-cells and regulatory T-cells which control the conversion of B-lymphocytes into plasma cells and are involved in the process of self-recognition.

Monoclonal antibodies

Antibodies have for many years been used in protein identification since they have the advantage of species specificity and can, for example, distinguish between the blood of humans and that of other species. However, methods based on the immune response have, until recently, been unpredictable because of the heterogeneity of the antibody preparations. The reasons for this are twofold. (1) Most macromolecules possess a number of different antigenic groups or *antigenic determinants* and stimulate the expansion of a number of different B-lymphocyte clones (page 308) and (2) a single antigenic determinant can stimulate several B-lymphocyte clones which synthesize antibodies with slightly different specificities, i.e. the response is polyclonal and a number of different antibodies are produced. Recently, however, by using *cell hybridization*, i.e. cell fusion techniques, it has been possible, in certain instances, to produce large amounts of homogeneous antibody derived from a single B-lymphocyte clone which is committed to the production of a single type of antibody molecule.

B-lymphocytes are obtained from the spleen of an animal, usually a mouse, which has been previously inoculated with an appropriate highly purified antigen. These are then incubated with myeloma cells which are a cell line of neoplastic (cancerous) B-lymphocytes maintained in pure culture in the laboratory. Under appropriate conditions, the spleen and myeloma cells fuse together to produce a hybrid cell called a *hybridoma*. The culture conditions are such that the unfused spleen and myeloma cells die leaving a variety of hybridomas each capable of producing antibody. A single hybridoma which produces antibody to the original antigen can be identified by reaction with radiolabelled antigen, and then isolated and grown in pure culture to produce a clone. Large quantities of antibody can then be produced by large-scale cell culture.

Monoclonal antibodies have now been produced against a wide range of medically important antigens such as serum proteins, enzymes, cell surface receptors, hormones, drugs, viruses and tumour-specific antigens. Their extreme specificity means that the antibody will react with only one particular target molecule such as a drug or hormone, which can then be identified in very low concentrations in the tissues.

Haemostasis

In higher animals the evolution of a cardiovascular system in which the circulation of the blood is maintained by large pressure differences brings with it the hazard of fatal haemorrhage if the wall of a blood vessel should be ruptured. As a consequence the simultaneous evolution of means for stopping excessive loss of blood became essential for survival and the higher vertebrates have evolved extremely sophisticated *haemostatic mechanisms*. The control of haemorrhage is the result of three different types of response, namely the vascular response which comes in the province of physiology rather than biochemistry and will not be dealt with here, the platelet response and the clotting of the blood.

The latter solidification process, which occurs when blood comes into contact with virtually any surface other than the endothelial lining of the blood vessels, takes about 5 min at room temperature and rather less at body temperature.

The *fibrin* that constitutes the fibrous material of the clot is formed from its precursor *fibrinogen*, a protein occurring in normal plasma at a level of about 0·3%. It is remarkable that a soluble protein present in such low concentration is nevertheless able, in a matter of a few minutes, to become transformed into a finely ramified insoluble meshwork which causes a local conversion of the blood into a smooth firm jelly. The conversion of fibrinogen into insoluble fibrin, in fact, provides a good model of fibre formation in the body.

The platelet response

When a blood vessel is ruptured the platelets respond very rapidly and form a platelet plug. Blood normally contains about 250 000 platelets mm^{-3} and they have a life-span of 8–10 days. Platelets are anucleate cell fragments 2–4 μm in diameter which are derived from the megakaryocytes. They are disc shaped and contain many granules that store physiologically active substances. When the endothelial lining of the blood vessels is intact the platelets circulate freely but, when the endothelium is damaged, they attach to the foreign surfaces and notably to exposed collagen fibres. This attachment causes the release within 1–3 s of a number of active substances, including ADP which causes the platelets to change shape and send out sticky processes so that they clump together and adhere to the wounded area. They also produce *serotonin* (5-hydroxytryptamine) and *thromboxane* which cause constriction of the blood vessels and thus restrict the flow of blood. The thromboxane facilitates further platelet clumping so that the whole process is self-promoting and very rapid, a platelet plug being formed within 10–20 s. The time taken for the formation of such a plug after submitting a patient to a standardized cut is known as the *bleeding time* and is used to test for abnormalities of haemostasis.

The platelets release further substances including a *platelet-derived growth factor* (page 366) and *clot retraction factor* (page 392). The importance of the platelets is apparent from the seriousness of the condition of *thrombocytopenia* in which they are deficient.

The fibrin clot

The platelet plug is fragile and only a temporary means of arresting the flow of blood and its formation is rapidly followed by the production of a fibrin clot. During the clotting process *fibrinogen*, which is very soluble, undergoes partial proteolysis and the resulting *fibrin* molecules then associate spontaneously to form a meshwork which encloses the blood corpuscles and serum. *Serum* may be defined as the pale yellow liquid that can be expressed from clotted blood.

Fibrinogen is formed in the liver and is found in the globulin fraction of the plasma proteins. It is a large dimeric protein (molecular weight 333 000) with a high axial (length/width) ratio and a considerable content of α-helix. Under the electron microscope the molecules appear as three globules strung together, the central globule being smaller than the terminal ones.

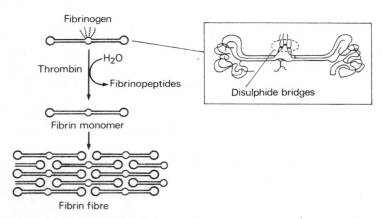

Figure 25.10 Fibrinogen and its conversion to fibrin

The monomers, which are joined together in the central globule, are made up of three polypeptide chains (αA, βB and γ) linked together by disulphide bonds (Figure 25.10). Each end of the molecule carries a strong negative charge so that the individual molecules repel one another. Fibrinogen is converted into fibrin by the enzyme *thrombin* which is a serine protease (page 86) and is similar to trypsin, chymotrypsin and elastase not only in its overall molecular shape and composition but also in the amino acids that constitute the active site. During the conversion of fibrinogen into fibrin, four -Arg-Gly- bonds are cleaved and two pairs of *fibrinopeptides* (A and B) are released from the terminal globules. The fibrinopeptides removed from the αA and βB chains constitute about 3% of the original fibrinogen molecule. They contain a number of glutamic, aspartic and sialic acid residues and, once these have been removed from the molecules, their strong negative repelling charge is lost. Fibre formation then occurs spontaneously as a result of the end-to-end and side-to-side aggregation of the newly formed fibrin molecules.

Fibrin stabilization

When the fibrin molecules first aggregate the clot is soft and can be fairly readily dispersed; thus fresh fibrin differs appreciably in character from the stable and insoluble material of the typical clot. Studies on highly purified fibrinogen solutions have shown that a factor known as the *fibrin-stabilizing factor*, FSF or Factor XIII$_a$, is necessary for the formation of the covalent bonds that give fibrin its characteristic properties. Factor XIII$_a$ is present in plasma in precursor form (Factor XIII) and is activated by thrombin in the presence of Ca^{2+}. Its action is to join the ε-amino group of a lysine residue in one fibrin molecule in peptide linkage with a glutaminyl residue in an adjacent molecule (Figure 25.11). Factor XIII$_a$ is therefore a trans-amidase which unites the fibrin monomers into a branched polymeric network of great insolubility and tensile strength.

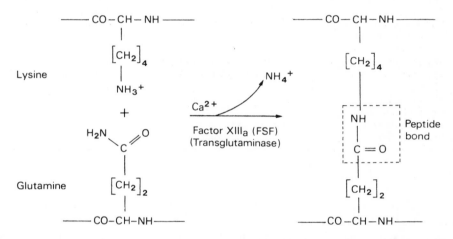

Figure 25.11 The stabilization of fibrin by the formation of peptide bonds between lysyl and glutaminyl side chains

The clotting cascade

For a clot to be formed, sufficient thrombin (Factor II$_a$) must be present at the site of injury but, at the same time, active clotting factors cannot circulate in the blood in concentrations that would allow clotting to occur. The dilemma is solved by having many of the clotting factors present in an inactive precursor form which is activated only as and when required. The clotting process is an *enzyme cascade* involving a series of hydrolytic reactions in which the product of one reaction acts as the enzyme for the next.

The process is confined to the area of the wound because at a number of points the reactions take place on surfaces provided by the everted phospholipid membranes of activated platelets and damaged endothelial cells.

A list of the numerous enzymes and cofactors involved in blood clotting is given in Table 25.3. These are usually known by a factor number using roman numerals and, since both an active and an inactive form exist, the active form is given the subscript a. This terminology has already been used for the fibrin-stabilizing factor, Factor XIII$_a$, and for thrombin, Factor II$_a$. Sometimes a factor has an alternative name which is usually either that of the patient in which a defect in the factor was first recognized or the worker who first described the defect. Where such names are

Table 25.3 Summary of human blood-clotting factors

Factor		Function of active form	Deficiency disorder
I	Fibrinogen	Precursor of fibrin	Hypofibrinogenaemia Afibrinogenaemia
II	Prothrombin	Hydrolyses fibrinogen Activates Factors XIII, V, VIII and Protein C	Hypoprothrombinaemia
III	Tissue Factor Tissue thromboplastin	Lipoprotein complex needed to bind Factors VII_a and X	—
IV	Calcium ions	Cofactor for several reactions	—
V	Proaccelerin	Protein cofactor for Factor X_a	Parahaemophilia
VII	Proconvertin	Hydolyses Factor X	Hypoproconvertinaemia
VIII	Antihaemophilic Factor	Protein cofactor for Factor IX_a	Classic haemophilia Haemophilia A
IX	Plasma thromboplastin component (PTC) Christmas Factor	Hydrolyses Factor X	Haemophilia B Christmas disease
X	Stuart Factor	Hydrolyses prothrombin	—
XI	Plasma thromboplastin antecedent (PTR)	Hydrolyses Factor IX	Haemophilia C PTA defect
XII	Hageman Factor Contact Factor	Hydrolyses Factor XI	Hageman trait
XIII	Fibrin-stabilizing Factor (FSF)	Catalyses the cross-linking of fibrin molecules	—

Notes: (1) Factor III is not a single factor
(2) There is no factor VI

sometimes used they are shown in the table. Fibrinogen, thrombin and tissue factor are exceptions to the above terminology and are commonly known as such.

The series of activating reactions that is ultimately responsible for the conversion of fibrinogen to fibrin produces a major amplification effect, which can be explained as follows.

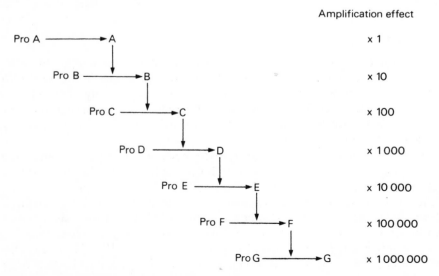

	Amplification effect
Pro A → A	× 1
Pro B → B	× 10
Pro C → C	× 100
Pro D → D	× 1 000
Pro E → E	× 10 000
Pro F → F	× 100 000
Pro G → G	× 1 000 000

Figure 25.12 The amplification effect of an enzyme cascade

Since one molecule of enzyme usually catalyses the transformation of a number of substrate molecules, the reactions of such a sequence progress geometrically. If one assumes that in each case 1 molecule of enzyme acts on 10 molecules of substrate, it can be seen from Figure 25.12 that, after a two-stage process, 1 molecule of initial enzyme A would be responsible for the production of 100 molecules of product C while after a six-stage process one million molecules of active substance G would be produced. This effect would explain the relatively long latent period before clotting takes place and then the sudden explosive production of fibrin.

All the enzymes involved in the formation of the initial fibrin clot are serine proteases with substrate specificities that are much higher than those of trypsin and chymotrypsin. They are synthesized and circulate in the blood in zymogen form.

The intrinsic pathway

The intrinsic pathway is so called because all the factors involved are present in the plasma in an active or inactive form. Initiation of the pathway occurs when a blood vessel is damaged and the exposed subendothelial surface binds the zymogen, Factor XII (*Hageman factor*). The contact causes the protein to undergo a conformational change which enables it to convert *prekallikrein* to *kallikrein*. Kallikrein is a protease which is complexed in plasma with a protein cofactor known as *HMW Kininogen* (high molecular weight kininogen). The enzyme–cofactor complex acts upon Factor XII cleaving it into a large unreactive peptide and the smaller serine protease Factor XII$_a$. Factor XII$_a$ then converts Factor XI into its active form (Factor XI$_a$). HMW Kininogen is also complexed to Factor XI in the circulation and stimulates the activation. Once it has been activated the surface-bound Factor XI$_a$ cleaves Factor IX (*Christmas Factor*) to produce its active form in a reaction that requires Ca^{2+} ions.

Factor IX$_a$ is responsible for activating Factor X in a reaction that is enhanced some 10^4–10^5 times by the presence of three accessory factors. These are a charged phospholipid surface, e.g. everted platelet membrane, Ca^{2+} ions and a very large auxiliary protein, Factor VIII$_a$ (*antihaemophilic factor*) which circulates in the blood in an inactive form. This complex of proteins, Ca^{2+} and phospholipids is sometimes referred to as *tenase* since it converts Factor X into its active form (Factor X$_a$).

Factor X$_a$, in combination with Factor V$_a$ and Ca^{2+} and in the presence of a phospholipid membrane, acts as a *prothrombinase* which finally converts prothrombin to thrombin (Figure

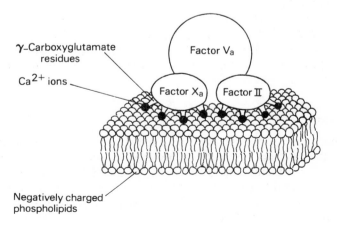

Figure 25.13 The role of phospholipids in the conversion of prothrombin to thrombin

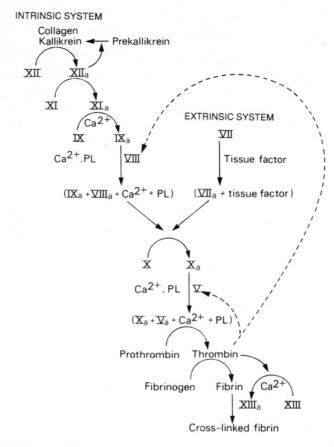

Figure 25.14 Cascade mechanism of blood coagulation. PL, phospholipid

25.13). Factor V, like Factor VIII, is not an enzyme but a very large protein cofactor that requires cleavage before it becomes functional.

It can be seen from Figure 25.14 that, apart from its major role in the conversion of fibrinogen to fibrin, thrombin has an activating effect on both Factor V and Factor VIII and in this way stimulates its own production. Thrombin is also a platelet activator and increases both the size of the platelet plug and the release of platelet constituents. It also activates the fibrin-stabilizing factor (XIII) in the presence of Ca^{2+} ions.

The extrinsic pathway

There is a second means by which Factor X can be activated known as the extrinsic pathway. The name derives from the fact that the pathway involves a *tissue factor* (Factor III) which is not present in the blood. Tissue factor is shed by the membrane of damaged cells and is a lipoprotein complex which provides a protein cofactor and also a surface on which Factor VII can activate Factor X in the presence of Ca^{2+} (Figure 25.14). Factor X_a increases its own production by activating Factor VII.

Clot formation mediated by the extrinsic pathway occurs much more rapidly than when mediated by the intrinsic pathway. Normally, of course, the two pathways operate in conjunction and are connected since Factor VII$_a$ can activate Factor IX as well as Factor X.

As mentioned on page 160, vitamin K is needed for the formation of the active forms of Factors II (prothrombin), VII, IX and X. The plasma of vitamin K-deficient animals usually contains normal levels of their zymogens but clotting is, nevertheless, impaired. The clotting abnormality is due to the inability of the deficient animals to convert certain glutamate molecules in the zymogens into γ-carboxyglutamate. This has a double negative charge and high affinity for Ca^{2+} ions. As stated above, Ca^{2+} ions and membrane phospholipids or lipo-proteins are necessary for the formation of the tenase, prothrombinase and Factor VII–tissue factor complexes. The formation of γ-carboxyglutamyl residues clustered at one end of the protein molecules enables them to bind tightly to the membrane through a calcium link (Figure 25.15) and hence to increase the rate of activation.

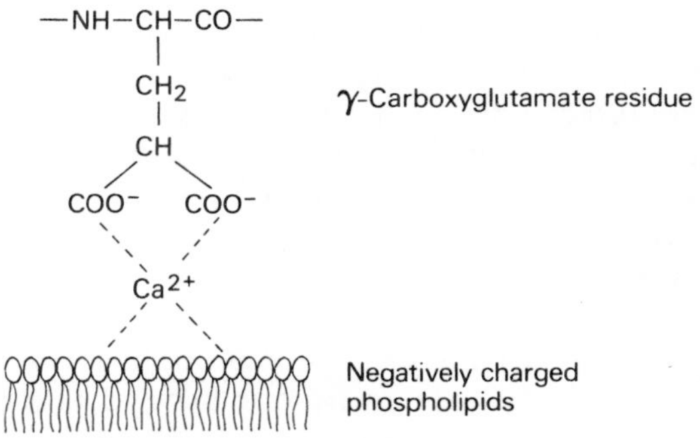

Figure 25.15 Binding of proteins containing γ-carboxyglutamate to phospholipids

Switching off the clotting process

Clot formation takes about 5 min depending on the size and position of the wound after which it is necessary to stop the process. Switching off the production of fibrin is achieved by negative feedback, i.e. inactivation of the activated factors. Thrombin, the last protease in the cascade, binds to a receptor protein known as *thrombomodulin* present on the endothelial wall of the blood vessels. This alters the thrombin so that it can no longer activate fibrinogen but instead activates another vitamin K-dependent serine protease known as *Protein C*. This, in the presence of Ca^{2+} and a protein cofactor, binds to a phospholipid membrane and forms a complex which inactivates Factors V$_a$ and VII$_a$ both of which are needed for the production of thrombin.

A further means of inactivating the proteases of the clotting cascade is provided by a number of protease inhibitors which are present in circulating blood. The two most important are *antithrombin*, which binds tightly to thrombin and can also scavenge Factors IX$_a$, X$_a$ and XI$_a$ when free in solution, and α-*antitrypsin*, which will inactivate Factor X$_a$ even when it is bound to a phospholipid membrane. Activated clotting intermediates may also be removed by the liver and to a lesser extent by other tissues.

The prevention of blood clotting

Any calcium chelating agent, e.g. citrate or EDTA, added to blood or plasma will prevent clotting as it prevents the formation of the necessary protein–phospholipid complexes. Such substances are useful for the prevention of clotting *in vitro*. Sodium citrate is also used in the preservation of blood for transfusion purposes. Clotting may also be prevented by certain natural anticoagulants such as *hirudin* which is obtained from the mouth glands of the leech and some snake venoms. Clinically the most commonly used anticoagulant is *heparin* which is a highly sulphated, and therefore acidic, polysaccharide related to chondroitin sulphate (page 408). Heparin is formed and stored in the mast cells present in the walls of blood vessels and in the connective tissue surrounding capillaries. It can be used either *in vivo* or *in vitro*. It is very powerful and acts very quickly but it has to be given by injection at fairly frequent intervals. A valuable feature, however, is that, should the patient show a dangerous tendency to haemorrhage, the heparin can be neutralized by injection of protamine sulphate which carries a strong positive charge. *Ancrod*, which is obtained from the Malayan pit viper and some other snake venoms, is slower acting than heparin. Ancrod removes fibrinopeptide A from the αA chain of fibrinogen but has no effect on the βB chain. Consequently very small clots are formed which are easily degraded by an enzyme present in the venom. In this way the level of fibrinogen in the blood is lowered and the risk of unwanted stable clot formation is reduced. A daily injection of the venom is required for this type of therapy.

Heparin and ancrod are direct-acting anticoagulants which must be given by injection. For long-term therapy certain coumarin derivatives may be given by mouth. One of these, namely *dicoumarol*, was identified as the factor present in spoiled sweet clover that is responsible for a haemorrhagic disease of cattle. The coumarin derivatives do not prevent clotting *in vitro* but they act as antagonists of vitamin K and, if given orally, prevent the formation of the essential γ-carboxyl groups on glutamyl residues in prothrombin and Factors VII, IX and X. Coumarin derivatives are widely used in the treatment of thrombosis, but, since their effects are cumulative and there is no antidote, they need to be used with considerable caution. The synthetic vitamin K antagonist *warfarin* is used clinically and also as a rat poison.

Wound healing and fibrinolysis

Blood clots when first formed are soft and jelly-like but they gradually contract to about half their original size, serum being expressed in the process. Clot retraction is promoted by a factor released from the platelets which causes a sort of knotting effect at the intersections of the fibrin network. The activated platelets also release a *platelet-derived growth factor* that induces the tissues surrounding the wound to proliferate thereby healing the lesion. When this has occurred the fibrin clot or *thrombus* must be removed. Fibrin is very insoluble and resistant to most proteolytic enzymes but it is attacked by a special serine protease called *plasmin*. Its zymogen *plasminogen* is present in serum and is thought to be preferentially adsorbed on to the fibrin clot where it is activated by a substance released from the endothelial cells that is also preferentially bound by fibrin. The plasmin breaks down the fibrin meshwork and any plasmin that escapes from the thrombus is quickly inactivated by combination with the inhibitor *antiplasmin*.

Plasminogen may also be activated by the enzymes *urokinase* and *streptokinase* found respectively in urine and in streptococcal extracts. These are used clinically as *fibrinolytics* in cases of pathological thrombosis. Here again caution is necessary since they may activate any free unbound plasminogen and excessive fibrinolytic activity will cause degradation of circulating fibrinogen so that there may be a risk of haemorrhage.

Just as normal blood contains substances which act as anticoagulants so it contains others that act as antifibrinolytics, and the system for removing clots seems to be almost as complicated as that which is responsible for their formation. However, perched as the higher vertebrates are on a knife edge between death from haemorrhage and death from thrombosis it is not surprising to find such complex systems of checks and counterchecks.

Inherited disorders of blood clotting

Production of defective clotting factors, cofactors or inhibitors due to genetic lesions results in clotting disorders of varying severity. When a blood vessel is damaged, the existence of the two separate pathways might be expected to ensure the formation of Factor X_a and hence of thrombin, even if one of the pathways is defective, but this is not the case. The well known condition of *haemophilia* is caused by lack of functional Factor VIII_a which suggests that only the intrinsic pathway should be affected but, nevertheless, severe haemorrhages may result from minor injuries such as tooth extractions. The condition is notable in that Queen Victoria who was a carrier of the disease, which is due to a faulty X-linked recessive gene, appears to have introduced the gene into the Russian and Spanish Royal families. Although three of her daughters and four of her granddaughters were carriers of the gene for haemophilia, her son, Edward VII, did not inherit it and so was unable to transmit it to his descendants.

Plasma lipids

Lipids are poorly soluble in water and special mechanisms are required for their transport from one tissue to another. More than 90% of the plasma fatty acids are present in the form of esters such as triglycerides, phospholipids and cholesteryl esters and these, associated with protein, form the *plasma lipoproteins*. The small amounts of fatty acids which remain unesterified, the so-called *free fatty acids* (FFA), are present complexed with albumin. Tissues other than the brain can take up these fatty acids and use them directly as a source of energy or convert them into some form of esterified lipid.

Plasma lipoproteins

Four main classes of plasma lipoprotein can be recognized from their densities and electrophoretic mobilities. They are all large complexes that contain triglycerides, phospholipids, cholesterol, cholesteryl esters and protein in varying proportions (Table 25.4) and consist of a hydrophobic core surrounded by a shell of proteins and phospholipids. The proteins are known as *apolipoproteins* or *apoproteins*. These are formed in the liver and small intestine and are of many different kinds. Some of them act as enzyme activators.

Table 25.4 The approximate percentage composition of plasma lipoproteins

	Chylomicrons	VLDL	LDL	HDL
Triglycerides	85	55	10	3
Cholesterol	2	8	8	3
Cholesteryl esters	4	8	36	18
Phospholipids	7	20	23	23
Protein	2	9	23	53
Density g ml^{-1}	0.94–1.006	1.006–1.019	1.019–1.063	1.063–1.21
Function	Transport of TGs from the small intestine	Transport of TGs from the liver	Cholesterol transport	Cholesterol transport

The four clearly recognized groups of plasma lipoproteins are *Chylomicrons* (page 250). These represent the largest of the lipoprotein complexes and have the lowest density, being mainly composed of triglycerides. They are synthesized in the intestinal mucosa and are responsible for carrying dietary lipids to the liver. They are hydrolysed by *lipoprotein lipases* present on the surface of the capillaries of the liver, muscles and adipose tissue. Low density lipoproteins may be formed from the remnants of chylomicrons. *Very low density lipoproteins (VLDL)*: complexes serve to transport the triglycerides that are synthesized in the liver to the peripheral tissues where, like the chylomicrons, they are acted upon by lipoprotein lipase. The plasma concentration of VLDL remains relatively constant. *Low density lipoproteins (LDL)* contain most of the plasma cholesterol chiefly in the form of cholesteryl esters. The apoprotein consists almost entirely of *apoprotein B (β-lipoprotein)*. LDL are normally responsible for the delivery of cholesterol to the extrahepatic tissues where they are taken up by endocytosis (page 266). Anything which causes LDL to accumulate is likely to contribute to the development of atherosclerosis. *High density lipoproteins (HDL)* are synthesized in the liver and intestine and are believed to facilitate the breakdown of chylomicrons and VLDL. They are especially important as scavengers which remove excess cholesterol from tissues. Those people who have high levels of HDL in their plasma are less likely to develop atherosclerosis and the LDL/HDL ratio may give some indication of a person's liability to develop the disease.

Urine

The main channel for excretion of substances other than carbon dioxide is the urine produced in, and excreted by, the kidneys which play a major role in homoeostasis. The fluid filtered off in the glomerulus is a simple protein-free filtrate of plasma but, as it passes through the tubules, its composition is greatly modified. Materials that are of value to the body are reabsorbed while others, for which it has no use, are eliminated. The tubular cells which guard the main exit route from the body show many similarities with the intestinal epithelial cells which guard the main route of entry. Control of the composition of the body fluids is, however, exerted more by the selective retention of substances by the kidney than by the intestinal cells which are less selective in what they absorb. The kidneys regulate the water and electrolyte content of the body as well as playing a part in maintaining the acid–base balance.

Although in the adult the kidneys account for only about 0·5% of the body weight, they receive 20–25% of the blood leaving the heart. About 125 ml of glomerular filtrate are formed each minute ($\equiv$ 180 litres in 24 hours) but the average amount of urine produced is only about 1 ml per minute ($\equiv$ 1·44 litres in 24 hours). Thus more than 99% of the water filtered off in the

Table 25.5 The composition of blood plasma and urine

	Plasma	*Urine* (average values)
pH	7·4	6·0
Specific gravity	1·026	1·016
Protein (g/100 ml)	7	—
Glucose (mg/100 ml)	90 (fasting)	—
Urea (mg/100 ml)	25	1300
Uric acid (mg/100 ml)	4	45
Creatine (mg/100 ml)	0·4	—
Creatinine (mg/100 ml)	0·9	100
Ammonia (mg/100 ml)	—	34
Bicarbonate (mM)	27	—
$Na_2HPO_4 : NaH_2PO_4$	4 : 1	1 : 6

glomerulus is reabsorbed in the tubules. The amounts of the other plasma constituents that are reabsorbed vary according to their nature and the conditions operating at the time but, as a result of the tubular processes, as shown in Table 25.5. the composition of normal urine is totally different from that of the plasma from which it is derived. While the figures given for the composition of plasma can be taken as fairly reliable, those given for urine represent average figures and show wide variations depending on such factors as the water and salt intakes, amount of exercise, climatic conditions and composition of diet.

Water balance

By excreting urine of different solute content the kidney is able to maintain the osmotic pressure of the body fluids within normal limits. About four-fifths of the water filtered off in the glomeruli are reabsorbed in the proximal tubules regardless of whether a dilute or concentrated urine is being produced, but the amount of water reabsorbed from the fluid reaching the distal convoluted tubule varies according to the degree of hydration. When the body is dehydrated the raised salt concentration, and/or reduced blood volume, stimulate specific osmo- and volume receptors in the hypothalamus and trigger the release of *antidiuretic hormone* (*vasopressin*) from the posterior pituitary into the bloodstream. The vasopressin increases the permeability of the distal convoluted tubules and collecting ducts to water, and more is reabsorbed. Lack of vasopressin causes the condition of water diabetes or *diabetes insipidus* in which the subject may secrete between 5 and 12 litres, or even more, of very dilute urine (sp. gr. 1·002–1·005) per day.

When body water is in excess, sodium ions are actively removed from the fluid present in the distal tubule (see below), but are not accompanied by appreciable quantities of water to which the tubules are relatively impermeable. In this way a hypotonic urine is produced and the excess water is removed.

Electrolyte balance

Since the reabsorption of water and Na^+ ions are intimately connected, in order to maintain a normal extracellular fluid volume, it is essential that the content of sodium chloride should also be normal. Reabsorption of Na^+ ions in the distal tubule is regulated by *aldosterone* which is released from the adrenal cortex when the concentration of Na^+ ions in the blood reaching the gland is reduced, and also in response to a fall in blood volume. Aldosterone increases the reabsorption of Na^+ ions and, although there appears to be no active transport for Cl^- ions, these are drawn along with the Na^+ ions by their electric charge.

Potassium ions are exceptional in being subject both to reabsorption from and secretion by the tubules. Secretion seems to involve an ion-exchange reaction in which Na^+ ions are reabsorbed and H^+ ions compete with K^+ ions. Anything that enhances H^+ ion excretion is likely to decrease the excretion of K^+ ions.

Acid–base balance

As already mentioned, the body has three lines of defence against alterations in the reaction of the body fluids.

1. Physicochemical mechanisms which include both dilution and buffering effects. Any acid produced is rapidly diluted by distribution throughout the whole of the extracellular fluid and most of the H^+ ions are removed by the blood buffers. There is inevitably a small decrease in the base/acid ratios of each of the buffer systems present and correspondingly a small reduction in pH.

2. Respiratory adjustment. The slight fall in pH is sufficient to stimulate the respiratory centre in the brain and cause an increase in pulmonary ventilation which causes extra CO_2 to be lost from the lungs until the normal $NaHCO_3/H_2CO_3$ ratio, and pH value, are restored. The *total* $NaHCO_3$ may, however, still be depleted as a result of its decomposition by non-volatile acids and restoration of this is a function of the kidneys.
3. The renal contribution. With the exception of lactate, which is converted to glycogen in the liver, the conjugate bases of the non-volatile acids are excreted as salts in the urine. Elimination of the H^+ by the kidney is a complex process the intricacies of which are still far from clear. In simple terms it may be divided into three processes: (i) reabsorption of $NaHCO_3$, (ii) excretion of increased amounts of NaH_2PO_4, (iii) the formation and excretion of ammonia.

(i) Reabsorption of bicarbonate

When an acid urine is excreted an amount of $NaHCO_3$ equivalent to that which has been filtered from the plasma is returned to the blood by the kidney tubules. Although this might appear to be a straight reabsorption, evidence suggests that the process is indirect and that the HCO_3^- which enters the blood is derived from metabolic CO_2 produced within the tubule cells. Because of the presence of carbonic anhydrase this is rapidly converted to H_2CO_3, which dissociates into H^+ and HCO_3^-. The HCO_3^- is reabsorbed and, by a neat piece of ion exchange, the H^+ is secreted into the lumen of the tubules while valuable Na^+ is reabsorbed from the tubules into the blood. How this process is effected is still somewhat of a mystery but it appears to be analogous to the secretion of HCl by the oxyntic cells of the gastric mucosa.

(ii) Excretion of titratable acid

As can be predicted from its pH, the Na_2HPO_4/NaH_2PO_4 ratio in plasma is about 4 : 1 which is the ratio in which the salts appear in the glomerular filtrate. However, as H^+ is secreted into the tubular lumen, the following reaction takes place

$$Na_2HPO_4 + H^+ \rightarrow NaH_2PO_4 + Na^+$$

and Na^+ is made available for reabsorption. In this way the amount of acid phosphate is increased at the expense of the basic salt and at pH 6·0, as can be calculated from the Henderson–Hasselbalch equation, the Na_2HPO_4/NaH_2PO_4 becomes 1 : 6·3 and at pH 5·4 it becomes 1 : 25.

The quantity of H^+ excreted in the form of NaH_2PO_4 can be readily determined by titrating the urine to the pH of blood, i.e. 7·4, with 0·1 M NaOH. This gives what is known as the *titratable acidity* of the urine.

The overall results of processes (i) and (ii) may be summarized as follows:

$$H_2CO_3 + Na_2HPO_4 \rightarrow NaHCO_3 + NaH_2PO_4$$
$$\text{reabsorbed} \quad \text{excreted}$$

(iii) Excretion of ammonium salts

It has long been known that in metabolic acidosis the excretion of ammonium salts by the kidney is significantly increased. The ammonia has been shown to be formed in the proximal tubules during the hydrolysis of glutamine by *glutaminase* which increases in amount in metabolic acidosis. Until recently it was believed that the ammonia formed in the reaction diffused into the lumen of the tubules where it combined with H^+ ions to form NH_4^+ ions. In this way excretion of NH_4^+ ions together with anions such as Cl^- and SO_4^{2-} allowed the H^+ ions to be excreted without a corresponding increase in the acidity of the urine.

$$\begin{array}{ccc}
\begin{array}{c} \text{CONH}_2 \\ | \\ [\text{CH}_2]_2 \\ | \\ \text{CHNH}_3{}^+ \\ | \\ \text{COO}^- \end{array}
& \xrightarrow{\text{Glutaminase}} &
\begin{array}{c} \text{COO}^- \\ | \\ [\text{CH}_2]_2 \\ | \\ \text{CHNH}_3{}^+ \\ | \\ \text{COO}^- \end{array}
\quad + \quad \text{NH}_4{}^+
\end{array}$$

This explanation for the increased excretion of ammonium salts is now being questioned. It has been pointed out that the hydrolysis of glutamine produces glutamate ions and ammonium ions rather than free ammonia. Furthermore most of the glutamate produced is converted into glucose in the kidney and the reactions involved in the conversion result in the uptake of two H^+ ions. This is equivalent to the production of two $HCO_3{}^-$ ions per molecule of glucose formed. Thus, for every two molecules of glutamine metabolized two $NH_4{}^+$ ions are excreted and two $HCO_3{}^-$ ions become available and help to compensate the acidosis.

An alternative view is gaining favour. In acidosis as the excretion of ammonium ions increases, that of urea decreases. Since $HCO_3{}^-$ ions are used in urea formation (page 283), the decrease in urea synthesis results in a sparing of $HCO_3{}^-$ ions which help to counter the acidosis. According to this view the increase in $NH_4{}^+$ ion excretion is seen as a mechanism for removing toxic ammonia which escapes conversion to urea. The classical explanation for the increased excretion of $NH_4{}^+$ ions by the kidney during acidosis is now believed to be a considerable oversimplification.

Although the urine is usually acid, an alkaline urine may be secreted by subjects whose diet contains large amounts of vegetables and fruit which produce alkaline salts in the body. A slight temporary increase in the alkalinity of the blood and urine may also accompany the secretion of gastric juice and is known as the *alkaline tide*. An alkaline urine contains bicarbonate and the Na_2HPO_4/NaH_2PO_4 ratio is increased. The excretion of ammonium salts is reduced.

The composition of urine

In order that the composition of the other body fluids may be kept constant, that of the urine must be able to vary widely. For this reason, even in a normal individual, the composition of the urine may be quite different according to the times and circumstances and, since the composition of samples collected over short periods may differ significantly from the average, a complete 24 hour sample should be analysed in order to obtain reliable values for the output of its various constituents. In the normal adult the volume excreted is of the order of 1000–2000 ml per day and 1500 ml is usually taken as the average figure. The quantity depends on the water intake, the external temperature and the diet as well as on the mental and physical state.

Urine is a clear yellowish fluid the depth of colour of which depends largely on its concentration. The colour is due principally to the pigment *urochrome* the origin of which is unknown.

Organic constituents

The chief organic constituents of urine are urea, uric acid and creatinine but an enormous variety of other organic substances are present in very small amounts, including various enzymes, hormones and vitamins.

Urea is the principal end product of protein metabolism in mammals (page 282) and the amount excreted is directly related to the protein intake. Normally urea comprises 80–90% of the total urinary nitrogen but, on a low-protein diet, the percentage is less because the quantity of the other nitrogenous constituents is not much affected by dietary changes. A normal adult in nitrogen balance who is consuming 65–70 g of protein will excrete about 11 g of nitrogen per day from which it follows that his urea output will be about 20 g. The output is increased in fever and other conditions in which protein catabolism is accelerated.

Uric acid (2,6,8-trioxypurine) which is the end product of purine metabolism is only slightly soluble in water. It is derived from the breakdown of both endogenous and dietary nucleoprotein. Normal adults excrete about 0·7 g per day.

Creatinine is an anhydride of creatine which is present in muscle in the form of phosphocreatine (page 331). Phosphocreatine is relatively unstable, the phosphate group being split off, and the creatine converted to creatinine.

$$HN{=}C\begin{array}{l} NH_2 \\ N-CH_2 \cdot COOH \\ CH_3 \end{array} \qquad HN{=}C\begin{array}{l} HN-CO \\ N-CH_2 \\ CH_3 \end{array}$$

Creatine   Creatinine

Creatine itself does not occur in any appreciable amount in the urine of adult males although it is found in the urine of children and sporadically in the urine of women. It is present, regardless of sex, in conditions in which there is wasting of the muscles. The amount of creatinine excreted by any normal individual remains remarkably constant from day to day. It is related to muscular development and not directly to the amount of exercise taken. In the average male it is of the order of 1–2 g.

Inorganic constituents

The chief cations present in urine are Na^+, K^+ and NH_4^+; Ca^{2+} and Mg^{2+} are present in lesser amounts. The corresponding anions are chloride, phosphate and sulphate. *Chlorides* are mainly excreted as sodium chloride and, since most of this is of dietary origin, the output varies with the intake. The amount of NaCl excreted per day is usually of the order of 10–15 g, but this is reduced in excessive sweating or in any condition in which water is retained in the body or is lost by a path other than the kidneys.

The urinary *phosphates* are derived from ingested inorganic phosphate as well as from the breakdown of phosphoprotein and cellular material such as phospholipid and sugar phosphates. In an alkaline urine in which base is being excreted by the kidney, phosphate excretion may be

Table 25.6 Amounts of urinary constituents normally excreted in 24 hours

	Average value	*Range*
Volume (ml)	1500	800–2000
Total nitrogen (g)	11	7–15
Urea (g)	22	10–35
Uric acid (g)	0·5	0·2–2·0
Creatinine (g)	1·7	0·8–2·0
Ammonia (g)	0·5	0·2–1·2
Sodium chloride (g)	12	8–15
Total phosphorus (g)	1·0	0·5–1·5
Total sulphur (g)	0·7	0·6–1·7
Calcium (g)	0·15	0·1–0·2

increased above the normal level of about 1.0 g P ($\equiv 2.5$ g P_2O_5) per day. In such urines a heavy cloud of insoluble calcium and magnesium phosphates tends to appear on standing. This readily dissolves when the urine is acidified.

The *sulphates* appearing in urine are mainly the end products of the metabolism of the S-containing amino acids, although inorganic sulphate absorbed from the food also contributes. Normally about 90% of the sulphate excreted is in the form of inorganic sulphates and only about 10% as organic or 'ethereal' sulphates.

As described above, some of the H^+ ions produced in the course of metabolism are converted to NH_4^+ in the kidney and excreted in the form of *ammonium* salts. The output of ammonia in this form is usually about $0.5–1.0$ g per day but this is increased in acidosis.

The amounts of various urinary constituents normally excreted in 24 hours are shown in Table 25.6.

Chapter 26
Epithelium

Epithelia are essentially surface tissues of ectodermal origin. The epidermis covering the surface of the skin on the outside of the body is a typical epithelium. However, epithelia cover the surfaces of other tissues and are not necessarily confined to the outside of the animal; oral epithelium and the epithelial lining of the intestine are examples of epithelia that line the wall of the alimentary canal and are kept moist by the secretion of mucous glands embedded in them. The functions of an epithelium are those that are clearly related to a superficial tissue, namely protection, absorption and secretion. The relative degree of development of these three functions varies considerably in different epithelia so that it is possible to classify these tissues according to which function predominates.

Protective epithelia

The best known protective epithelia are the epidermis of the skin together with related structures such as nails, hair and feathers, as well as analogous tissues, including some of specifically dental interest, such as the oral and gingival epithelium. Protective epithelia are often keratinized though not necessarily so. Thus, while the masticatory gingival epithelium is covered by a layer of keratin, the neighbouring crevicular gingival epithelium and the alveolar mucosal epithelium are not.

Epithelia usually form a covering to connective tissue from which they are separated by a *basement membrane* (Figure 26.1). Since epithelium has no blood supply of its own, it derives its nutrients from, and disposes of its waste products into, the neighbouring connective tissue which contains capillaries. There is considerable interaction between epithelial and connective tissue cells which influence each other's division and differentiation and this interaction presumably takes place across the basement membrane. This structure stains strongly with the periodic acid–Schiff reagent which indicates the presence of glycoprotein which contains unsubstituted sugar residues. The basement membrane is shown by the electron microscope to consist of two distinct parts, a deeper layer consisting of *reticulin* and a more superficial part, which can in turn be divided into the *lamina densa* and the *lamina lucida*. Histologically, reticulin appears as a fine branching network which stains black when treated with solutions containing silver salts, probably as a result of the reducing behaviour of sugar residues in glycoprotein.

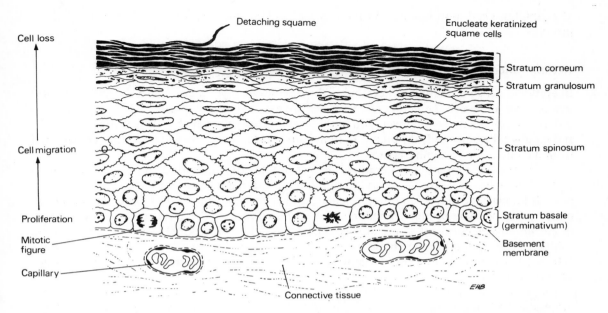

Figure 26.1 Succession of cells in lightly keratinizing stratified squamous epithelium. Keratinized squames are shown in black with the width of intercellular spaces exaggerated

Chemical characterization of reticulin is difficult because it usually occurs rather sparsely and mixed with a variety of other tissue components. However, purified reticulin from the cortex of human kidneys has been shown to consist of a combination of collagen, carbohydrate (probably glycoprotein) and possibly lipid. It is thus a complex made up of high molecular weight substances. The lamina densa may influence the transfer of molecules between connective tissue and epithelium and hence would be expected to exert control over the epithelium. It has been suggested that both connective tissue and epithelium collaborate in building up the basement membrane and that the epithelial cells behave atypically by secreting a proline-rich protein into its outer layers.

The layer of epithelial cells in contact with the basement membrane is known as the *stratum basale* or *germitivum*. These basal cells undergo division to replace those that are continually shed from the outer surface of the epithelium (Figure 26.1). Differentiation also begins in the basal layer, most probably as a separate process. As cells differentiate they move away from the basement membrane and become flattened in a direction at right angles to their movement. The rate of cell division in the basal layer balances the rate at which cells are shed from the surface, and it has been suggested that this is controlled by a feedback mechanism involving a water-soluble heat-labile substance or *chalone* (page 366) produced in the outer layers which suppresses mitosis in the stratum basale.

As the cells are pushed towards the surface by cell multiplication in the basal layer, changes occur in their morphology. In both keratin-forming and non-keratinizing epithelia a *prickle cell layer* is first formed known as the *stratum spinosum*. In this layer the cells of the non-keratinizing crevicular gingival epithelium are slightly smaller than those in the same layer of the keratinizing masticatory gingival epithelium. The polygonal cells in this non-keratinizing epithelium then undergo a rapid further transition to a final layer of flattened cells parallel with the tooth surface. The attachment to the tooth enamel is by means of a glycoprotein 'glue' rather than by any visible structural element. Keratinization, on the other hand, involves a further series of changes affecting both cell morphology and the physical and chemical properties of the predominant proteins.

Keratinization

In epithelia which are about to keratinize, the prickle cell layer merges into the flatter *stratum granulosum* in which *keratohyalin* granules appear in the cytoplasm. The final stage of differentiation results in the formation of the *stratum corneum*, which is the keratin layer itself. It contains fully cornified, shrunken, flattened and featureless cells and is sharply demarcated from the underlying granular layer.

The systematic formation of keratin as an end product of many protective epithelia suggests that it is a highly organized process but, although the general nature of the changes that take place is known, the details and, in particular, the mechanism by which such changes occur are not understood. The primary function of keratin is to protect the surface with a layer that is physically strong, coherent and relatively impervious to both microorganisms and substances in solution. The chief difference between keratins and the underlying connective tissue proteins is that the structural elements of keratins are intracellular, whereas those of connective tissues are extracellular.

The keratin molecule in its native or *α-keratin* form is essentially long, thin and highly orientated and, as revealed by X-ray diffraction studies, contains long stretches of *α*-helix (page 57) which, unlike the collagen helix, consists of a single chain. However, the helices do not occur singly or in straggling bundles but in a highly systematic arrangement. Two or three discrete helices are twisted together to form a cable (*protofibril*) and a number of such cables are then arranged to form a *microfibril* of about 7 nm diameter. This is of the same order of size as the *tonofilaments* present in the basement cells, a fact of possible significance in the subsequent keratinization. The arrangements of cables within a microfibril may vary from one kind of epithelial tissue to another.

The microfibrils are embedded in an amorphous protein cement or matrix which is believed to consist of relatively short polypeptide chains with high proportions of serine, threonine, proline and especially cystine.

A second form of keratin, known as *β-keratin*, is produced by stretching the *α*-keratin in hair to about twice its original length. The X-ray diffraction pattern of *β*-keratin is similar to that of silk fibroin (page 56) and its structure, like that of fibroin, is based on the *β*-pleated sheet. There is a difference, however, in that polypeptide chains are in a parallel (Figure 5.2a) and not an antiparallel arrangement.

The main change during keratinization is the conversion of the intracellular protein from a hydrated structure, compatible with the life of cells, to a tough highly insoluble protein which fills the region inside the shrunken cells more or less completely. Keratinization appears to accompany cell lysis, both of which take place in the region where hydrolytic enzymes are present in largest amounts. This seems to indicate that, at a certain stage, non-keratinizable components of the cell are rapidly removed, leaving the keratinized periphery as the main component of the keratin layer. The action of hydrolytic enzymes implies a degree of cellular control. An alternative view is that the changes that accompany keratinization are brought about by the fall in pH which occurs when the cells have migrated a sufficient distance from the neighbouring connective tissue for the supply of nutrients to be small and for metabolites to accumulate.

The highly insoluble keratin which remains as an end product contains a high proportion of S–S bridges joining the different polypeptide chains together and giving the structure great mechanical strength. If these bridges are broken, for example by reduction with thioglycollic acid, there is an increase in solubility and a decrease in tensile strength. Use is made of this in the permanent waving of hair when temporary reduction of the sulphur bridges renders the fibres more pliable and enables them to be reorientated in the stretched β-pleated sheet form; subsequent reoxidation fixes them in place. Histochemical evidence that the sulphydryl groups of cysteine are converted to the disulphide linkages of cystine during keratinization is less satisfactory, especially for gingival epithelium where some authors report an increase of sulphydryl bonds, some of disulphide and some of both types. However, the extraction from epidermis of a soluble *prekeratin* of molecular weight 640 000 having sulphydryl groups but no disulphide linkages is strong evidence that the formation of disulphide linkages is an essential step in the formation of insoluble keratin. Conversion of soluble prekeratin to insoluble keratin involves a kind of polymerization and probably takes place in the granular layer.

The amino acid composition of keratins, particularly those of different tissues in the same animal (Table 26.1), shows more variation than does the composition of other structural proteins such as collagen and elastin. In particular the content of the sulphur-containing diamino acid cystine varies enormously. It is very high in hair (12–18%), high in nail, much lower in the epidermis and lower still in the oral epithelium. High- and low-sulphur keratins from different tissues are sometimes referred to as hard and soft keratins respectively as the proportion of cystine bridges affects the physical properties. Apart from the high cystine content of some forms, the overall amino acid composition of keratins lacks any striking features.

Keratin considered as the bulk protein of the stratum corneum is a heterogeneous material with several levels of structural organization. Thus the proteins of the cell membranes have a different composition from that of the material that they enclose. They have a lower mechanical strength than the intracellular keratin and are more susceptible to attack by proteolytic enzymes to which keratin itself is enormously resistant. On the other hand, the cell membrane protein is not readily dissolved by oxidizing and reducing agents to which keratin is unusually susceptible.

Table 26.1 Amino acid composition of some epithelium proteins (values given as amino acid residues per 1000 total residues)

	Keratin from			Secreted protein (parotid saliva component)
	Oral epithelium	Epidermis	Nail	
Aspartic acid	82·4	73·8	69·4	53
Threonine	53·0	34·4	66·7	6
Serine	74·1	173	113·3	48
Glutamic acid	128·3	120·9	132·7	194
Proline	38·8	16·5	61·4	353
Glycine	99·2	209	67·8	203
Alanine	80·2	42·8	54·9	12
Half-cystine	10·7	33·0	92·7	—
Valine	63·6	29·5	59·2	8
Methionine	20·7	9·6	8·4	1
Isoleucine	48·4	33·0	34·7	5
Leucine	98·9	59·5	79·4	11
Tyrosine	29·5	31·8	29·0	3
Phenylalanine	36·4	25·1	22·8	2
Histidine	14·6	16·3	9·4	16
Lysine	61·6	39·9	31·9	47
Arginine	59·5	51·8	66·6	43
Amide	69·9	82·2	94·6	—

By enclosing a substance of great mechanical strength within frail but specifically resistant membranes, a combination is obtained which resists not only mechanical trauma but also microbiological attack.

The epidermis contains substantial amounts of various lipid substances which may play an important part in building up the keratin structure and maintaining the integrity of epithelial tissues. It would seem likely that lipids also act as lubricants and water-proofing agents. Skin cells often have incomplete sets of enzymes for cholesterol synthesis and, in the human epidermis, the synthesis goes as far as 7-dehydrocholesterol but does not reach cholesterol.

Secretory epithelium

The gums or gingiva are the soft tissues surrounding the teeth and consist of vascular connective tissue covered by stratified squamous epithelium, known as *gingival epithelium*. While this epithelium is of a keratinizing type, whether it keratinizes or not depends upon its precise location (Figure 26.2). The oral epithelium beyond the gingival margin keratinizes whereas the junctional epithelium does not. The oral sulcular epithelium which connects these zones does not keratinize near the junctional epithelium but has an increasing tendency to do so towards the gingival margin, where it joins the oral epithelium.

The *salivary glands*, which occur in various parts of the mouth, are composed of typical secretory epithelium, but differ both in size and the composition of their secretions. The epithelial cells of these glands do not keratinize but actively pour out aqueous secretions which contain not only sodium, chloride, calcium, magnesium and phosphate ions but also amylase and high molecular weight glycoproteins. Salivary glycoproteins are typical glycoproteins (page 479) and their composition is very different from that of the intracellular keratins. The glycoprotein of human parotid saliva has an extremely high content of proline which accounts for more than one-third of the total amino acid residues (Table 26.1). The secretions of the of salivary glands differ considerably in composition. They are discussed in more detail in Chapter 33.

Dental enamel, although essentially a structural and mechanical element, has some claim to be considered as a product of secretory rather than protective epithelium. The ameloblasts which

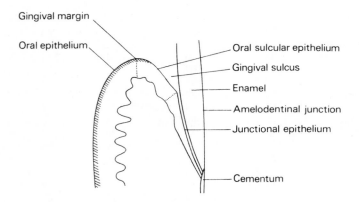

Figure 26.2 The dentogingival junction showing three types of gingival epithelium, oral, oral sulcular and junctional, and the diminishing degrees of keratinization (as denoted by diagonal hatching)

produce enamel are epithelial cells whose main initial function is to secrete a concentrated protein solution, in which large crystals of hydroxyapatite subsequently grow. The solution contains two groups of proteins: the more abundant group (*amelogenins*) are removed from the enamel via the ameloblasts as the enamel undergoes maturation, leaving the less abundant *enamelins* behind in the mature enamel. At the end of their short lives ameloblasts degenerate without striking changes in their intracellular proteins. However, the enamelins have some of the characteristics of low-sulphur keratins, and, in this respect, enamel in its final state has some resemblance to other protective epithelia. Enamel is discussed more fully in Chapter 32.

The epithelium of the gastric mucosa is remarkable in producing a high concentration of hydrochloric acid without destroying itself. There is a large difference between the pH of the blood (pH 7·4) and that of the gastric secretion (pH 1·1) which means that the concentration of H^+ in the latter is 1 000 000 times that of blood. The cells that secrete hydrochloric acid have a very high rate of respiration; this is necessary to provide energy for the chemical work involved in the active transport of hydrogen ions. The chloride ions are transported from blood to gastric juice by a passive mechanism which maintains neutrality of total electrical charge in the solutions. Chloride ions lost from the blood are replaced by bicarbonate ions from the carbon dioxide produced in the course of metabolism. The process is catalysed by carbonic anhydrase and has certain similarities to the chloride shift which occurs when carbon dioxide is taken up from the tissues by the blood (page 376).

Absorptive epithelium

The epithelium lining the intestines can be regarded as both secretory and absorptive since most of the small molecules that constitute the ultimate food supply of the animal enter through its cells. Contact with the external biochemical environment is more nearly approached at this point than anywhere else in the body, since the composition of air which bathes skin and lungs is relatively constant, while the food and fluid intake is constantly changing.

While epithelia are basically simple arrangements made up of single (in *simple epithelia*) or several (in *stratified epithelia*) layers of characteristically shaped, e.g. *cuboidal*, *columnar* or *squamous* (i.e. flattened) cells, they are capable of modification to serve a variety of functions in different organs. Thus the epithelial cells in the small intestine have numerous finger-like *microvilli* projecting from their surfaces. These microvilli greatly increase the surface area and are correlated with the absorptive function of the tissue.

Microvilli are also found on the free surfaces in the proximal convoluted tubules of the kidney. Renal epithelium takes on a great variety of morphological forms to fulfil a range of functions. The epithelial cells or *podocytes* of Bowman's capsule have little feet or pedicels which interdigitate with those of neighbouring endothelial cells of blood capillaries, along a basal lamina to form an efficient filter mechanism, the slit membranes being an effective barrier to all but the smallest molecules. In the thin segment of the loop of Henle, the epithelium is of the simple squamous type, whereas in other parts of the kidney tubules, simple cuboidal epithelium interdigitates tortuously with neighbouring cells, so as to provide maximum surface contact for exchange of solutes.

Chapter 27
Connective tissue

Living organisms are not merely random collections of cells; each organism grows according to a detailed pattern which determines both the structure and the functions of its many constituent parts, and ensures that they are all integrated with one another both anatomically and biochemically. One of the objects of this book is to emphasize the molecular basis of life and, further, that chemical and anatomical structures merge into each other, these terms merely serving to distinguish different orders of size and perhaps complexity. There can be no better illustration of the merging of these two orders of structure than the connective tissues.

One of the basic requirements for systematic arrangement within tissues is a mechanical one – a means of maintaining the cells in appropriate relationship to each other despite the various forces which act upon them, including gravity, externally applied physical stress and the internal movements of the organism itself which result from growth and exertion.

Two contrasting systems for organizing their mechanical structures are employed by multicellular organisms. These systems differ in whether the mechanical elements that determine the rigidity of the structure are closely associated with cells or frankly extracellular. A good example of a mechanical system of the former type occurs in higher plants where the cells secrete a strong thick layer around themselves, the cell wall, which resists the internal pressure exerted against it by the cell itself. As a result, the individual cells are rigid like inflated motor tyres and thus form the basis of a rigid multicellular structure. The main building material of plant cell walls is cellulose, a homopolymer composed of bundles of chains each of which contains about 5000 glucose units. Another kind of cell-based mechanical organization occurs in the keratinous epithelia of higher animals (Chapter 26).

The cellular type of mechanical organization has certain limitations and is suitable mainly for static tissue situations. Animals lead active lives and their mechanical structures are adapted to various dynamic requirements, both in the stresses they have to meet and in the changes which tissues undergo in the course of a lifetime. As a result, in many animal tissues, the cells have lost their primary mechanical function and occupy a very much smaller proportion of the total volume of the tissue than in plants. In animal tissues the mechanical function is taken over by extracellular tissue elements, comprising protein fibres embedded in a polymeric aqueous gel. The restriction of mechanical function to extracellular tissue components permits larger spaces between cells and makes possible a greater freedom in tissue pattern. Thus more than one type of cell may occur in the same tissue and there is scope for continuous reorganization to meet the needs of growth, repair, changing stress and cell replacement, without loss of the original tissue characteristics. All these features are seen in an extensive but unified family of tissues found in vertebrates, known as the connective tissues.

Occurrence and characteristics of connective tissues

Connective tissues fulfil many functions but their primary function is a mechanical one, connective tissue elements being responsible for maintaining cells, tissues and organs in proper relationship to one another. They also provide the animal firstly with support, usually by means of a rigid skeleton, to which the softer tissues are attached and, secondly, with a system for the transmission of mechanical force, so that the contractile power of the muscles can be harnessed to the skeletal framework and used to move the animal as a coordinated whole. Connective tissues are essentially mesodermal in origin being derived from the primitive mesenchyme, a layer of the early embryo. They all contain the fibrous protein *collagen*, as their most important and characteristic constituent. Typical forms are tendon, the corium layer of the skin, loose connective tissue, cartilage and the basement membranes of various tissues. In a mineralized form connective tissue is present in calcified cartilage, bone, dentine and cementum, which are described in Chapter 29. Connective tissues thus include many of the tissues of specific dental interest such as the oral subepithelium (corresponding to the corium of skin), the periodontal membrane or periodontal ligament, the alveolar bone of the tooth socket, cementum, dentine and the dental pulp.

The main components of connective tissues are shown in Table 27.1. The *fibroblasts* are responsible for the synthesis of the remaining non-living extracellular components, and, when actively laying down collagen fibres in soft connective tissues, are typically amoeboid cells which protrude spiky processes. They may become differentiated as in bone, where the *osteocytes* become embedded throughout the mineralized tissue, and in dentine, where *odontoblasts* remain near the boundary between the mineralized dentine and the pulp with their processes passing through the thickness of the dentine. The connective tissue cells first lay down the *ground substance* as a gel containing various kinds of macromolecule. This contains a relatively large volume of water and provides a suitable environment for the subsequent deposition of the fibrous proteins. These are secreted by the fibroblasts as macromolecules which are further assembled extracellularly, and eventually give rise to large insoluble fibrous aggregates, which, as the connective tissue matures, fill most of the extracellular space and give the tissue great mechanical strength.

Table 27.1 Components of connective tissues

Cells	Fibroblasts in more or less differentiated forms, e.g. chondroblasts, odontoblasts, osteocytes, osteoblasts, etc.
	Fat cells, macrophages, plasma cells, mast cells and leucocytes
Interfibrillar matrix or ground substances (molecules, often high polymers)	Proteoglycans (glycosaminoglycans)
	Glycoproteins
	Phospholipids
	Water
Protein fibres	Collagen
	Reticulin
	Elastin

Although the most common and characteristic type of connective tissue cell is the fibroblast many other types of cell are present in loose connective tissue. These mostly have a protective role. They include *fat cells*, *macrophages*, *plasma cells*, *mast cells* and *leucocytes*. The macrophages and some of the leucocytes are phagocytic and are able to engulf cellular debris, bacteria and inert foreign matter; the plasma cells are derived from B-lymphocytes and produce immunoglobulins while the mast cells produce heparin and histamine and also, in some species, serotonin (5-hydroxytryptamine).

The ground substance

A great variety of complex substances, of high molecular weight which contain both sugar and amino acid units, are associated with the fibrous elements of connective tissues. These are collectively described as *mucosubstances* or *glycoconjugates*, and may be divided into two categories known as *proteoglycans* and *glycoproteins*. Some lipid material is also present.

The proteoglycans contain heteropolysaccharides known as *glycosaminoglycans*, an unwieldy term that emphasizes their content of hexosamines and uronic acids. Formerly glycosaminoglycans were known as *mucopolysaccharides*. The best known members of this group are the *chondroitin sulphates* and *hyaluronic acid*. Though they are characterized by the structure of their polysaccharide chains, these are almost invariably associated with protein, hence the term proteoglycan.

Proteoglycans

The most characteristic structural feature of the proteoglycans is the possession of very highly polymerized carbohydrate chains (with 150 to several thousand sugar residues) having only two kinds of modified sugar residue alternating along the whole length of the chain. One of these is usually a hexosamine and the other, a hexuronic acid. Hexosamines are derived from hexose sugars by replacement of the hydroxyl group on C-2 by an amino group. Sometimes this amino group is modified by having an attached acetyl group so that the resulting structure ($-NH \cdot CO \cdot CH_3$) does not ionize and cannot acquire a positive charge. Hexuronic acids resemble the hexose sugars but differ from them in having C-6 as a carboxyl group instead of a primary alcohol group. Provided that the carboxyl group is unsubstituted, it confers weakly acid properties. In some proteoglycans, a molecule of sulphuric acid is attached in ester linkage to an oxygen atom from one of the hydroxyl groups of the hexosamine. Ionization of the ester sulphate group gives such proteoglycans strongly acidic properties, which are responsible for their specific staining reaction with the dye *Alcian Blue*. Thus proteoglycans are large polyvalent anions, and are able to attract and bind cations, usually Na^+ and K^+, referred to as *counterions* which maintain both electrical and chemical neutrality.

With the exception of keratan sulphate, which contains galactose residues in place of uronic acid, the composition of connective tissue glycosaminoglycans shows variations on the theme described in the previous paragraph (Table 27.2). Hyaluronic acid is only weakly acidic, whereas the chondroitin sulphates have strongly acidic sulphate groups.

Glycosaminoglycans are nearly always associated with a smaller amount of protein. At one time this was thought to be a loose electrostatic association, but recently it has been shown that the polysaccharide is usually covalently linked through an alkali-labile *O*-glycosidic bond to a serine group on the protein. This gives a very large molecule, with a single protein chain, *the core protein*, to which many long carbohydrate chains are covalently attached (Figure 27.1).

Table 27.2 Features of the composition of glycosaminoglycans from connective tissues

Polysaccharide	Hexosamine	Uronic acid (or hexose)
Hyaluronic acid	N-Acetyl-D-glucosamine (1 : 3 linkage, SO$_4$ absent)	D-Glucuronic acid (1 : 4 linkage)
Chondroitin 4-sulphate	N-Acetyl-D-galactosamine (1 : 3 linkage, 4-SO$_4$)	D-Glucuronic acid (1 : 4 linkage)
Dermatan sulphate	N-Acetyl-D-galactosamine (1 : 3 linkage, 4-SO$_4$)	L-Iduronic acid (1 : 4 linkage)
Chondroitin 6-sulphate	N-Acetyl-D-galactosamine (1 : 3 linkage, 6-SO$_4$)	D-Glucuronic acid (1 : 4 linkage)
Chondroitin	N-Acetyl-D-galactosamine (1 : 3 linkage, SO$_4$ absent)	D-Glucuronic acid (1 : 4 linkage)
Heparan sulphate	N-Acetyl-D-glucosamine (partially sulphated)	D-Glucuronic acid
Keratan sulphate	N-Acetyl-D-glucosamine (1 : 4 linkage, 6-SO$_4$)	D-Galactose (1 : 3 linkage)

Hyaluronic acid occurs widely in connective tissues but is most easily isolated from synovial fluid which acts as a lubricant for the cartilage of joints, or from umbilical cord where it exists as a complex containing 25–30% of protein. The association is a loose one as removal of protein does not cause a marked fall in the high viscosity of synovial fluid. The particle weight of hyaluronic acid is very high being $1\text{–}4 \times 10^6$, the structure consisting of a single very long polysaccharide chain. Mutual electrostatic repulsion between the negatively charged carboxyl groups on the uronic acid residues causes the molecule to form a loosely tangled skein or net in intimate contact with the extracellular water. Like other proteoglycans, it does not possess a unique configuration, the flexible molecules having 'average' shapes.

Chondroitin sulphate is also found in small amounts in many connective tissues and is a major

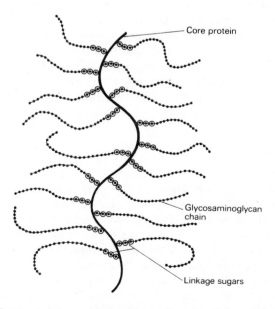

Figure 27.1 Arrangement of a proteoglycan molecule with protein core and glycosaminoglycan chains

constitutent of cartilage. The material from cartilage has a molecular weight of $1–5 \times 10^6$ and the molecule consists of a protein core with 30–60 polysaccharide chains, each of molecular weight approximately 50 000, covalently attached. Mutual repulsion of the negatively charged carbohydrate chains makes the core behave like a rigid rod 3700 Å (370 nm) in length.

Glycoproteins

Glycoproteins are conjugated proteins having one or more short irregular heterosaccharide side chains bound covalently to the polypeptide chain. In some respects therefore they resemble proteoglycans of the chondroitin sulphate type but differ from them in the shortness of their polysaccharide chains (2–20 units long) which do not contain a regularly repeating disaccharide unit. The carbohydrate content is usually lower than in proteoglycans. Glycoproteins vary enormously in the number, composition and size of their carbohydrate side chains. Like glycosaminoglycans, they possess acetylhexosamines but uronic acids are not present in glycoproteins. *Mannose* and *galactose* and the methyl pentose, *fucose* (6-deoxy-L-galactose), occur commonly, but the most characteristic constituent is *N-acetylneuraminic acid (sialic acid)* which often terminates the free ends of the carbohydrate chains. Sialic acid is both a sugar and an amino acid and its strongly acid carboxyl group (pK 2·6) gives it acidic properties throughout a wide range of pH, which it confers on the glycoprotein as a whole. Glycoproteins which contain sialic acids are known as *sialoproteins*. The polar nature of sialic acid makes this group of proteins strongly hydrophilic, stretching out the side chains in an aqueous environment. Glycoproteins are present in saliva and are responsible for its surface active and 'spinnbarkeit' properties. They probably occur in the ground substance of many connective tissues but in rather small proportions. The best characterized connective tissue glycoprotein is *bone sialoprotein* (page 439).

The glycoproteins, as mentioned in Chapter 5, are a most interesting and varied group of proteins and are of special importance in oral biology as constituents of both saliva and the capsules of many bacteria. The rigid wall of these bacteria is composed of the glycopeptide *murein*, which is elaborately cross-linked so that it forms a single bag-shaped molecule. This is responsible for the shape and mechanical strength of the cell wall (page 205) and its importance is illustrated by the lethal effects of penicillin, which interferes with its synthesis (page 480). Its carbohydrate component is susceptible to the antibacterial enzyme *lysozyme*.

The main classes of lipid identified in connective tissues include neutral fats, fatty acids, phospholipids and sterols, especially cholesterol. Very few investigations have been made on lipids in soft connective tissues, except for their deposition in porous foreign bodies implanted in these tissues. These experiments suggest that all four types of lipid can be synthesized by fibroblasts.

Functions of the ground substance

An essential function of the proteoglycans in the ground substance of connective tissues is to provide an extracellular environment which facilitates the laying down and maturation of fibres during tissue development. Newly formed tissues, whether in the embryo or young animal or the granulation tissue in healing wounds, have larger proportions of water and carbohydrate and smaller amounts of protein, especially collagen fibres, than older tissues. This may explain why it is difficult for sutures to hold in young and healing tissues.

The higher water content of young tissues provides a clue to one of the most important properties of proteoglycans, which enables them to form the intial extracellular milieu for fibre deposition. Their molecules being polyanionic spread out in net-like form, each strand being associated with a comparatively large quantity of water. This is hydrogen bonded to the hydrophilic hydroxyl groups and loosely held by 'solvation' of the fixed ionized groups on the proteoglycan chains (see Chapter 3). Because they have very open structures the proteoglycans will hold an enormous weight of water per unit weight of organic material and, although soft tissues contain up to 70% of water, no fluid seeps out when they are punctured.

The small molecules of nutrients and waste products can diffuse freely, through the water held by proteoglycans, but diffusion of macromolecules, such as tropocollagen (page 44), is restricted to those regions that are fairly remote from the individual strands of this hydrated net. Such molecules are therefore channelled through the free water, either within the large holes in the network or between the larger sheets of netting. Presumably the restriction to free diffusion resulting from the size and spatial distribution of these holes affects the distribution and orientation of newly laid down collagen fibres.

Evidence for the existence of proteoglycan nets, the strands of which are surrounded by water envelopes, was obtained by subjecting a gel of soluble collagen to ultracentrifugation. This produced a compact pellet of collagen containing very little water, but when the experiment was repeated with the addition of a very small proportion of hyaluronic acid to the collagen, a much larger pellet with a higher water content was obtained. It was calculated that the thin chains of hyaluronic acid are normally surrounded by an envelope of water having a radius of 50 Å (5 nm) from which the soluble collagen was excluded. Chondroitin sulphate has an even greater effect than hyaluronic acid and can retain ten times more water than a pellet containing collagen alone. It has been suggested that collagen may become entangled in the fine polysaccharide side chains of chondroitin sulphate.

At present it is not possible to account for the specific behaviour of each of the various proteoglycans occurring in tissues. The kinds and proportions of different mucosubstances vary greatly between tissues and even change in the same tissue as it ages. Thus cartilage is rich in *chondroitin 4-sulphate* and *dermatan sulphate*, whereas *chondroitin 6-sulphate* and *keratan sulphate* are dominant in the cornea. Skin contains hyaluronic acid, dermatan sulphate and chondroitin 6-sulphate, which predominate in turn as the embryonic tissue grows older. As rib cartilage ages, the chondroitin sulphate is replaced by keratan sulphate. The proportion of fibrous protein to proteoglycan also varies in different tissues and, as already mentioned, increases with age. Since collagen is the principal fibrous protein and characteristically contains a high proportion of hydroxyproline (page 35), the hydroxyproline/hexosamine ratio is a convenient index of the extent to which the ground substance has been impregnated with fibres. Values for this index vary considerably, e.g. 2·8 for cartilage, 12·2 for skin and 30 for tendon.

The various constituents of connective tissues are structurally integrated and do not act in isolation. Thus although cartilage is characteristically rich in proteoglycans, very little can be extracted with water but, if the tissue is finely ground to destroy the structure, as much as 60–80% of the total chondroitin sulphate can be extracted. The remaining polysaccharide is firmly bound to the collagen and can only be removed by reagents that break bonds between carbohydrate and protein. These bonds help to anchor proteoglycans in position within the tissue.

The connective tissue glycosaminoglycans are readily broken down within the body and numerous data on the turnover rates of hyaluronic acid and the chondroitin sulphates have shown their half-lives to vary from 2 to 4 days depending on the type of glycosaminoglycan, the organ and the age of the animal.

Enzymes known as *hyaluronidases* are widely distributed in animal tissues and, in several cases, have been shown to have acid pH optima and to be localized in the lysosomes. Experiments carried out *in vitro* have, in fact, shown the lysosomes to contain a full complement of the enzymes needed to convert hyaluronic acid and the sulphated glycosaminoglycans to their monosaccharide constitutents. The enzymes of this hyaluronidase group are able to depolymerize the glycosaminoglycans *in vivo*, so facilitating movement of both water and polysaccharide through the tissue spaces. By locally breaking down this attenuated structure the hyaluronidases increase the permeability of the tissue and when present in animal venoms and bacterial toxins they act as 'spreading factors'. The oligosaccharides produced by the action of hyaluronidase may subsequently be acted upon by various exoglycosidases.

Some disorders of proteoglycan metabolism, e.g. *Hurler's syndrome*, have been shown to be enzyme-deficiency diseases in which a lysosomal enzyme is missing (page 203).

Fibronectin

The fibronectins are a family of glycoproteins of high molecular weight which are found in cells, extracellular fluids and tissues, including connective tissues. They are involved in the adhesion of cells to extracellular matrices, the coagulation of blood and wound healing. Loss of fibronectin from the surfaces of cells is associated with changes in cell morphology, and deficiency of fibronectin on malignant cells may be associated with increased invasiveness, as cells no longer cluster together.

Fibronectin is present in plasma at a concentration of 250 μg ml^{-1}, where it exists mainly as a polypeptide dimer of molecular weight 220 000. It has an asymmetrical elongated structure with several globular domains, joined by sections that are susceptible to proteolysis. Fibronectin also has regions which are capable of binding specifically to a variety of molecules, including fibrin, Factor XIII, heparin, actin, collagen and surface structures of various species of micro-organisms. Because of its ability to interact with cell surfaces as well as collagen fibrils, fibronectin probably plays an important part in the organization of the larger-scale structural patterns of individual connective tissues.

The protein fibres

The extracellular protein fibres are the most important and characteristic constituents of connective tissues. As already mentioned, the protein molecules are synthesized by the fibroblasts and secreted into the watery ground substance where they become organized into fibres by aggregation of the individual macromolecules under the action of physicochemical forces. The macromolecules thus can be regarded as prefabricated building units, designed for rapid self-assembly into much larger structures. Once assembled, the resulting fibrils and fibres give the connective tissue enormous mechanical strength compared with that of the ground substance alone.

Three main kinds of fibrous protein are found in connective tissues, *collagen*, *reticulin* and *elastin*. Collagen is the most abundant protein of mammals and accounts for 25–30% of their total protein content. Reticulin, although a histologically defined entity, is built up from collagen units, together with carbohydrate and possibly lipid, as described in Chapter 26. Elastin, on the other hand, is an entirely different protein; it is more restricted in its occurrence and is found abundantly where great mechanical strength together with elasticity is required, as in the major arteries.

Collagen

The name collagen comes from the Greek, meaning a glue producer. When this white insoluble fibrous protein is heated with water it gradually breaks down to produce the soluble derived

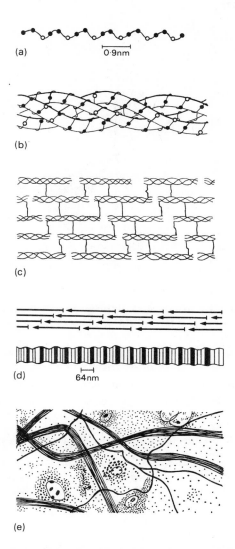

(a)

0·9nm

(b)

(c)

(d)

64nm

(e)

Figure 27.2 Features of collagen structure at increasing orders of size. (a) Single helical chains of protocollagen. (b) Triple helix. (c) Portion of a collagen fibril. N.B. The individual triple helices are considerably foreshortened so that the cross-linkages may be shown. (d) Part of a collagen fibre at a lower magnification than (c) showing (1) quarter staggering effect and (2) striated appearance of a stained fibril. (e) Bundles of collagen fibrils as they appear in connective tissue

protein, *gelatin* (animal glue). Gelatin resembles collagen in composition but the systematic structure has been disarranged so that gelatin is soluble in water in which it forms a gel.

Collagen occurs throughout the vertebrate subphylum and also in slightly varied forms in several invertebrate phyla. Only arthropods, which have the polysaccharide chitin as an alternative constructional material, lack collagen. It seems that collagen appeared early in evolution and its composition and structure have changed relatively little, suggesting that its design has approached optimum efficiency.

Application of refined methods of chemical analysis, X-ray diffraction and electron

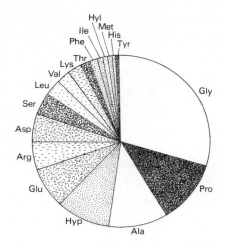

Figure 27.3 Composition of collagen. The area of the sectors corresponds to the relative abundance of the amino acids

microscope techniques have built up a picture of the structure of collagen fibres ranging from the atomic level to that of the connective tissues themselves (Figure 27.2).

Chemical composition

The amino acid composition of a typical mammalian collagen is summarized in Figure 27.3, while Table 27.3 includes values from a wider range of animals. There is a remarkably constant

Table 27.3 Amino acid composition of various vertebrate collagens (values given as residues per 1000 total residues)

	Toad skin	Python skin	Whale skin	Human	
				Skin	Bone
Alanine	98	125	111	115	114
Glycine	301	315	326	324	319
Valine	22	20	21	25	24
Leucine	29	26	25	25	26
Isoleucine	14	12	11	10	13
Proline	110	119	128	125	123
Phenylalanine	19	14	13	13	14
Tyrosine	6	2	4	4	5
Serine	66	44	41	37	36
Threonine	26	18	24	18	18
Cystine	—	—	—	—	—
Methionine	9	6	5	7	5
Arginine	49	50	50	49	47
Histidine	7	5	6	5	6
Lysine	29	28	26	27	28
Aspartic acid	55	48	46	47	47
Glutamic acid	78	62	70	78	72
Hydroxyproline	78	102	89	91	100
Hydroxylysine	4	4	6	6	4

pattern throughout mammalian tissues. Slightly larger variations occur among the vertebrates as a whole, although certain features are common throughout. The main features of composition in mammalian collagens are as follows.

1. The most abundant residue is *glycine*, which, instead of a hydrocarbon side chain, has a second hydrogen atom attached to the backbone carbon atom. Glycine makes up almost exactly one-third of all the amino acids of collagen, and sequence studies show that, along the greater part of the collagen chain, every third residue is glycine.
2. Collagen contains two amino acids, *hydroxyproline* and *hydroxylysine*, that are not found in other animal tissue proteins. Although hydroxyproline is present in concentrations of about 1 residue in 10 in mammalian collagen, hydroxylysine occurs as only 1 in 200 (Table 27.3). During the biosynthesis of collagen, hydroxyproline and hydroxylysine are incorporated into the *protocollagen* chain (page 416) as proline and lysine and are specifically

$$HO-HC-CH_2$$
$$H_2C \quad CH-COOH$$
$$NH$$

4-Hydroxyproline

$$CH_2NH_2$$
$$CHOH$$
$$CH_2$$
$$CH_2$$
$$HOOC-CHNH_2$$

δ-Hydroxylysine

hydroxylated only after the polypeptide chain has been formed. Hydroxyproline is derived from proline, the commonly occurring imino acid of proteins, by substitution of a hydroxyl group in its heterocyclic pyrrolidine ring. Hydroxylysine is formed by addition of a hydroxyl group to the penultimate carbon atom in the side chain of lysine. The other 16 amino acids found in collagen occur in most proteins.
3. The total *imino acid content* of collagen is higher than in most other proteins. Proline and hydroxyproline together account for two-ninths of the residues. Wherever an imino acid unit occurs there is a loss of free rotation about successive bonds in the polypeptide chain because of the influence of the rigid planar pyrrolidine ring (Figure 27.4). In consequence the chain is both stiff and bent at this point.
4. Collagen is a *hydrophilic protein* having a relatively high proportion of amino acids with polar side chains and a relatively low proportion with lipophilic side chains. Hydroxyproline and hydroxylysine enhance this effect and, as a consequence, in an aqueous environment the collagen molecule remains extended and does not fold up on itself like globular proteins.
5. Unlike keratin, collagen has *large amounts of a few kinds of amino acids* and only small amounts of the remainder. Four amino acids, glycine, alanine, proline and hydroxyproline, together occupy two-thirds of the positions in the polypeptide chain (Figure 27.3).
6. The total of amino acids with basic side chains slightly exceeds those with free carboxyl groups. Collagen is thus a *basic protein* with an isoelectric point in the region of pH 9·4.
7. Glucose and galactose are covalently bound to both soluble and insoluble vertebrate collagens and together account for 0·4% by weight, so collagen may be regarded as a *glycoprotein* with an exceptionally low content of carbohydrate.

Structure of the collagen macromolecule

The individual polypeptide chains of collagen each contain approximately 1000 amino acid residues while the *tropocollagen* macromolecule contains three polypeptide chains, twisted

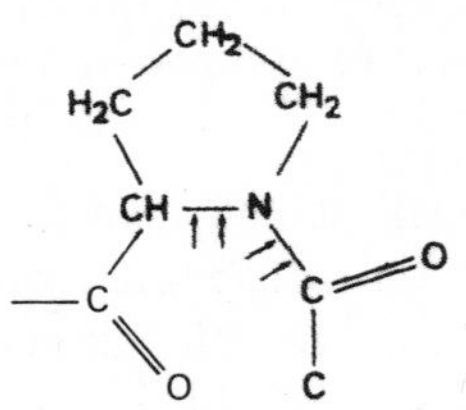

Figure 27.4 The ring structure of an imino acid showing how it restricts the conformation of polypeptide chains. No free rotation can occur about the two bonds in the main chain indicated by arrows. Atoms in the shaded area are coplanar

round each other like a three-stranded rope. The resulting molecule is long (280 nm) and narrow (1·35 nm). It is shaped like a thin rod and, unlike its component chains, is stiff or only very slightly flexible.

The detailed spatial structure has been worked out using X-ray diffraction data, together with the clue that glycine occupies every third position. The main structural features of the collagen macromolecule are shown in Figure 27.5.

Each of the three chains is wound round its own (chain) axis in a simple left-handed helix of pitch approximately 0·9 nm and having three amino acid units per turn, as shown in Figure 27.5(a). It will be noticed that every third residue comes vertically above each other in a stack. In the diagram glycine residues are denoted by white circles and other residues by black circles; the stack of glycine residues is on the right-hand side in Figure 27.5(a).

Now consider three such simple helices placed with their chain axes parallel to each other along the edges of an equilateral triangular prism. The axis of the molecule (shown as a broken arrow in Figure 27.5b) passes through the centre of the prism and parallel to the chain axes. Each chain is arranged with its stack of white glycine residues pointing inwards towards the molecular axis, and the helices are staggered by a distance of 0·3 nm so that the glycine units are equally spaced along the axis. Since the glycine residues have no side chains, this allows the closest possible packing of the three simple helices (Figure 27.5b). The actual structure of the collagen

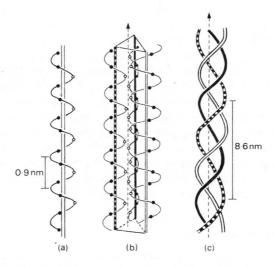

Figure 27.5 Arrangement of the polypeptide chains in the collagen macromolecule

molecule is easily derived from this by giving the system a slight twist so that the chain axes themselves form gentle right-handed helices of pitch 8·6 nm round the straight central axis of the macromolecule (Figure 27.5c).

The three chains in the collagen macromolecule are held together by hydrogen bonds between NH and CO groups in the backbones of different polypeptide chains. Studies with molecular models show that these sets of hydrogen bonds can only be formed if the three chains approach one another as closely as possible. In addition to the part played by glycine residues, the presence of so many imino acids in collagen assists the close approach of chains because of the appropriate bending in the polypeptide chain, wherever they occur. Moreover, the lack of free rotation in this region enhances molecular stability. Fish collagens, which have lower contents of imino acids than mammalian collagens, are less stable as shown by their lower temperatures at which the molecules are denatured. Two hydrogen bonds can be formed for every three amino acid residues since the imino acid residues, proline and hydroxyproline, are unable to form hydrogen bonds as they have no hydrogen attached to their nitrogen atoms.

Soluble collagen and the α subunits

A small proportion of the collagen in tissues, particularly those from young animals or healing wounds, will dissolve in cold salt solutions. This *soluble collagen* has all the characteristics of collagen *in situ*, including the capacity to form fibres. Neutral sodium chloride solution is able to dissolve some 1%, and acid citrate buffer approximately 5%, of the collagen from calf skin. Soluble collagen has been shown to be the most recently formed collagen and consists of isolated tropocollagen macromolecules in free solution. If such a solution is heated above 40°C, thermal forces denature the macromolecules by breaking the hydrogen bonds, which hold the polypeptide chains together in the triple helix and so allow the chains to separate and form random coils. The solution containing the free polypeptide chains is referred to as *parent gelatin*. The three chains derived from each macromolecule are referred to as α subunits; in most tissues, two of the three chains appear to be identical and are designated α1, the third being α2.

Collagen biosynthesis

The synthesis of collagen presents a number of unusual and interesting features, since the polypeptide chains undergo extensive modification during or after their synthesis. So-called *protocollagen* chains which contain unhydroxylated proline and lysine are assembled on the ribosomal complexes of the fibroblasts, and hydroxylation of certain of the proline and lysine residues occurs after they have been built into the chain, possibly while the nascent chains are still attached to the ribosomes. This point has still to be decided. The hydroxylation of proline is catalysed by *protocollagen proline hydroxylase* which requires molecular oxygen, 2-oxoglutarate, ferrous iron and ascorbic acid for its activity. Ascorbic acid deficiency arrests collagen biosynthesis and causes scurvy. The factors that determine which proline residues shall be hydroxylated are not fully understood, but it has been found that the enzyme has no effect on free proline and will only hydroxylate residues that are situated on the amino side of a glycine residue, e.g. Gly–X–Pro–Gly–. A different enzyme appears to be responsible for the hydroxylation of lysine.

The protocollagen chains, as synthesized within the fibroblast, are about 20% longer than the α chains of tropocollagen and it is in this longer form that three of them come together to form a triple helix. Further modification occurs at this stage in that galactose or glucosyl galactose units become attached by glycosidic linkage to certain of the hydroxylysine residues. It is in this hydroxylated glycosylated extended triple helical form, which is known as *procollagen*, that the collagen building units appear ready to be secreted into the extracellular matrix where *fibrilogenesis* occurs. The additional *telopeptide* is removed from procollagen either as it leaves the cell or extracellularly, prior to the aggregation of the tropocollagen units, so formed.

Two reasons have been suggested for the existence of procollagen: firstly, that the extra lengths of chain that contain both cysteine and tyrosine in some way promote the formation of the triple helix and, secondly, that it prevents the molecules from aggregating into fibrils while they are still located within the cell.

The enzyme that causes the partial proteolysis of procollagen and removes the disposable 20% of residues may be present extracellularly, but so far it has not been identified.

Aggregation of macromolecules to form a fibril

The next largest element of collagen structure is the *fibril*, which is formed by the aggregation of many tropocollagen macromolecules. The collagen fibril is revealed by the electron microscope as a structure from 20 to 100 nm in width (varying according to the tissue and its age) and of indefinite length. The electron microscope shows characteristic cross-striations repeating every 64 nm. Fibrils are slightly flexible structures and usually follow a gently curving path through the tissue, perhaps following the track of the fibroblast which synthesized the macromolecules. Fibrils usually occur in parallel bundles which constitute the fibres visible with the optical microscope and give each connective tissue its own characteristic weave pattern (see Figure 27.2e).

Fibrilogenesis is an extracellular process involving side-by-side aggregation of tropocollagen units. Orientation and mutual attraction are brought about mainly by electrostatic forces between charged groups on the ionized side chains of neighbouring macromolecules. The main evidence for this is that 'native type' collagen fibrils have been reconstituted *in vitro* from solutions of soluble collagen simply by adjusting the electrolyte concentration.

The concentration and type of electrolyte have an important effect on whether fibrils are produced and their main characteristics. It seems likely therefore that the same effect should operate *in vivo*, where, in addition to small ions, polyelectrolytes such as hyaluronic acid and chondroitin sulphate are present in the ground substance of the developing connective tissue. In addition to electrostatic forces, hydrogen bonding and hydrophobic bonding probably help to hold the macromolecules together in a specific relationship to form the fibrils.

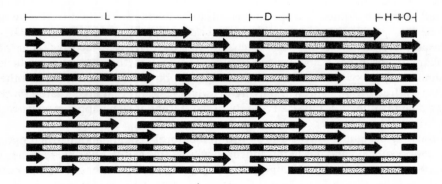

Figure 27.6 Aggregation of collagen macromolecules to form a striated fibril – the quarter staggered arrangement

The periodic fine structure of the fibril as seen in the electron microscope probably corresponds to repeated regions in which particular kinds of amino acid side chains predominating in specific parts of macromolecules are brought into register by aggregation.

Several attempts have been made to account for the observed periodicity. The earliest idea assumed that there is a systematic aggregation of macromolecules in *quarter staggered array*, each macromolecule overlapping its neighbour by one-quarter of its length (Figure 27.6). If the repeat distance of the fibril structure (64 nm) is designated D, the length L of the macromolecule (280 nm) works out at 4·4D and it is necessary to assume a hole having a length of 0·6D between the ends of successively aligned macromolecules so that the effective overlap O is only 0·4D, leaving a hole (H = 0·6D) between the head and tail of successive molecules.

Recently it has been pointed out that in the quarter staggered arrangement only a single plane of the fibril is considered and that, if three dimensions are taken into account, it is no longer possible to fit all the macromolecules into a quarter staggered system. In fact, for a collagen fibril of average diameter, only two-thirds of the molecules could be fitted into such a pattern and alternative possibilities have been suggested though none is completely satisfactory.

Formation of cross-linkages and the maturation of collagen

Up to the present, the only bonds that have been considered here as holding the three polypeptide chains together in the macromolecule and, on a larger scale, the macromolecules within the fibril, have been comparatively weak ones, namely hydrogen bonds, electrostatic forces and hydrophobic bonds. There is evidence that in mature collagen there are also covalent bonds between different polypeptide chains, and that, though these are relatively few and widely separated (Figure 27.2), they play a very important part in keeping the whole structure of the fibril firmly locked together. This is supported by the finding that only a small fraction of the collagen in tissues will dissolve in neutral sodium chloride solutions which break non-covalent bonds.

Similarly there is definite evidence for strong intramolecular bonds between the polypeptide chains within individual triple helices. It has already been mentioned that when solutions containing soluble collagen are heated, hydrogen bonds are broken and the three chains come apart; the mixture of chains can then be separated chromatographically. In addition to the α subunits, which represent single polypeptide chains, larger particles can be separated having slightly different chromatographic properties. These are the β and γ fractions. They represent combinations of two or three of the α chains joined by stable cross-linkages, e.g. β_{12} composed of one $\alpha1$ and one $\alpha2$ chain, β_{11} composed of two $\alpha1$ chains, and γ units, containing all three chains from a macromolecule.

It thus appears that when the macromolecule is first incorporated in the fibril it is held in position only by weak forces, and that, with the passage of time, covalent cross-linkages spontaneously form both intramolecularly within the triple helices and intermolecularly between neighbouring helices in the same fibril until the constituents of the whole fibril are firmly joined by covalent bonds, as shown in Figure 27.2(c). Only a few of these cross-linkages, perhaps only two or three per macromolecule, are necessary to stabilize the structure. This is because the structure is already highly ordered by weak bonds and thus requires only sufficient covalent cross-linking to prevent it from uncoiling and the chains slipping apart.

The gradual spontaneous formation of stable cross-linkages, known as the *maturation* or *ageing* of collagen, begins as soon as the fibril is laid down and continues slowly for many months. Thus as it ages, collagen gradually increases in mechanical strength and resistance to denaturation, and decreases in solubility. The turnover time for collagen is very long compared with most proteins but differs considerably for different collagen molecules within the same tissue. Newly laid down collagen is more soluble than the older highly cross-linked material and therefore more likely to be dissolved and replaced. This applies at all stages of maturation, the less cross-linked fraction turning over quite rapidly and the highly cross-linked one extremely slowly.

The nature of the stable cross-linkages in collagen has proved difficult to study because they are so few in number and are of an unusual type. Unlike the keratins, most mature collagens contain no cysteine so that disulphide bridges cannot be formed. Various possibilities have been suggested, but present opinion favours cross-linkages involving lysine and hydroxylysine.

At this point it should be mentioned that the first 16 residues of the α chains of tropocollagens do not have glycine in every third position and do not adopt the triple helical structure which starts at residue 17. The non-helical N-terminal region does, however, contain a lysine or hydroxylysine residue which, according to Piez, acts as a cross-linkage precursor. The first step in the cross-linkage process is the conversion of this and possibly other lysine (or hydroxylysine) residues to an aldehyde known as *allysine* (or *hydroxyallysine*) which then undergoes condensation with another molecule of hydroxylysine with the formation of a double bond and the elimination of water (Figure 27.7). Reduction of the double bond stabilizes this collagen cross-linkage.

The existence of a cross-linkage based on aldehydes also explains the aetiology of the rare condition of *lathyrism* which occurs in animals eating the seed of a sweet pea *Lathyrus odoratus* which contains a toxic agent (γ-glutamylaminopropionitrile). In this disease the connective tissues have a high water content and a brittle collagen, a high proportion of which is extractable. The condition can also be induced artificially by administering various organic nitriles such as aminoacetonitrile. Organic nitriles do not affect the synthesis and aggregation of the tropocollagen molecules but prevent the conversion of free amino groups of lysine to aldehydes and hence the formation of stable cross-linkages and maturation of the collagen. They have no effect on collagen that is already mature.

The importance of cross-linkages in maintaining the normal tensile strength and degree of extensibility of the connective tissues is illustrated by the *Ehlers–Danlos syndrome*, a hereditary disorder of connective tissue which is characterized by a hyperextensible skin, hypermobile joints, fragile tissues and a tendency to bleeding. The disorder appears in a variety of forms in

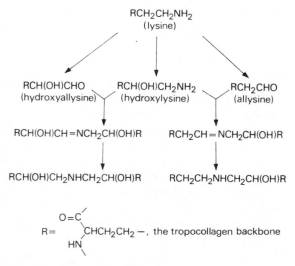

Figure 27.7 Formation of lysine-derived cross-links in collagen

one of which the collagen has been found to have an excess of lysine and a deficiency of hydroxylysine as a result of a functional deficiency of *lysyl hydroxylase*. Cross-linking is defective in collagen lacking hydroxylysine.

Another disorder resulting from a collagen abnormality is *dermatosparaxis* which occurs in cattle and is characterized by a very fragile skin. In this case the basic defect is a lack of *collagen protease*, the enzyme that removes the extra polypeptide segment which distinguishes procollagen from tropocollagen. The fact that the normal $\alpha1$ and $\alpha2$ chains are replaced by the longer pro-$\alpha1$ and pro-$\alpha2$ chains appears to prevent the collagen fibres from forming normal orderly bundles in the dermis.

Yet another connective tissue disorder which may result from a collagen abnormality is *osteogenesis imperfecta* where there is disruption of the normal collagen–apatite relationship. Among its most frequent manifestations are brittle bones, deafness, a thin skin, loose-jointedness and hernia. The teeth often have an abnormal coloration and, although the enamel is essentially normal, the dentine is defective and soft, and the root canals and pulp chambers tend to become obliterated.

Genetically distinct collagen types

It has recently been discovered that at least nine distinct types of collagen exist whose composition is genetically determined. The different types presumably have subtle variations of function, since different connective tissues vary as regards the presence or absence, as well as the relative proportions, of the types of collagen which they contain. Table 27.4 summarizes the kinds of α-chain which are present in the five most commonly occurring genetically determined types of collagen, together with the tissues within which each type is present in substantial amounts.

Table 27.4 Genetically determined types of collagen

Collagen	Constituent chain(s)	Tissues where present
Type I	$\alpha1(I), \alpha2(I)$	Skin, tendon, bone, dentine, placenta
Type II	$\alpha1(II)$	Hyaline cartilage
Type III	$\alpha1(III)$	Skin, vessel walls
Type IV	$\alpha1(IV), \alpha2(IV)$	Basement membranes
Type V	$\alpha1(V), \alpha2(V), \alpha3(V)$	Vessel walls, uterus
Type I – trimer	$\alpha1(I)$	

The amino acid composition of the nine kinds of constituent α-chains which make up type I to type V collagens is shown in Table 27.5. While all these α-chains conform to the typical collagen pattern already described (e.g. glycine 330–350, hydroxyproline 91–125 residues per 1000), there are substantial variations in some of the lesser amino acid constituents. In particular hydroxylysine varies from five residues per 1000 in $\alpha1(III)$ chains to 50 per 1000 in the $\alpha1(IV)$ chains of type IV collagen. Moreover no less than 44 of these 50 chains are glycosylated. Since type IV collagen is associated with basement membrane, which shows the characteristic staining reactions of reticulin with silver stains, clearly a special type of collagen is required to associate closely with the polysaccharide and lipid, known to be major constituents of reticulin.

Collagenase

Because of its unusual triple helical structure very few enzymes are able to attack collagen but it has been known for some time that specific *collagenases* are produced by certain bacteria notably the *Clostridia* group of anaerobes which cause gas gangrene. Although tissue collagenases are obviously necessary for the normal resorption and turnover of collagen in the body, attempts to demonstrate their presence in vertebrate tissues were for a long time singularly unsuccessful. However, a tissue culture technique in which metamorphosing tadpole tails are grown on reconstituted collagen gels has been developed and the presence of collagenase indicated by an area of collagen breakdown in the vicinity of the tissue. Using this technique a variety of mammalian tissues has been shown to produce collagenases and recently it has been possible to identify specific collagenases in tissue extracts and some biological fluids.

By definition, collagenases are enzymes which are capable of digesting native collagen fibrils under physiological conditions of pH, temperature and ionic strength and which act by cleaving

Table 27.5 Amino acid composition of the human collagen chains (residues/1000 total residues)

Amino acid	$\alpha1(I)$	$\alpha2(I)$	$\alpha1(II)$	$\alpha1(III)$	$\alpha1(IV)$	$\alpha2(IV)$	$\alpha1(V)$	$\alpha2(V)$	$\alpha3(V)$
Hydroxyproline	109	94	99	125	123	111	115	109	92
Aspartic acid	42	44	43	42	45	49	49	50	42
Threonine	16	19	23	13	19	30	21	29	19
Serine	34	30	25	39	38	30	23	34	34
Glutamic acid	73	68	89	71	78	65	100	89	97
Proline	124	113	120	107	85	73	130	107	98
Glycine	333	338	333	350	334	324	332	331	330
Alanine	115	102	103	96	30	47	39	54	49
Half-cystine	0	0	0	2	0	2	0	0	1
Valine	21	35	18	14	33	27	17	27	29
Methionine	7	5	10	8	15	14	9	11	8
Isoleucine	6	14	9	13	32	38	17	15	20
Leucine	19	30	26	22	52	56	36	37	56
Tyrosine	1	4	2	3	5	7	4	2	2
Phenylalanine	12	12	13	8	27	36	12	11	9
Hydroxylysine	9	12	20	5	50	36	36	23	43
Lysine	26	18	15	30	6	7	14	13	15
Histidine	3	12	2	6	6	6	6	10	14
Arginine	50	50	50	46	22	42	40	48	42
Gal-Hyl	1	1	4	—	2	2	5	3	7
Glc-Gal-Hyl	1	2	12	—	44	29	29	5	17

the helical part of the molecule. This definition excludes proteolytic enzymes such as trypsin and pronase which attack the non-helical part of the molecule. Tadpole and human skin collagenase, and probably other vertebrate collagenases, act by splitting all chains of the helix about three-quarters of the way from the *N*-terminus at a Gly-Leu bond. This produces long (TCA) and short (TCB) fragments the component chains of which separate spontaneously. The resulting single chains are then susceptible to digestion by non-specific tissue enzymes.

Collagenases have been demonstrated in bone, skin, synovial tissue, gingival tissue and polymorphonuclear leucocytes. They are most readily obtained from tissues where the rate of collagen breakdown is increased, either as a result of some normal process such as the involution of the postpartum uterus, or as a result of disease, e.g. in gingivitis, rheumatoid arthritis, or wound healing. While, for the most part, the enzymes from the various tissues share the same characteristics there are some differences of unknown physiological significance.

The presence of active collagenases poses a threat to the integrity of body structures so it is to be expected that their activity is closely controlled. Collagenases are readily inhibited by components of normal serum, notably by the α-globulin fraction as well as by cysteine and EDTA. While crude extracts of normal human skin have no collagenase activity, if the proteins are separated chromatographicallys some of the fractions are enzymically active having apparently been unmasked. One way in which collagenase activity may be regulated is apparently by controlling the concentration of protein inhibitors. There is also some evidence that collagenase is synthesized in an inactive precursor form. *Procollagenase* was first shown in tadpole tail, but human leucocytes also have been found to contain a procollagenase which can be activated by trypsin and by a constituent of the synovial fluid in rheumatoid joints.

Gingival collagenase

In periodontal disease there is destruction of collagen in the periodontal membrane and alveolar bone which support the teeth. Samples of gingivae from patients suffering from gingivitis produce lysis of collagen in culture plates. Since collagenase has been shown to be present in normal gingivae, it seems likely that both bacterial and endogenous collagenases may contribute to the breakdown of the tooth-supporting structures.

Breakdown of connective tissue in vivo

The collagen present in the various connective tissues is made up of a number of fractions of differing age and stability and although the newly formed fibrils are most readily degraded even the most stable forms are subject to resorption under certain physiological or pathological conditions.

Most of the work on collagenase has been carried out on pure preparations of collagen whereas the breakdown of connective tissue *in vivo* is a far more complex process in which a variety of lysosomal enzymes probably act synergistically with collagenase. Hyaluronidase may be initially necessary to depolymerize the matrix and allow the collagenase access to the collagen fibrils. Even then hydrolysis of collagen to the TCA and TCB fragments does not guarantee solubilization of the fibrils. The further steps needed to remove the fragments from the fibril can be effected either by collagenase itself or by other non-specific proteases. A problem arises since, whereas collagenase is active in the neutral pH range, the lysosomal proteases act best at pH 4·5–5·0. The presence of collagen fibres undergoing lysis within the vacuoles of macrophages in the involuting mouse uterus supports the idea that once fibrils have undergone partial breakdown they can be digested intracellularly by the connective tissue cells.

Elastin

Whereas collagen is found where a pliant but relatively non-extensible framework is required, for example in ligaments, tendons, fascia and joint capsules, elastin fibres are found in considerable quantities in the arteries, lungs and skin, as well as in the neck ligaments of grazing animals where they contribute to the elasticity of the tissues. The composition and properties of the yellow elastic fibres are quite different from those of collagen. Elastin, like collagen, contains a high proportion of glycine and also of alanine, valine and leucine which have non-polar hydrocarbon side chains. On the other hand, it contains exceedingly small amounts of amino acids with ionizable side chains. Hydroxylysine is altogether absent from elastin and hydroxyproline is present in much smaller amounts than in collagen.

Elastin, in contrast to collagen, is a highly lipophilic protein. The amino acids are attracted to each other by hydrophobic bonds rather than to environmental water. This probably accounts for the very great hydrothermal stability of elastin.

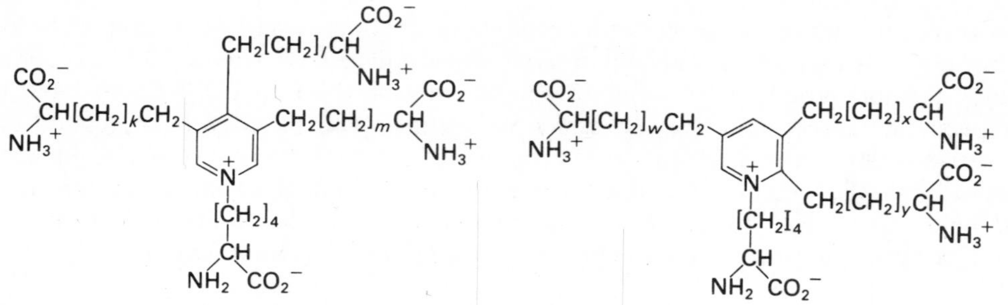

Figure 27.8 Desmosine and isodesmosine cross-links in elastin which connect four chains together to give a rubber-like elasticity

Elastin is highly cross-linked by a special type of structure whereby four polypeptide chains are connected together at one point giving rise to a stable system with a rubber-like elasticity (Figure 27.8). The structures responsible for cross-linking the chains have been isolated from acid hydrolysates of elastin. These desmosine units, which are much too bulky to fit into a systematic structure like collagen, are formed from lysine in a process analogous to the maturation of collagen. The relative lysine contents of soluble and mature elastin are shown in Table 27.6. Mature elastin is very insoluble and consequently cannot be subjected to extensive sequence analysis, but a soluble form has been isolated from the aortae of copper-deficient pigs which are unable to form normal cross-linkages. Data obtained on this soluble elastin show that it contains two different types of region namely (1) areas that are rich in alanine and lysine and are presumably concerned with cross-linking and (2) areas that are rich in glycine, proline and valine which may be concerned with extensibility. On the basis of these and other findings a model for the elastin molecule has recently been proposed but the validity of this model, which has many interesting features, has still to be established.

Table 27.6 Amino acid composition of soluble and mature elastin compared with that of collagen

	Human skin collagen (residues per 1000 residues)	*Elastin* (residues per 850 residues)	
		Soluble	*Mature*
Glycine	324	275	277
Alanine	115	196	197
Proline	125	95	86
Hydroxyproline	91	7·5	12
Valine	25	110	105
Isoleucine	10	15	16
Leucine	25	38	44
Tyrosine	4	12	14
Phenylalanine	13	24	27
Arginine	49	4·4	5·5
Lysine	27	38	6
Asp + Asn	47	2·7	7·5
Threonine	18	12	14
Serine	37	8	11
Glu + Gln	78	16	18
Hydroxylysine	6	—	—
Met + Cys + Trp + His	12	0	2·6

Section 7

Calcified tissues

Chapter 28
Biological mineral

Mineralized tissues consist of an inorganic phase and one or more organic components. Some idea of the range of organisms which possess mineralized tissues, together with the types of mineral and organic components they contain is given in Table 28.1. Vertebrate mineralized tissues all have a form of calcium phosphate as their main inorganic constituent, but other highly

Table 28.1 Some mineralized tissues found in various groups of living organisms

Group of organisms	Mineralized tissue	Inorganic component	Organic components
Diatoms	Shell	SiO_2	Polyuronic acids Amino acids Polyamines
Higher plants	Cell wall	$CaCO_3$ (calcite)	Cellulose Pectins Lignins
Radiolaria	Exoskeleton	$SrSO_4$	?
Brachipods (Lingula)	Shell	Hydroxyapatite	Chitin Protein
Molluscs Arthropods (Squila)	Exoskeleton Chellae	$CaCO_3$ { Calcite Aragonite Hydroxyapatite	Chitin Protein Chitin

Vertebrates	Epithelia
	  Balleen
	  Claws, nails, feathers
	Tooth
		Hydroxyapatite	Keratins
			'Intracellular mineralization'

	Enamel	Hydroxyapatite	Amelogenins
	Dentine Cementum Skeleton	Hydroxyapatite	Collagen
	Bone	Hydroxyapatite	Collagen
	Cartilage Pathological	Hydroxyapatite	Collagen + chondroitin sulphate
	Renal calculi	Ca salts	Glycoproteins

insoluble substances, such as silica, strontium sulphate and two forms of calcium carbonate, are found in plants and invertebrate animals. Thus, mineralization is not synonymous with calcification.

A great variety of organic components are present in mineralized tissues, but mainly they are substances of high molecular weight and many of them are polyions. The calcified tissues of vertebrates all have a protein as their main organic constituent, though the type of protein varies.

The mineralized tissues of vertebrates are bone, dentine, enamel and cementum, but these form only a small fraction of those found in the living world.

Biological apatite

The inorganic components of vertebrate mineralized tissues consist of extremely small crystals, mostly with dimensions of approximately 10–$20 \times 5 \times 5$ nm. A significant proportion of non-crystalline calcium phosphate may also be present. The crystals in dental enamel have a diameter of 40 nm and, although still too small to be clearly resolved by the optical microscope, are considerably larger than those of bone, dentine and cementum.

The crystalline mineral in bones and teeth is generally regarded as an imperfect *calcium hydroxyapatite*. Apatite minerals, principally *calcium fluorapatite*, are both abundant and ubiquitous and are the principal source of phosphate for fertilizers. Their abundance is probably an expression of the very high affinity which calcium and phosphate ions have for each other so that it is perhaps not surprising that, on account of its stability, calcium hydroxyapatite has been selected to play an important part, both structurally and physiologically, in many living things. Ions other than calcium, phosphate and hydroxyl are present in the crystallites in which the atomic ratio of calcium to phosphorus departs considerably from the theoretical value of $1 \cdot 67$ (Table 35.1).

The accurate determination of the spatial relationships of ions in a crystal lattice requires that large well-formed single crystals be studied using a variety of techniques including X-ray diffraction, spectroscopic and optical methods. The best apatite crystals for such studies are those of artificially prepared calcium fluorapatite and, the next best, articifically prepared calcium hydroxyapatite. The description which follows is therefore principally of calcium fluorapatite, but the structure of calcium hydroxyapatite will also be mentioned.

Crystal structure

A well-formed crystal of calcium fluorapatite is a prism which can be described as having a principal axis, c, about which there is hexagonal symmetry. Three axes of equal length can be drawn normal to the c axis and at an angle of 120° to each other. These are the a axes (Figure 28.1). The basic structure of the calcium fluorapatite lattice can be likened to the pattern of a honeycomb placed vertically and viewed from above, looking along the c axis. At each of the six corners of each cell of the honeycomb, there is a calcium ion (Figure 28.2). Two phosphate ions lie between each pair of adjacent calcium ions and are displaced somewhat to either side of a line joining the calcium ions. The phosphate ions are tetrahedral in shape with phosphorus at the centre and four oxygen atoms at the apices of the tetrahedron. The projection of the phosphate tetrahedron, when viewed along the c axis, is triangular. The structure envisaged so far is a series of hexagonal cylinders whose points of intersection are formed by calcium ions and whose walls are formed by phosphate ions which are, themselves, in a hexagonal array. Within each hexagonal cylinder or 'cell' there are more Ca^{2+} ions, and also F^- ions. The Ca^{2+} ions are placed

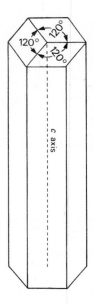

Figure 28.1 Diagram of an ideal crystal of fluorapatite showing the principal or *c* axis and the three equal *a* axes normal to it

at the apices of an equilateral triangle at the centre of which there is a F^- ion on the central *c* axis of the cylinder. *The Ca^{2+} ion triangles* are stacked on top of each other with the F^- ions directly above (or below) each other. Adjacent Ca^{2+} ion triangles are, however, rotated through 60° with respect to one another. The effect of this rotation is that when the Ca^{2+} ion triangles are viewed from above, that is, looking along the *c* axis, they appear as small hexagons (Figure 28.3). When the Ca^{2+} ion triangles, with their centrally placed F^- ions, are incorporated into the larger hexagonal cylinders, the resulting complete calcium fluorapatite structure appears as shown in Figure 28.4. The Ca^{2+} ions at the corners of the larger hexagons are referred to as *column Ca^{2+} ions*.

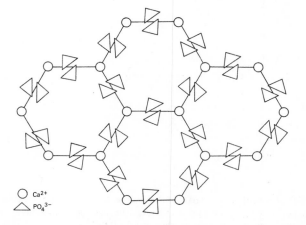

Figure 28.2 Basic structure of the calcium fluorapatite lattice. The large hexagonal 'cylinders' have been formed by joining the centres of Ca^{2+} ions in the crystal lattice. The projection of a phosphate tetrahedron is a triangle

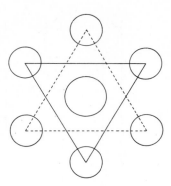

Figure 28.3 The Ca^{2+} ion triangles as they would appear superimposed when viewed along the *c* axis of the crystal lattice. At the centre of each triangle and in its plane is a F^- ion. Adjacent triangles are rotated through 60° with respect to each other giving a hexagonal outline when viewed along the *c* axis (Figure 28.4)

The unit cell

In order to simplify description of the ionic interrelationships in a crystal lattice, an entity known as the *unit cell* is used. The unit cell is a portion of a crystal which contains the least number of ions necessary to establish all of the ionic relationships which occur in the lattice. Even though a unit cell does not exist by itself, a crystal can be thought of as being built up of hundreds or even thousands of unit cells. The unit cell of calcium fluorapatite contains ten calcium ions, six phosphate ions and two fluoride ions, whilst the unit cell of calcium hydroxyapatite contains two hydroxyl ions instead of the fluoride ions. The ions within a unit cell of calcium fluorapatite and calcium hydroxyapatite can, thus, be written $Ca_{10}(PO_4)_6X_2$ where X is F^- in fluorapatite and OH^- in hydroxyapatite. However, since a unit cell has no separate existence, the shorthand expression above is not analogous to the formula for a chemical compound which exists as

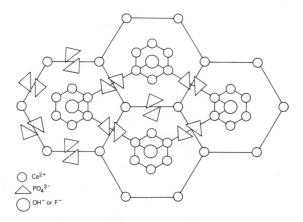

Figure 28.4 The relative positions of the ions in part of a crystal of fluorapatite as they would appear when viewed along the *c* axis. The ions do not all lie in the same plane. The small hexagonal outlines have been formed by joining the projection of ions in the 'calcium triangles'. The parallelogram is the boundary of a unit cell. N.B. It is not possible in a simple two-dimensional representation to show the relationship $Ca_{10}(PO_4)_6F_2$ quantitatively because fractions of ions are shared between different unit cells

Table 28.2 Unit cell dimensions (Å)

	a	c
Fluorapatite	9·367	6·884
Hydroxyapatite	9·418	6·880

discrete molecules. Whereas, for example, CH_3COOH states the composition of a discrete entity, i.e. a molecule, of undissociated acetic acid, $Ca_{10}(PO_4)_6(OH)_2$ states the composition of a repeating unit which does not exist on its own. The outline of a unit cell is shown in Figure 28.4 superimposed on the basic honeycomb pattern (Figure 28.2) which is the appearance if the lattice could be viewed along the c axis. The plane in which Figure 28.4 is drawn is at right angles to the c axis and is termed the ab plane. The lengths of the sides of the unit cell in the ab plane are termed a and b respectively, and the length of the unit cell along the c axis is termed c. In both fluorapatite and hydroxyapatite $a = b$. Values of a and c for fluorapatite and hydroxyapatite are given in Table 28.2. The positions of ions along the c axis, or axes parallel to it, are given as the fraction or percentage of the unit cell c dimension by which the particular ion lies above the ab plane. For example, the Ca^{2+} ions at the corners of large hexagonal units which go to make up the honeycomb structure shown in Figure 28.2 are repeated throughout the crystal lattice at intervals of one-half of the c axis distance of a unit cell. This is expressed as $c/2$ or 0·5 or 50(%). Such a value is termed a z *coordinate*. The z coordinates for fluoride and for hydroxyl ions are given in Table 28.3.

Table 28.3 The z coordinates (fraction of c) for hydroxyl and fluoride ions in hydroxyapatite and fluorapatite respectively

Fluorapatite	0·25	0·75
Hydroxyapatite	0·19	0·69
	0·31	0·81

In Figures 28.1, 28.2, 28.3 and 28.4, the relative sizes of the ions are reasonably correct but, for clarity, the distances between them are shown as being much greater than they are in a real crystal where they are packed closely together.

Fluorapatite and hydroxyapatite

It can be seen from Table 28.3 that F^- ions are situated one-quarter and three-quarters of the distance along the c axis of a unit cell. This is the same distance along the c axis as the Ca^{2+} ion triangles. The F^- ions in fluorapatite, therefore, lie in the same plane as the Ca^{2+} ions in the Ca^{2+} ion triangles (Figure 28.5a). In hydroxyapatite, however, the OH^- ion does not lie in exactly the same plane as the Ca^{2+} ions in the Ca^{2+} ion triangles, but is displaced either above or below the plane triangles (Figure 28.5b). In a unit cell, both OH^- ions will be displaced. Consequently, there are two possible sets of z coordinates for the OH^- ions according to whether they are displaced upwards or downwards. It can be seen that the structure of hydroxyapatite is less regular and compact than that of fluorapatite. This may help to explain why the former is more readily dissolved by acid.

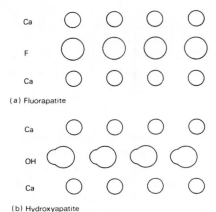

(a) Fluorapatite

(b) Hydroxyapatite

Figure 28.5 Ca^{2+} ion triangles viewed at right angles to the c axis. In fluorapatite (a) the F^- ions lie in the same plane as the Ca^{2+} ion triangles. In hydroxyapatite (b) the slightly larger OH^- ion is displaced to one side or the other of the plane of the Ca^{2+} ion triangles. The c axis is parallel with the top of the page

The variable composition of biological apatite

Although the atomic ratio of calcium to phosphorus in biological apatites may vary in either direction from the ideal value of 10:6, they all give diffuse X-ray diffraction patterns with apatite characteristics. Apart from variations in the Ca:P ratio, biological apatites include variable and often considerable quantities of 'foreign' ions. Thus, on a dry weight basis, they may contain 5% of carbonate, 1–2% of citrate, 1–2% of sodium, 0·5–1% of magnesium, 0·2–0·5% of potassium and chloride, small amounts of fluoride, and traces of zinc, manganese, molybdenum, iron, copper, lead, strontium, tin, aluminium and boron.

This variation in chemical composition, whilst the basic lattice remains unaltered, requires explanation. The diffuse nature of the X-ray diffraction pattern was attributed, some fifty years ago, to the size of the crystals which are so small that each one contains only a few hundred unit cells. More recent studies by both X-ray diffraction and electron microscopy have suggested that, in addition to the minute hydroxyapatite crystals, bone mineral contains a substantial proportion of small particles which do not give a systematic diffraction pattern but only diffuse scattering. This component, *amorphous calcium phosphate* (ACP), has been estimated to form as much as 68% of the mineral in the femur of very young rats, some 35% in adult rats and about 40% in human adults. When prepared in the laboratory, it exists as minute spheroids, about 20 nm in diameter, each with a denser outer shell enclosing a less dense central portion. Little is known about the arrangement of ions within them, except that the structure is not apatite. The Ca:P ratio is about 1·5. When such an amorphous component is present, it will give the mineral a lower overall Ca:P ratio than that of an ideal calcium hydroxyapatite (1·67).

Other ways in which the Ca:P ratio could be caused to depart from the ideal include: (1) the presence of an additional crystalline compound, octacalcium phosphate, whose unit cell composition is $Ca_8(HPO_4)_2(PO_4)_4 \cdot 5H_2O$ and whose Ca:P ratio is 1:3·3, giving rise to the possibility that biological mineral may be an 'intercrystalline mixture'; (2) substitution of other ions for calcium in the crystal lattice. For example, hydroxyapatites prepared by precipitation from solutions of different pH have different Ca:P ratios. Substitution of hydronium ions for calcium ions causes a decrease in the Ca:P ratio; (3) adsorption of excess phosphate or calcium phosphate complexes on to the crystal surface.

The presence of 'foreign' ions in biological apatite is due, in part, to the stability and ionic nature of the apatite lattice which allows 'foreign' ions to exchange or substitute for the normal residents to a great degree. A few of the many such substitutions which may occur in calcium hydroxyapatite are given in Table 28.4. The main factor which determines whether or not one ion may substitute for another is their relative sizes. Differences in charge are less important provided electrical balance can be maintained by other compensatory substitutions.

Table 28.4 Some ions which can substitute for calcium, phosphate or hydroxyl ions are listed below each of them respectively

Ca^{2+}	PO_4^{3-}	OH^-
Mg^{2+}	CO_3^{2-}	Cl^-
Na^+	HCO_3^-	F^-
Sr^{2+}	HPO_4^{2-}	CO_3^{2-}

The composition of biological apatite can also be varied by adsorption of ions on to the crystal surface. Because of the extremely small size of the crystals they have a relatively large surface area and a considerable net electrical charge on their surface. The biological implications of these features are considered in the next section.

Reactivity of hydroxyapatite

In a classical experiment carried out some years ago, a small amount of phosphate containing radioactive phosphorus was added to a large volume of a buffered solution of calcium phosphate which was in equilibrium with solid calcium hydroxyapatite. Starting immediately after the radioactive phosphate had been introduced into the system, small samples of the solution were removed at intervals and their radioactivity was determined. The results are shown in Figure 28.6. Clearly, radioactivity disappears from solution at three quite different and decreasing rates. In order to explain these results, it is necessary to consider the nature of biological apatite. In the first place, the crystals are exceedingly small containing only a few hundred unit cells. This

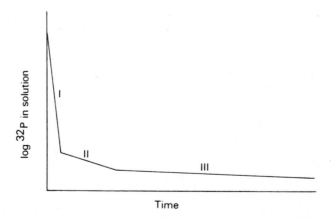

Figure 28.6 The disappearance of radioactive phosphate from a solution containing phosphate ions in equilibrium with those in solid calcium hydroxyapatite. Step I takes place in minutes, step II in hours and step III in days

means that many of the ions in the crystal lattice occupy surface positions where they produce a mosaic of positive and negative electric charges. Because the phosphate ion in the lattice is polarizable, that is to say, the distribution of its charge can be non-uniform, the negative charge on phosphate ions in surface positions will tend to shift towards neighbouring positively charged Ca^{2+} ions inside the crystal with a reduction in its negative surface charge. On the other hand, the Ca^{2+} ions are not polarizable so that those in surface positions retain their full positive charge. The result is a slight preponderance, at physiological pH values, of positive over negative charge at the crystal surface. Secondly, again because of the very small size of the crystals, they have a very large surface area. That of the hydroxyapatite of bone is of the order of $200–300\ m^2\ g^{-1}$.

The hydration shell

A further important feature of calcium hydroxyapatite is that it possesses substantial quantities of firmly bound water termed the *hydration shell*, and in the hydration shell of hydroxyapatite suspended in a dilute KCl solution, the concentration of calcium and phosphate ions is about $0.6\ \text{M}$ whilst that in the bulk solution is about $0.2\ \text{mM}$. The binding of water and other polarizable ions is a result of the high surface charge on the crystals and is the means by which this charge is neutralized. The effect of binding *polarizable* ions is a gradual dilution of the surface charge. Ca^{2+} ions in solution are hydrated ($Ca^{2+}\cdot 10H_2O$) and, unlike the Ca^{2+} within the crystal lattice, are polarizable. The interface between the crystal surface and its adjacent liquid is represented in Figure 28.7. Clearly, because of the gradual neutralization of surface charge by polarizable ions, the strength with which the ions, including those of the hydration shell itself, are attracted to the crystal surface decreases as the distance from the crystal surface increases.

   In order to answer the question 'where does the hydration shell finish and the bulk solution commence?', it is necessary to determine the size of the hydration shell. In a sense, this is arbitrary because it will depend on the means used and on the sample of hydroxyapatite. It has been shown, however, for an artificially prepared hydroxyapatite that, whilst some water may be removed by low-speed centrifugation, when the centrifugal force is increased substantially, a constant amount of water remains. This persistently retained water is regarded as the hydration shell and, for one particular sample of hydroxyapatite, each crystallite was found to have a hydration shell equivalent to twice its own volume.

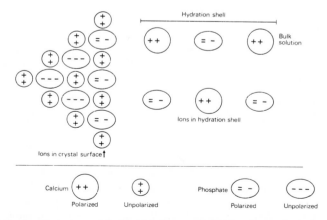

Figure 28.7 A diagram to show the nature of the interface between crystal surface and solution. The surface charge on the crystal is gradually diluted by large polarizable ions in the hydration shell

Exchange reactions

The presence of the hydration shell and the bound ion layer within it help to explain the data summarized in Figure 28.6. Whilst the ions in the hydration shell are attracted to the crystal surface, they are, nevertheless, in constant motion. Because of this movement, ions are continually shifting from the hydration shell to the bulk solution, and vice versa, in a continuous rapid process of exchange. This exchange accounts for the initial rapid loss of radioactivity, radioactive phosphate ions in the bulk solution exchanging with non-radioactive phosphate ions in the hydration shell. The second slower loss of radioactivity can be explained by an exchange of radioactive phosphate in the hydration shell with phosphate ions in the surface of the crystal, this being reflected as a slower exchange between ions in the hydration shell and those in the bulk solution. The third and slowest loss of radioactivity is explicable as an exchange of radioactive phosphate ions in the crystal surface with non-radioactive ions in the interior of the crystal. This exchange will be reflected, in turn, by exchange between ions in the crystal surface and the hydration shell, and those in the latter and the bulk solution which is where the loss of radioactivity is finally sustained and detected. The four regions between which ions are exchanged are shown diagrammatically in Figure 28.8 and related to the curve in Figure 28.6.

Exchange among any of the four compartments is not limited to calcium and phosphate ions but may include any other species present in the bulk solution. Depending on the ion, it will be more or less concentrated in the hydration shell and will, or will not, be able to exchange with ions in the crystal lattice. Monovalent ions such as Na^+, F^- and K^+ enter the hydration shell but do not become concentrated within it. Equilibrium is established between the ions in the bulk solution and those in the hydration shell. The polarizable ions include hydrated ions, especially multivalent ones, such as calcium, carbonate, citrate, magnesium and strontium, which, because of their ability to neutralize the surface charge on the crystals, tend to concentrate in the hydration shell where they are known as the *bound ion layer*. These ions are freely mobile, however, and can exchange readily with ions in the bulk solution.

Mention has already been made of substitution within the crystal lattice. A 'foreign' ion, provided that it is similar in size to the ion which it replaces, may exchange for a normal hydroxyapatite constituent. This process is called *heteroionic exchange*, whereas the exchange of like ion for like is called *isoionic exchange*. There are, thus, two ways in which ions other than calcium, phosphate or hydroxyl may become part of the structure of biological apatite. Firstly,

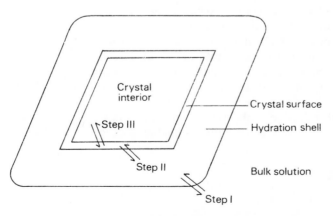

Figure 28.8 A diagrammatic representation of the four regions among which ions in solution may exchange with those in the crystal lattice of apatite. Step I is a rapid reaction which accounts for part I of the curve in Figure 28.6. Steps II and III account for parts II and III respectively in Figure 28.6

foreign ions of suitable size present in the liquid in which the mineral forms may be built in as the solid phase accumulates and, secondly, ions existing in mineral will exchange with foreign ions in the liquid bathing it. The chemical composition of biological apatite will therefore, to some extent, reflect the composition not only of the fluid in which it was formed, but also that of the fluid by which it is bathed. It is thus possible, either deliberately or accidentally, to vary the composition of the mineral slightly, although ions occupying internal lattice positions undergo exchange reactions only to a very limited extent.

Fluoride incorporation

Fluoride is often deliberately incorporated into the dental enamel in order to confer resistance to dental caries. The fluoride content of the mineralized tissues can be increased by ensuring that the teeth develop in a fluid containing fluoride ions at an optimal level. In this way, they are built more or less permanently into the crystal lattice. This can be achieved by adding fluoride in the correct amounts to public water supplies (page 149). It is also possible to incorporate a certain amount of fluoride into fully formed dental enamel by placing various phosphate- and fluoride-containing gels on the teeth. Exchange reactions enable fluoride ions to replace hydroxyl ions in surface positions. There will also be a limited exchange of hydroxyl ions in the enamel for fluoride ions in the saliva, ingested liquids and fluoride-containing toothpastes (Chapter 36).

The contribution of biological apatite to electrolyte and acid–base balance

The large surface area of the skeletal mineral is of considerable physiological significance because it enables the mineral to act as a reservoir which resists sudden changes in electrolyte concentrations in the serum or extracellular fluid (ECF). For example, a sudden fall in serum (and therefore ECF) sodium causes the rapid movement of sodium ions from the skeleton into the ECF to restore the previously existing equilibrium. The converse is also true. The bone mineral is therefore an important factor in stabilizing the electrolyte composition of the body fluids, including their acidity. Dissolution and reprecipitation of bone mineral are occurring all the time but, under conditions of increased acidity, the reaction

$$2PO_4^{3-} + 3H^+ \rightleftharpoons HPO_4^{2-} + H_2PO_4^-$$

is driven to the right and dissolution exceeds reprecipitation. The acid is neutralized but some bone mineral dissolves. Bone, therefore, represents a vast reserve of alkali.

In an adult human, not all of the mineral is readily accessible because of the continued deposition of bone during which the internal regions become more remote from the ECF and increasingly highly mineralized so that movement of ions through the densely packed mineral becomes very restricted. Even so, the skeletal mineral has a reactive surface area of about $90\,000\,m^2$!

Biological mineral thus not only confers an appropriate degree of hardness on the tissues in which it occurs, but also acts as a readily accessible reservoir of electrolytes.

Chapter 29
Bone, dentine and cementum

The calcified collagens

The mesodermal tissues bone, dentine and cementum are all similar in chemical composition and may be regarded as calcified collagens, since their predominating organic component is the protein collagen. Cartilage, another mesodermal tissue which undergoes calcification, also contains collagen but differs from the other three in having a much higher content of chondroitin sulphate. The mineral constituent of all these tissues occurs as a separate phase of biological apatite crystals together with amorphous calcium phosphate.

The extracellular substance of bone, dentine and cementum is thoroughly and fairly uniformly impregnated with tiny crystallites of apatite between, on the surface of and within the collagen fibrils, wherever there are small spaces between organic components. The apatite crystals are much smaller than those of enamel (see Chapter 28).

The collagen fibrils are laid down in the ground substance by specialized types of fibroblast – osteoblasts, odontoblasts and cementoblasts – at the developing edge of the tissue. At first the fibrils are uncalcified and the newly laid down *osteoid tissue* or *predentine* is distinguished from older calcified bone or dentine by its position as well as by the absence of crystals. Soon, amorphous calcium phosphate and, shortly afterwards, hydroxyapatite make their appearance. The initial tiny amorphous clusters rapidly grow to crystals of limited size, their growth slowing down as this size is approached. The crystals also multiply in numbers, with the result that the recently formed tissue cannot be readily distinguished from the neighbouring heavily mineralized area, laid down shortly beforehand. The *osteoblasts*, which laid down the osteoid, become embedded in the mineralized bone, and are then known as *osteocytes*, which are connected to one another by cytoplasmic processes. In dentine, *odontoblasts* move away from the amelodentinal junction and persist as a row of cells near the junction of the predentine and pulp, leaving behind long processes penetrating the thickness of the dentine.

The origins and functions of calcified mesoderm

In the mammalian embryo, cartilage precedes bone and a good deal of the skeleton is first laid down in a cartilaginous model by the process of *endochondral ossification*.

The skeleton provides mechanical support for the body, a rigid framework for muscle attachment and a system of levers which enable different parts of the body, e.g. limbs and jaws, to be moved by muscular contraction.

Dentine, which constitutes the main body of a tooth, also gives mechanical support by acting as a tough but elastic cushion for the enamel which covers the crown. The *cementum* encasing the roots holds fast the uncalcified collagen fibres of the *periodontal membrane* or *ligament*, which anchor the teeth in the jaw. The biochemical functions of these tissues are also important, the skeleton functioning throughout life as a large reservoir for calcium and phosphate ions as well as the metabolically important ions lactate and citrate. In this way bone plays a crucial role in calcium and phosphate homoeostasis.

Interchange between tissue fluid and the inorganic phase in bone, with regard to these two ions, takes place at two levels.

1. The first level, which is entirely *physicochemical*, occurs at the crystal surfaces. Here two distinct types of interaction, which differ in their time scale and reversibility, take place.
a. A fast exchange reaction occurs at the mineral surface, where there is a small, labile reserve of inorganic ions, including about 6 g of calcium, which is loosely adsorbed on the mineral surface and so can be augmented or diminished, without affecting the structure of the bone. Studies with radioisotopes have shown that complete exchange between plasma calcium and this reserve calcium takes place within about 1 min in young animals and 5 min in older animals.
b. A much slower irreversible reaction also occurs between tissue fluid and bone, and results in the gradual laying down of stable parts of the apatite lattice. Since the plasma and tissue fluids are normally supersaturated with respect to apatite (Chapter 31), this results in a steady drift of calcium and phosphate ions from solution in the blood to the solid calcium phosphates of bone. The degree of mineralization of a given piece of bone tissue will continue to increase indefinitely by this process, but as time goes on the rate of increase slows down as the crystals approach their maximum size and fill up all the available space within the tissue.
2. The second level involves two kinds of cellular participation: resorption of existing bone by osteoclasts and deposition of new bone by osteoblasts. Over short periods these two processes, acting at different sites, approximately balance each other. Acting in conjunction, they not only continuously remodel the surface contour of the bone but also play a major part in the control of calcium and phosphorus metabolism for the whole organism. Co-ordination at this second level is achieved through hormonal mediation of calcium and phosphate homoeostasis which ensures that the concentrations of these ions in the plasma and tissue fluid remain constant (Chapter 30).

Preparation of calcified tissues for analysis

Before a tissue can be analysed, it must be completely separated from neighbouring tissues which would otherwise contaminate it and invalidate the results. This is difficult with calcified tissues since they are hard and cannot be cut or broken readily without generation of heat which may cause decomposition; moreover, they are frequently in close juxtaposition to other tissues. Thus in addition to bone tissue the bones contain cartilage, periosteum (an uncalcified connective tissue), and fatty or haemopoietic marrow. Compact (cortical) bone is easily isolated in a relatively pure state from a long bone, such as a femur, of a large animal like the cow.

Dentine and cementum present greater difficulty since they are very firmly joined together and the dentine is also joined to the even harder enamel. After powdering the whole tooth, dentine and enamel can be separated by making use of the considerable difference between their densities (dentine 2·14; enamel 2·95). The main disadvantage of this is that both tissues may be contaminated by 'junction particles' of intermediate density. Cementum (density 2·03) and dentine do not differ sufficiently in density to permit a clear-cut separation.

Another method, which permits finer control, is to cut a longitudinal section through the tooth by means of a slicing machine with a diamond-impregnated disc and then systematically to dissect the section by hand. By using this technique it is possible to investigate how a given consituent varies in amount in differing areas of dentine.

Chemical balance sheets for the composition of bone and dentine

Carefully 'purified' samples of mineralized tissue have been analysed in attempts to account for the whole of their weight as known substances. In this way, chemical 'balance sheets' can be drawn up for particular tissues. Tables 29.1 and 29.2 show the results of analyses of purified cow bone and human dentine, respectively. Information regarding the composition of cementum is limited but suggests that it closely resembles bone.

Table 29.1 Composition of air-dried compact bone tissue (bovine femur diaphysis)

	Percentage by weight	
Inorganic matter		70
Insoluble in hot water	68·7	
Water-soluble	1·25	
Organic matter		21·73
Collagen	18·64	
Resistant protein material	1·02	
Citrate	1·0	
Proteoglycan (chondroitin SO₄) } Sialoprotein Mucoprotein }	1·0	
Total lipid	0·07	
Water (lost below 105°C)		8·18

Table 29.2 Composition of normal human dentine

	Percentage by weight	
Inorganic matter		75
Ash	72	
Carbon dioxide	3	
Organic matter		20
Collagen	18	
Resistant protein	0·2	
Citrate	0·89	
Lactate	0·15	
Chondroitin sulphate	0·4	
Lipid	0·2	
Unaccounted for (water retained at 100°C, errors etc.)		5

Comparison of the two tables shows that the composition of bone and dentine is extremely similar with some 70–75% of inorganic matter, most of which is calcium phosphate in the form of crystalline apatite, some 20% of organic matter of which 90–95% is collagen, and a certain amount of associated water. The living tissues contain substantially more water than is shown in the tables, probably within the range 15–20%.

The percentage of inorganic matter in bone increases with the length of time for which each particular piece of tissue has been laid down. Thus the degree of mineralization varies in the same bone, e.g. the femur, according to both the species of animal and age of the individual. It also differs from one bone to another within the same animal and even within different parts of the same bone. In microradiographs of tranverse sections of compact bone neighbouring Haversian systems (*osteons*) vary in radiolucency according to their age, the older ones being highly calcified and the newly formed ones less mineralized. A given region of bone continues to increase in its content of inorganic matter until it is eventually removed by resorption. The calcium phosphate content of an entire bone must be the sum of its constituent parts, which themselves vary in histological age because of continuous remodelling. Dentine does not necessarily undergo remodelling and so reaches a great histological age when it attains a degree of calcification of approximately 75% (Table 29.2) which is close to the maximum inorganic content for a mineralized collagenous tissue. This value is approached but seldom reached in areas of bone which persist for a long period before resorption. The values for inorganic matter given in Tables 29.1 and 29.2 are expressed on a weight basis and on account of its high density necessarily overemphasize the inorganic phase.

The reactivity of bone mineral

Some but not all of the apatite present in the body can take part in physicochemical exchange and substitution reactions. The proportion of the inorganic phase of bone which can participate in such reactions decreases as the bones become more highly mineralized. In adult animals about two-thirds of the skeletal mineral has been shown to be stable and unreactive.

When hydroxyapatite crystals have been formed, provided the solution remains super-saturated, the crystals will continue to form and grow until some physical factor becomes limiting. As mineral is deposited, water is lost so that eventually the film of water remaining between the mineral particles, or between the apatite crystal surface and the surrounding collagen, becomes so thin that it will not allow any further influx of mineral ions. When this happens crystal growth ceases. At the same time loss of mineral ions is prevented. Consequently the mineral which is deposited in calcifying tissues becomes progressively more isolated and the only reactive mineral in the adult animal results from the continual creation of new surfaces by cellular remodelling processes.

The presence of reactive mineral has an important physicochemical buffering effect on the ionic composition of the body fluids. An even greater contribution by the skeletal mineral to the control of the electrolyte level in the body fluids is achieved by the hormonal regulation of cellular processes (Chapter 30).

If some two-thirds of the apatite (mostly within cortical bone) is 'out of reach' of the body fluids and ions, it seems legitimate to regard this fraction of bone as inert stony material which does nothing more than serve a mechanical function. There is, however, a sinister feature of this non-reactive bone mineral since dangerous radioactive elements can replace ions in the apatite lattice during its formation. By taking up permanent residence there they may damage the surrounding soft tissue components through the radiation they emit when they decay. This is particularly true of strontium-90 which can replace calcium in the lattice. Radioisotopes are potentially much more dangerous to young growing animals, where the element can become incorporated into a large proportion of the mineral, some of which is eventually destined to become unreactive, than to mature individuals where it can react only with the exchangeable mineral.

Hard tissue collagens

Since the collagen of mineralized connective tissues is the predominating organic constituent, it might be expected to differ substantially from the collagen of soft tissues, such as skin and tendon. In fact, hard and soft tissue collagens are surprisingly alike in their main structural aspects and amino acid composition.

The electron microscope shows that both hard and soft tissue collagens occur as fibrils with regular striations at 64 nm intervals. The fibrils of bone and dentine collagens are arranged more haphazardly than those of soft tissues and require higher magnification to reveal the individual fibrous elements. By measuring the volume of water which is inaccessible to ^{14}C-labelled polyethylene glycol and assuming that this water is all intrafibrillar but extramolecular, the extramolecular volume of collagen fibrils in demineralized bone and dentine ($1\cdot26$–$1\cdot41$ ml g^{-1} of dry collagen) has recently been shown to be almost twice as great as that of tendon ($0\cdot70$ ml g^{-1}). This suggests that, within the fibril, the collagen molecules in hard tissues are separated laterally from their nearest neighbours by a $0\cdot6$ nm gap, whereas the corresponding gap in soft tissues is only $0\cdot3$ nm. Thus a phosphate ion, approximately $0\cdot4$ nm in diameter, would be able to penetrate between the molecules in a hard tissue but not in a soft tissue. Furthermore, there is sufficient space within the collagen fibrils of bone to accommodate all the hydroxyapatite crystallites, and, because of the limited extrafibrillar space, at least 56% of them must be within the fibrils.

Collagens from bone and dentine are more stable than those of soft tissues. It is extremely difficult to extract soluble collagen from bone collagen, even after demineralization. Dentine collagen shows a tremendous resistance to swelling in acid solutions. Whereas skin collagen shows swelling amounting to several hundred per cent in the region of pH 2–2·5, swelling cannot be detected in dentine collagen within the range pH 0·5–5·0, even in the presence of urea.

The greater stability of hard tissue collagens probably results from their being more highly cross-linked than collagens in soft tissues. Thus collagens from dentine and cementum have especially large numbers of hydroxyallysine–hydroxylysine cross-linkages (page 419) as well as enhanced amounts of the cross-linkage between allysine and hydroxylysine.

Non-collagenous proteins

The calcified collagenous tissues contain up to 10% of their organic content (approximately 2% of their total weight) as proteins other than collagen and other mucosubstances such as proteoglycans. Some of these non-collagenous organic substances are believed to be specifically concerned in the local mechanisms which determine calcification (page 457). The high degree of organization of mineralized tissues suggests that mineralization is not simply the precipitation of apatite crystals in a biological environment that happens to contain certain organic molecules, but rather that it is specifically induced by the organic matrix. However, up to the present, none of these components has been demonstrated to have a clearly defined role in mineralization.

In bone

Calcified cartilage is different from woven and lamellar bone which contain *bone sialoprotein*, a substance of molecular weight 25 000. Bone sialoprotein contains 20% of sialic acid which

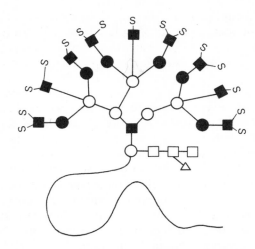

Figure 29.1 Structure of bone sialoprotein. S, sialic acid; ○, glucosamine; ●, galactosamine; ■, galactose; □, mannose; △, fucose

renders the molecule highly acidic as does the unusually high proportion of aspartic and glutamic acid units in its single polypeptide chain. It has a single highly branched polysaccharide side chain (Figure 29.1) containing a variety of monosaccharide units and with every branch terminating in sialic acid. The acidic nature of bone sialoprotein is shown by its ability to stain with the dye Alcian Blue, but with Coomassie Blue only after the sialic acid residues have been removed with neuraminidase. A second type of bone sialoprotein has recently been discovered in developing bone which has a molecular weight of 75 000 and is able to stain directly with Coomassie Blue.

Osteocalcin or *bone Gla protein* (BGP, page 161) contains three residues of γ-carboxy-glutamic acid (Gla) all of which are critical for the binding of this protein to calcium ions from solution and to hydroxyapatite. The periodic spacing of these Gla residues at 0·54 nm intervals is considered to be complementary to the 0·545 nm spacing of calcium in hydroxyapatite. The second carboxyl group becomes attached to the carbon atom of the glutamic acid residues as the result of vitamin K-dependent post-translational carboxylation. The rate of synthesis of osteocalcin by osteoblasts is accelerated by 1,25-dihydroxycholecalciferol. The amount of osteocalcin in the bone of different animal species varies up to a maximum of 2% of bone protein but human bone contains only about one-tenth of this level. Gla-containing protein is found circulating in blood at low levels, the amount being raised in diseases with increased bone turnover such as Paget's disease, primary hyperparathyroidism and renal osteodystrophy. The presence of increased levels is of diagnostic value for this type of disease. A second type of Gla-containing protein, known as *matrix Gla protein (MGP)*, has recently been discovered in bone; it contains 5 Gla residues per molecule.

Bone contains several phosphoproteins in which phosphate groups are linked as phosphoserine and phosphothreonine. The best known is *osteonectin* an acidic glycoprotein of molecular weight 32 000. Osteonectin binds strongly to hydroxyapatite and also to denatured collagen, although the collagen binding is inhibited by small amounts of fibronectin. The binding of osteonectin to biological apatite is so strong that it cannot be extracted without demineralization. Osteonectin has separate domains for binding to collagen and mineral, both low- and high-affinity sites being responsible for calcium binding. Osteonectin interacts five times more strongly with biological apatite than does osteocalcin. Three other less well characterized phosphoproteins of molecular weight 75 000, 62 000 and 24 000 have been isolated from bone. All three are acidic with large amounts of aspartic and glutamic acid residues. The two larger ones are glycoproteins. The smallest phosphoprotein has no oligosaccharide chains but six residues of hydroxyproline are present per molecule.

Bone contains small proteoglycans of molecular weight 70 000–150 000 in contrast to the large proteoglycans (molecular weight >1 000 000) found in calcified cartilage. The glycosaminoglycan associated with the proteoglycan of bone is almost entirely chondroitin 4-sulphate.

In dentine

Only approximately 10% of the matrix of human *dentine* is non-collagenous and 70% of this dissolves on demineralization with EDTA, the remaining 30% being associated with collagen. Of the non-collagenous part of the matrix about 5% consists of proteoglycan, mainly chondroitin 4-sulphate with a very acidic protein core; albumins and globulins account for a further 2·6% and dialysable peptides 4·2%. The major part of the non-collagenous matrix consists of three types of high molecular weight component: less-acidic glycoproteins, anionic glycoproteins and phosphoproteins.

The *less-acidic glycoproteins* of dentine have been separated into 12 homogeneous fractions of which four are major components, comprising 80% of the whole. Their molecular weights range from 12 000 to 26 500 and they consist of some 80% of protein with smaller amounts of sialic acid, hexosamine and sugars, including fucose. They represent the most abundant constituents of the non-collagenous part of the human dentine matrix but nothing is known of their biological function.

Three *anionic glycoproteins* have been separated from dentine, two of which are similar in amino acid composition and differ mainly in carbohydrate content. They are strongly acidic with a total of 390 aspartic and glutamic acid residues per 1000 and a high content of serine. Together they account for 14% of the non-collagenous part of the dentine matrix.

Phosphoproteins have been studied mainly in bovine, rat and rabbit dentine where they are claimed to account for more than half of the non-collagenous matrix proteins. They are also known as *phosphophoryns* a unique class of proteins in which aspartic acid and serine together account for approximately 80% of the amino acid residues. From 50 to 95% of the serine residues are phosphorylated, the proportion increasing from fetal to permanent teeth. The phosphophoryns are relatively large proteins, ranging in molecular weight from 38 000 to 150 000 depending on the source. A role has been proposed for phosphoproteins in the mineralization of dentine. The most newly laid down part of the dentine, known as *predentine*, is not mineralized and it has been suggested that phosphophoryns secreted at the junction of predentine with dentine bind to collagen and shuttle Ca^{2+} ions along to the mineralization sites.

Other organic constituents

Citrate

Both bone and dentine contain about 1% of citrate and since the weight of the skeleton is considerable, this accounts for the greater part of the citrate stored in the body. Citrate forms complexes with calcium ions and seems to be mainly associated with the inorganic phase since it is co-precipitated with calcium phosphates under neutral conditions and dissolves when bone is demineralized with acid or neutral EDTA.

It is far from clear whether the incorporation of the citrate ion into calcified tissues is merely a consequence of the stability and solubility properties of calcium citrates or whether it plays an essential part in the mineralization process. It increases the solubility of apatite and inhibits alkaline phosphatase. Citrate accumulation in bone is influenced by both parathormone and vitamin D. High levels of vitamin D appear to stimulate osteocytes to produce citrate and this may play some part in the subsequent increase in resorption. Despite these observations no clear picture of the role of citrate in mineralization has emerged.

Lipids

Small amounts of lipids, mainly triglycerides and cholesterol, are present in compact bone and a wide range of saturated and unsaturated straight chain fatty acids are found in glycerides from human dentine. Small amounts of many phospholipids are present in both bone and dentine.

Chapter 30
The metabolism of calcium and phosphorus

Calcium and phosphorus are among the most abundant elements in the body and it is appropriate to consider them together since they constitute the greater part of the mineral phase of the hard tissues. A 70 kg man contains some 1150 g of calcium and about 700 g of phosphorus, representing about 1·7 and 1·0% respectively of the total body weight.

Some 600 g of phosphorus are located in the skeletal and dental tissues as inorganic (ortho)-phosphate while the remaining 100 g are present in various forms in the soft tissues and extracellular fluids. Apart from the inorganic phosphates, which make an appreciable contribution to the buffering capacity of the extracellular fluids, phosphorus-containing derivatives of carbohydrates, lipids and proteins all have important functions in the body. Furthermore, phosphoric acid is an essential constituent of nucleotides including the high-energy di- and tri-phosphates and the nucleic acids.

As much as 99% of the total calcium is found in the hard tissues while the remaining 1% is present in soft tissues, mainly in the extracellular fluids where it exerts powerful physiological effects. For this reason the concentration of extracellular Ca^{2+} ions is maintained within very close limits by mechanisms which will be described later in this chapter. Ionic calcium is essential for muscular contraction, transmission of nerve impulses, neuromuscular irritability and for maintaining the integrity of cell membranes; it is also necessary for the clotting of blood and milk.

Calcium is almost entirely extracellular in its distribution in contrast to phosphorus, which is more abundant than calcium in soft tissues and is largely intracellular.

Calcium and phosphorus metabolism

Vitamin D and calcium metabolism

Vitamin D has long been recognized as an essential factor in the absorption of calcium from the gut. As mentioned in Chapter 12, deficiency of this vitamin in infants and children causes rickets, which is characterized by abnormal endochondral calcification, resulting in bones that are hypocalcified and soft. Rickets can be induced experimentally in rats fed on diets lacking vitamin D or low in phosphorus.

Though the mechanism by which vitamin D exerts its effects on calcium metabolism has only comparatively recently been elucidated, it has long been realized that the vitamin is intimately concerned with movement of calcium across the intestinal wall. This was shown to be an active process by experiments *in vitro* using everted gut sacs from healthy animals. Calcium ions were found to be moved from the mucosal to the serosal surface against a concentration gradient, provided that a metabolizable carbohydrate and oxygen were both present. The mechanism is fairly specific for calcium although strontium can be transported competitively but at a much slower rate. This discrimination against strontium is fortunate since it minimizes uptake of the radioactive fission product strontium-90, from the 'fall-out' of nuclear weapons, and so lessens damage to cells by radiation from this isotope.

Transport of calcium across the gut wall completely stops in animals that have been depleted of vitamin D but begins again, after a definite time-lag, when vitamin D is restored to their diet. However, if vitamin D is added *in vitro* to the everted gut sac from an animal starved of the vitamin, it has no effect in stimulating transport of calcium against a concentration gradient. This apparent paradox was resolved by a series of investigations, the success of which depended upon, firstly, the ability to produce labelled cholecalciferol with a sufficiently high specific activity for it to be studied at physiological dose levels and, secondly, the development of chromatographic techniques for the separation and subsequent identification of nanogram (10^{-9} g) levels of steroids and related compounds. By means of these techniques it has been shown that cholecalciferol is first converted in the liver to 25-hydroxycholecalciferol (25-HCC) (Figure 30.1), which is more biologically active than cholecalciferol itself. This substance is then hydroxylated further, in the kidney, to produce 1,25-dihydroxycholecalciferol (1,25-DHCC), the most potent antirachitic substance known. Furthermore, 1,25-DHCC, unlike cholecalciferol itself, can stimulate calcium transport in isolated gut sacs *in vitro*. The 1,25-DHCC finds its way

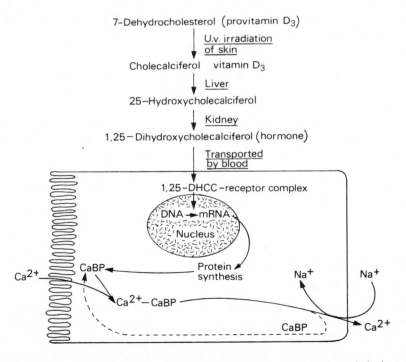

Figure 30.1 The mechanism of the action of vitamin D on the absorption of calcium through the intestinal wall

to the nucleus of the surface intestinal cells, where it unmasks a specific gene which, by transcribing the appropriate mRNA, codes for a *calcium-binding protein* CaBP. This protein is located in the intestinal brush border and effects transport of calcium across the wall of the intestine. The need for two successive hydroxylations of cholecalciferol in the liver and kidney and the subsequent migration of the 1,25-DHCC to the target cells, followed successively by unmasking, transcription and protein synthesis, accounts for the time-lag observed before cholecalciferol produces its effect in deficient animals. Administration of *actinomycin D*, an inhibitor of protein synthesis, has been shown to block the physiological response to vitamin D by preventing the synthesis of the calcium-binding protein.

Dihydroxycholecalciferol is able to act on a number of tissues with columnar epithelial cells, including intestinal mucosa, kidney tubules, the shell gland of birds and probably also various types of bone cell where it may assist the synthesis of osteocalcin (page 161). Its mode of action is very similar to that of steroid hormones (Figure 30.1). In this respect its precursor, vitamin D_3, may be considered to function as a *prohormone* rather than a vitamin. The ability of 1,25-DHCC and other metabolites of vitamin D_3 to act on bone and kidney cells, as well as those of the intestine, means that vitamin D plays a key role in calcium and phosphorus metabolism (Figure 30.2).

The kidney cells are adaptable in that they can hydroxylate 25-HCC in alternative positions according to the need of the body for calcium. When the plasma calcium concentration tends to be low, the highly active 1,25-DHCC is formed but in normal and hypercalcaemic conditions the isomer 21,25-DHCC is produced instead. The latter is less active in promoting absorption of calcium but acts on the kidney to increase calcium excretion.

A practical outcome of these discoveries concerns the treatment of patients suffering from *vitamin D-resistant rickets*, who respond only to huge doses of the vitamin. This condition can result from chronic renal failure or from an inherited metabolic defect affecting the enzyme responsible for hydroxylating 25-HCC at the 1-position. Consequently the kidney cells are

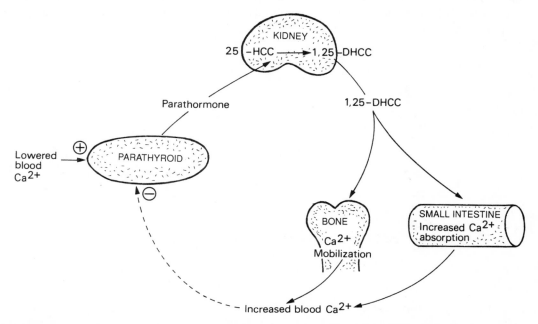

Figure 30.2 The action of parathormone and 1,25-dihydroxycholecalciferol in controlling blood calcium level

unable to produce 1,25-DHCC. Minute doses of this active metabolite are able to alleviate the failure of calcium absorption, bone disorders and muscular weakness. Unfortunately 1,25-DHCC is at present in short supply; however, synthetic 1-HCC is almost as effective as 1,25-DHCC to which it is probably converted in the body.

Excretion of calcium and phosphorus

Most of the calcium that is lost from the body is excreted in the faeces, this being mainly unabsorbed dietary calcium. However, the digestive secretions all contain small amounts of calcium, and individuals on a calcium-free diet continue to excrete faecal calcium. The normal daily excretion is of the order of $0 \cdot 1$–$0 \cdot 3$ g ($2 \cdot 5$–$7 \cdot 5$ mmol). The quantity of phosphorus excreted daily varies with the dietary intake. As with calcium an appreciable proportion of ingested phosphorus remains unabsorbed and is eliminated in the faeces. Phosphorus is also excreted in the urine, almost entirely in the form of orthophosphates (e.g. NaH_2PO_4 and Na_2HPO_4). Their role in the regulation of acid–base balance is discussed on page 395. Urinary excretion of phosphate is increased in hyperparathyroidism.

Blood calcium

The total concentration of calcium in blood, or more specifically in plasma (since little calcium is present in the cells), is maintained within very narrow limits. The mean value is 10 mg dl^{-1} ($\equiv 2 \cdot 5$ mM) and the range of variation is only 9–11 mg dl^{-1}. The calcium is present in three different forms.

1. Ionic calcium. This is the physiologically active form of calcium; it is diffusible and dialysable and accounts for about half of the total (Figure 30.3). A reduction in the level of ionized calcium in the plasma causes increased neuromuscular irritability and the condition of *tetany*. Such a reduction may result from an increase in the pH of the blood or inadequate calcium absorption.

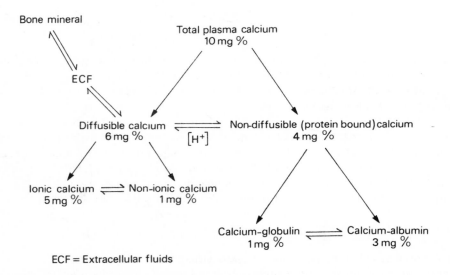

Figure 30.3 The relationship of plasma calcium 'compartments'

2. Protein-bound calcium. This is non-diffusible and accounts for a further 40% of the total. This fraction is distributed between the plasma albumin and the globulins in a ratio of about 3 : 1. The calcium is electrostatically bound and the amount held increases with pH because the net negative charge on the plasma proteins increases.
3. Diffusible non-ionic calcium. The remaining 10% of calcium is probably present in the form of complexes with citrate, phosphate and bicarbonate; although non-ionic it is dialysable.

The three forms of calcium are in equilibrium with each other and alterations in the amount of one form result in adjustments of the other forms, so that at constant pH the relative proportions are maintained. The relationships of the various plasma calcium compartments are shown in Figure 30.3. The plasma calcium concentration shows no diurnal variation and is unaffected by age or the calcium content of the diet.

The extreme stability of the plasma calcium concentration is illustrated by the fact that, when an amount of calcium greater than that normally present in the whole of the extracellular fluids was injected into experimental animals, there was only a transient increase in the plasma calcium concentration, even though only half of the calcium was excreted during the experimental period. Conversely, alternate bleeding of experimental animals and transfusion with calcium-free blood merely causes a hypocalcaemia of short duration. Such experiments show that very efficient mechanisms exist for adding calcium to blood when the level falls and removing it when the level rises.

Blood phosphorus

The phosphorus content of the blood is more variable than that of calcium. Several kinds of phosphorus compound are present (Table 30.1).

1. Inorganic phosphates. These are present in plasma, where they occur in adults at a concentration of 2·5–4·5 mg P dl^{-1} ($\equiv$0·8–1·5 mM). In children the level is significantly higher (4–7 mg P dl^{-1}). Although absolute concentrations differ from one species to another, similar age differences are apparent.
2. Phosphate esters. These are essentially cellular constituents and are almost entirely absent from plasma. Whole blood contains 20–27 mg per 100 ml. This is accounted for by phosphate intermediates of glycolysis, various nucleotides and nucleic acids.
3. Lipid-soluble phosphorus. Phospholipids are present in both cells and plasma, giving a concentration of 10–12 mg of lipid-soluble P per 100 ml^{-1} of whole blood. The phosphorus content of blood, unlike that of calcium, varies with the dietary intake. A low intake is associated with a low plasma P level and it is relatively easy to induce rickets in rats by feeding them a diet low in phosphorus.

Table 30.1 Distribution of phosphorus in the blood of an adult

| | *Blood phosphorus concentration* (mg%) | | |
	Whole blood	*Cells*	*Plasma*
Total	35–40	70–80	12–14
Inorganic	2–3	0–2	3–4
Ester	20–27	50	0·5
Phospholipid	10–12	20	5–10

From G. N. Jenkins (1978) in *The Physiology and Biochemistry of the Mouth*, 3rd edn, Blackwells, Oxford

Calcium and phosphorus homoeostasis

Because of the close dependence of neuromuscular activity on the concentration of calcium ions in the body fluids, it is essential that this level should be kept constant within very narrow limits. Control of phosphate ion concentration is also important, although rather larger variations can be tolerated for phosphate than for calcium. These levels are controlled mainly by the various dynamic relationships that exist between the dissolved ions in the extracellular fluids and the solid phosphates of bone (page 438). The very rapid exchange reaction involving a small labile reserve of calcium and phosphate ions is purely physicochemical in nature and consequently limited in scope, yet it enables the plasma calcium concentration to be rapidly adjusted, equilibrium being established in about 4 min.

A more positive control of calcium ion concentration is brought about by the cell-mediated resorption or deposition of stable bone material. These adjustments are slower, but quantitatively greater, than the simple exchange reaction. They take place with great precision with regard to the sites in the bone where resorption and deposition occur, their timing and the constancy of plasma ion concentration achieved. The process thus provides for both the continuous remodelling of bone and for the calcium–phosphorus homoeostasis of the blood and tissue fluids. The former depends on the position on the bone surface of various stimulated cells and the latter on the net result of stimulation of cells in bone, intestine and kidney by parathyroid hormone, calcitonin and vitamin D. The mode of action of these substances and the interplay of their various effects are complex.

Parathyroid hormone

The importance of the parathyroid glands in calcium metabolism was recognized many years ago when it was shown that their removal from animals resulted in *hypocalcaemia*, accompanied by *tetany*, a condition characterized by convulsions and muscular spasms. Shortly afterwards, it was shown that, when an extract of bovine parathyroid tissue was injected into parathyroidectomized dogs, it restored the normal plasma calcium concentration and abolished tetany. The same extract produced marked elevation of plasma calcium when administered to normal dogs. In Man the parathyroid glands which produce *parathyroid hormone* or *parathormone* (PTH) are two pairs of pea-sized bodies situated close to or within the capsule of the thyroid gland. No tropic hormone is involved in stimulating production of PTH. The parathyroid glands monitor the calcium concentration of the blood passing through them and, by a negative feedback mechanism, regulate their rate of PTH secretion accordingly. There is a reciprocal relationship between the concentration of PTH and calcium in the circulating blood: the lower the calcium concentration the greater the rate of hormone secretion. The action of the hormone on bone cells results in an increase in blood calcium, and, when the calcium level rises sufficiently, the parathyroids produce less PTH so that the blood calcium level rises no further.

The calcium ion concentration of blood is controlled very precisely at a level of $5·2\,mg\,dl^{-1}$ ($\equiv 1·3\,mM$) corresponding to a total calcium concentration of 10 mg per 100 ml mainly as a result of the action of parathormone. In normal people variations from this level are virtually undetectable, which suggests that the monitoring mechanism of the parathyroids is extremely sensitive to changes in the calcium ion concentration of the blood. In fact, the calcium level maintained by the action of PTH is approximately twice the concentration that would result simply from the solubility of bone mineral. In this sense the operation of parathormone can be regarded as continuously 'boosting' what would otherwise be the equilibrium level for fluids in contact with solid calcium phosphate.

The primary mechanism by which parathormone raises the calcium concentration of plasma is its effect on osteoclasts, causing them to proliferate and resorb the neighbouring bone. The parathormone acts on the cells by increasing the activity of membrane-bound adenylate cyclase and hence the intracellular production of cAMP. As a result, the osteoclasts not only dissolve the stable inorganic phase and release calcium and phosphate ions into the blood, but also through the secretion of acid hydrolases, including presumably a collagenase, dissolve the organic matrix completely. Thus pronounced osteoclastic activity is accompanied by the appearance of hydroxyproline, which is unique to collagen, in the urine. The effect of PTH on bone cells is not immediate but is apparent in from 30 min to 2 h, with a maximum after 6 h, as judged by the blood calcium concentration.

It might be expected that increased bone resorption through the agency of PTH would also cause an increase in plasma phosphate concentration. In fact this does not occur because the hormone has an independent effect on the kidney, causing a decrease in phosphate reabsorption by the tubules and consequently an increase in its excretion. On the other hand, parathormone increases the reabsorption of calcium by kidney tubules and so reduces excretion, thus conserving the plasma calcium (Figure 30.4).

In addition to its effects on bone and kidney cells, PTH affects the transport of calcium in the cells of the intestine and the lactating mammary gland. The hormone increases the absorption of calcium from the gut and its secretion in milk. Thus parathormone resembles vitamin D in regulating calcium transport in various kinds of cell. It too may act by regulating the biosynthesis of a specific protein, since actinomycin D prevents the action of PTH on osteoclasts which results in mobilization of bone mineral. Actinomycin D, however, does not affect the increased phosphate excretion by the kidney caused by PTH, so presumably a different mechanism is involved.

Parathyroid hormone consists of a single polypeptide chain of 84 amino acid residues. All the residues are necessary for maximum calcium mobilization and phosphaturic effect but the part of the molecule containing only the 34 *N*-terminal residues has some activity.

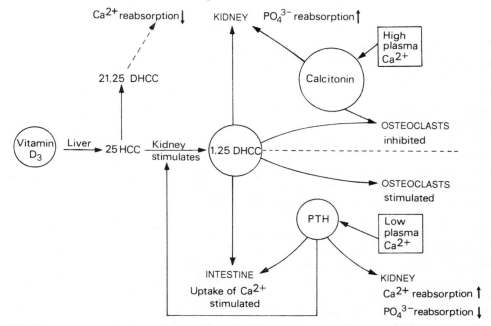

Figure 30.4 The complementary roles of parathormone, calcitonin and vitamin D in controlling calcium and phosphate metabolism

Calcitonin

For many years it was accepted that the plasma calcium concentration was regulated solely by the negative feedback mechanism involving PTH. However, if such a feedback system is all that is involved, the plasma calcium concentration might be expected to fluctuate round a mean value and this is not so. As already stated, the plasma calcium stays very steady and it was Copp, in 1962, who first questioned the adequacy of PTH to explain this close regulation. He was puzzled to find that when bovine PTH was injected into rats a consistent small decrease in the plasma calcium concentration occurred prior to the expected hypercalcaemic response. This suggested the possibility of a calcium-lowering factor in the parathyroid extract.

To determine the origin of the hypocalcaemic factor the effect of independent perfusion of the thyroid and parathyroid glands with high-calcium blood was examined but discrepancies were found in the results of different workers, which arose from technical difficulties in the independent perfusion of the two glands. Subsequently experiments carried out on pigs which have parathyroids well separated from their thyroid gland confirmed that perfusion of the thyroid with high-calcium blood produces a hypocalcaemic response, presumably as a result of secretion of Copp's hypothetical calcium-lowering hormone which he had already designated *calcitonin*.

Calcitonin is produced in the parafollicular or C cells of the thyroid gland which are homologous with the ultimobranchial body of birds and fish. The hormone has been isolated from a variety of species and always consists of a single chain of 32 amino acids, although there are considerable variations in its amino acid composition and relative activity when administered to rats.

$$\underset{2}{Ser} \qquad \underset{6}{Thr}$$

H$_2$N—Cys (1) —S—S— Cys(7)-Val-Leu(9, 8)

2Ser   Thr6

3Asp—Leu—Ser (4, 5)

All forms of calcitonin contain a 1,7-disulphide ring structure of the type shown. This is reminiscent of other hormonal ring structures in insulin, vasopressin, oxytocin, growth hormone and prolactin.

Although the thyroid gland is probably the most important source of calcitonin, the parathyroid glands and the thymus, which contain C cells as vestiges of the ultimobranchial body, also produce the hormone.

The principal effect of calcitonin is to inhibit bone resorption by osteoclasts and this is reflected in a decreased excretion of hydroxyproline in the urine. Like PTH it acts on the stable calcium pool. Tissue culture preparations of bone, to which PTH has been added, show resorption but, if calcitonin is also added, resorption is inhibited. There is no evidence to support the idea that calcitonin promotes the deposition of bone.

The secretion of calcitonin, like that of PTH, is probably governed solely by blood calcium concentration, since there is no evidence for the existence of a trophic hormone that stimulates its release. The dual control system represented by PTH and calcitonin exerts rigorous control over the plasma calcium concentration and is much more efficient than PTH would be acting alone. Calcitonin is somewhat quicker acting than PTH and may be involved in rapid adjustments when the plasma calcium concentration might otherwise 'overshoot'. It has been suggested that while PTH is really the main regulator for plasma, calcitonin is somehow concerned with the balance between bone formation and resorption.

The dual control system is analogous to, but more efficient than, the regulation of blood glucose by the pancreatic hormones insulin and glucagon. The major effects of PTH and calcitonin on bone and kidney are summarized in Figure 30.4.

The relationship of vitamin D, parathormone and calcitonin

In addition to its role in the intestinal absorption of calcium, vitamin D also directly influences bone and kidney cells. This interaction with parathormone and calcitonin affects the metabolism of calcium and phosphate in a complex manner which is still not completely understood.

Vitamin D is essential for the action of parathormone on osteoclasts whereby bone resorption and a hypercalcaemic response are induced. For this reason parathormone is comparatively inactive in patients with rickets. The mechanism of this synergistic effect is not clear but, since actinomycin D blocks the hypercalcaemic activity of vitamin D, it may be that the vitamin induces the formation of a calcium-binding protein in osteoclasts in a similar manner to its behaviour in the intestine. Certainly excess of vitamin D has effects on bone cells similar to those of PTH in that it mobilizes bone calcium and produces hypercalcaemia. In vitamin D deficiency, production of PTH is greatly increased in an attempt to compensate for the chronic hypocalcaemia.

In the kidney, the effect of PTH in promoting phosphate excretion does not depend on the presence of vitamin D. The vitamin itself, however, promotes retention of phosphate by reabsorption. High levels of vitamin D therefore enhance the blood levels of both calcium and phosphorus on account of the action of the vitamin on osteoclasts and kidney cells, respectively. Recent work suggests that the enzyme system which converts 25-HCC to 1,25-DHCC in the kidney is regulated by PTH rather than being controlled directly by the blood calcium level. It has been suggested that the formation of 1,25-DHCC may also be affected by the phosphate concentration in the kidney cells.

The antagonistic effects of calcitonin on bone resorption also appear to require the presence of vitamin D. Thus the vitamin is necessary for the action of both PTH, which promotes resorption, and calcitonin, which inhibits it. This is just one more aspect of the complex interplay of mechanisms involving these three substances which ensure the stability of blood calcium and the proper maintenance of the calcified tissues through continuous remodelling.

Once the dental hard tissues have been formed and mineralized, vitamin D, parathormone and calcitonin have little or no effect on them. In young animals, however, vitamin D deficiency and hypoparathyroidism have been shown to be associated with hypomineralization of these tissues, especially dentine, although calcitonin has not so far been found to influence them.

Chapter 31
The mineralization process

Hydroxyapatite crystals are usually confined to areas where there is a need for high mechanical strength, rigidity or hardness as in bone, dentine and enamel. They do not normally occur at all in 'soft tissues', the only other site of occasional local occurrence being within such epithelial keratins as hard claws and beaks.

The restriction of hydroxyapatite crystals to certain kinds of tissue suggests that some mechanism (or mechanisms) exists for their deposition in tissues where they are functionally useful and nowhere else. The nature of this mechanism is still not completely understood. An idea that persists is that one or more of the organic components of hard tissues is specifically concerned with deposition of minute apatite crystals and this is sometimes referred to as the *organic matrix* or nucleator of the crystallites.

The term 'matrix' is also often used more loosely in a histological context to denote a continuum that fills spaces between discrete entities. Thus the continuous material, rich in proteoglycans and collagen, that fills the spaces between the cells of cartilage, is referred to as the 'cartilage matrix', despite the fact that the cells have themselves produced this intercellular material rather than been produced by it. This is not in accord with the strict definition of a matrix as 'the place or medium in which something is bred or developed', which is applicable to the deposition of inorganic crystallites that occurs during mineralization and suggests that a true hard tissue matrix should: (1) be in existence before whatever is bred, i.e. the crystals, (2) participate in their development and (3) enclose them spatially.

Though the idea of an organic matrix for such tissues as bone and enamel is widely held, the exact manner in which the matrix participates in the development of crystallites still needs to be demonstrated. Other important problems concern why mineralization occurs only at specific sites, and what physicochemical principles govern the equilibrium between hydroxyapatite and its ions in solution.

Difficulties arise, not so much in explaining why mineralization readily and regularly occurs in certain tissues, but rather why other tissues, which resemble them in many ways, do not normally mineralize. Thus it is relatively easy to explain how crystals of a very sparingly soluble substance such as hydroxyapatite can be formed in bone, on the basis of the concentrations of calcium and phosphate ions present in blood; these are sufficiently high to permit small crystals of biological apatite to grow at the expense of ions in solution. It is more difficult to appreciate why, under apparently similar conditions, a tissue such as skin which, like bone, contains collagen as a major constituent, does not mineralize, except rarely after injury. A complete explanation of mineralization should indicate what factors determine where it will occur, what limits its spread and how its timing in different regions of bone is coordinated.

An early theory of mineralization – the alkaline phosphatase hypothesis

Although it has now been almost completely abandoned, Robison's alkaline phosphatase theory formulated in 1923, emphasizes some of the essential problems that must be solved by any satisfactory theory of mineralization. Robison noticed that sites of mineralization frequently contain an enzyme operating at high pH values which is capable of hydrolysing organic phosphate esters with the release of inorganic phosphate ions:

$$\left.\begin{array}{l}\text{Hexose monophosphate}\\ \text{Hexose diphosphate}\\ \text{Glycerophosphate}\end{array}\right\} \xrightarrow[\text{phosphatase}]{\text{Alkaline}} HPO_4^{2-}$$

He suggested that in mineralization a possible function of this alkaline phosphatase is to raise the local concentration of inorganic phosphate ions and thus to cause the precipitation of calcium phosphate, when its solubility product is exceeded.

$$Ca^{2+} + HPO_4^{2-} \rightleftharpoons \text{solid } CaHPO_4 \rightleftharpoons \text{Apatite}$$

A number of objections raised to this theory led to its gradual abandonment. Firstly, it was argued that the concentration of organic phosphate in plasma was too low for this to serve as an effective source of phosphate ions. Robison conceded this point but suggested that a store of organic phosphate was built up at the calcification site by the alkaline phosphatase acting in reverse, before calcification began. A second criticism was that some other sites, such as the kidney, which do not normally calcify, contain considerably higher concentrations of alkaline phosphatase than the calcification sites themselves. Thirdly, it was pointed out that the inorganic phase is more highly organized than can be accounted for by simple precipitation, since the apatite crystallites are regular in size, distribution and orientation. To answer this, Robison proposed a 'second mechanism', necessary for smooth deposition of inorganic crystals, which partly anticipated the later *epitactic concept* (page 456). Finally, it appeared that there is no necessity for the phosphate ion concentration to be raised for deposition of solid calcium phosphate to occur. Slices of cartilage from rachitic rats became mineralized when incubated in solutions containing the same concentration of calcium and phosphate ions as those found in the serum of young normal rats. The same conclusion can be reached on the theoretical grounds discussed in the following section.

Solubility product of some calcium phosphates

When a sparingly soluble salt is placed in water, both anions and cations leave the surface of the solid and dissolve. This process continues until the solution is saturated with respect to the salt; at this point a dynamic equilibrium is established in which the same number of ions are deposited on the surface as leave it in a given time. Once saturation has been reached, there is no net gain or loss of the solid phase. Conversely if the solid salt is placed in an aqueous solution, which is supersaturated with respect to the solid, there will be a net deposition of ions on the surface of the solid until equilibrium is reached at the same solute concentration as before. This concentration will be constant for a given substance at a specified temperature. Furthermore, the product of the ionic concentrations will be constant at a value known as the *solubility product*. Thus considering the case of the sparingly soluble salt, calcium sulphate, the solubility product can be defined as follows:

$$K_{sp}(CaSO_4) = [Ca^{2+}] \times [SO_4^{2-}] = 2\cdot3 \times 10^{-4} \, (\text{g-ion} \, l^{-1})^2$$

The solubility product is measured in units corresponding to the square of concentration; the less soluble a substance the smaller will be its solubility product.

Biological apatite, the crystalline phase of bone, dentine and enamel, consists essentially of hydroxyapatite modified by the presence of carbonate, small amounts of magnesium, sodium, and possibly citrate, either within the lattice or adsorbed on the crystal surfaces (page 430). The theoretical possibilities for ionization of hydroxyapatite are complex because more than one calcium ion and more than one phosphate ion can arise per unit of $Ca_{10}(PO_4)_6(OH)_2$. In addition the pH (which controls hydroxyl ion concentration), the carbonate concentration and the presence of macromolecules all affect the solubility product. The concepts used to describe the solubility characteristics of simple salts are therefore not easily applied to biological apatite. Furthermore, the formula given for hydroxyapatite probably has little meaning in relation to particles of molecular size, since such small aggregates of calcium and phosphate ions are known to be very unstable. Fortunately, experiments on the solubility of hydroxyapatite have shown that the simplest of all possible solubility products, namely $[Ca^{2+}] \times [HPO_4^{2-}]$, best describes the actual solubility behaviour of this substance. The solubility products of hydroxyapatite itself, biological apatite and calcium hydrogen phosphate at pH 7·4, an ionic strength of 0·16 and 37°C (i.e. under physiological conditions) may therefore be considered as simple products of the calcium ion concentration and the concentration of the monohydrogen phosphate ion HPO_4^{2-}, which is the most abundant phosphate ion under these conditions.

The solubility product of biological apatite has been determined by suspending fresh defatted powder from cortical bone in an artificial solution containing inorganic ions at the concentrations present in an ultrafiltrate of normal serum. When equilibrium had been established the solution was removed and replaced by a fresh portion which was equilibrated, removed and analysed. Solutions obtained by repeating this procedure several times were found, after the first few changes, to have the same calcium and phosphate levels and these were used to calculate the solubility product for biological apatite.

$$K_{sp}(\text{biological apatite}) = [Ca^{2+}] \times [HPO_4^{2-}] = 0\cdot69 \, (\text{mmol} \, l^{-1})^2$$
$$= 8\cdot5 \, (\text{mg Ca and P} \, dl^{-1})^2$$

When determined using crystals of pure hydroxyapatite and solutions containing only calcium and phosphate ions, i.e. in the absence of carbonate, magnesium, sodium or citrate ions, the solubility product is less than $0\cdot013 \, (\text{mmol} \, l^{-1})^2$. The presence of these additional ions clearly increases the solubility of biological apatite. Small pH changes in the region of pH 7 cause large changes in the solubility of hydroxyapatite which is also influenced by the solid-to-solution and calcium-to-phosphate ratios. As the solid-to-solution ratio increases, the solubility increases (Kelvin effect).

Hydroxyapatite is the most stable and, at neutral pH, least soluble calcium phosphate. Calcium hydrogen phosphate, which is readily formed by precipitation, is considerably more soluble.

$$K_{sp}(CaHPO_4 \cdot 2H_2O) = [Ca^{2+}] \times [HPO_4^{2-}] = 2\cdot6 \, (\text{mmol} \, l^{-1})^2$$
$$= 32 \, (\text{mg Ca and P} \, dl^{-1})^2$$

Serum concentrations of calcium and phosphate in relation to the solubility of biological apatite

There has been some uncertainty concerning the concentration of free calcium ions in serum because a substantial proportion of the total calcium is bound to plasma protein or is present in non-ionizable forms (page 446), but the concentration of ionized calcium in normal serum is now well established as approximately $1 \cdot 3 \, \text{mM}$ $(5 \cdot 0 \, \text{mg dl}^{-1})$. The concentration of free mono-hydrogen phosphate ions in serum varies from approximately $0 \cdot 8 \, \text{mM}$ $(2 \cdot 5 \, \text{mg dl}^{-1})$ in fasting adults to a maximum value almost twice as great in well-fed infants. The ionic product of any solution is the product of actual concentrations of ions present in that solution whereas the solubility product is the special case of the ionic product for a saturated solution.

The ionic product for calcium and phosphate in human serum can therefore be calculated in the same units as for the solubility product.

$$[Ca^{2+}] \times [HPO_4^{2-}] = \begin{matrix} \text{Fasting} \\ \text{adult} \\ 1 \cdot 05 \end{matrix} \quad \text{to} \quad \begin{matrix} \text{Normal} \\ \text{infant} \\ 2 \cdot 0 \end{matrix} \quad \begin{matrix} \text{Mean} \\ \text{value} \\ 1 \cdot 5 \end{matrix} \, (\text{mmol l}^{-1})^2$$

$$= \quad 13 \quad \text{to} \quad 25 \quad 18 \quad (\text{mg Ca and P per 100 ml})^2$$

The normal range for the ionic product for serum of 13–25 (mg Ca and P per 100 ml)^2 greatly exceeds the solubility product of $8 \cdot 5$ (mg Ca and P per 100 ml)^2 for biological apatite (see above). Normal serum is thus supersaturated (or metastable) with respect to the solid inorganic phase of bone, dentine and enamel, but undersaturated with respect to calcium hydrogen phosphate.

The concepts of crystal growth and nucleation

Homogeneous nucleation

It now remains to explain the apparent paradox that the ionic product for calcium and monohydrogen phosphate ions in serum exceeds the solubility product of both hydroxyapatite and biological apatite and yet crystals of these substances are not formed in the bloodstream. Of the several reasons for this, the most basic one can be demonstrated by a simple experiment.

A solution containing Ca^{2+} and HPO_4^{2-} ions and having the same ionic product as serum (18 (mg per 100 ml)^2) in a clean container can be kept indefinitely without the separation of crystals. If, however, apatite crystals are introduced into the solution, they grow in size at the expense of ions from solution and the ionic product of the solution falls until it is equal to the solubility product for hydroxyapatite, at which point crystal growth stops.

If, on the other hand, a series of similar solutions of Ca^{2+} and HPO_4^{2-} ions with gradually increasing ionic products from 18 (mg per 100 ml)^2 upwards is made up, it is found that no solid separates until the ionic product reaches approximately 35 (mg per 100 ml)^2, when crystals form. Curiously enough these do not consist of hydroxyapatite but of the more soluble calcium hydrogen phosphate $CaHPO_4.2H_2O$, which has a solubility product of 32 (mg per 100 ml)^2. However, this substance is unstable above pH $6 \cdot 2$ and its crystals are completely converted in the solid phase to hydroxyapatite, within a few hours

$$10CaHPO_4 + 4OH^- \rightarrow Ca_{10}(PO_4)_6(OH)_2 + 2H_2O + 4H_2PO_4^-$$

The apatite crystals then act as templates and bring about precipitation and growth of more apatite.

These experiments suggest two important ideas. (a) *Homogeneous nucleation* (i.e. the formation of the first solid where no solid existed before) is more difficult to achieve than the growth of existing solid; (b) there is some special difficulty in nucleating crystals of hydroxyapatite in homogeneous solution. This is shown by the fact that it is easier to nucleate another and more soluble calcium phosphate. It appears that clusters containing the 18 constituent ions of hydroxyapatite, and resembling the apatite lattice in pattern, occur infrequently and are very unstable. There seems to be a critical size of cluster which must be built up before it is able to grow spontaneously and in order to build up such critical clusters, some sort of energy barrier has to be overcome. One way of doing this is to add crystals of apatite.

Heterogeneous nucleation – epitaxy

While experiments with artificial solutions go some way towards explaining why apatite crystals are not formed in blood, despite the fact that blood is supersaturated with respect to hydroxyapatite, they do not explain how the first crystals arise in mineralizing tissues. To do this it must be realized that conditions within these tissues are not the same as in artificial solutions, since the tissues contain the organic matrix as a pre-existing solid.

It is well known that solid surfaces tend to promote the formation of new crystals from a supersaturated solution. Thus, the presence of a foreign solid, even for example dust, will assist the crystallization of a substance from solution. Any solid surface will have some effect in promoting nucleation, but if the solid surface has a similar structural pattern to that of the new solid to be formed, it will be a more effective *nucleator*.

The concept of *epitaxy* (Greek = on-arrangement) was suggested as the promotion of the growth of one crystalline substance on a different crystalline material having similar lattice spacings. This phenomenon is widely established for inorganic substances and Neuman was the first to suggest that the organic matrix of mineralizing tissues may act as an epitactic agent for the formation of the first hydroxyapatite crystals. The basic assumption is that somewhere in or upon one of the organic constituents of bone there is a pattern of charges that matches the ionic lattice of hydroxyapatite and can act as a nucleation centre for the formation of the crystals. Calcium and phosphate ions are presumably held by electrostatic forces on the surface of the epitactic nucleator so as to form a pattern similar to that of the hydroxyapatite lattice. The presence of the organic nucleator thus reduces the energy barrier for small aggregates of ions that would otherwise be unstable. Such stabilized aggregates are then able to grow in size at the expense of ions from the supersaturated solution surrounding them and produce larger and more stable aggregates which grow to form the hydroxyapatite crystallites of the mineralized tissue.

The need for an organic seeding agent may explain why apatite crystallites are not formed in soft tissues. The only difficulty is that the epitactic grouping, forming the nucleation centre on the organic matrix of mineralizing tissues, has never been identified with certainty.

Possible organic nucleators

Collagen

This has been widely held to be the most likely organic nucleator of apatite crystallites. Like apatite, collagen is abundant and uniformly distributed in bone, dentine and cementum. Recent evidence suggests that most, if not all, the apatite crystallites are actually inside the collagen fibrils, probably within the 'holes' which are a consequence of the mode of aggregation of collagen molecules into fibrils (page 418) and which provide potential sites for nucleation and subsequent crystal growth. One of the most convincing arguments for collagen acting as a specific nucleator is the demonstration that, of the various kinds of reconstituted collagen, only the 'native' type with the 64 nm spacing can bring about nucleation of apatite from solutions with calcium and phosphate concentrations close to those in plasma. Presumably the fibril with 64 nm spacings is the only type with the correct juxtaposition of ionized groups, perhaps in regions bordering the 'holes' within it. This is supported by the finding that the initial mineralization takes place at definite points on the sub-bandings of the fibrils, within the 64 nm periodicity. It has also been claimed that the crystallites, which subsequently form, are orientated parallel with the fibrils and are regularly arranged with respect to the 64 nm spacing. However, this is disputed and it has been suggested instead that the orientation is mainly with respect to cell surfaces.

Two difficulties which, until recently, have prevented collagen from being accepted as an epitactic agent are, firstly, failure to demonstrate relevant differences between collagens from soft and mineralized tissues, and, secondly, failure to demonstrate the nature of the epitactic centres in collagen. However, the finding (page 439) that the collagen molecules within the fibrils of bone and dentine are more widely separated than those in tendon suggests that inorganic phosphate ions can penetrate the interior of fibrils in hard tissue collagens to reach the interior 'holes' and form apatite crystallites there. This is not possible in tendon fibrils, where the collagen molecules are too close together to allow phosphate ions to enter. New evidence has been obtained that the epitactic centres of collagen consist of sets of ionized carboxyl groups at specific sites in the macromolecule. When the carboxyl groups are chemically blocked, mineralization fails to take place, whereas blocking of other types of ionizable groups of collagen does not affect its ability to nucleate apatite. If this is correct, it suggests that the epitactic centres of collagen attract an appropriate pattern of calcium ions, and that these in turn combine with phosphate ions to build up the apatite lattice.

Proteoglycans

While some workers have claimed that glycosaminoglycans such as chondroitin sulphate inhibit the mineralization of soft connective tissues, others have put forward the view that, acting in conjunction with collagen, they give rise to a 'local factor', capable of initiating mineralization. Here too the action is considered to depend on the electrostatic binding of calcium ions, in this instance by sulphate groups. It is not yet settled whether glycosaminoglycans promote or inhibit mineralization or even whether they are directly involved.

Lipids

Sites in bone and dentine that are currently undergoing mineralization show various specific histochemical reactions. One of these is staining by Sudan Black after treatment with pyridine, which has been attributed to lipid material.

Bone sialoprotein

Two other kinds of histochemical staining found near sites of mineralization are metachromasia and periodic acid–Schiff (PAS) staining. Since bone sialoprotein (page 439) is strongly PAS positive, this may indicate its presence at mineralization sites and its possible participation in epitaxy. The sialoprotein is highly acidic and has an abundance of carboxyl groups which might participate in ionic binding of calcium at epitactic centres.

Bone morphogenetic factor

In spite of considerable research no particular chemical structures have been found to have a clear-cut epitactic function for the nucleation of biological apatite crystals. A *bone morphogenetic factor* has been postulated but, although active extracts have been prepared from cultures of mineralizing bone, no specific substance has yet been isolated.

It has been assumed that a non-collagenous protein is responsible for influencing the local mechanisms of mineralization, and attention has recently been focused on several compounds of this class, including osteocalcin and osteonectin in bone (page 440) as well as less-acidic and anionic glycoproteins and phosphoproteins in dentine. As yet, however, no non-collagenous protein from any mineralized tissue has had its biological function unambiguously determined.

Inhibition of mineralization

Mineralization is a potentially dangerous process because the supersaturated state of the plasma could lead to rapid deposition of hydroxyapatite at unsuitable sites should it become accidentally nucleated. A widespread inhibitory system exists which forms a second line of defence against this happening, the first being the restriction of active nucleation to the hard tissues.

Urine and plasma contain a powerful inhibitor of mineralization, which is probably present in most tissues. It has been identified as the inorganic pyrophosphate ion $(P_2O_7^{4-})$ which presumably attaches itself to the growing crystal surface of apatite, competing for sites in the lattice pattern normally occupied by the inorganic phosphate ion (HPO_4^{2-}). Further growth of the ion cluster then ceases because the pyrophosphate ion is too large and has an unsuitable charge distribution to fit into the apatite lattice.

Although intracellular pyrophosphate is rapidly destroyed by pyrophosphatase (page 211), pyrophosphates may be widely distributed in the body fluids and the question arises how mineralization can take place in the hard tissues when this inhibitor may be present. The answer probably lies in the extracellular alkaline phosphatases, the main function of which in mineralization was at one time suggested to be to supply phosphate ions. Recently it has been shown that alkaline phosphatases from mineralization sites have a marked pyrophosphatase activity, splitting the pyrophosphate ion into two orthophosphate ions. Thus there exists at the mineralization sites, an enzyme capable of breaking down an inhibitor of mineralization and simultaneously of increasing the inorganic phosphate concentration. The main function of alkaline phosphatase at mineralization sites is therefore now believed to be the destruction of pyrophosphate, as it diffuses into mineralizing bone, rather than liberation of inorganic phosphate as suggested by Robison.

The direct involvement of cells in the initiation of mineralization

Following the initial failure to identify the epitactic agent, attention was turned to the possibility of the direct involvement of cells in initiating hard tissue mineralization. Large amounts of calcium and phosphate have been detected in bone cells, the calcium probably being concentrated in the mitochondria by an energy-requiring active transport mechanism. Electron microscopy has shown that bone, cartilage and dentine, which are undergoing mineralization, all produce vesicles or globules, which originate from cells and apparently pass through the plasma membrane into the extracellular region. These vesicles initially contain comparatively high concentrations of phosphate and calcium ions, derived from the cytoplasm and probably concentrated by the mitochondria. After losing their connection with cells, the hitherto amorphous electron-dense contents change to needle-shaped crystals, similar to those associated with collagen fibrils in the fully mineralized tissue. It is assumed that water is lost through the membrane of the vesicle, with a resultant increase in the concentration of ions. At a sufficiently high concentration, precipitation of solid occurs, not as hydroxyapatite but perhaps as amorphous calcium phosphate $(Ca_3(PO_4)_2 \, xH_2O)$ which is known to be present in substantial amounts in bone, especially young bone. The amorphous calcium phosphate may then be converted to the more stable hydroxyapatite by solid state transition. This mechanism may account for the initial formation of apatite which can then lead to further apatite formation by crystal growth and seeding. However, it is not easy to envisage how this process could lead directly to crystallite formation in the interior of the collagen fibrils, since access between collagen molecules is limited to particles of ionic dimensions.

Mineralization – a synthesis of ideas concerning an unsolved mystery

Clearly the last word on mineralization has yet to be spoken. There are many aspects of this phenomenon, and ideas which have previously been rejected have tended to reappear in a slightly different guise. Thus the hypothesis that alkaline phosphatase is involved, although not found to be necessary to explain an increase in phosphate concentration, has returned in modified form to account for the local destruction in mineralizing bone of the pyrophosphate ion which inhibits mineralization. Likewise while epitactic properties could not be demonstrated for proteoglycans or initially for collagen, it is now believed that osteocalcin, osteonectin, phosphoproteins and specific arrangements of carboxyl groups in collagen may play crucial roles in mineralization mechanisms. Similarly the concentration of calcium by cells and its secretion in vesicles may be locally important even if it does not occur in all mineralizing tissues.

It is possible to build up a picture of mineralization from these various concepts which has not yet been completely proved. It is suggested that at sites where mineralization is to take place, the cells secrete alkaline phosphatase, which breaks down pyrophosphate ions, which would otherwise inhibit the growth of crystal surfaces. The supersaturated levels of calcium and phosphate ions in the tissue fluid (page 455) then enable all existing biological apatite crystal surfaces to grow spontaneously.

The thermodynamic probability of new crystals being created spontaneously is vanishingly small but two suggestions have been made to overcome this difficulty and each may play a part in different circumstances.

The first is that calcium, and probably phosphate ions as well, are concentrated by hard tissue cells, and subsequently secreted in matrix vesicles. In this way the (calcium × phosphate) ion product may be boosted above the solubility level of the more soluble, but spontaneously nucleable, calcium phosphates, such as amorphous calcium phosphate. Under appropriate conditions, this substance may undergo solid phase transformation to biological apatite, which cannot itself be formed by homogeneous nucleation. This type of mineralization may occur in extrafibrillar situations at an early stage of the process, e.g. calcospherites may be formed where maximum ordering of the inorganic phase has not yet been reached.

The second means for the production of biological apatite crystals is by epitaxy, and the more recently discovered minor organic constituents of hard tissues, including the phosphoproteins, now have to be considered as possible nucleators, as well as collagen itself. This kind of nucleation may be associated with more regularly arranged crystals than occur as a result of solid phase transformation. This is the case whether crystallization occurs very rapidly as in dental enamel, where it may be assisted by enamelins, amelogenins or phosphoproteins, or very slowly inside the collagen fibrils of bone or dentine, most probably in the holes between the molecules. The more rapid but less systematic initial extrafibrillar mineralization by the first mechanism may be reorganized architectonically by the organic matrix via solution of calcium and phosphate ions.

The final result is a pattern of biological apatite crystals which is appropriate to the mechanical functions of the particular tissue. While the same general principles apply, the details of the process will vary between different mineralized tissues producing their characteristic structures.

Chapter 32
Enamel

Dental enamel is a unique biological system that provides a hard surface for the teeth, and enables them to reduce food to particles sufficiently small for effective attack by the digestive enzymes. Provided that it remains free from disease, human enamel can withstand a lifetime of crushing work without becoming fractured or completely worn away. Enamel is capable of performing this function only because of its most abundant constituent, hydroxyapatite, which gives it a hardness intermediate between that of iron and carbon steel.

If enamel were hard but brittle, as it would be if it was formed from a single crystal of apatite, it would fracture when brought into contact with the enamel on the surface of the opposing tooth, during mastication. This does not occur because enamel has a very high elasticity for a material of its hardness. This elasticity primarily depends upon its being composed of a large number of crystallites, which are in close contact but are not crystallographically continuous, and are arranged in definite patterns. The elasticity of enamel depends on both its own structure, and that of the whole tooth.

Three main aspects of tooth structure determine how physical stress is distributed within enamel. Firstly, the gross morphology of the *enamel cap* defines the shape of both the *occlusal surface* and the *amelodentinal junction*. Secondly, forces within the enamel are transmitted to the underlying dentine, which is softer and more elastic than enamel and acts as a firm cushion. Thirdly, the internal structure of enamel at histological and ultrastructural levels has an important bearing on its elastic behaviour. This concerns the division of enamel into prismatic structures, the shapes, directions and mutual interlacing of the prisms and finally the arrangement of the crystallites within the prisms (Figure 32.1).

In freshly secreted enamel, crystals first appear near the *ameloblasts* and, as soon as they do so, the enamel takes on the pattern of its final form, an intricate beautifully arranged two-phase system which may not only last throughout life, but may survive in fossil form for millions of years.

Histological structure

Electron micrographs of mature enamel show that most of its volume is occupied by inorganic crystallites. Though these are discontinuous, they are in such close contact that the second phase, which consists mainly of water with some organic matter, occupies only narrow gaps

460

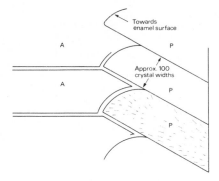

Figure 32.1 The arrangement of hydroxyapatite crystals within enamel prisms. A, ameloblasts; P, prisms

between the crystals. Early in development the crystals form as long thin ribbons or plates and at this stage a higher percentage of the volume is occupied by the organic phase. The two-phase concept is important (i) in relation to the growth of the inorganic crystallites in the surrounding organic phase during maturation of the enamel and (ii) to the concept of 'spaces', which are responsible for the microporous properties of mature enamel.

At a larger order of size, enamel has a prismatic structure, the enamel prism or rod representing the most obvious histologically defined entity. In cross-section its dimensions are approximately the same as those of an ameloblast but it is extremely long and may extend from the amelodentinal junction to the enamel surface. Adjacent prisms are approximately parallel but show local changes of direction. The prisms are formed as the result of the activity of ameloblasts, and one ameloblast may contribute to several prisms, while each prism receives material from more than one cell. In the outermost layer of fully formed human enamel the prisms merge into each other and a thin surface layer is produced. This layer resembles reptile enamel which is less than 1 mm thick and is not prismatic but continuous.

Most of the hydroxyapatite crystals have their long axes approximately parallel to each other and almost parallel to the prism direction (Figure 32.1). Near the edges of the prisms the directions of the crystallites progressively deviate, the ends of the crystallites which are nearer the enamel surface being turned outwards away from the prism axis and towards the prism boundary. As a result of this progressive deviation there is, at the boundary, an abrupt change of crystallite orientation from one prism to the next. The prism boundaries are rendered visible under the microscope by this discontinuity of crystal orientation, rather than as was at one time thought, by a solid prism sheath of organic matter. However, electron micrographs of the earlier stages of enamel maturation do show that the region near the prism boundary contains fewer crystallites and consequently more of the organic phase than within the prisms.

The composition of mature enamel

The physical properties and chemical resistance of enamel are quite different from those of bone, dentine and cementum. At first this appears surprising since all four tissues are mineralized with hydroxyapatite but there are two important differences between enamel and the other tissues. Firstly, whereas bone, dentine and cementum contain some 20% by weight of collagen, mature enamel has only approximately 0·6% of organic matter (Table 32.1) while apatite accounts for approximately 99% of its dry weight. Secondly, the apatite crystals in

Table 32.1 A chemical balance sheet for mature human enamel

		Percentage by weight	
Total inorganic matter			95·0
Ash (700°C)		91·7	
Carbonate		2·9	
Total organic matter			0·6
Total proteinaceous material		0·35	
Low molecular weight material	0·06		
Enamelins, etc.	0·29		
Citrate		0·02	
Lactate		0·01	
Carbohydrate		0·0016	
Fatty acid		0·01	
Total water			4·0
'Free' water, lost at 100°C, *in vacuo*		2·2	
'Bound' water, lost between 300 and 400°C		0·83	

enamel are approximately ten times wider and thicker (approx. 50×50 nm) and much longer than those that impregnate the calcified collagens, so that their volume is at least 1000 times greater. Such large crystals of apatite cannot be produced in synthetic systems at normal temperatures and pressures.

Accurate values for the composition of enamel depend upon the preparation of enamel powder, free from contamination by dentine, surface cuticle, plaque, etc. Contamination is especially serious for investigations of the organic constituents in mature enamel which are present at a very low level. Thus, if enamel with a true content of only 0·5% of organic matter is contaminated by only 1% of its weight of dentine containing 20% of collagen, its apparent content of organic matter would be raised to 0·7%. For this reason the figure of 0·6% for total organic matter in enamel may be slightly high. The value of approximately 0·35% for total 'true enamel protein' has been corrected for contaminating collagen on the basis of its hydroxy-proline content.

The small amounts of citrate and lactate that are present may be associated with the inorganic phase. The level of carbohydrate in mature enamel is extremely low, the chief sugar components being galactose, glucose and mannose. The fatty acids consist chiefly of palmitate, stearate and oleate in approximately equal amounts.

The water content of enamel is uncertain because of the difficulty of determining the most firmly bound fraction, which is lost only at high temperatures, at which other constituents begin to be decomposed. A total value of 4% by weight for water in mature enamel *in vivo* is probably realistic. Nuclear magnetic resonance studies have provided evidence for the existence of 'freely tumbling' or loosely bound water within the 'spaces' of enamel.

Local variations in composition in different regions of the same tooth have been investigated by systematic micro-dissection of $100\,\mu$m thick sections of enamel and microanalysis of pieces from specific regions. Another approach is to dissolve the enamel systematically, layer by layer, from the exposed surface and to analyse the resulting solutions. The composition of enamel varies considerably particularly through its thickness. Thus the density of human enamel falls from approximately 3·01 at the surface, where mineralization is highest, to 2·89 near the amelodentinal junction, although local irregularities occur. The inorganic content varies directly, and the organic content inversely, with the density. Carbonate content is also inversely related to density rising from approximately 2·25% at the enamel surface to 3·9% near the amelodentinal junction. Apatite crystals of high carbonate content are less stable than those of low carbonate content as the pH is reduced. This local variation in carbonate content may have some bearing on the pattern of carious attack. Another important local factor affecting caries susceptibility is the distribution of fluoride. This is present at high concentration in the original enamel surface, where it may reach several hundred parts per million, and falls rapidly with depth to 20–50 parts per million in the interior enamel.

The values given in Table 32.1 are expressed on a weight basis whereas in terms of volume about 87·1% is occupied by the inorganic phase, 11·5% by water and 1·4% by organic matter. Mature enamel thus resembles a sintered mass of crystallites with the small spaces between them occupied by water. The small proportion of organic matter is mainly associated with the water in these spaces rather than with the crystallites. Although the aqueous phase occupies a relatively small part of the total volume, it is nevertheless, the continuous phase and is probably in communication throughout the enamel. All the same, in terms of hardness and behaviour under compressive loads, enamel behaves almost as though the inorganic phase were continuous, at least in contrast to dentine and bone where the crystallites are definitely separated by collagen, resulting in these tissues being softer and more deformable under load than enamel.

Gross composition of developing enamel and its changes during maturation

An understanding of the nature of mature enamel and of the protein matrix of enamel can best be obtained by considering (1) the composition of enamel shortly after it has been laid down by ameloblasts and (2) the maturation process which subsequently changes it.

When a tooth first begins to form the enamel appears as a pink jelly-like layer but soon changes to a chalky white mass which, though it looks highly mineralized, is actually quite soft and can be easily cut with a knife or gently scraped away from the more coherent underlying dentine. The enamel remains friable for some time but continuous increase in its degree of mineralization results in its becoming extremely hard before the tooth erupts.

During enamel development several processes occur. Firstly, there is *secretion* of the organic phase by the ameloblasts, followed by its *mineralization*; this involves two processes, *crystallite formation*, occurring soon after secretion of the matrix, and *crystal growth*, which occurs in several stages. The overall change by which the newly secreted organic phase becomes mineralized is known as *maturation*.

The changes in composition that developing enamel undergoes during maturation were first studied by Deakins in 1942. He dissected pieces of enamel from pigs' teeth at various stages of mineralization and measured their contents of inorganic matter, water and organic matter in relation to the increasing density of the enamel, as maturation proceeded.

Table 32.2 Gross composition of pig enamel at the lowest and highest degrees of mineralization

	Lowest mineralization (Very soft; density 1·45)			Highest mineralization (Very hard; density 2·76)		
	$mg\,mm^{-3}$	% by weight	Volume*	$mg\,mm^{-3}$	% by weight	Volume*
Inorganic	0·54	37·0	0·16	2·62	95·0	0·82
Organic	0·27	19·0	0·20	0·05	1·8	0·04
Water	0·64	44·0	0·64	0·12	4·3	0·12
Total	1·45	100·0	1·00	2·79	101·1	0·98

* Volume in mm³ occupied by each constituent, calculated assuming densities of 3·18 for inorganic and 1·31 for organic material

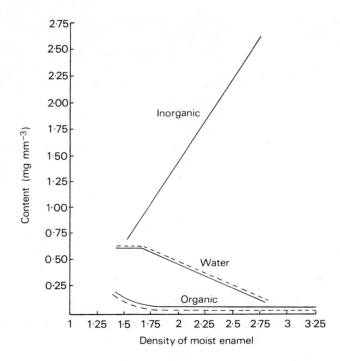

Figure 32.2 Changes in the inorganic, water and organic matter content of enamel with density during maturation. The full lines represent Deakins' original values including his correction for carbonate. The dotted lines include an additional correction for 1·2% of bound water

The composition of enamel at the beginning and end of maturation is given in Table 32.2, while the values for inorganic matter, water and organic matter in various intermediate stages of maturation are plotted against density in Figure 32.2.

Clearly there is a continuous gain in the inorganic phase and a reciprocal loss of water and organic matter during maturation. Furthermore, as judged by the weight lost per unit volume of enamel, these losses are not simply the result of dilution by the newly forming inorganic crystals but represent the actual removal of both water and organic matter from the tissue. The removal of organic matter during maturation is also apparent from and supported by experiments in which the whole of the enamel from complete deciduous dentitions of human fetuses and newly born infants was separated. It was shown that the total *weight* of protein present rose to a maximum of approximately 100 mg, 1 month after birth, and then decreased to a steady value which was only one-tenth of this.

The bulk protein of human fetal enamel was subsequently characterized and found to account for 20% of the weight, a value almost equal to that obtained by Deakins for the total organic matter of the youngest pig enamel. Thus the organic matter of young enamel is mainly proteinaceous, only small quantities of other organic constituents, viz. 0·23% of carbohydrate and 0·06% of phospholipid, having been detected.

The total protein of developing enamel has an unusual amino acid composition (Figure 32.3) which distinguishes it from collagens, keratins and the protein of mature enamel. Possession of a unique protein system during its formative stages and the subsequent differential loss of its major protein components during maturation are characteristic features of enamel development which distinguish it from other tissues. The term *amelogenins* is used to designate those proteins

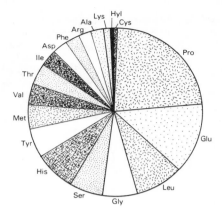

Figure 32.3 The amino acid composition of total protein from human developing enamel

that predominate in newly secreted enamel and which are removed during maturation of the enamel, a process which accompanies its transition from a material with the softness of jelly to one with the hardness of rock. The minor protein components of newly secreted enamel, known as *enamelins*, are not removed during maturation and largely persist in the fully mature enamel (Figure 32.4). Amelogenins and enamelins contrast strikingly in amino acid composition (cf. Tables 32.4 and 32.5).

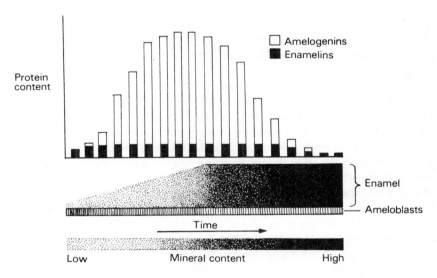

Figure 32.4 Changes of amelogenin and enamelin content during maturation of enamel compared with the increasing thickness of enamel and mineral content. (From L. W. Fisher and J. D. Termine (1985) *Clinical Orthopaedics*, **200**, 363, by permission)

The inorganic phase

Early analyses showed that mature enamel consists largely of calcium phosphates, and the existence of biological apatite in dental enamel was first recognized by the similarity of its

Table 32.3 Inorganic constituents of mature human enamel (values given as % by weight)

	Thermal neutron activation analysis Sound	Chemical analysis	
		Sound	Carious
Ca	37·4	36·75	35·95
P	18·3	17·41	17·01
CO_2	—	2·42	1·56
H_2O	—	2·02	3·07
Na	1·16	(0·25–0·9)	—
Mg	0·36	0·54	0·40
Cl	0·65	(0·19–0·30)	—
K	—	(0·15–0·30)	—
F	—	0·012	0·058
Ca/P (weight)	2·04	2·09	2·08

composition and physical properties to those of fluorapatite. It is now generally agreed that the apatite lattice is a good, though approximate, representation of the structure of the inorganic phase of enamel. The proportions of the more abundant constituents of the inorganic portion are summarized in Table 32.3.

The extreme hardness of enamel (6·5 on Moh's scale) results from the intrinsic hardness of apatite (Knoop hardness 430 kg mm^{-2}). The density of mature enamel approaches 3·01 g ml^{-1} compared with 3·1 g ml^{-1} for hydroxyapatite.

The larger size of the crystals in enamel, compared with those in bone and dentine, affects not only its physical properties but also reduces the surface of the inorganic phase rendering it less reactive. Enamel crystallites dissolve more slowly and less completely than those of dentine when exposed to solutions below pH 6; this has an important bearing on the stability of enamel under conditions tending towards incipient caries. The *c* axis of the lattice is parallel to the length of the crystals, which in turn is approximately parallel to the prism axis. Different crystal faces are dissolved by hydrogen ions at different rates, so attack is selective. Chelating agents also dissolve different crystal faces selectively but the pattern of attack is different from that of acid.

Taking mineral hydroxyapatite (100) as a standard, the crystallinity of human enamel (70) is more perfect than that of bone (35). This difference may, however, have been exaggerated by the greater scattering of X-rays by the organic components of bone.

Crystal development in enamel takes place in three stages each with a different mechanism. The first stage involves the initiation of a small crystal 'seed' *de novo*. It takes place near the surface of the ameloblasts soon after they have begun to secrete the organic phase immediately after the first dentine has been laid down. No more is known about the mechanism of the initiation in enamel than in other mineralized tissues (Chapter 31). It may occur on one of the enamel proteins, possibly the enamelin, or perhaps on the neighbouring dentine collagen.

The second stage involves growth of the crystal seeds to form long thin ribbons which grow rapidly in length in the prism direction towards the retreating ameloblasts, as they lay down newly synthesized matrix proteins. This has been observed with the electron microscope and attributed to formation of a single unit-cell thickness of octacalcium phosphate, growing in two dimensions only (i.e. in length and width but not in thickness).

The third or maturation stage consists of the subsequent slower growth of the crystallites in the third dimension, in which there was no increase at all during the second stage. This growth in thickness probably occurs in two steps. In the first a layer of octacalcium phosphate one unit cell in thickness is deposited on the 100 face of the crystal. In the second step a unit-cell thickness of octacalcium phosphate is hydrolysed and takes up Ca^{2+} ions to produce a layer of hydroxyapatite two unit cells thick.

$$Ca_8H_2(PO_4)_6 \cdot 5H_2O + 2Ca^{2+} \rightleftharpoons Ca_{10}(PO_4)_6(OH)_2 + 4H^+ + 3H_2O$$

These mechanisms explain the rapid colonization of newly laid down enamel by the thin ribbon-like crystals and the slower maturation step, during which the ribbons grow steadily in thickness and cause a continuous increase in the degree of mineralization. Neighbouring crystals grow towards one another, so that the inorganic phase gradually encroaches more and more on the continuous aqueous and organic phase. This explains why, but not how, protein and water are lost during maturation.

Fluoride ions have an important effect on the formation of the inorganic phase in enamel since they act as a catalyst for the conversion of octacalcium phosphate to hydroxyapatite. This has been demonstrated for extremely low levels of fluoride *in vitro* and it has also been shown that the presence of fluoride during hydroxyapatite formation improves the perfection of the crystals.

Fluoride is tenaciously held by the inorganic phase of enamel. In solution at concentrations of less than 100 ppm it replaces hydroxyl ions in the apatite lattice, which is partially converted to fluorapatite. Above this level a second phase of calcium fluoride is formed. These substances have been demonstrated, both *in vitro* and on the enamel surface where the concentration of fluoride is highest, to be for practical purposes less soluble in slightly acid solutions than is unsubstituted hydroxyapatite. Fluoride likewise becomes concentrated in regions of local demineralization such as enamel defects and areas of incipient caries. Here it replaces hydroxyl ions on the surface of damaged hydroxyapatite crystals, the fluorapatite surface so formed being less vulnerable to further acid attack than if it had remained as hydroxyapatite. Thus in both healthy and carious enamel, fluoride effectively decreases solubility and promotes re-mineralization of the inorganic phase.

Until recently it was thought that when the apatite lattice contains fluoride, it is more stable in the presence of acid than when fluoride is not present. However, experiments showed that enamel *initially* dissolves in acid at the same rate, whether it contains fluoride or not. When fluoride is present in enamel, however, the rate of solution of enamel falls very rapidly with time compared with the rate for enamel which does not contain fluoride. It therefore appears that fluoride ions are only effective in reducing enamel solubility when in solution. The uptake of fluoride by the enamel surface and by carious enamel is especially important in protecting these vulnerable areas by forming a local immobilized store some of which will be released in the presence of acid and will protect the enamel in its immediate neighbourhood from further attack by the acid.

When biological apatite is exposed to hydrogen ions, the solubility equation

$$Ca_{10}(PO_4)_6(OH)_2 \rightleftharpoons 10Ca^{2+} + 6(PO_4)^{3-} + 2OH^-$$

$$\qquad\qquad H^+ \updownarrow \qquad\qquad \updownarrow H^+$$

$$\qquad\qquad HPO_4^{2-} \qquad\quad H_2O$$

$$\qquad\qquad H^+ \updownarrow$$

$$\qquad\qquad H_2PO_4^-$$

moves to the right because the hydrogen ions remove both phosphate and hydroxyl ions. Fluoride in solution probably protects by playing the same part as the hydroxyl ions, since fluoride is likely to be present at a higher concentration than hydroxyl. At the *critical pH* (pH 5·5) the hydroxyl ion concentration is only 10^{-8} g-ions per litre, whereas 1 ppm fluoride solution contains 5×10^{-5} g-ions per litre. Since the pK of HF is several pH units below that of water, hydrogen ions are much less effective at removing fluoride as HF than hydroxyl ions as water at pH 5·5.

The organic phase

Proteins of young enamel

Amelogenin proteins are present in high proportions in the developing enamel of mammals. The amino acid composition of amelogenins from various species is shown in Table 32.4 from which it can be seen that, as compared with most proteins, they have a high content of proline, glutamic acid, histidine and methionine. Cystine, hydroxylysine and hydroxyproline are completely lacking or present in minimal amounts.

Table 32.4 Amino acid composition of amelogenins from various species (values given as residues per 1000 total residues)

	Human	*Pig*	*Ox*
Aspartic acid	30	39	33
Threonine	38	39	27
Serine	63	50	49
Glutamic acid	142	152	159
Proline	251	218	253
Glycine	65	69	54
Alanine	20	24	22
Valine	40	35	38
Methionine	42	54	55
Isoleucine	33	38	34
Leucine	91	95	95
Tyrosine	53	51	47
Phenylalanine	23	25	26
Lysine	18	16	16
Histidine	65	71	73
Arginine	23	20	19

The low glycine content and the virtual absence of hydroxyproline distinguish young enamel proteins from collagen. The amelogenins are also quite different in composition from proteins in the keratin group (page 402) especially as regards the predominance of histidine over the other basic amino acids. Cystine in enamel protein is substantially lower than in skin or oral epithelium which have the lowest levels of cystine of any recognized keratins (see Table 26.1). Amelogenins resemble protein components of parotid saliva one of which has a high proline content and another being rich in histidine. Enamel and salivary proteins are both products of actively secreting epithelial cells and may therefore possibly belong to the same broad family group. If this is so, it would be logical to regard enamel as a highly specialized calcified secretion rather than a tissue.

The protein from young enamel has been shown by various electrophoretic and chromatographic techniques to be heterogeneous. On starch–urea gels, seven components are separated, one of which is present in high concentration in the youngest enamel but rapidly diminishes in amount relative to other components as the enamel matures. Electrophoresis on a concentrated polyacrylamide gel has shown as many as 17 bands, five of which represent major protein components.

Amelogenins behave as a mixture of substances of different chemical composition, the molecules of which are capable of aggregating with their own and possibly other species to form a variety of more complex molecular aggregates of higher molecular weight. Recently some of the major amelogenin components have been prepared in a pure state and their amino acid sequences determined. It is now clear that enamelins are also present in developing enamel, in fact their synthesis begins slightly in advance of amelogenin secretion (Figure 32.4). Unlike amelogenins which are lost during maturation, enamelins largely persist in mature enamel.

Proteins of mature enamel

Proteins are much less abundant in mature than in young enamel. Water-soluble material of low molecular weight, is probably distributed throughout the thickness of mature enamel, adsorbed on the hydroxyapatite. After demineralization, ribbons of an acid-insoluble protein, apparently of high molecular weight, are demonstrable mainly in the inner third of enamel from human molars. The insoluble protein probably represents mainly enamelins which have persisted in the mature enamel. The protein integument, acquired by the outer surface of the enamel after eruption, is clearly not a true enamel constituent.

The soluble protein material accounts for only one-quarter to one-eighth of the total protein in human incisors and molars respectively. The separation of uncontaminated protein from the middle portion of human mature enamel has proved more difficult than with bovine enamel because the small size and convoluted shape of human teeth offer greater difficulty to microdissection. The preparation, the composition of which is given in Table 32.5, has some eight residues per 1000 of hydroxyproline suggesting that it contains some 8% of degraded collagen, which is probably a contaminant. The amino acid pattern of the soluble proteinaceous material is otherwise similar to bovine preparations which have been obtained completely free from collagen. It is present in a degraded condition, largely as peptides and amino acids. Though its function is not entirely clear it probably consists of the last traces of proteins which were abundant in the young enamel and were subsequently broken down and lost during maturation.

Insoluble protein is distributed unevenly within enamel with the greatest concentration near the amelodentinal junction, where enamel spindles and tufts occur. After demineralization, the insoluble protein remains in the form of ribbons, floss and amorphous powder. The composition of this insoluble protein differs little between ribbons and floss, which appear to be related and serve to fill up 'spaces' of different shapes and sizes between the inorganic crystallites. There is also a resemblance between the insoluble protein of enamel, enamelin, and the low sulphur keratin of human oral epithelium (Table 26.1, page 402). If the resemblance is based on a true relationship between these proteins, it would suggest that the insoluble proteins of mature enamel and the enamelins belong to a group once known as 'pseudo-keratins'. If, as appears likely, the insoluble ribbons are products of ameloblast activity, the ameloblasts, in addition to their main function as secretors of amelogenin, would seem to retain a primitive characteristic of protective epithelium by producing small amounts of an insoluble 'keratin'. However, if this is so, it does not appear to be produced by the usual route of intracellular keratinization since the ameloblasts remain active long after its formation.

Late in maturation, the ameloblasts degenerate and, soon after eruption of the tooth, are replaced on the enamel surface by an integument, acquired from external sources. The integument covers the entire exposed enamel surface and may, in places, be overlaid by plaque containing bacteria and extracellular polysaccharides (Chapter 34). This plaque can be stained with basic fuchsin and removed by scrubbing with detergent solution. The underlying

Table 32.5 Amino acid composition of proteinaceous material from mature human enamel (values given as residues per 1000 total residues)

	Water-soluble	*Insoluble ribbons*	*Acquired pellicle*
Cystine (half)	4	20	13
Hydroxyproline	8	2	0
Aspartic acid	54	79	71
Threonine	42	52	43
Serine	119	82	46
Glutamic acid	106	136	133
Proline	137	81	44
Glycine	193	62	81
Alanine	53	69	146
Valine	32	52	53
Methionine	34	22	12
Isoleucine	19	23	30
Leucine	66	111	64
Tyrosine	23	51	14
Phenylalanine	33	49	29
Hydroxylysine	4	6	0
Lysine	26	40	51
Histidine	19	27	19
Arginine	28	36	42
Ornithine			26
Muramic acid			21
Diaminopimelic acid			4
Hexosamines			53

integument, which is left intact, can then be detached after demineralizing the surface enamel with dilute acid. Acquired pellicle separated in this way contains approximately 50% of protein with a composition intermediate between the proteins of precipitated salivary mucin and bacterial cell wall (Table 32.5).

Patterns in the development and maturation of enamel

The deposition and maturation of enamel progress in a series of patterns both in space and in chemical composition. Such patterns vary from the relative simplicity of a continuously erupting rabbit incisor to the elaborate mineralization pattern of a human molar, which may involve initially independent and latterly overlapping mineralization from as many as five cuspal centres.

The pattern of mineralization can be followed by microradiography of thin sections and is related to the pattern of enamel protein secretion. In human incisor teeth, a zone of high radiodensity begins to spread from the tip of the amelodentinal junction, under what will become the cusp of the tooth (Figure 32.5). It increases rapidly as a narrow band along the junction and simultaneously spreads through the thickness of the enamel at the cusp, until it reaches the outer surface of the enamel (Figure 32.5b). Having traversed the thickness of the enamel, the radio-opaque zone spreads progressively towards the root, with the portion adjoining the amelodentinal junction considerably, and that part near the enamel surface slightly, ahead of that in the mid-enamel so that the front of high mineralization is characteristically concave (Figure 32.5c).

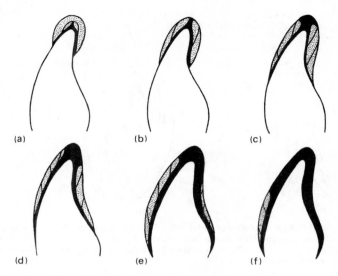

Figure 32.5 The pattern of mineralization in the enamel of an incisor tooth. The partially mineralized matrix is shown stippled and the final mineralization, moving outwards from the amelodentinal junction, is shown black

The pattern of increasing mineralization in enamel also corresponds to the changes that occur in enamel proteins during maturation. Figure 32.6 shows the percentages of protein in various regions of two teeth of different dental age from the same full-term human deciduous dentition. Comparison of Figure 32.5 with Figure 32.6 shows that the spatial patterns for inorganic matter and protein are inversely related. Since it was necessary to take rather large samples of enamel for the determination of proteins, only the broader features of the pattern of protein distribution are shown by chemical analysis.

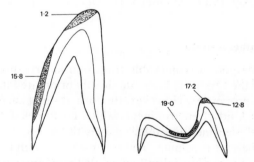

Figure 32.6 The protein content (% of dry weight) in various regions of enamel in a central incisor and a second molar from the same full-term human deciduous dentition

Staining techniques also show that the protein pattern complements that of inorganic matter even in the minute details. The cut surface of partially mineralized enamel when treated with Papanicolaou EA 65, a solution containing eosin and light green SF, is differentially stained in a pattern resembling the microradiographs which show the distribution of inorganic phase within enamel. The same pattern is obtained in sections of enamel where the teeth have been partially demineralized by treatment *in situ* with acetate buffer at pH 4·5. These solutions have the effect

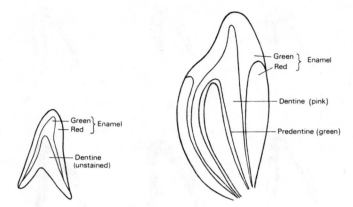

Figure 32.7 An early developing human incisor (left) and a developing human incisor at a later stage. When stained with Papanicolaou EA 65 stain, the youngest enamel matrix, which is only slightly mineralized, stains red, while the staining changes abruptly to green in areas where maturation has occurred, owing to the deposition of (green staining) hydroxyapatite and loss of (red staining) protein (cf. Figure 32.5)

of selectively dissolving part of the apatite, so that even fully mature enamel can be sectioned after embedding the tissue in paraffin wax. The eosin component stains the initially laid-down lightly mineralized enamel red, while the light green SF stains the more mature enamel near the cusp and amelodentinal junction. Figure 32.7 shows incisors of successive stages in which the enamel is only partially mature. Near the crown of the tooth it stains green while the cervical regions stain red. Independent chemical evidence shows that the red staining material is enamel protein while the material that stains green is mainly hydroxyapatite.

Analysis of dental enamel at successive stages of maturation shows also that there are changes in the relative proportions of the amino acids, and that during maturation the various protein components present in newly formed enamel are not all lost at the same rate.

The nature and role of enamel protein

As enamel matures it undergoes a remarkable transition in structure and physical properties resulting in the growth of the relatively large and highly orientated apatite crystals which give mature enamel its unique properties. However, the formation of such crystals is dependent on the existence of a specific kind of environment, which facilitates deposition of relatively few crystals, as compared with dentine, and then enables them to grow in such a way that they ultimately fill up nearly the entire volume. The organic or protein phase thus acts as a matrix for these large crystals and has a crucial influence on the manner in which enamel develops and matures.

Evidence is rather conflicting with regard to the extent to which enamel protein is fibrillar in the sense that collagens and keratins are. Early electron microscope studies suggested that a fine fibrillar network was present in the organic phase during maturation and it was also proposed that organic sheaths occur on the surface of inorganic crystallites. However, this appearance could also result from the growing crystallites compressing the protein into the diminishing channels between them. Fearnhead prepared enamel protein by five different methods designed to cause minimum alteration to organic components and so avoid artefact formation, and could find no evidence for fibrils by electron microscopy, infrared absorption or X-ray diffraction studies. It therefore seemed likely that the organic components of developing enamel have an amorphous structure, these physical observations being consistent with a gel-like matrix. Certainly a gel can be prepared from the main protein components of developing enamel. Electron microscopy of immature rat enamel has been reported to show double helices with a variable pitch running parallel to the prism direction. They are considered to be wound around the inorganic crystals, the structure being stabilized laterally by multiple links between adjacent parallel helices. If the existence of this relatively organized extracrystalline structure is confirmed, it may prove to represent the more persistent enamelin components as distinct from the transitory gel-like amelogenins. There are differences of opinion concerning the structural configuration of the protein chains in the bulk protein of young enamel as revealed by X-ray diffraction analysis but if a regular structure is present it is certainly not conspicuous.

In developing enamel the organic phase is mobile and constantly changing. This is clear from the manner in which radioisotopes of amino acids, such as glycine, proline and histidine, are incorporated into the enamel, as shown by radioautography. Rapid incorporation occurs through the ameloblasts into the secreted organic phase but, instead of the labelled material remaining as a sharp line as it does in dentine, in regions where proteins are undergoing synthesis at the time of administration, the label soon spreads widely and eventually penetrates the entire thickness of the enamel, even to areas that were laid down before the label was injected.

This suggests that the organic phase of maturing enamel is more mobile and perhaps more labile than the collagen fibres of dentine. Thus if the labelled isotopes are used for synthesis of new enamel proteins, these must be capable of some degree of movement under the influence of either concentration or pressure gradients through the less mineralized channels in the newly laid down enamel. Crystal growth occurs rapidly in these regions, so the protein may be involved in the transport of inorganic ions through the considerable distance from the enamel surface to the growing crystals. Perhaps histidine, which is abundant in early enamel protein and has been implicated in the binding of metal ions by other proteins, provides a mechanism whereby ions can be alternately taken up near the ameloblasts and released at the apatite crystal surface. This could operate by the imidazole side chain alternately changing from an uncharged to a charged state as a result of small physiological pH changes (page 36).

There is, at present, little definite information concerning the mechanisms for the systematic loss of protein during maturation, but it has been suggested that either an enzymic or a rheological mechanism may be involved. Proteins are first removed from enamel in a region that is remote from the ameloblasts (Figures 32.5–32.7). This region becomes highly mineralized at a relatively early stage and forms an impermeable barrier between the cell processes of the odontoblasts and the mid-layers of enamel which are the next to become heavily mineralized and lose protein. In many tissues removal of protein is accomplished by the action of proteolytic enzymes but in enamel the pattern of protein loss is such that it is not likely to result from a soluble enzyme diffusing into the enamel from either ameloblasts or odontoblasts. Clearly, once enamel has become separated from the ameloblasts by its own thickness, it is no longer under direct cellular control. The mechanisms for maturation, i.e. for crystal growth and protein removal, are therefore presumably built into the structure of enamel when it is formed. One possibility is that intact lysosomes are released from the cells at the same time as the enamel proteins; this would provide a means by which proteolytic enzymes might remove proteins from the enamel in the observed pattern. It would, however, be necessary for the lysosomes to remain intact in those parts of the enamel where maturation was incomplete and later to break down and release their contents in regions where mineralization was reaching a high level. The resulting fragments of enamel proteins would be more diffusible and would leave the enamel more readily than their native precursors. Latent enzyme activation could conceivably occur as a result of a time-controlled mechanism.

A rheological mechanism for the loss of protein is also attractive since it is capable of being built into the structure of the secreted enamel which, given a simple motive influence, such as a continued influx of calcium and phosphate ions, could proceed through a series of physicochemical changes. The water and proteins which constitute the continuous phase occupy a series of branching channels between the crystals. These channels are very narrow in the most mature enamel nearest the dentine, where the apatite crystals approach one another more closely than in regions nearer the surface, where the enamel is less mature and has wider channels. Thus there will be a clear pathway for proteins leaving the mature zone to pass back towards the ameloblasts at the enamel surface. If the protein phase is a viscous sol, the increase in pressure and reduction of volume available to the sol, which would result from the growth of crystals, would tend to squeeze out the protein through the labyrinth of channels towards the enamel surface. Moreover, if the enamel protein were in the form of a thixotropic gel (i.e. one that melts when pressure is applied to it and gels again when the pressure is reduced), this would be liquefied where pressure was greatest in the zone of largest crystals and would tend to flow towards regions of lower pressure near the enamel surface. Electron micrographs suggest that degraded proteins do in fact leave enamel via the ameloblasts. Both ameloblasts and the enamel organ contain a variety of hydrolytic enzymes that would presumably be capable of breaking down the expelled protein. Enzymes that have a limited specific action on amelogenins have recently been demonstrated in developing enamel.

The discovery that amelogenins exist as a hierarchy of aggregates which readily dissociate and reaggregate, according to local conditions, may be relevant to the rheological behaviour of enamel protein during maturation. Thus changes in pH and the concentration of inorganic ions will affect the interactions between polypeptide chains.

Another explanation for the mechanism of protein breakdown in the enamel matrix centres round the high proline content of amelogenins. By preventing free rotation about bonds in the protein backbone (page 415) the proline increases the rigidity of the molecule so that force applied to it, for example by the pressure of growing crystals, may be transmitted along the polypeptide chain and result in disaggregation and consequent reduction in the viscosity of the solution.

The protein system of young enamel is complex and many different mechanisms operate at the various sites and levels concerned with crystal growth and protein dispersal in maturation. Future progress depends upon clarification of the relationship between the organic and inorganic phases of enamel. Dental histology and electron microscopy have provided abundant information concerning the apatite crystallites but, until recently, very little about enamel proteins. The importance of these was revealed by analytical biochemistry, which has also provided some indication of their role in building up the enamel structure.

Whatever the origin of the hydroxyapatite crystals, the protein sol or gel provides an excellent medium for their growth to an abnormally large size, compared with what is possible elsewhere in living organisms. Their initial rapid growth in the prism direction presumably depends on the orientation of protein molecules, probably resulting from their extrusion by the ameloblasts. The enamelins would seem to be implicated for this role as they remain rather firmly bound to the inorganic crystals throughout maturation. The subsequent growth of the crystals in thickness may, in turn, rely upon provision by the protein of a mechanism for maintaining the supply of calcium and phosphate ions from the enamel surface to the growing crystal. Last but not least in importance is the capacity for the amelogenins to disaggregate and leave the enamel. Like a good mother this matrix protein not only nurtures her progeny in infancy but eventually leaves them to face the rigours of post-eruptive existence and possible palaeontological immortality.

Section 8

Biology of the mouth

Chapter 33
The oral environment

The oral cavity shows many of the biological characteristics of the gut as a whole. However, because of its exposed position at the beginning of the alimentary canal, its intrinsic biological properties are continually modified by environmental factors, particularly by contamination with microorganisms and by the intake of food. The bacteria which inhabit the mouth constitute a *community* of many different species and the study of their interactions with the tissues of the oral cavity is necessary for an understanding of oral biology in health and disease.

Organisms and their surroundings together constitute an *ecosystem* and each ecosystem has physical, chemical and biological properties that determine the composition of the community and dictate which organisms will dominate the system and which will fail to survive. In the mouth, those populations for which it has favourable nutritional and physiological characteristics survive and unsuited species fail to become established, so that the community is maintained in balance by the operation of natural selection. Each organism has a particular biological role or *niche* within the community so that species with identical biological properties will compete for the same niche; a mixed community becomes stable only when each organism has a different role to play thus avoiding competition.

The mouth, together with the rest of the gut, constitutes a natural open system and the oral cavity can be regarded as a fermentation chamber providing a suitable environment for the continuous culture of microbial populations. Relatively constant conditions are ensured by the flow of saliva which, in association with a frequent intake of food, provides a regular source of fresh substrates. At the same time, soluble products of microbial activity are continually removed and swallowed, so that their concentrations do not rise to any significant extent. The mouth is at a constant temperature, and the flow of saliva not only keeps it moist but also serves to remove many of the bacteria as well as helping to maintain the pH and ionic composition within a limited range. In other words, the mouth can be considered to contain a mixed bacterial culture preserved in a *steady state*. The bacteria, in turn, modify the physical and chemical composition of their surroundings and establish a commensal relationship with their host and a stable, interspecies relationship among themselves.

So far the mouth has been considered as a single entity; it can, however, be subdivided into a number of small independent ecosystems, each with a unique set of organisms selected on the principles already described. The main problems confronting the dentist involve the relatively restricted regions of the tooth surface and its supporting tissues, since the bacterial populations in these areas modify their environment in a manner that may lead to disease. The relationship between the tooth surface and the rest of the mouth can be summarized as follows:

$$\text{Enamel + environment} \left\{ \begin{array}{l} \text{mixed saliva} \\ \text{diet} \\ \text{bacteria} \end{array} \right. \longrightarrow \text{Dental plaque} \left\{ \begin{array}{l} \text{specific bacteria} \\ \text{matrix} \\ \text{fluid} \end{array} \right.$$

Dynamic interactions between the saliva, diet and oral bacteria lead to the accumulation of material on the tooth surface. This is known as *dental plaque* which can be defined as the deposit which forms on the tooth in its natural environment and, unlike food debris, cannot be removed by a water spray. It is composed of localized concentrations of bacteria specific to this surface together with some degraded mammalian cells. These are surrounded by a matrix containing both protein and polysaccharide and the whole is bathed in a fluid derived from the saliva. On this basis, plaque can be said to have the characteristics of a simple tissue.

Plaque is almost always found on the non-occluding surfaces of the teeth which are only subject to abrasion if the teeth are brushed. Plaque may be present in healthy mouths and does not necessarily lead to pathological changes. However, it is recognized as the common factor in the two main dental diseases, namely *dental caries* and *periodontal disease*.

Dental caries is characterized by the loss of calcified material from the tooth while periodontal disease is a chronic inflammatory process that leads to the gradual destruction of the supporting tissues of the tooth and is often associated with the deposition of calculus.

Saliva

Saliva is a mixed secretion more than 90% of which is produced by the parotid, submandibular and sublingual glands. The remainder is contributed by accessory glands present on the soft palate and on the internal surfaces of the lips and cheeks. The type of secretion varies according to the gland and, whereas parotid saliva is serous or watery in consistency, that from the submandibular and sublingual glands contains different glycoproteins and is much more viscous. Their viscosities relative to water at (1·0) 37°C are parotid 1·3, submandibular 2·6 and sublingual 11·0.

The volume of saliva secreted each day is difficult to determine. An average value of between 1·0 and 1·5 litres is often cited but this may well be an overestimate. Under resting conditions, the rate of flow is about $0·3 \, \text{ml min}^{-1}$ (range $0·05-1·8 \, \text{ml min}^{-1}$) and this increases to about $2·5-5·0 \, \text{ml min}^{-1}$ on stimulation. On this basis, since during sleep the flow is negligible, it may be calculated that between 700 and 800 ml are produced each day so that over a period of weeks or months the surfaces of the teeth are exposed to large volumes of saliva.

Estimates suggest that about 1·0 ml of saliva is present in the mouth at any one time. It has been found that the average volume required to initiate the swallowing reflex is 1·1 ml and that 0·8 ml remains after swallowing, thus removing about 0·3 ml each time. Because the estimated surface area of the teeth and soft tissues is very large, about 200 cm^2, it follows that these surfaces are covered by a film of saliva, no more than 100 μm thick. This allows rapid exchange between the saliva and the underlying surface and favours the deposition of salivary macromolecules providing a more dynamic relationship between the enamel and saliva than is generally realized. Assuming a daily salivary volume of 700–800 ml it follows that the 1·0 ml pool of saliva is replaced 700–800 times each day, requiring about 2500 swallows in the process! This high dilution rate is essential for the effective removal of food debris and prevents the accumulation of excessive numbers of bacteria. The average adult swallows between 1·0 and 2·5 g of bacteria each day and defective salivary flow quickly results in microbial overgrowth and oral stagnation.

The functions of saliva

Saliva has many functions the most important of which are as follows.

Protective

The epithelial surface of the whole of the gastrointestinal tract is covered by a continuously flowing layer of mucus so that the environment of these surfaces is largely independent of the chemical composition of the contents. The glycoproteins in saliva provide both mechanical and chemical protection. Also, because of its large volume and continuous flow, saliva flushes away large numbers of bacteria and accumulating toxins. If the flow of saliva is suppressed, pathological changes may supervene and excessive dryness leads to *stomatitis*, i.e. inflammation of the mouth and an increase in dental caries.

The properties of saliva which make it a good lubricant also help to protect the soft tissue surfaces from physical damage which might otherwise be caused by hard textured foods or excessive temperatures. Similarly, buffers present in saliva help to protect both hard and soft tissues from chemical damage resulting from bacterial acid production. Protection against the damaging effects of bacteria may also be provided by such specific components as immunoglobulins and lysozyme (page 409), which break down the coat polysaccharides of certain types of bacteria.

Repair

The precipitation of a film of proteins and glycoproteins rich in calcium and phosphate on the enamel surface is believed to be essential for the effective remineralization of an early carious lesion.

Digestive

Lubrication with saliva helps to soften the food and aids the formation and swallowing of a food bolus. The rate of removal of substances from the mouth depends on factors such as the rate of saliva flow, the adhesive properties of the food and the activity of salivary enzymes, notably *amylase*. This enzyme initiates the digestion of starch (page 224) and the breakdown and consequent removal of residual material commonly found around the teeth.

Control of water balance

When the body is dehydrated water is conserved by cutting down the rate of salivation which, in turn, causes thirst so that under normal circumstances the fluid is replaced by drinking.

Miscellaneous

By lubricating the lips and tongue saliva facilitates speech and, since it acts as a solvent, it also aids *gustation*. Saliva may perhaps be considered to play a role in excretion since heavy metals such as mercury and lead are secreted into it; this does not, however, provide a final solution to the problem of their disposal since they are subsequently swallowed and may be reabsorbed. Lastly, to the great convenience of the dentist, the rheological* properties of saliva help to retain dentures in position although this can hardly be part of Nature's grand design!

* Rheology concerns the flow and deformation of matter.

The composition of saliva

Saliva, for experimental work, can be collected with special cannulae directly from the ducts of the glands. This material is pure and sterile and truly representative of the secretion of the gland in question. However, *mixed saliva*, which is usually collected from the mouth during paraffin wax stimulation, is of very variable composition. In addition to fractions from each gland, it contains food debris, plaque, bacteria, degraded mammalian cells and possibly some gingival sulcus fluid. In spite of its heterogeneity and variability, the composition of mixed saliva is of great importance since it is this fluid which gives rise to the acquired enamel integuments (page 490). Some idea of the composition of a normal average sample of mixed saliva can be obtained from Table 33.1.

The secretion of saliva appears to be an active process as its composition is very different from that of the plasma and also, when the ducts are ligated, secretion continues even when the

Table 33.1 The average composition of mixed human saliva and normal values for plasma

Water	94·0–99·5%	
Solids	0·5 (stimulated)–6·0% (unstimulated)	
Specific gravity	1·002–1·008	
pH (average)	6·7	
pH (range)	6·2–7·6	
	Saliva (mM)	*Plasma* (mM)
Inorganic		
Ca^{2+}	1–2	2·5
Mg^{2+}	0·2–0·5	1·0
Na^+	6–26	140
K^+	14–32	4
NH_4^+	1–7	0·03
$H_2PO_4^- + HPO_4^{2-}$	2–23	2
Cl^-	17–29	103
HCO_3^-	2–30	27
F^-	0·001–0·005	0·01
SN^-	0·1–2·0	—
Organic		
Urea (adults)	2–6	5
Urea (children)	1–2	—
Uric acid	0·2	3
Amino acids (free)	1–2	2
Glucose (free)	0·05	5
Lactate	0·1	1
Fatty acids ($mg\,l^{-1}$)	10	3000
Macromolecules ($mg\,l^{-1}$)		
Proteins	1400–6400	70000
Glycoprotein sugars	110–300	1400
Amylase	380	—
Lysozyme	109	—
Peroxidase	3	—
IgA	194	1300
IgG	14	13000
IgM	2	1000
Lipid	20–30	5500

pressure in the ducts is about twice that of the normal blood pressure. Stimulated mixed saliva contains 99·0–99·5% water, and the solid matter is composed of approximately equal amounts of organic and inorganic matter. Saliva is hypotonic and has a specific gravity of 1·002–1·008. The pH varies from 5·6 to 8·0 but the average value is about 6·7.

Inorganic constituents

Although the ions present are similar to those found in plasma the relative concentrations of Na^+, K^+, Ca^{2+}, Mg^{2+}, Cl^-, SO_4^{2-}, $H_2PO_4^-$ and HPO_4^{2-} show clearly that saliva is not a simple ultrafiltrate of blood plasma. Thus, while the sodium, calcium, magnesium, chloride and bicarbonate levels are lower than those of plasma, the phosphate and particularly the potassium levels are higher. Other organic constituents may include thiocyanate, iodide, fluoride and traces of copper, iron, manganese, cobalt and molybdenum. The importance of thiocyanate as an antibacterial agent is discussed on page 527.

Saliva does not contain enough ionic calcium and phosphate to give spontaneous precipitation but is able to support crystal growth in the presence of a suitable nucleator (page 456). Recent investigations show that, as all of the phosphate and more than 90% of the calcium is in an ionic state, saliva at normal pH values must be supersaturated with respect to all the biologically important calcium phosphate solid phases (Table 35.1) including dicalcium phosphate dihydrate which acts as a precursor of hydroxyapatite during calcification (page 455). This supersaturation is maintained by specific molecules in parotid and submandibular saliva which bind to calcium phosphate surfaces and prevent spontaneous precipitation and crystal growth. These include anionic proline-rich proteins and the phosphopeptide *statherin* which act in much the same way as other macromolecules which are known to inhibit bone formation. They may help to maintain the integrity of the enamel surface during acid attack and prevent undesirable calcification from taking place within the salivary glands and their ducts. Statherin is unusual in that all but one of the charged amino acids it contains is present in the *N*-terminal third of the molecule, the remainder of the molecule being relatively hydrophobic. This uneven distribution allows it to bind to apatite surfaces while presenting a hydrophobic face to the surrounding water, preventing further crystallization.

Organic constituents

The major organic constituents of saliva are the proteins which amount to 0·15–0·25 g per 100 ml. Sensitive methods of protein separation such as gel electrophoresis have shown that a great variety are present, and that many of them are glycoproteins which are responsible for the viscosity and lubricating properties of saliva. The glycoproteins contain one or more heterosaccharide side chains, covalently bonded to a protein backbone. The side chains may be branched and contain a relatively small number of sugar residues; they lack a serially repeating unit and often end with a sialic acid residue. The structure of a typical *salivary glycoprotein* is shown in Figure 33.1. The carboxyl group of sialic acid (pK 2·6) is fully ionized at physiological pH values and confers a strong negative charge on the molecule. The intramolecular electrostatic repulsion caused by the close proximity of these charges on neighbouring side chains (and steric hindrance effects due to the bulkiness of the oligosaccharide chain) help to maintain the molecules in an extended configuration. The long rod-like structures of the glycoprotein molecules and their tendency to aggregate in solution are responsible for the characteristic physical properties of saliva and other secretions which contain them.

Other soluble glycoproteins present in saliva include antibodies, mainly IgA and the blood group substances, i.e. the A, B and O agglutinogens. These are found in about 80% of the

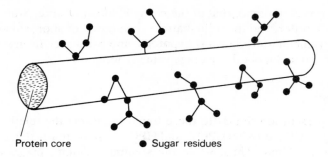

Figure 33.1 The structure of a typical glycoprotein

population who are known as *secretors* and in whom the concentration is several hundred times that of the red blood corpuscles. This is of some medicolegal significance since the blood group of a secretor may be determined from traces of saliva left on drinking vessels or cigarette ends.

Saliva contains a variety of enzymes including α-amylase in relatively large amounts and also carbonic anhydrase and lysozyme as well as peroxidase and phosphatase activities. Many of the enzymes found in mixed saliva are derived from oral bacteria.

Apart from its macromolecular constituents, saliva contains small amounts of lipid, a variety of amino acids, urea and a number of vitamins. The amino acid pool is rich in alanine, glycine and glutamic acid but is low in proline and the sulphur-containing amino acids. Analyses show that there is a poor correlation between the free amino acid composition of saliva and that of plasma and the plaque fluid; this indicates selectivity in secretion and the existence of concentration gradients in the mouth. Urea diffuses freely across cell membranes and the urea content runs parallel with that of blood. Free carbohydrate is present only in very small amounts in uncontaminated saliva but may, of course, be present in high concentrations after starch or sugars have been eaten.

Over the years, many attempts have been made to relate the composition of the saliva to both the nature of the diet and the incidence of caries, but it is now realized that so many factors influence its composition that, unless these are strictly controlled, it is not possible to correlate one set of findings with another. If any such relationship exists, the rate of flow and hence the buffering power of the saliva would appear to be the factors most likely to affect the ability of bacterially produced acids to attack the mineral elements of the teeth.

The buffering action of saliva

Although proteins exert a buffering action, the main buffering effect of the salivary proteins is exerted only below pH 5 which is beyond the physiological range, and the pH and effective buffering properties of saliva depend mainly on its bicarbonate content (Figure 33.2). The concentration of carbonic acid in freshly secreted saliva is about the same as that in plasma, namely 1·3 mM and, because of the stability of the carbonic acid concentration in plasma which is in equilbrium with the alveolar CO_2, it does not alter very much when the flow rate is increased. On the other hand, the bicarbonate is derived partly from the plasma and partly from the metabolic activity of the glands themselves which contain carbonic anhydrase. It will be remembered (page 27) that the pH of the buffer system is defined by the Henderson–Hasselbalch equation:

$$pH = pK + \log[HCO_3^-]/[H_2CO_3]$$

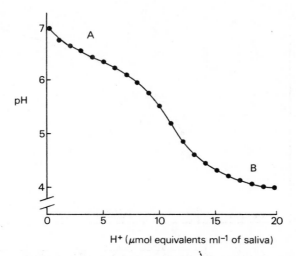

Figure 33.2 The titration of mixed saliva with acid. Buffering regions: A, mainly bicarbonate and phosphate; B, due to salivary protein. Note the poorly buffered region between pH 6·0 and 4·5

so, at resting flow rates when little metabolic CO_2 is produced and bicarbonate is reabsorbed in the ducts, the pH value approaches the pK value of 6·1 (Figure 33.3). Moreover, the buffering capacity is low since the total concentration of H_2CO_3 and HCO_3^- is only 2–3 mM. Stimulation causes an increased flow of saliva and decreases the reabsorption of bicarbonate with a consequent increase in the $[HCO_3^-]/[H_2CO_3]$ ratio and in the pH. When the flow rate increases

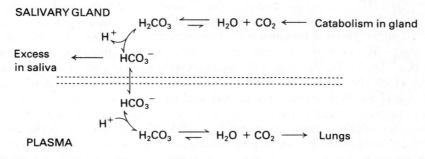

Figure 33.3 The production of bicarbonate in the saliva

to about 1 ml min^{-1} the bicarbonate concentration rises to about 30 mM and at higher flow rates may increase to as much as 60 mM. These concentrations of bicarbonate produce pH values of 7·5 and 7·8 respectively (Figure 33.4). Thus bicarbonate provides an effective buffer against acid provided that the rate of flow of saliva is high.

If, after collection, the saliva is left exposed to the atmosphere, the concentration of carbonic acid falls as CO_2 is lost. The reaction is catalysed by the carbonic anhydrase present and the pH can rise to a value of 8·5–9·0 if the saliva is left undisturbed.

Saliva also contains inorganic phosphates which contribute to its buffering power. The pK value for the dissociation

$$H_2PO_4^- \rightleftharpoons H^+ + HPO_4^{2-}$$

is 6·8 and, since the pH of unstimulated saliva is usually in the region of 6·1 and the total phosphate concentration is about 5mM, it can be seen from the Henderson–Hasselbalch

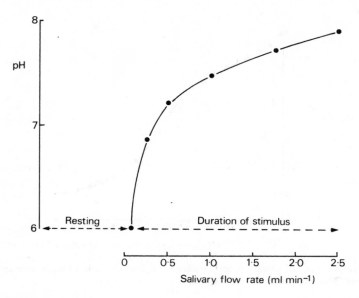

Figure 33.4 The effect of stimulation for 3 min on the flow rate and the pH of parotid saliva. The unstimulated (resting) pH is shown for comparison

equation that the concentration of $H_2PO_4^-$ must be greater than that of HPO_4^{2-}. An increase in the rate of flow which raises the pH to 7 or above causes the total phosphate concentration to fall to about 2 mM. The HPO_4^{2-} ion now becomes the predominant member of the buffer pair even though, because of the reduction in total phosphates, its concentration is not much greater than in unstimulated saliva. The relative constancy of the concentration of HPO_4^{2-}, despite variation of flow rate, is significant because the solubility of hydroxyapatite appears to be governed by the ion product $[Ca^{2+}] \times [HPO_4^{2-}]$ (page 455) which determines the *critical pH*. This is defined as the pH at which the fluid at the tooth surface becomes undersaturated with respect to hydroxyapatite and allows the removal of calcium and phosphate from the enamel.

Attempts to raise the concentrations of calcium and/or phosphate in saliva with a view to decreasing enamel solubility have not been successful. The calcium ion is the most closely regulated of the plasma electrolytes and remains constant in spite of variations in dietary intake. Neither supplementation of the diet of rats with moderate amounts of inorganic phosphate nor infusion of human subjects with sufficient phosphate to bring about a threefold increase in blood levels caused an appreciable change in the phosphate concentration of saliva. Nevertheless, rats fed a phosphate supplement showed a marked reduction in caries, presumably as the result of a local effect.

Factors affecting salivary composition

The relative contributions from the various glands

Appreciable differences occur in the proportions of its constituents according to the source of the saliva. For instance, parotid saliva is rich in amylase and phosphate and poor in mucus and calcium compared with submandibular and sublingual secretions. The minor mucous glands secrete saliva which contains traces only of phosphate and have chloride as their main anion.

The flow rate

This is subject to physiological regulation and has a marked effect on the composition of the saliva. The flow is increased not only by direct stimulation of taste and olfactory receptors but also by other forms of oral stimulation, such as those experienced during dental treatment. The exact nature of the stimulus also affects the composition.

The flow rate is also affected by the *circadian rhythms,* i.e. regular fluctuations in bodily functions occurring over a 24 hour period and, as already mentioned, saliva flow is low or absent during sleep. When required for comparative studies saliva must be collected at a fixed time of day.

Nausea, which is usually associated with vomiting, causes increased salivation and sweating. On the other hand, fear causes a dry mouth, and dehydration and general anaesthesia are also accompanied by low rates of flow.

In general, if the flow rate is increased above the unstimulated rate the sodium, calcium, chloride, bicarbonate and protein concentrations and pH increase, whereas the phosphate, magnesium and urea concentrations decrease while potassium shows little change. At very high rates of flow the composition of saliva, which is normally hypotonic, tends to approach that of plasma.

The nature of the stimulus

While working on dogs Pavlov found that the composition of the saliva depended on the nature of the stimulus and that, whereas dry food or sand evoked a copious watery secretion, the secretion produced by meat was much thicker and richer in mucosubstances. It has also been found that the consumption of a high-carbohydrate diet is followed by a rise in the amylase content of mixed saliva. It seems likely that alterations in response to different forms of stimulation result mainly from differential alterations in the rate of flow of various glands. It is possible, however, that different stimuli can alter the composition of saliva from a particular gland without affecting the rate of flow.

The diet

During mastication food is shredded and broken up into small fragments which are mixed with saliva and formed into a bolus. This causes dissolution of soluble constituents, facilitates swallowing and initiates the digestion of starch by salivary amylase. What happens after the bolus has been swallowed is only of indirect interest to the dentist. However, although the nutrients mentioned in Section 3 are necessary for the health of the body as a whole, certain dietary constituents are believed to have a direct effect on the tooth–saliva–bacteria relationship and the incidence of dental disease. Chief among these are sugars, fluoride, calcium and vitamin D which are considered in more detail in other sections of the book.

Dietary composition

Sugars

A definite relationship exists between the frequency of consumption of refined sugars, the proportion of acidogenic organisms in the plaque and the incidence of caries. In man, sucrose is particularly damaging both on account of the large quantities consumed (page 133) and the manner in which it is metabolized by the oral bacteria (page 495). Sugars affect bacterial metabolism within the plaque in two ways. Firstly, they are used for energy production, which, under the localized anaerobic conditions prevailing in the plaque, results in the formation of a variety of organic acids. Secondly, they may act as substrates for the formation of both intracellular and extracellular polysaccharides. The latter include glucans and fructans which are readily formed from sucrose and play an important part in determining the consistency and thickness of the plaque film.

Human diets also contain a high proportion of starchy foods but these have a relatively low cariogenic potential compared with the sugars, although the products of their breakdown by amylase, namely maltose, isomaltose and small amounts of glucose, also act as substrates for the plaque bacteria.

Proteins and protein derivatives

Saliva collected directly from the ducts possesses no proteolytic activity. However, oral bacteria produce a wide range of proteases and peptidases and these are found both in mixed saliva and in the dental plaque where they are responsible for the liberation of peptides and amino acids from protein. Under physiological conditions, these enzymes appear to be slow acting and are unlikely to have any significant effect on the dietary protein except at sites where meat or fish fibres are retained, e.g. between the teeth.

Apart from acting directly as a substrate for bacterial action, dietary protein may have other effects. For example, there is a tendency for dietary as well as salivary proteins to be deposited on the surface of the teeth. The accumulation of this material may reduce the solubility of the enamel and provide a measure of protection against the onset of caries. Caseinogen, the phosphoprotein present in milk, has a particularly high affinity for calcium and may initiate the formation of a calcium–protein complex on the enamel surface.

In normal subjects, protein-rich diets do not cause a rise in the blood urea level but the blood urea level does tend to rise with age and causes a corresponding increase of the level in the saliva. Urea is an important substrate for bacterial metabolism and is converted into ammonia which plays a part in regulating the acid–base balance within the plaque (page 505). This could be a contributory factor in the higher incidence of periodontal disease in older subjects.

Fats

The presence of fat in the diet has been shown to reduce the incidence of caries in experimental animals, although a similar effect has not been demonstrated conclusively in Man. Various reasons have been suggested for the effect of the fat, such as protection of the enamel surface by the formation of a hydrophobic molecular film, the increased availability of fat-soluble vitamins in the plaque or the possibility that fat has antimicrobial properties, but the real reason is not known.

Vitamins

Dietary vitamins may help to provide the needs of the oral flora. However, many of the bacteria are themselves capable of synthesizing vitamins, if suitable sources of nitrogen and energy are available. Bacteria that are unable to synthesize the vitamins that they require probably exist in symbiotic relationship with others that do.

Although most vitamins have little effect on the tooth–saliva–bacteria relationship, vitamin B_6 deserves individual mention since it may promote amino acid metabolism and in so doing reduce acid production in the plaque. Despite earlier expectations, however, it does not exert a caries-protective effect in Man.

Trace elements

Evidence exists that certain trace elements can reduce the incidence of caries. Systemically administered fluoride appears to favour the deposition of apatite with a reduced solubility in acid (page 429) and also to be essential for maturation of the enamel and the remineralization of an early carious lesion (page 511). Even after the teeth are fully developed, the presence of fluoride in the oral fluids is beneficial because fluoride ions are adsorbed on the enamel surface and have an adverse effect on bacterial metabolism (page 500).

Manganese, molybdenum, vanadium and strontium are also said to reduce caries. Their mode of action is not known but they may reduce enamel solubility.

Organic phosphates

Certain foods such as unrefined cereals and sugar cane juice contain organic phosphates, e.g. phytate (inositol hexaphosphate), which reduce enamel solubility, apparently by reacting with calcium phosphate salts on the enamel surface. The view that this type of compound has a caries-inhibiting effect is supported by observations that dietary supplements of calcium glycerophosphate reduce caries in rats and monkeys. At the same time, the calcium-binding properties of phytate may adversely affect the absorption of calcium from the intestine (page 143).

Other dietary considerations

Frequent eating may increase the degree of caries associated with a particular diet since this increases the time that substrate is available for the oral bacteria, whereas the same amount of food, if eaten all at once, is only available for a limited time. Furthermore, the way in which food is prepared can influence the degree of retention. Liquid foodstuffs provide nutrients in solution; these are freely available to the bacteria but are rapidly removed by swallowing. Uncooked foods are often fibrous and require vigorous chewing so that the increased salivary flow promotes rapid clearance; acidic and spicy foods also act as salivary stimulants. Dry gritty foods are cleared quickly but may become impacted in the fissures of the teeth while sticky foods, especially cooked starch, are retained on surfaces, particularly between the teeth as was shown in the Vipeholm experiment (page 133). The most damaging effects result from the consumption of sticky foods at frequent intervals.

The oral flora

The mouth of the newborn infant is entirely devoid of microorganisms but, within hours of birth, possibly at a time coincident with the first feeding, it shows evidence of bacterial colonization. Successful colonization of any particular site depends on the ability of the pioneering species:

1. To obtain all their nutrients from the saliva and the diet.
2. To tolerate the physical variables such as changes in pH, oxygen tension and ionic strength, to which they may be exposed.
3. To overcome the defence mechanisms of the host, for example, salivary lysozyme, transferrin, the peroxidase system and salivary antibodies.

4. To grow at a rate which, at least during early colonization, is as great as that of any other invading species.
5. To resist other bacteria which may act as predators or parasites or may produce toxins.
6. To adhere to surfaces.

This last property is of special importance in relation to the oral flora since cells tend to be swept away by the flow of saliva so that only organisms which are able to adhere to surfaces will become established.

The only surfaces available for colonization in the edentulous infant are epithelial surfaces and bacteria are continually removed from these by the shedding of surface cells. The pioneer organisms are aerobes or facultative anaerobes, usually streptococci and lactobacilli. Once invasion has occurred, the complexity of the oral communities increases during the next few months, particularly on the new surfaces provided by the eruption of the teeth. A list of common oral organisms together with some of their properties is shown in Table 33.2.

The enamel is a unique non-shedding hard surface which acquires its own pioneering organisms. For example, in contrast with *Streptococcus salivarius* which is mainly found in the saliva and on the soft tissues, *Streptococcus mutans* and *Streptococcus sanguis* only appear when the teeth erupt. Differences also occur in the distribution of *Actinomyces*. *A. naeslundii* can be

Table 33.2 Some typical microorganisms of dental plaque

Gram-positive organisms

(1) *Type*   *Cocci*
    Species   *Streptococcus*
    Examples   *S. mutans*
                 S. sanguis
                 S. mitior
                 S. milleri
                 S. salivarius (saliva and mucosal surfaces only)

   Commonest oral bacteria and can represent up to 70% of plaque organisms. Strongly acidogenic, fermenting sugars and other dietary carbohydrates to organic acids which can reduce the external pH to 4–5. Produce intracellular and extracellular polysaccharides which act as carbohydrate reserves and enhance surface colonization. Frequently isolated from carious plaques and produce caries in experimental animals, especially *S. mutans*.

(2) *Type*   *Filaments*
    Species   *Actinomyces*
    Examples   *A. israelii*
                 A. viscosus
                 A. naeslundii
                 A. odontolyticus

   High proportions in plaque (4–80% of total organisms); especially common in the gingival region. Weakly acidogenic but can cause root caries and periodontal disease in animals. Form 'basic plaque community' along with streptococci. *A. israelii* causes actinomycosis.

(3) *Type*   *Rods*
    Species   *Lactobacillus*
    Examples   *L. casei*
                 L. acidophilus

   Acidogenic, producing mainly lactic acid, and acid tolerant. The pH optimum for growth is 5·5 which is sufficiently low to inhibit most other bacteria. Found in very low concentrations in plaque but predominate in active carious lesions. Require a source of B vitamins.

Table 33.2 continued

Gram-negative organisms

(1) *Type*   *Cocci*
   Species   *Neisseria*

Aerobic organisms, early colonizers of the enamel surface but reduced in number as the plaque develops and becomes anaerobic.

(2) *Type*   *Cocci*
   Species   *Veillonella*
   Examples   *V. alcalescens*
                V. parvula

Strictly anaerobic and unable to metabolize carbohydrates. Found in association with streptococci and derive energy from the fermentation of lactate to propionic acid, acetic acid, carbon dioxide and hydrogen. Represent 0–60% of plaque bacteria, also common on tongue.

(3) *Type*   *Cocco–bacilli* (short rods)
   Species   *Haemophilus*
   Example   *H. influenzae*

Low pathogenic potential, found on all surfaces and require haemin and NAD^+ for growth.

(4) *Type*   *Rods*
   Species   *Bacteroides*
   Examples   *B. melaninogenicus*
                B. oralis
                B. ruminicola

Strictly anaerobic, nutritionally demanding and derive growth factors from gingival fluid. Found in high numbers (0–66%) in gingival plaque and periodontal pockets. Proteolytic organisms fermenting amino acids to formate, acetate and succinate. May produce collagenase, hyaluronidase and chondroitin sulphatase. Probable periodontal pathogens.

(5) *Type*   *Filaments*
   Species   *Fusobacteria*
   Example   *F. nucleatum*

Strictly anaerobic, common in plaque and associated with adult periodontitis. Ferment amino acids.

(6) *Type*   *Spiral*
   Species   *Spirochaetes*
   Examples   *Treponema denticola*
                T. macrodentium
                T. oralis

First appearance in early teens and associated with periodontal disease. Anaerobic metabolism obtaining essential nutrients from the blood and gingival fluid, e.g. putrescine, spermine and isobutyrate. Also ferment amino acids to acetate, ammonia, hydrogen sulphide and carbon dioxide. Invade tissues and are highly pathogenic. Represent 2% of total organisms in healthy tissues and about 40% in periodontal disease.

(7) *Species*   *Yeasts*
   Example   *Candida albicans*

Not bacteria but fungi, generally in low numbers but increase following antibiotic therapy. Colonize epithelial surfaces and can cause candidosis (thrush).

isolated from toothless children whereas *A. viscosus* only appears after eruption of the teeth. The colonization of an individual surface is an example of *ecological succession* in which there is increasing species diversity, leading finally to a *climax community* in which each niche is occupied. This is not static but a highly dynamic and self-regulatory system in which the metabolic activities of the various species complement each other, a good example being the mutual interdependence of streptococci and *Veillonella* (page 505). It should be noted that although saliva contains 10^7–10^8 organisms per ml it is not considered to have its own flora, the organisms being derived from the colonized surfaces.

The climax plaque community in children is similar to that found in adults except that the numbers of *Bacteriodes* and oral spirochaetes increase in the region of the gingival crevice during adolescence, probably because of the extremely anaerobic conditions and provision of specific growth factors in the gingival crevice fluid.

A detailed description of the microbial populations at different sites in the mouth and on the tooth surface is beyond the scope of this book, but, reference should be made to the concept of a basic plaque community. Studies on plaques from a number of animals and reference to Table 33.2 indicate that the streptococci and *Actinomyces* are the best adapted of the oral bacteria and that a mixture of the two species forms the basis of a plaque composition common to all mouths. Other populations are then superimposed on this basic mixture, depending on local conditions. The relative proportions of streptococci and *Actinomyces* depends on the nature of the diet, a sugar-rich diet favouring the streptococci, particularly those which have the ability to produce extracellular polysaccharides from sucrose and to ferment carbohydrates to acid.

The many strains of non-pathogenic bacteria that are normally present in the gastrointestinal and upper respiratory tracts help to ward off attack by other invasive organisms. This may be due to a direct effect on the pathogenic organism or to some modification in the host. Thus *gnotobiotic* (germ-free) conditions or the use of antibiotics and antiseptic mouthwashes may have the effect of removing this form of microbial defence. Furthermore, disturbances of the normal balance of the oral flora may allow minor strains, such as the yeasts, to become predominant and may lead to pathological changes. As might be expected, germ-free animals often succumb to organisms not usually considered to be pathogenic.

The role of bacteria in the formation of dental plaque and their implication in dental caries and periodontal disease are considered in more detail in the following chapters. These diseases are still not fully understood even though a hundred years have elapsed since Miller first suggested that caries results from the accumulation of acids produced within the plaque. Early workers considered plaque to be a 'gelatin-like' substance formed on the tooth by the 'caries fungus'. However, experimental evidence was lacking and it was not until it had been shown that (*a*) in the rat, caries could be prevented by penicillin, and (*b*) caries could be induced by infecting germ-free rodents with bacteria, that the relationship between caries and bacteria was conclusively proved. Subsequently work on gnotobiotic animals, maintained on diets containing a high proportion of carbohydrate, showed that, if their mouths were inoculated with single strains of streptococci isolated either from rats with active caries or from human plaque, they developed carious lesions, although the high-carbohydrate diet alone did not lead to caries.

In conclusion, even though the precise relationship between plaque bacteria and the initiation of caries and periodontal disease is not fully understood, it is clear that these diseases do not involve the introduction of new microbes in the mouth but result from a localized imbalance in the bacterial composition of the plaque, which allows the proliferation of selected members of the community with pathological results. When normal commensal bacteria produce disease in this way they are called *opportunist pathogens*. The disease itself can then lead to new sites becoming open to colonization and the evolution of different and usually more extreme communities. The carious cavity and the periodontal pocket are examples of this; the former encourages the proliferation of highly acidogenic bacteria such as *S. mutans* and the acid-tolerant lactobacilli, while the latter favours the growth of strictly anaerobic Gram-negative rods and spirochaetes.

Chapter 34
The formation and properties of dental plaque

When a tooth is brushed with an abrasive agent it is possible to remove all the organic material that has accumulated on the surface and expose the 'naked' apatite crystals. If the tooth is then allowed to interact with saliva, either naturally in the mouth or in a bacteria-free artificial system, a thin acellular surface film forms within a few minutes. This material is known as the *acquired pellicle*. Examination under the electron microscope has shown that this integument is about $10\,\mu$m thick and consists of a surface and subsurface layer. Initially, the surface is gelatinous but it hardens with time and may become calcified.

Pellicle stains positively for carbohydrate and protein and appears to be derived from the salivary proteins. Its amino acid composition is similar to that of a typical glycoprotein and it contains hexoses, hexosamines and fucose. However, the glucose/galactose ratio differs from that in saliva and it has been suggested that the pellicle consists of a specific salivary glycoprotein fraction whose oligosaccharide side chains are resistant to enzymic degradation.

Calcium and phosphate ions are thought to be involved in the precipitation of salivary proteins to form the pellicle and the protein matrix of plaque. It is well established that proteins bind to calcium phospate surfaces, especially hydroxyapatite crystals. Experiments have shown that a pure hydroxyapatite surface carries a net positive charge due to the protonation of some of the phosphate groups, but gains an overall negative charge following treatment with saliva. This surface modification by salivary proteins may be due to binding of these proteins to the apatite surface or to a tightly held water layer by direct ionic links, ion–dipole interactions and hydrogen bonding. Calcium and phosphate may each form ionic bonds with oppositely charged groups in the salivary proteins and this may lead to the co-precipitation of protein with insoluble calcium phosphate salts. Plaque contains high concentrations of calcium and phosphate as compared with saliva, and salivary glycoproteins have been found to be rapidly and selectively bound by hydroxyapatite powder and powdered enamel, the adsorbed material having a similar electrophoretic mobility to protein collected from extracted teeth.

The mechanism of pellicle formation is far from clear but there is no doubt that it forms rapidly on all enamel surfaces. Although there is justification for regarding it to be normal for a tooth to be covered with pellicle, there is considerable controversy as to whether this integument has any function. It may protect the teeth against acid attack, and abraded areas of enamel are undoubtedly more susceptible to decalcification, but it has not been proved whether this is due to removal of the pellicle or of some other components of the enamel surface. The presence of

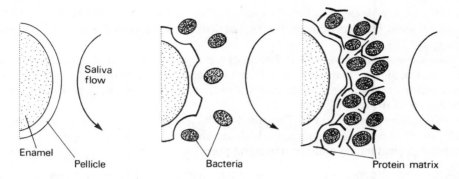

Figure 34.1 Three successive stages in the colonization of a pellicle-covered enamel surface by bacteria during early plaque formation

the protein–calcium phosphate complex increases the resistance of enamel to dissolution and, since enamel defects are often filled with insoluble protein, pellicle formation may assist in subsequent recalcification (page 513). Another suggestion is that, because it provides a continuous layer of protein at the enamel–gingival interface, it may be implicated in the adhesion of the gingival epithelium to the tooth.

Newly formed pellicle is quickly invaded by bacteria (Figure 34.1) derived from the saliva, the adjacent soft tissues and any defects in the enamel surface, and their growth produces discrete colonies which eventually fuse to produce a bacterial mass. At first the bacteria rest on top of the pellicle but soon come to lie in saucer-shaped depressions, which suggests that the pellicle is being actively metabolized. During colonization a matrix of protein is deposited around the bacteria and, in time, the bacterial–protein complex becomes detectable as dental plaque. This is particularly noticeable around the gingival margins and can be demonstrated by the use of suitable *disclosing solutions*, such as erythrosine or basic fuchsin. Crystals of calcium phosphate may form within mature plaque but take weeks to appear; plaque which is obviously calcified is called *calculus* (page 514).

Plaque, like pellicle, can form in the absence of food and, perhaps surprisingly, the rate of plaque formation is greater during periods of fasting than immediately after meals. Consequently, plaque will form overnight and be present in detectable amounts the following morning. This type of plaque has a relatively loose texture and only when it is exposed to foodstuffs, particularly sucrose, does it become thick and gelatinous. It may then extend over the gingival two-thirds of the tooth. Once formed, plaque remains in sheltered areas almost indefinitely so that the mouth can contain plaque in many different stages of maturity. This is reflected in its bacterial composition and metabolism, as well as in the texture and properties of the matrix.

The plaque flora – cell adhesion

It is generally recognized that the adhesive properties of microorganisms determine whether or not they can colonize particular sites. Thus the ability of cells to adhere to surfaces and to one another is responsible for bacterial colonization, and the interactions between a solid surface and a bacterium in the supernatant fluid can be considered as occuring in three stages.

1. The initial *reversible deposition* (or capture) of a single cell on to the surface. This depends on non-covalent physicochemical forces, particularly ionic interactions and Van der Waals' forces (page 15).
2. The time-dependent *irreversible adhesion* of the captured cell. Surface stabilization depends on calcium bridging, hydrophobic interactions and the formation of covalent bonds with surface groups at distances of less than 0·4 nm, or the establishment of polymer bridging at distances up to 10 nm.
3. The *colonization* of the surface. This involves the growth and multiplication of cells and the development of cell-to-cell contacts which are characterized by the appearance of bacterial extracellular products, mainly proteins and polysaccharides.

Deposition experiments at pH 6·5, using a pure hydroxyapatite surface and non-aggregated single-cell cultures of streptococci suspended in KCl solutions, showed a very strong and non-selective affinity of all the strains to the surface. Prior incubation of the hydroxyapatite and the

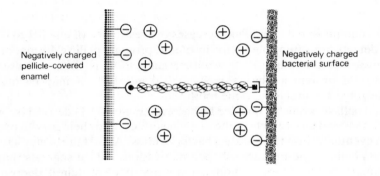

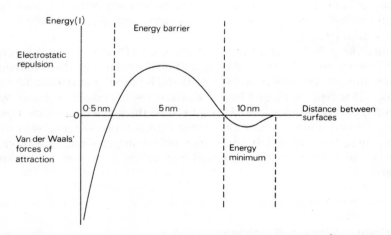

Figure 34.2 Cell–surface interactions. The total energy of interaction (I) of a negatively charged bacterial cell with a negatively charged pellicle-covered enamel surface is shown as a function of separation distance in an aqueous solvent of moderate ionic strength. The cell is temporarily held in an energy minimum about 10 nm from the surface and is subsequently stabilized in this position by polymers which specifically interact with each surface. The polymers could be an integral component of the cell structure or be produced by bacterial metabolic activity or be a salivary component. They could also promote bacterial cell–cell interactions in the same manner. Key: –(●–, –[■–, specific recognition sites; ⊃⊂⊗⊃⊂, polymer bridge; –⊖, fixed negative charge on surface; ⊕, adsorbed counter ions in medium

cells separately in saliva before the experiments not only reduced subsequent deposition by more than 90% but also increased the selectivity; bacteria with relatively hydrophobic surfaces such as *S. sanguis* and *S. mitis* deposited more readily than did *S. mutans* and *S. salivarius* which are relatively hydrophilic.

Hydroxyapatite at pH 6·5 carries a net positive charge and readily attracts bacteria, most of which have an overall negative charge on their surface owing to their outer covering of *teichoic acid*, a polymer of glycerol or ribitol units joined by phosphodiester bonds. The binding of salivary proteins to the hydroxyapatite converts the positive surface to a negative one and treatment with saliva makes the bacteria slightly less negative, both surfaces now having a degree of hydrophobic character. Deposition of bacteria under these conditions will depend on a balance between negative charge repulsion, Van der Waals forces of attraction and hydrophobic interactions between specific groups on the bacterial and salivary-coated hydroxyapatite surfaces. Successful 'capture' holds the cell in a minimum-energy position about 10 nm from the surface (Figure 34.2) on which it may become stabilized by bridging the gap with polymeric material, usually protein, or by bacterial 'appendages' which include flagellae, pili and fimbriae. Adhesion may be increased by the presence of aggregating molecules in the saliva. However, saliva-induced aggregation may also serve to prevent surface attachment by forming bacterial clumps which are more readily removed by salivary flow, in much the same way that immunoglobulins help to immobilize invading bacteria (page 381). It may be concluded that saliva reduces overall deposition and encourages the attachment of organisms which are part of the 'normal' plaque flora rather than 'opportunistic' pathogens such as *S. mutans*. The enamel surface, once it is colonized, unlike other epithelial surfaces such as the tongue and oral mucosa, is unable to shed its bacterial load by surface desquamation. Consequently, the rate of initial deposition is roughly proportional to the rate of colonization and the bacteria remain in place more or less permanently unless they are removed by the forces of mastication or vigorous toothbrushing. Plaque films several millimetres in thickness can develop on inaccessible surfaces and in stagnation sites.

Plaque matrix

Formation in the absence of food

The extracellular matrix of plaque formed in the absence of food is thin and relatively porous and it is thought to consist largely of insoluble calcium phosphate–protein complexes together with modified salivary glycoproteins. Until recently no satisfactory explanation could be offered for the precipitation of the latter from saliva. Glycoproteins which contain sialic acid are known as *sialoproteins* and characteristically have a low isoelectric point; consequently they are unlikely to precipitate at physiological pH values. However, if the sialic acid is removed the isoelectric point rises and precipitation becomes more likely; it also makes the molecules more susceptible to proteolysis. Removal of other non-terminal sugars reduces their viscosity still further and contributes to the loss of their extended configuration.

The reduction in viscosity of saliva which occurs on standing is thought to be due to the presence of hydrolytic enzymes in the oral fluid. Plaque does not contain either sialic acid or fucose, which are the characteristic terminal sugars of the oligosaccharide chains of the salivary glycoproteins, and these sugars are known to be rapidly metabolized when added to mixed saliva or aqueous suspensions of plaque. On the other hand, if saliva is collected directly from the ducts under sterile conditions it remains as a clear aseptic liquid and the glycoproteins remain intact, but, if oral bacteria are added to this sterile saliva, either as mixed saliva or as a suspension of plaque bacteria, and the mixture is incubated, then almost all the sugars are lost leaving a

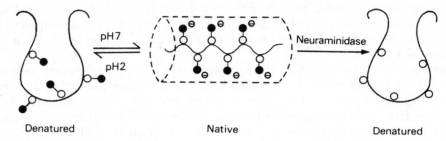

Figure 34.3 The denaturation and collapse of an elongated sialoprotein molecule either by enzymic removal of the negatively charged sialic acid or by charge neutralization at low pH. Only the latter process is reversible. ●, Sialic acid; ○, *N*-acetylgalactosamine; ~, protein core

precipitate of protein. Saliva collected directly from the mouth is already contaminated by bacteria and within a few hours loses all its sialic acid and fucose and about half of the remaining sugars.

These observations suggest that the oral bacteria produce extracellular enzymes which split off sugars sequentially from glycoprotein side chains. The release of sugars is catalysed by *bacterial glycosidases* and sialic acid by *neuraminidase*. The presence and later removal of the terminal negatively charged sialic acid residue could explain how the degraded glycoproteins can be precipitated out of saliva and their protein residues (Figure 34.3) incorporated onto the surface of the developing plaque. This theory is consistent with the observation that plaque can form during fasting and suggests that, in the absence of other easily metabolizable carbohydrates, the bacteria use sugars derived from glycoproteins. Subsequent proteolysis of the denatured protein produces peptides and free amino acids which then act as bacterial substrates.

Formation in the presence of food

Human volunteers fed on a high-protein high-fat diet developed a thin structureless plaque on their teeth which was little altered when glucose was added but, when the glucose was replaced by sucrose, their teeth became covered with thick gelatinous plaque. This suggests that there is a direct relationship between the consumption of sucrose and the presence of certain polysaccharides which give the plaque, formed under these conditions, its sticky adhesive quality. While animals fed sucrose-rich diets produce large amounts of plaque and develop severe caries, substitution of the sucrose by other sugars or by starch leads to the formation of a less well-defined plaque and, at least in short-term experiments, to the development of significantly less caries.

Further support for the role of sucrose in the formation of a gelatinous plaque comes from *in vitro* experiments carried out with mixed oral flora. When either plaque bacteria or contaminated saliva were incubated with sugars, copious amounts of an adhesive carbohydrate-containing precipitate were found in the tubes containing sucrose. Significantly less material was found in the tubes containing glucose, fructose or lactose although appreciable amounts were sometimes found in the presence of maltose.

The matrix formed in the presence of carbohydrates may be compared with the extracellular matrix of connective tissues. However, the plaque polysaccharides are not glycosaminoglycans but glucans and other high molecular weight homo- and hetero-polysaccharides which are interspersed with the protein component. Examination of the extracellular polysaccharides produced by cariogenic and non-cariogenic streptococci grown in sucrose media showed that the total amount of material was about the same in the two groups but that the cariogenic group produced a heavy tenacious deposit on the walls of the culture vessels, while the non-cariogenic group produced little or none. This suggests that differences occurring between the two groups lie not in the quantity but rather in the quality of the polysaccharides produced.

Chemical analysis has shown that the extracellular carbohydrate is composed mainly of polymers of glucose i.e. *glucans* in which the residues are joined by α-1 : 6, α-1 : 3 and α-1 : 4 linkages. Glucans in which the α-1 : 6 linkages predominate are known as *dextrans* whereas a polymer containing mainly α-1 : 3 linkages is called a *mutan*. Lesser amounts of *levan*, a β-2 : 6-polyfructose (Figure 34.4) are also present.

A considerable amount of information is now available about substances of this type since they have been extensively investigated in relation to problems caused in the sugar-refining and citrus fruit industries by bacteria which convert sucrose to dextrans. In general, dextrans which have a high proportion of α-1 : 6-linked glucose residues and levans with β-2 : 6-linked fructose residues are water-soluble whereas mutans which have a high proportion of α-1 : 3-linked glucose residues are insoluble in water. Different transferase enzymes are thus required to catalyse the formation of the different links and the enzymes *dextran sucrase* and *levan sucrase* (also known as *glycosyltransferase* and *fructosyltransferase* respectively) have been obtained from sucrose cultures of plaque streptococcal strains. *S. mutans*, for example, produces mainly α-1 : 3-linked glucose polymers and this is believed to contribute to the pathogenicity of this strain. Both enzymes show a high substrate specificity for sucrose and their equilibrium constants favour polymerization. The ΔG^0 for levan formation is about $-8 \cdot 4 \, \text{kJ mol}^{-1}$ while that for dextran formation probably exceeds $-16 \cdot 8 \, \text{kJ mol}^{-1}$. The enzymes are either extracellular or

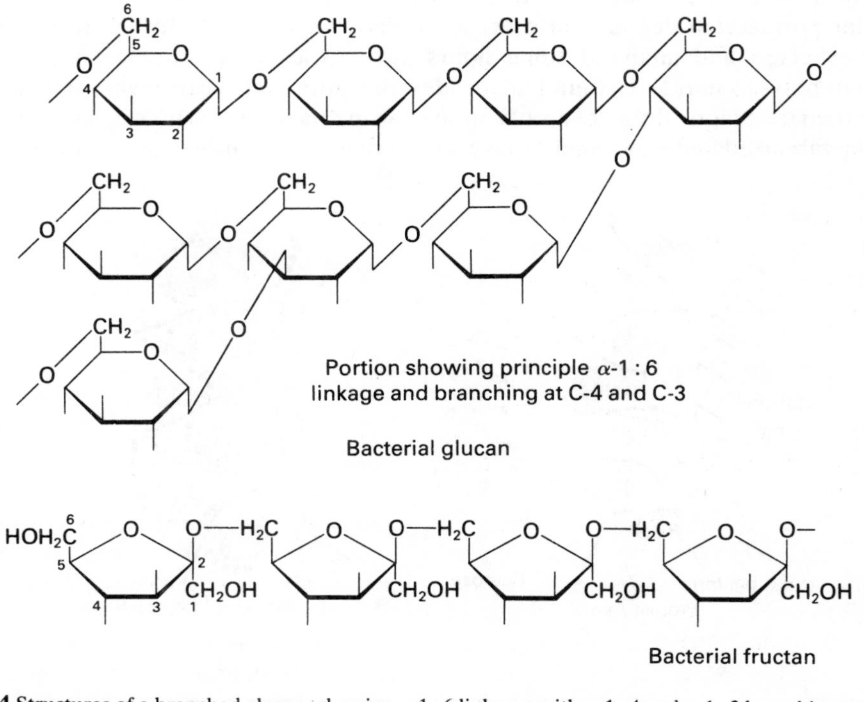

Portion showing principle α-1 : 6
linkage and branching at C-4 and C-3

Bacterial glucan

Bacterial fructan

Figure 34.4 Structures of a branched glucan, showing α-1 : 6 linkages with α-1 : 4 and α-1 : 3 branching and a straight chain fructan with β-2 : 6 linkages

bound to the bacterial surface and catalyse the transfer of glucose or fructose units directly from sucrose to the growing polyglucose and polyfructose chains.

$$\text{Sucrose(G–F)} \xrightarrow[\text{(G)}_n \text{ primer}]{\text{Dextran sucrase}} \text{dextran (G)}_{n+1} + \text{fructose}$$
$$\alpha\text{-1}:6\text{-links and }\alpha\text{-1}:4\text{ and }\alpha\text{-1}:3$$
$$\text{branch points}$$

$$\text{Sucrose(G–F)} \xrightarrow[\text{(F)}_n \text{ primer}]{\text{Levan sucrase}} \text{levan (F)}_{n+1} + \text{glucose}$$
$$\beta\text{-2}:6\text{ linkages}$$

The enzymes are very similar in catalytic activity to glycosidase (page 95) except that one of the saccharide units is transferred to a preformed primer rather than to water.

The polymerization is different from glycogen synthesis since no phosphorylated intermediates or high-energy compounds are involved. However, in sucrose the potential reducing groups of both constituents (carbon-1 in glucose and carbon-2 in fructose) are involved in the linkage and its free energy of hydrolysis is about $-29 \cdot 3 \text{ kJ mol}^{-1}$ which is of the same order as that of ATP, and it is suggested that the enzymes are able to use this energy for the polymerization reaction. The free energy of hydrolysis of maltose and lactose is much lower (about $-16 \cdot 8 \text{ kJ mol}^{-1}$) and consequently they are less effective glycosyl donors. This may explain why sucrose has been found to promote greater extracellular polysaccharide production by the oral bacteria.

Regarding the role of the extracellular polysaccharides in plaque formation and metabolism, it is generally believed that the production of gel-like polymers increases the bulk of developing plaque (Figure 34.5) and that, as these sticky and relatively insoluble materials accumulate, they restrict the free movement of molecules between the plaque fluid and the saliva. This results in increasingly anaerobic conditions, and enhances the production of acid metabolites. The extracellular polysaccharides may also act as reserve carbohydrate for bacterial use. When plaque is collected and analysed some hours after exposure to sucrose, the bulk of the extracellular polysaccharide is found to be dextran, although both levan and dextran are produced when the plaque flora are grown on sucrose media *in vitro*. This suggests that the levan is rapidly metabolized and experiments have shown that levan is more susceptible than dextran

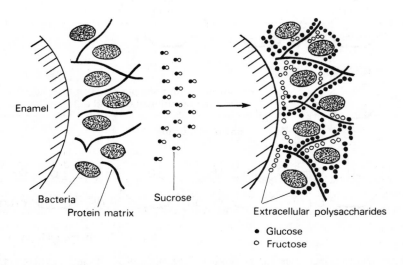

Figure 34.5 Extracellular polysaccharide formation from dietary sucrose by bacteria within dental plaque

to degradation by the oral bacteria. Human plaque collected after an overnight fast contains very little levan, but its levan content rises within a few minutes if the mouth is rinsed with a sucrose solution and then falls to its former level within 1 hour.

These experiments lead to the conclusion that plaque microorganisms respond to dietary sucrose by the rapid formation of both dextran and levan and that, after removal of the sucrose, the levan is rapidly broken down. When levan is metabolized within the plaque, free fructose is released. Furthermore, many bacteria and, notably, cariogenic strains carry an intracellular store of glycogen-like molecules which, during periods of carbohydrate deprivation, may be used for the provision of energy.

If oxygen is not freely available, breakdown is incomplete and these substances will lead to the production of acid. It appears therefore that sucrose may not only be directly responsible for acid production within the plaque but also, indirectly, when its intracellular and extracellular derivatives are metabolized.

The ability of a bacterial species to produce extracellular polysaccharides does not necessarily mean that it will be cariogenic. Several levan-producing strains of *Streptococcus salivarius* and dextran-producing strains of *S. sanguis* fail to produce carious lesions in gnotobiotic rats. In addition to glucans and fructans, various other hetero- and homo-polysaccharides are formed particularly under conditions of limited growth. Cariogenicity seems to depend on the specific saccharide produced and this in turn depends on such factors as the nature of the sugar, the strain of bacteria and the length of time the bacteria are exposed to the sugar.

The development and properties of mature plaque

In newly formed plaque the matrix has a relatively loose and open structure but as the plaque ages the matrix forms a compact meshwork of entangled protein and polysaccharide with limited space for penetration by other molecules (Table 34.1). As the molecular weight of the polysaccharide components increases the permeability decreases and larger molecules are excluded. Molecular exclusion is responsible for an unequal partition of molecules in the mouth. The cells and large molecules already present are retained within the mesh-like structure of the plaque but the soluble salivary proteins are prevented from entering.

Table 34.1 Typical composition of plaque

Water: 80% of wet weight	50% intracellular
	30% extracellular
Organic material: 20% of wet weight	10% bacterial in origin
	6% extracellular protein
	2% extracellular polysaccharide
	+ variable inorganic component*

* This is mainly calcium and phosphate which can become a considerable proportion of the total when plaque becomes calcified

The matrix proteins act as polyelectrolytes and their ionization will depend on the pH of the local environment. Thus the matrix acts both as a gel filtration system and as an ion-exchanger and the movement of charged ions will depend on the local charge density. Small neutral substrate molecules such as sugars and urea will easily diffuse into the plaque, whereas small charged molecules such as organic acids and ammonium ions, which are common products of bacterial metabolism, may be retained by the matrix (Figure 34.6a). In addition, the matrix of mature plaque is an effective barrier to the bulk flow of water so that water is partially immobilized within the plaque and constitutes a large part of its weight. This physical retention

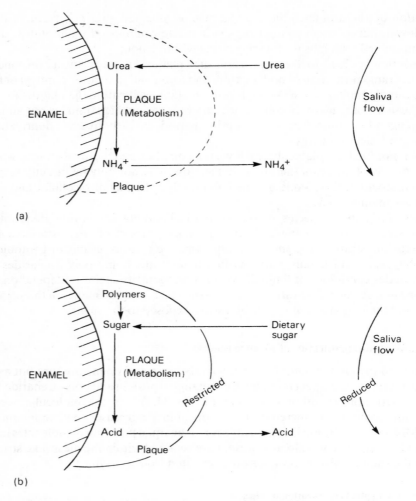

Figure 34.6 The movement of metabolites between the saliva and plaque fluid. (a) An *open plaque* representing the thin bacterial–protein aggregate formed on all surfaces in the absence of dietary carbohydrates. The entry of small uncharged molecules from the saliva, such as urea, is unrestricted provided that a concentration gradient is present. The charged products of bacterial metabolism such as the ammonium ion and bicarbonate resulting from urea hydrolysis tend to be retained owing to the ion-exchange capacity of the plaque. However, high internal concentrations are avoided owing to continuous removal by salivary flow. (b) A *closed plaque*, that is one which is usually associated with a carbohydrate-rich diet. This forms thick polysaccharide-containing deposits at inaccessible sites and is isolated from salivary flow. The organic acids produced by bacterial carbohydrate metabolism can be retained within the plaque for a considerable time. This can lead to gradients of up to 3 pH units between the interior fluid and external saliva.

of water enables the bacteria to exist in partial isolation from the rest of the mouth. The degree of isolation will be governed by regional variations in the composition of the plaque which largely depend on variations in its age and thickness (Figure 34.6b).

Plaque supernatant fluid, separated from the bacteria and insoluble matrix by high speed centrifugation, contains a wide range of soluble organic and inorganic ions (Table 34.2). The latter are present at much higher concentrations than in the saliva, suggesting that they must be concentrated in some way; potassium is probably derived from lysed bacterial cells and the high calcium and phosphate ion product is important in maintaining saturation at the enamel surface.

Table 34.2 Average composition of plaque fluid. Average salivary values are given for comparison

	Plaque fluid (mM)	*Saliva* (mM)
Calcium	6·5	1·5
Magnesium	3·7	0·3
Sodium	35	13
Potassium	62	20
Inorganic phosphate	14	5
Ammonia	30	4
Urea	0	4
Lactate		
fasting	60–150	0·1
5 min after sugar	350–900	—

In summary it may be said that the plaque which forms in the absence of dietary carbohydrate is relatively thin and has a matrix which is almost entirely derived from the salivary proteins. This provides a relatively porous structure into which oxygen and fluids, e.g. saliva, gingival fluid and dietary liquids, can penetrate. It is also permeable to the bacterial products that form within it, which are readily lost by diffusion. It is the thicker gelatinous anaerobic plaque, formed in the presence of dietary sugars, notably sucrose, which excludes saliva and hence is responsible for the formation and accumulation of acid, that is conducive to the development of caries (Chapter 35). The marked effect of plaque thickness on the diffusion times of plaque acids is shown in Figure 34.7.

Fluoride in plaque

Even when obtained from people living in areas where the fluoride content of the water is low, plaque always contains this element. Fluoride analyses on plaque obtained from such people after 24 hours without brushing their teeth have given values of up to 10 ppm. In another survey of plaque fluoride, a range of 6–180 ppm was reported, the values being related to the fluoride content of the drinking water. However, water and food are not the only immediate sources of plaque fluoride and contributions may be expected from both saliva and the enamel surface. In the neutral pH range, uptake of fluoride by apatite is virtually irreversible but, if the enamel is exposed to acids, fluoride will be released. However, if the enamel were a major source of plaque fluoride it might be expected that the fluoride content of the enamel surface would diminish in people who remove plaque daily by cleaning their teeth. The fluoride content of enamel may, in fact, decrease, but the change is slow and is greatest near the occlusal surface, where least plaque forms, so that the loss is more likely to be due to abrasion and attrition than to dissolution. On the other hand, increasing age is accompanied by a steady increase in the fluoride content of the enamel near the gingival crevice where the accumulation of plaque is greatest.

Opinion favours the steady flow of saliva as the main source of plaque fluoride, even though saliva contains only 0·01 to 0·02 ppm of fluoride or even less. Smaller amounts are believed to be derived from the intermittent exposure of the plaque to food and drink. Calculations show that the absolute amounts of fluoride in plaque are very small; for example, the total amount present in 10 mg of plaque containing 20 ppm is equivalent to that present in only 10–20 ml of saliva or 0·2 ml of fluoridated water.

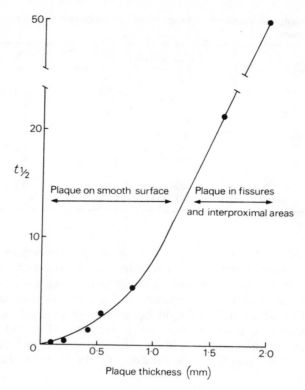

Figure 34.7 The effect of plaque thickness on the outward diffusion of free acid. $t_{1/2}$ is the time for 50% of the free acid to diffuse out

Since the concentration of fluoride in the plaque is so much greater than that of the saliva, it is clear that most of it must be present in a bound form and measurements made with a fluoride electrode suggest that less than 5% of plaque fluoride is present as free ions. Experiments were undertaken by Jenkins to determine whether the plaque fluoride is bound to the inorganic or organic constituents of the matrix or to the bacteria. Most of the fluoride was found in the bacteria which had been separated from the matrix by extraction with alkali, and several species of bacteria, including some derived from plaque, were shown to take up and concentrate fluoride from the medium in which they were grown. Pure cultures of bacteria, isolated from plaque and grown on a fluoride-containing medium, were slower to produce acid from sugar than similar organisms grown on a fluoride-free medium. Plaque obtained from subjects living in towns with fluoride in their water supply produced less acid from sugar than did plaque from unfluoridated areas. Difficulty was experienced in ensuring that the experiment was adequately controlled since the reduction of caries in the group exposed to fluoride might be responsible for a reduction in the acid production. However, comparison of plaque from subjects living in Newcastle and the neighbouring city of Durham in the periods immediately before and after fluoridation of the Newcastle water showed that, whereas before fluoridation samples of plaque from the two cities showed identical pH changes on exposure to sugar, in the weeks immediately after fluoridation the pH fall in the plaque on exposure to sugar of the Newcastle subjects was appreciably less than that of the Durham subjects.

Thus, even though fluoride may exert its main beneficial effects by reducing the solubility of enamel in acid, it also reduces bacterial acid production. Furthermore, fluoride may affect the proportions of the various types of plaque bacteria and cause a reduction in those that store intracellular polysaccharides which can act as a source of acid.

The effects of fluoride are discussed more fully in Chapter 36.

Chapter 35
Plaque metabolism and dental disease

Dental plaque is particularly noticeable in the sheltered areas provided by fissures, the points of tooth contact and the gingival margins. These are the areas which encourage food retention and are susceptible to carious attack. Caries only occurs to a limited extent on other surfaces which are accessible and subject to self-cleansing, and the incidence of caries at any particular site appears to be inversely related to its exposure to saliva. The lower anterior teeth which are continually bathed in saliva are, in general, caries-resistant, whereas the upper anteriors which have a limited saliva access are caries-prone. On the other hand, regions that are exposed to saliva, especially the lingual side of the lower incisors and the buccal side of the upper molars, tend to develop *supragingival calculus* in later life.

Experiments have shown that the presence of food or food residues in the oral cavity is not necessary for plaque formation since the amount of plaque deposited on the teeth of rats, dogs and monkeys, fed by stomach-tube was about the same as in normally fed animals. Furthermore, it was found that animals fed a cariogenic diet by stomach-tube failed to develop caries. It appears therefore that a carious attack on the teeth must result from interaction between the oral bacteria and the food, and only those bacteria which (1) can adhere effectively to the tooth surface and (2) produce appreciable amounts of acid will cause demineralization; and the types of the bacteria present and their metabolic activities depend on the properties of plaque.

If plaque is not removed soon after it is formed, it thickens and becomes less permeable. This limits the supply of oxygen and the number of anaerobic organisms increases at the expense of the aerobic types, although the streptococci, which are *facultative anaerobes*,* remain relatively constant. The bacterial composition of mature plaque is quite different from that found elsewhere in the mouth. Plaque which is a week old contains cocci, rods, filaments, vibrios and spirochaetes among many others. The bacteria are closely packed and often dominated by filamentous organisms which lie at right angles to the enamel surface. Coccal forms have been observed in close association with the filaments, and the outer layers of the plaque contain large numbers of Gram-positive and Gram-negative cocci (Table 33.2). Distinct regions may be observed within the plaque, each of which is dominated by a particular bacterial type, and this results in the existence of a variety of physical and chemical gradients which may affect bacterial growth and survival. Adjacent sites may be very different, not only with respect to the type and

---

* Microorganisms which can obtain energy and grow either in the presence or absence of oxygen.

amount of nutrients available, but also in their oxygen content, pH, ionic strength and content of toxins. Consequently, although it is convenient to regard the plaque as a single metabolic entity, it actually consists of many relatively independent *micro-territories* whose biochemical properties may be appreciably different from those of the plaque as a whole.

From the metabolic point of view, plaque bacteria can be divided into two main groups, namely, those which utilize nitrogenous materials and produce basic substances which tend to cause a rise in pH, and those which convert carbohydrates into organic acids and tend to lower the pH. Although the metabolism of a particular microorganism may be primarily based on one or other type of activity, many bacteria use both kinds of substrate. However, in any given situation within plaque, the type of micro-organism that predominates will depend to a large extent on the supply of substrates. These may either be exogenous, i.e. transient substrates of dietary origin, or endogenous substrates, which are present in the plaque fluid at virtually all times. This fluid is mainly derived from the saliva but, in the gingival regions, the gingival fluid makes a significant contribution. The substrates include urea, amino acids, peptides, proteins, glycoproteins and cell debris, as well as extracellular glucans and fructans. How these various materials are utilized will depend on the types of organism present and the existing conditions. In a developing plaque, where energy is required for biosynthetic reactions, glucose will be broken down by glycolysis but the fate of the pyruvate will depend on the availability of oxygen. Aerobic conditions, which allow the pyruvate to be completely oxidized to carbon dioxide and water via the citrate cycle and respiratory chain, are found only at the outer surface of the plaque. In the interior of a thick, rapidly growing plaque the inwardly diffusing oxygen is rapidly exhausted and in the resulting anaerobic conditions the pyruvate is converted into lactate. Other organic acids, such as acetic, butyric, formic and propionic, are produced as well and are

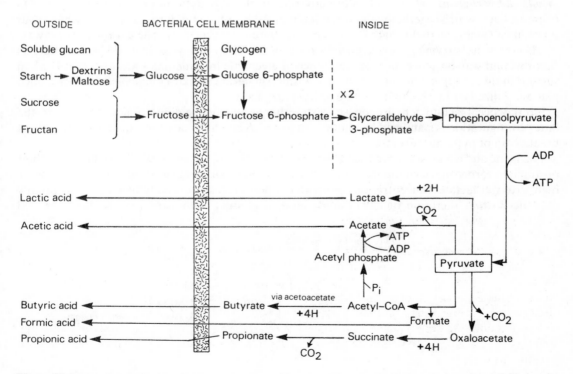

Figure 35.1 Bacterial fermentation of various carbohydrates. A simplified scheme to show how organic acids may be produced in the dental plaque

responsible for the low pH values often found in dense plaque. A simplified scheme showing how these acids may be derived from pyruvate in anaerobic bacterial systems is given in Figure 35.1.

Sugar metabolism and acid production

Streptococci are the most important organisms in terms of acid production and special features of their metabolism are worth mentioning. They can take up sugars from the surrounding medium by a high-affinity transport mechanism which is energized by phosphoenolpyruvate (page 534) and is known as the *phosphotransferase system*. It is specific for individual sugars and operates at neutral pH values. This allows the organism to survive at low sugar concentrations and neutral pH values, conditions which are found naturally in the saliva and on the enamel in the absence of food. In addition, streptococci have a second, low affinity sugar uptake system which is activated by a *protonmotive force* (pmf) (page 221). This operates maximally in *S. mutans* at pH 5·5 and allows the organism to take advantage of the pH gradient generated when the extracellular pH is low compared to the intracellular pH. Consequently, the cell can continue to transport and metabolize sugars under acidic conditions which are unfavourable to other bacteria. This adaptation to a sugar-rich environment and a low pH make it a dominant organism in cariogenic plaques.

Streptococci do not contain enzymes of the citrate cycle, nor do they possess cytochrome systems but, instead, they rely on anaerobic glycolysis for their energy. The fate of pyruvate produced by this pathway is then determined by the overall availability of sugars. The enzyme *lactate dehydrogenase* is allosterically activated by the glycolytic intermediate fructose 1,6-bisphosphate, which together with glyceraldehyde 3-phosphate tends to accumulate when sugar is readily available so that lactate formation is favoured (Figure 35.2). The alternative pathway, catalysed by the enzyme *pyruvate formate lyase*, is inhibited by glyceraldehyde 3-phosphate so that this pathway only becomes operative when glycolytic intermediates are low, that is when sugar is in short supply. This allows the organism to generate an extra molecule of ATP for each glucose utilized, from the intermediate acetyl phosphate.

Streptococcal lactate dehydrogenase exists either as an inactive dimer or active tetramer; the latter configuration is stabilized by binding fructose 1,6-bisphosphate thus increasing the rate of breakdown of pyruvate sevenfold.

The lactic and acetic acids produced by these pathways are transported out of the cell in their protonated forms and accumulate in the external medium, often at very high concentrations. A high external lactate concentration, generated when glucose is readily available, eventually prevents further secretion of lactate and causes a gradual acidification of the bacterial cell

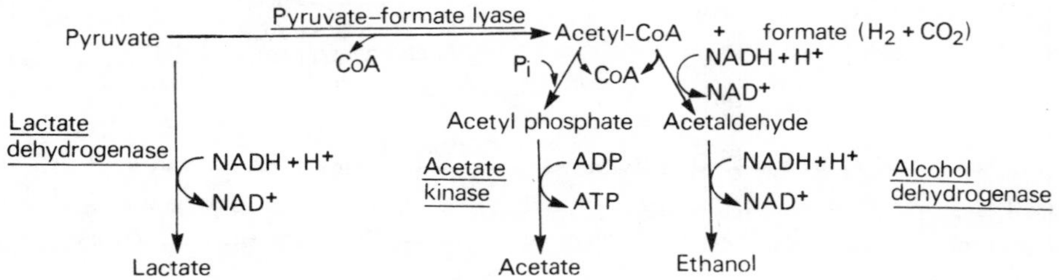

Figure 35.2 The formation of acids from pyruvate by streptococci showing the alternative pathway taken when sugar is in short supply

interior so that the cell ceases to metabolize. *Veillonella*, organisms that utilize lactic acid, benefit from this plentiful supply of substrate and aid the streptococci by the removal of an unwanted waste product. *Veillonella* metabolize lactate by the following reactions:

$$\text{Lactate} + H_2O \rightarrow \text{acetate} + CO_2 + H_2$$
$$\text{Lactate} + H_2 \rightarrow \text{propionate} + H_2O$$

Propionic and acetic acids have higher pK values than lactic acid and so tend to act as buffers at higher pH values, thus raising the pH of the medium.

In practice, it is not possible to equate plaque acid production directly with the presence of any one type of bacterium. Analyses of organic acids in overnight fasting plaque before exposure to dietary sugar showed a predominance of acetic acid with some propionic, butyric and formic acids. The total acid concentration increased immediately after exposure to sugar, mainly due to the formation of lactic acid, while the concentration of the other acids tended to decrease. Fasting plaque has a neutral or slightly alkaline pH, and Stephan in 1940, using a micro pH electrode, demonstrated that the application of a sugar solution caused the intraplaque pH to fall rapidly to about pH 5.5 within 2–3 min, corresponding to the maximum rate of lactic acid production. It took up to 40 min for the pH to return to resting conditions, as lactic acid was slowly replaced by the other organic acids. Modern techniques using indwelling electrodes fixed in the dentition allow plaque pH to be measured continuously and values as low as pH 4·0 have been measured in response to sucrose. Acid is produced from a range of carbohydrate-containing foods, fruits and juices and this technique is used to determine the potential cariogenicity of foodstuffs. pH changes vary from site to site depending on salivary access and plaque thickness and typical *Stephan curves* are shown in Figure 35.3.

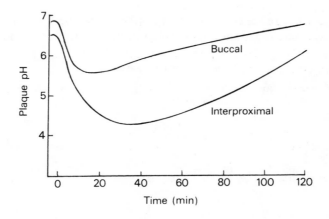

Figure 35.3   Typical Stephan curves showing the response of human dental plaque to sucrose. Plaque was allowed to accumulate for 72 h. At 0 time the subject rinsed with 5 ml of a 10% sucrose solution for 60 s

Nitrogen metabolism and base production

The provision of a source of nitrogen is just as important for bacterial growth as the provision of a source of energy and reference of Table 33.1 (page 478) shows that salivary urea is the most readily available source. Plaque possesses a high urease activity and a number of different reactions are known by which microorganisms incorporate ammonia into amino acids, namely:

1. 2-Oxoglutarate + NH$_3$ $\xrightleftharpoons[\text{Glutamate dehydrogenase}]{\text{NAD(P)H + H}^+ \quad \text{NAD(P)}^+}$ L-glutamate + H$_2$O

2. Pyruvate + NH$_3$ $\xrightleftharpoons[\text{Alanine dehydrogenase}]{\text{NADH + H}^+ \quad \text{NAD}^+}$ L-alanine + H$_2$O

3. L-Glutamate + NH$_3$ $\xrightarrow[\text{Glutamine synthetase}]{\text{ATP} \quad \text{ADP}}$ L-glutamine + P$_i$

4. 2-Oxoglutarate + glutamine $\xrightarrow[\text{Glutamate synthetase}]{\text{NADH + H}^+ \quad \text{NAD}}$ 2 L-glutamate + H$_2$O

Subsequent transamination reactions then provide the other amino acids needed for protein synthesis. Glutamine serves as a –NH$_2$ donor in a number of biosynthetic reactions and Figure 35.4 shows how carbohydrate and nitrogen metabolism may be interrelated in the plaque. An additional source of amino acids within the interior may be provided by hydrolysis of matrix proteins.

Free amino acids, if not required for protein synthesis, can be fermented under anaerobic conditions. Generally, these reactions produce organic acids as well as ammonia and, therefore,

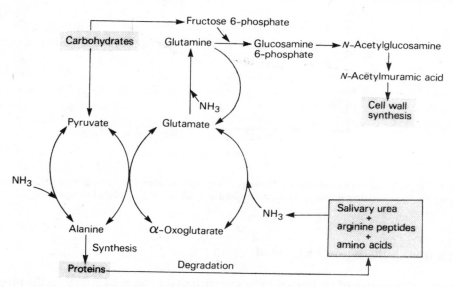

Figure 35.4 Integration of bacterial carbohydrate and nitrogen metabolism. The simultaneous incorporation of pyruvate and ammonia may reduce the extent to which these metabolites accumulate

are unlikely to have a marked effect on plaque pH. Arginine and arginine-containing salivary peptides are a special case, however, since they act as substrates for base-producing reactions by the *arginine deiminase pathway*:

$$\text{Arginine} \rightarrow \text{citrulline} + NH_3$$
$$\text{Citrulline} + P_i \rightarrow \text{carbamoyl phosphate} + \text{ornithine}$$
$$\text{Carbamoyl phosphate} + ADP \rightarrow ATP + CO_2 + NH_3$$

This pathway which is widely distributed in bacteria, acts as an energy source under anaerobic conditions, and produces a marked *pH-rise effect* due to the production of NH_3. It is induced by arginine supplementation. It also acts as a source of ornithine which can subsequently be decarboxylated, particularly at low pH values, to produce an increase in the pH (page 508) and the evil-smelling amine putrescine which occurs in decaying meat.

$$\text{Ornithine} + H^+ \rightarrow \text{putrescine} + CO_2$$

NADH is produced by the energy-producing anaerobic oxidation of many amino acids according to the scheme:

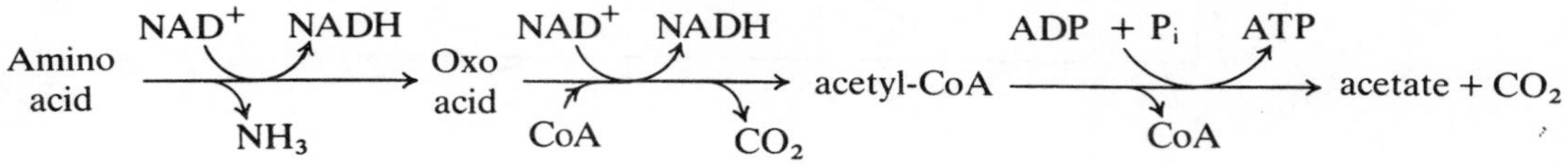

The NADH can be reoxidized to NAD^+ either by the reductive deamination of ornithine or by the reductive cleavage of a proline ring to produce 5-aminopentanoic acid $CH_2NH_3^+[CH_2]_3COO^-$.

These reactions were first described by Stickland and this δ-amino acid may account for up to 25% of the total amino acids in plaque fluid. *Stickland reactions* are usually associated with amino acid-fermenting anaerobic organisms which are commonly found in the region of the gingival crevice and in periodontal pockets. Tissue destruction and proteolytic activity in this region would generate an excess of free amino acids thus favouring 5-aminopentanoic acid accumulation.

In a long-established plaque, when bacterial growth is limited, more ammonia may be produced than is required for amino acid production. Accumulation of either ammonia or organic acids will influence the acid–base ratio and hence the pH of the plaque. However, when the system is an open one and there is a good flow of saliva, pH changes will be resisted since the bacterial waste products are able to diffuse away from their site of origin (Figure 35.5a). This is the situation in the thin loosely aggregated type of plaque which contains little or no extracellular polysaccharide. However, if plaque is allowed to accumulate, through inadequate oral hygiene, formation of extracellular polysaccharides, especially when sucrose is readily available, will lead to the formation of closed plaque which retains organic acids and ammonium salts within its matrix (page 497). The accumulation of these charged metabolites is greatest at sites where access for saliva is poor, resulting in pronounced changes in the pH which only returns slowly to normal after the supply of substrate has been exhausted (Figure 35.5b). Sometimes a new steady state may be established at a higher or lower pH value and this may provoke a long-term modification in the plaque flora which will cause pathological changes in the host.

Certain factors tend to counteract changes in plaque pH.

1. As shown in Figure 35.5(a) ammonia produced at acid pH values will tend to neutralize accumulated acid, while acid that is produced under alkaline conditions will neutralize accumulated base.

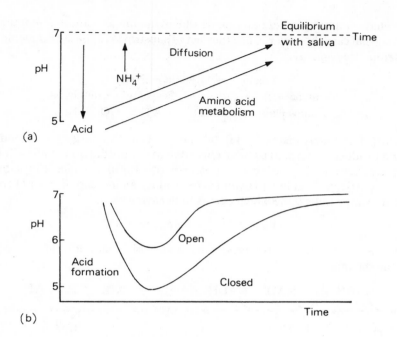

Figure 35.5 (a) Factors influencing changes in plaque pH with time; (b) The extent to which the site and therefore the open or closed nature of the plaque controls its pH

2. Pyruvic and 2-oxoglutaric acids may take up ammonia to form amino acids (page 280), thereby removing both acidic and basic metabolites. This could explain the relatively high levels of alanine and glutamic acid found in aqueous extracts of plaque.
3. Metabolites produced by one type of bacterium may be used by another type; for example, *Veillonella* are unable to break down carbohydrates but utilize lactic acid as an energy source instead. Their numbers have been found to increase with the number of streptococci.
4. The availability of arginine-containing substrates.

Decarboxylation reactions

Extracts of plaque have been shown to contain γ-aminobutyric acid, putrescine, cadaverine, agmatine and histamine which are the amines corresponding to glutamic acid, ornithine, lysine, arginine and histidine respectively. The presence of these compounds is believed to result from the decarboxylation of amino acids by plaque bacteria at low pH values:

$$R \cdot \underset{\underset{COO^-}{|}}{CHNH_3^+} + H^+ \xrightarrow{\underset{\text{decarboxylase}}{\text{Bacterial}}} R \cdot CH_2NH_3^+ + CO_2$$

Below pH 5·5 carbon dioxide is released and the net effect is the loss of the carboxyl group and removal of a proton so that the pH of the medium tends to rise. The free amino acids which act as substrates for the reaction are derived from (1) the saliva and gingival fluid, (2) the hydrolysis of proteins present in the plaque matrix, and (3) bacterial syntheses. The bacterial decarboxylases have pH optima on the acid side of neutrality (pH 4·5–6·0). They are inducible enzymes and are synthesized only when amino acids are present and the pH is low. This has led to the interesting suggestion that the reaction constitutes a natural neutralization mechanism; thus, if the pH value of a bacterial culture should fall, its decarboxylase activity will increase and the consequent production of amines will tend to restore the pH to its former value (Figure 35.5a). Attempts to test the effectiveness of this mechanism have shown that decarboxylation reactions have a significant acid-neutralizing effect only when the plaque glucose concentration is low. Therefore, although the acid produced from a 'natural' diet containing starchy foods and non-refined sugars, such as are present in fruits, might be neutralized by amines produced as a result of bacterial decarboxylation reactions, they would be insufficient to deal with the high concentrations of sucrose found in a typical Western diet.

In summary, it may be said that bacterial metabolism causes pH changes which, in an open plaque, are subject to controlling factors which tend to resist the change. On the other hand, should the plaque become closed because it develops at a site with poor saliva access, the pH changes may be sufficient to cause alterations in calcium phosphate solubility which result in clinical changes at the tooth surface.

Calcium phosphate solubility and plaque disease

Dental caries causes a reversal of the physicochemical processes involved in the maturation of the dental hard tissues. A similar reversal occurs in periodontal disease which eventually leads to loss of the alveolar tissue supporting the teeth. Both conditions may result from the persistent accumulation of plaque, which, in some situations is often converted into calculus as a result of the deposition of insoluble calcium phosphates within it.

Calcium phosphate exists in a variety of solid forms or phases (Table 35.1). The nature of the dominant phase is determined chiefly by the relative concentrations of calcium and phosphate ions and the pH of the medium. When exposed to acid, any calcium phosphate present as a solid phase will be converted to a new and more soluble phase with a lower molar ratio of calcium to phosphate, and calcium ions will be released into the medium. Conversely, exposure to a more alkaline environment causes the formation of a different phase with a lower solubility and a higher calcium to phosphate molar ratio. At the same time phosphate ions are released. As a result, the pH regulates both the nature of the solid phase and its biological properties. The most important salt is hydroxyapatite and Figure 35.6 illustrates how, by altering the local pH, the metabolism of cells at a solid–fluid interface can control calcium and phosphate interchange between the solid and the tissue fluids. Whereas in bone, cellular activities are well regulated and the pH is kept within the range of pH 6·5–7·5, in plaque, as a result of the metabolic activities of the microorganisms present, the pH ranges widely between pH 4·5 and 8·5. When the pH falls

Table 35.1 Calcium phosphate salts

Salt	Formula	Ca/P	Molar ratio
Phosphoric acid	H_3PO_4	$Ca_0(PO_4)H_3$	0
Monocalcium phosphate	$Ca(H_2PO_4)_2$	$Ca_{1/2}(PO_4)H_3$	0·5
Dicalcium phosphate*	$CaHPO_4$	$Ca_1(PO_4)H_1$	1·0
Octacalcium phosphate	$Ca_8(PO_4)_4(HPO_4)_2 \cdot 5H_2O$	$Ca_{4/3}(PO_4)H_{1/3}$	1·33
Tricalcium phosphate	$Ca_3(PO_4)_2$	$Ca_{3/2}(PO_4)H_0$	1·5
Hydroxyapatite	$Ca_{10}(PO_4)_6(OH)_2$	$Ca_{5/3}(PO_4)OH_{1/3}$	1·67

* Brushite is the dihydrate of dicalcium phosphate

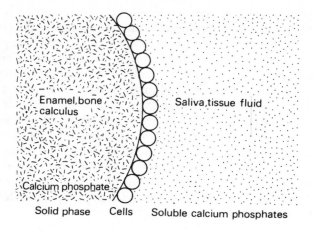

pH range :   Bone cells   6·5 −7·5
             Plaque   4·5 − 8·5

Figure 35.6 Calcium phosphate solubility at a solid–fluid interface. Cellular metabolic activity, by producing a local change in the pH, determines the distribution of calcium and phosphate between the solid phase and tissue fluid

towards the lower end of the range, hydroxyapatite is converted by rapid reaction with acid to a more soluble salt with a lower calcium to phosphate ratio:

$$Ca_{10}(PO_4)_6(OH)_2 + 8H^+ \rightarrow 6CaHPO_4 + 2H_2O + 4Ca^{2+}$$

Reduction in pH and dental caries

Although under mildly acidic conditions dicalcium phosphate ($CaHPO_4$) is the most stable of these salts, it gradually dissociates into its constituent ions which being soluble may be lost into the saliva

$$CaHPO_4 + H^+ \xrightarrow{\text{Slow}} Ca^{2+} + H_2PO_4^-$$

A critical factor in the solubilization process is the area of the exposed surface. The dicalcium phosphate forms a protective coating to the underlying hydroxyapatite since is is removed relatively slowly, the rate depending on the concentration of calcium and phosphate ions to which it is exposed at the tooth surface. The process is shown in Figure 35.7 (period A) in which calcium phosphate solubility is related to pH.

As the acid is neutralized by its reaction with the hydroxyapatite and by mechanisms discussed previously, the plaque pH rises and steady state conditions tend to be restored. This means that the dicalcium phosphate is exposed to increasingly alkaline conditions which tend to convert it back into a salt with a higher calcium to phosphate ratio (Figure 35.7, period B) and ultimately to hydroxyapatite, since this is the most stable form in the neutral pH range. This process is described by the reaction:

$$10CaHPO_4 + 8OH^- \rightarrow Ca_{10}(PO_4)_6(OH)_2 + 4HPO_4^{2-} + 6H_2O$$

but the complex structure of hydroxyapatite makes it unlikely that this reaction will occur directly, and many theories have been put forward to explain how the initial aggregation barrier is overcome under physiological conditions. It is thought that dicalcium phosphate may undergo

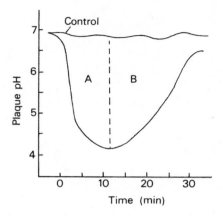

Figure 35.7 The relationship between the pH in plaque at the different stages of the Stephan curve and the solubility of calcium phosphates. A, period of increased calcium phosphate solubility. Solubilization proceeds readily in young immature enamel which is rich in magnesium and carbonate but is reduced in older fluoride-containing enamel. B, period of calcium phosphate precipitation. Remineralization is favoured by the catalytic effect of fluoride ions

molecular reorientation to form a non-crystalline amorphous calcium phosphate which acts as an intermediate in the process.

Analysis of synthetic amorphous calcium phosphate indicates that it is composed of 1 nm diameter $Ca_9(PO_4)_6$ clusters which close-pack randomly to form 30–80 nm spheres. These take up calcium and hydroxyl ions to form crystalline apatite and the following stepwise sequence of reactions can be envisaged:

$$Ca^{2+} + HPO_4{}^{2-} \rightarrow CaHPO_4 \tag{35.1}$$
$$3CaHPO_4 \rightarrow Ca_3(PO_4)_2 + HPO_4{}^{2-} + 2H^+ \tag{35.2}$$
$$3Ca_3(PO_4)_2 \rightarrow Ca_9(PO_4)_6 \tag{35.3}$$
$$Ca_9(PO_4)_6 + Ca(OH)_2 \rightarrow Ca_{10}(PO_4)_6(OH)_2 \tag{35.4}$$

Reactions 35.2 and 35.4 tend to lower the pH by the production of H^+ ions and removal of OH^- ions, respectively; consequently the maintenance of a high pH helps to drive the reaction and favours reprecipitation, particularly in the presence of fluoride ions (page 529).

Since in normal calcification the whole process is probably directed and controlled by the organic matrix, it is not surprising that solubilization and reprecipitation fail to re-form the well-ordered structure that existed in the original enamel. Instead a disorganized electron-dense modified apatite is produced on the tooth surface (Figure 35.8a). After frequent and prolonged exposure to acid attack, the process is no longer completely reversible and gradually leads to a permanent loss of calcium and phosphate from the enamel particularly in the more soluble regions rich in magnesium and carbonate (Figure 35.8b). A *zone of cavitation* or decalcification forms immediately beneath the electron-dense surface layer and is clinically apparent as white spot formation (Figure 35.8c). Eventually the irregular and permeable surface layer breaks down, bacterial invasion takes place and more plaque is formed within the shelter of the cavity which, under conditions approximating to a closed system, causes further severe acid attack and the ultimate destruction of the enamel.

A diagrammatic representation of the chemistry of subsurface demineralization is shown in Figure 35.9. The lactate anion $CH_3CHOH.COO^-$ is represented as L^- and the calcium lactate complex as CaL_2. It is thought that acid attack deep within the enamel is favoured by the ability

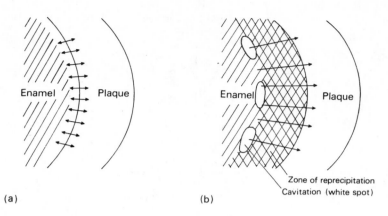

(a)

(b)

Zone of reprecipitation
Cavitation (white spot)

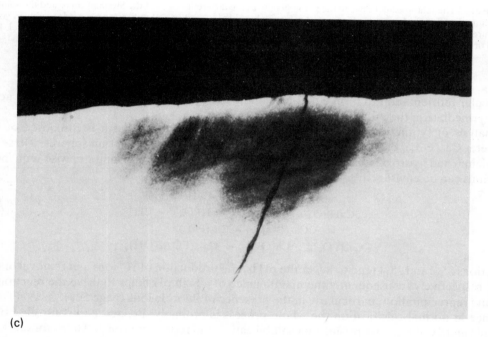

(c)

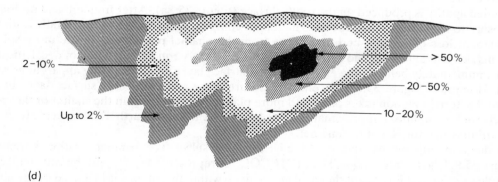

2-10%

Up to 2%

>50%

20-50%

10-20%

(d)

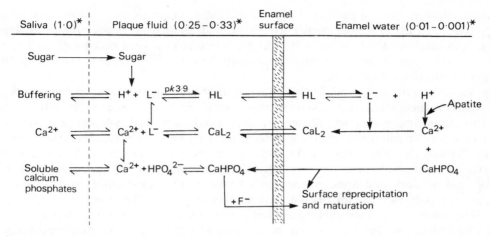

Figure 35.9 Interchange of molecules between the saliva, plaque fluid and enamel water. It is assumed that interchange depends on concentration gradients and that charged species diffuse less readily than neutral molecules. Heavy arrows indicate the overall direction of reactions involved in the carious process. See the text for explanation of abbreviations

of the uncharged and undissociated form of lactic acid $CH_3CHOH.COOH$ (LH) to pass into the enamel water before redissociating and lowering the internal pH. Similarly, ionic calcium can be lost from the enamel as uncharged CaL_2.

Changes in calcium phosphate solubility in plaque have been summarized by Kleinberg who put forward a unifying theory which distinguishes between (1) a 'normal' plaque maintained at or near salivary pH values which is supersaturated but metastable with respect to calcium phosphate solubility; (2) a 'cariogenic' plaque which has a lower than average pH, is less saturated and favours dissolution at pH values below 5·0; (3) a 'calculogenic' plaque with a higher than average pH leading to spontaneous precipitation.

Increased pH and calculus formation

The plaque matrix contains high concentrations of calcium and phosphate, either as ions in solution or bound as a calcium phosphate–protein complex. This is particularly evident in areas close to the ducts of the salivary glands. The ability of the matrix to concentrate these ions from the saliva favours calcium phosphate precipitation at high pH values. A precipitate of dicalcium phosphate can, as we have seen, mature and undergo crystal growth to give a salt of a higher calcium to phosphate molar ratio so that the plaque itself tends to mineralize:

$$\text{Aggregate of organic material rich in } Ca^{2+} \text{ and } P_i^- \text{ ions} \longrightarrow \text{Organic matrix containing amorphous calcium phosphate} \xrightarrow[\text{high pH}]{\text{Time}} \text{Crystalline calcium phosphates}$$

Figure 35.8 (a) Ionic exchange between the enamel surface and the plaque fluid to produce a highly substituted surface layer. (b) An incipient carious lesion. Severe acid attack on the enamel surface produces a subsurface decalcification, a relatively dense outer layer due to reprecipitation and a net migration of ions out of enamel. (c) A microradiograph of an early carious lesion in enamel (× 140). The striae of Retzius, prisms and cross striations appear enhanced because of selective demineralization. A well-mineralized 30–40 μm wide surface zone is present. The crack running through the lesion was created during preparation. (d) A contour map of the same lesion which gives the percentage pore volume distribution throughout the lesion. The outer line represents the demarcation between altered translucent enamel and normal tissue. The centre of the lesion is about 130 μm below the surface

Areas in which there is a persistent deposit of plaque make gingival debilitation an added factor. The destruction of host tissue is associated with an increase in bacterial proteolysis and amino acid catabolism which leads to a higher pH and promotes precipitation. The whole process is analogous to bone formation, the essential differences being in the type of matrix and the lack of effective cellular control.

The haphazard nature of calculus formation is illustrated by its heterogeneous composition. Supragingival calculus that is at least 6 months old contains 70–80% mineral, mainly apatite, but with substantial amounts of octacalcium, tricalcium and some dicalcium phosphates. It is made up of very small crystals that coalesce to form a calcifying front throughout the body of the plaque. Initially the calcified material is laid down around the bacteria but these eventually die and become fossilized to give a heterogeneous structure with islets of mineralization within the plaque and non-calcified areas within the calculus itself. Calcification of plaque is not a continuous process because the pH is always tending to revert to the steady state value and this favours re-solution, but it should be regarded as resulting from an overall high pH.

Epidemiological studies have shown that, in people over 30, the amount of calculus and the frequency with which it occurs rise with age. The amount of plaque, however, is more or less constant for all age groups, and consequently the relationship between the occurrence of plaque and the onset of calcification is difficult to define. Perhaps it is simply that the longer the plaque is in the mouth the more likely it is to calcify, although it would seem that there must be qualitative changes in the plaque in older subjects, for example a higher pH in association with increased concentrations of calcium and phosphate. The presence of a calcified mass on the tooth surface does not appear to affect the integrity of the enamel and cementum. The mineralization process itself may, in fact, have a beneficial effect by hardening the enamel and possibly by recalcifying acquired pellicle or plaque within an early carious lesion. Calculus, however, presents an extremely rough and irregular surface which is ideal for the attachment and proliferation of bacteria and it is always found to be covered by a softer layer of plaque.

There are two main types of calculus.

1. *Supragingival dental calculus*. This is a mineralized plaque which occurs above the gum margins, usually on teeth situated near the orifices of the salivary glands. It is a white to yellow moderately hard deposit, about 35% by volume mineralized and covered superficially by a layer of vital plaque.
2. *Subgingival dental calculus*. On the other hand, subgingival dental calculus is a very hard mineralized plaque which occurs on the root surface below the gum margin. It is structurally dissimilar to supragingival calculus, containing more calcium phosphate crystals, mainly as tricalcium phosphate, and fewer bacteria and is stained dark brown to greenish–black. It occurs primarily in areas that are chronically inflamed, is about 60% mineralized and it too is covered superficially with vital plaque.

A microbiological study of both types of calculus showed a complex bacterial population,

Table 35.2 Predominant bacteria in gingival margin plaque

	Health	*Gingivitis*	*Periodontitis*
Streptococci	40	27	6
Actinomyces	45	26	19
Gram-negative rods (mainly *Bacteriodes*)	13	25	74
Spirochaetes	2	—	38

qualitatively similar to the flora of gingival margin plaque (Table 35.2), the chief difference being a lack of *S. mutans* and an increased prevalence of *S. sanguis*. It appears that vitality is not essential for mineralization and may even retard the process; it is also possible that some bacteria are more calculogenic than others, for example, *Bacterionema matruchotii* readily produces intracellular apatite crystals in calcium phosphate media at pH 7·4.

Gingivitis and periodontal disease

Plaque and calculus are both key components of a vicious spiral which leads eventually to chronic periodontal disease:

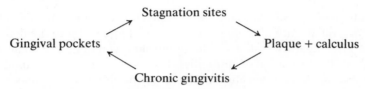

The frequency, amount and severity of gingivitis and periodontal disease, like the amount of calculus, increases with age. Studies have indicated that the occurrence of gingivitis is due only to the presence of plaque and that calculus is a secondary factor which reduces the effectiveness of oral hygiene. Acute gingivitis can be produced by allowing plaque to accumulate, and can be cured by its subsequent removal. It is now accepted that the transition from chronic gingivitis to periodontal disease involves the spread of inflammation from superficial to deeper tissues, i.e. periodontal disease is caused by inadequate control of plaque-induced gingivitis which is often associated with a failure of the host defence mechanisms. Histologically this transition is observed as a break in the attachment of the fibres of the periodontal membrane to the tooth, allowing apical migration of the crevicular epithelium. Ultimately a periodontal pocket is formed, associated with an inflammatory reaction and bone resorption.

Periodontal disease can become established wherever there is a deposit of plaque at the gingival margin, but other factors which encourage bacterial stagnation or debilitation of the gingival epithelium make infection more likely. These include trauma, food impaction, carious cavities, faulty restorations, badly designed dental appliances, tooth malalignment, missing teeth and lack of adequate function of unopposed teeth. The severity of the attack appears to be proportional to the number of bacteria, and microbiological samples of gingival plaque, collected as the disease develops, show an increasing predominance of anaerobic Gram-negative rods especially *Bacteroides* species and spirochaetes (Table 35.2).

Although this type of study does not prove that these organisms are directly responsible for the disease, they both have great potential for tissue destruction. *Bacteroides melaninogenicus* produces collagenase, hyaluronidase and proteolytic enzymes; it generates H_2S and NH_3 during metabolism, and certain of its capsular components act as endotoxins (see below). Spirochaetes are seen in large numbers at the front of the advancing pocket, they are capable of invading the tissues and can cause a reduction in the numbers of polymorphonuclear leucocytes, lymphocytes and fibroblasts as well as the destruction of the epithelial attachment to the root surface. However the precise manner in which the bacteria destroy the integrity of the crevicular epithelium and periodontal tissues is still in dispute. Direct tissue invasion by spirochaetes can be observed in some acute forms of gingival disease but it is not a consistent feature of chronically inflamed gingivae and the most likely cause is a continuing liberation, by superficially situated bacteria, of harmful substances which penetrate the intact epithelium.

Bacterial toxins

Exotoxins

These are generally extracellularly liberated proteins, some of which are among the most potent tissue poisons known. Classic examples include botulinum, tetanus, diptheria and *Shigella* neurotoxins; less potent are the *haemolysins* and *leucocidins*, produced by various streptococcal and staphylococcal species, which destroy red and white blood corpuscles, respectively. It is suggested that plaque bacteria may produce similar exotoxins although no substances specifically responsible for periodontal disease have been identified.

Endotoxins

These are lipoprotein–polysaccharide complexes which form an integral part of the cell walls of Gram-negative bacteria and are liberated at cell death. If injected into the dermis they rapidly produce a severe inflammatory response; the lipoprotein component is toxic while the polysaccharide stimulates the formation of antibodies. Prior sensitization of the tissues enhances the subsequent response to a later application of the same endotoxin and increases the capacity of the neutrophils to phagocytose microorganisms. This hyperactivity may, however, harm the tissues following the release from lysed white cells of lysosomal enzymes and collagenase which modify tissue proteins. These modified proteins are themselves antigenic, and give rise to further antibody–antigen reactions, migration of T and B lymphocytes, discharge of lysosomal enzymes and more modified tissue protein. A vicious spiral of persistent chronic inflammation is thereby established. The sera of humans suffering from periodontal disease have been found to contain higher levels of antibodies to oral bacterial endotoxins than those from healthy individuals.

Enzymes

The plaque bacteria produce hydrolytic enzymes which, if allowed to act, will destroy connective tissue. These are collectively known as *spreading factors*, and include hyal-uronidase, chondroitin sulphatase, glycosidases, collagenase and various other proteolytic enzymes. However no matter how great their potential for damaging tissue components, these enzymes cannot be considered as direct pathogenic factors until it has been shown that they act on the tissues *in vivo* to produce a pathological response.

Low molecular weight components

Peptides, glycopeptides, oligosaccharides, amines, hydrogen sulphide, methyl mercaptan (CH_3SH), organic acids and ammonium salts are present in aqueous extracts of plaque. Such compounds produce an inflammatory response and cell damage in experimental models and may be among the agents responsible for disease. Many of these agents are both readily diffusible and lipid soluble and, therefore, capable of penetrating the intact crevicular epithelium. Before an inflammatory agent can be positively implicated, it must be shown to have a toxic effect at the concentrations found in plaque from diseased mouths. One substance which, under certain conditions, fulfils these requirements is ammonia. Cells can tolerate large quantities of ammonia when it is administered slowly because of the efficient detoxifying mechanisms which convert it into urea, glutamine or asparagine. However, when total ammonia concentrations and the extracellular pH are high in periodontally involved plaque, the ammonium ion dissociates into a hydrogen ion and an uncharged lipid-soluble species:

$$NH_4^+ \xrightarrow{\text{p}K = 9.02} NH_3 + H^+$$

Since the hydrogen ion penetrates lipophilic membranes at a slow rate, the pH gradient between the plaque and tissue fluids allows the NH_3 species to enter the cell sufficiently rapidly to overwhelm the cell buffering systems and cause a rise in the internal pH and consequent cellular damage. The pH and volume of gingival fluid has been shown to increase as the severity of the disease increases; pH values as high as 9.0 were recorded in extreme cases. Amines, organic acids and other compounds with a state of charge which is a function of pH can enter the cell in a similar manner as shown:

$$RNH_3^+ \rightleftharpoons H^+ + RNH_2 \xrightarrow{\text{Cell wall}} RNH_2 + H^+ \rightleftharpoons RNH_3^+$$

Plaque   Cell wall   Cell interior

Cell buffering

Biochemical aspects of cell damage

The products of plaque metabolism can inflict a prolonged chemical attack on the tissues which may lead to dental caries or to periodontal disease. The final manifestation of both conditions is tissue death resulting from disturbance of the finely balanced homoeostatic mechanisms that preserve the cells in their normal steady state. When the dental pulp is exposed to bacterial invasion by a carious lesion or the gingival tissues are infected by plaque, the cellular organization is sufficiently upset to provoke irreversible changes. Cell damage results within seconds in a fall in the ATP/ADP, NAD^+/NADH, and $NADP^+$/NADPH ratios and an increase in the lactate/pyruvate and glycerophosphate/dihydroxyacetone phosphate ratios. The oxidative phosphorylation sequence is disrupted and this soon becomes apparent from morphological changes in the mitochondria, endoplasmic reticulum, plasma membrane and nucleus. The polyribosomes dissociate, protein synthesis ceases and, if the damage is on a large enough scale, there is an increase in serum enzyme activities due to leakage from the damaged tissues. The cell is unable to repair itself and the accumulation of lactic acid causes an intra-cellular acidosis which leads to disruption of the membranes and, eventually, the hydrolytic enzymes in the lysosomes are released. Reduced ATP concentrations result in early failure of the sodium pump as this consumes a substantial proportion of cellular energy. Sodium ions pass into the cell, driven in by concentration and electrical gradients, and as the total intracellular cation concentration increases, it attracts water into the cell leading eventually to oedema.

The bacterial invasion also produces a complex *inflammatory reaction* which allows cells, proteins and water to pass from the blood into the tissues to react with the invading stimulus. The factors that trigger off this response are not fully understood but it is thought that the initial event is the release of histamine and 5-hydroxytryptamine (serotonin), which cause dilation of the blood vessels and an increased rate of blood flow. The vessel walls become permeable and allow the passage of fluid, immunoglobulins and other plasma proteins into the tissues. The increased water content of the tissues may be sufficient to cause swelling, while a second group of mediators appears slightly later and sustains the vascular leakage. These are polypeptides called *kinins*, which are released from inactive precursors or *kininogens*, present in the blood plasma, by enzymes known as *kallikreins*, found in both plasma and tissue fluids. Inflammation is also characterized by the emigration of phagocytes from the vessels to the infected site, attracted by the production of certain peptide chemotactic agents. The phagocytes engulf the invading bacteria and tissue debris but, if the invasion is great enough or the bacteria sufficiently toxic, large numbers of phagocytes are destroyed, their lysosomes being disrupted with release of enzymes into the tissues. Since these have acid pH optima, their activity is favoured by the earlier accumulation of acid and causes cellular macromolecules and extracellular structures to break down and form pus.

The probable relationship between plaque, calculus formation and the development of periodontal disease is summarized in Figure 35.10. Because of its toxic nature the presence of plaque near the gingival margin causes inflammation of the superficial gingival tissues. These become red, swollen and tender, the oedematous swelling causes stretching and glazing of the free gingivae and papillae, leading to pocket formation, stagnation and an increased area for retention of plaque. The associated exudate of gingival crevice fluid provides substrates for base formation (urea, amino acids, peptides and proteins), the pH tends to be high, and the presence of calcium and phosphate in the fluid creates conditions which are ideal for the proliferation of subgingival plaque and its subsequent calcification. The continual liberation of toxins by the plaque, the presence of subgingival calculus plus chronic inflammation, antigenic stimulation, hypersensitivity reactions and destruction by lysosomal and plaque enzymes not only prevent healing but encourage further tissue damage. The eventual development of a periodontal pocket causes further stagnation, deeper penetration of subgingival plaque and calculus which perpetuate the disease. The formation of supragingival calculus is shown in Figure 35.10 as an independent sequence of events, although its presence will cause an increased retention of supragingival plaque.

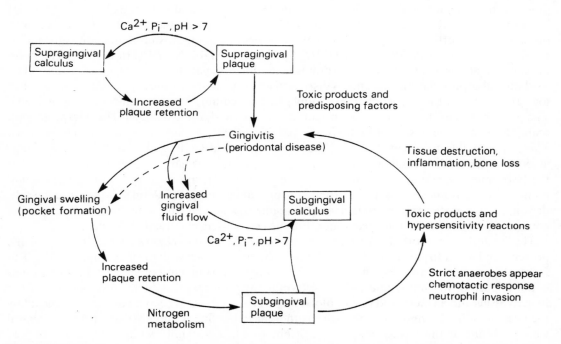

Figure 35.10 The sequence of events initiated by supragingival plaque in the development of gingivitis, subgingival plaque, subgingival calculus and periodontal disease

If there is a reduction in pH as a result of bacterial activity, the equilibrium

$$H^+ + HCO_3^- \rightleftharpoons H_2CO_3 \rightleftharpoons H_2O + CO_2$$

is displaced towards the right. The carbon dioxide which is evolved is only slightly soluble, and below pH 6·0–5·5 is released as a gas. When this is produced in a confined area such as the pulp, it, together with the effects of oedema, will cause the internal pressure to increase and produce the severe pain characteristic of *acute pulpitis*. If the pressure becomes greater than the arterial blood pressure, the blood supply will be sealed off at the constricted apex of the tooth and produce a closed system within the pulp. Cells which were previously undamaged will have their blood supply, and therefore oxygen and glucose, cut off and so be forced to metabolize their stored carbohydrate anaerobically. Lactic and citric acids then accumulate and together with acid produced by the bacteria will overwhelm the tissue buffering systems causing a fall in pH, lysosomal destruction and extensive cell death.

Pulpal destruction encourages the proliferation of the invading bacteria which eventually pass outwards through the apex and initiate the inflammatory changes which develop into a periapical abscess. In this site, however, response is modified by its more open nature and the presence of alveolar bone. An adequate blood supply reduces the closed system effect, while the local drop in pH during the initial stages, together with lysosomal activity, solubilizes the bone and destroys the matrix. The inorganic ions are redeposited in an irregular fashion in the less acid regions around the site of resorption to give the X-ray picture of a radiolucent area surrounded by a radio-opaque ring. Hopefully the bacterial invasion will remain contained and, if extraction or treatment of the tooth removes the primary site of tissue infection, the area will be filled with granulation tissue and eventually recalcified to replace the missing bone.

Chapter 36
The prevention of plaque-induced diseases

As mentioned earlier, good dental health is usual in primitive societies where a fibrous and abrasive low-sugar diet provides for vigorous mastication, increased salivary flow, self-cleansing and stimulation of the periodontal tissues. In contrast the majority of people in modern industrialized societies consume a soft sugar-rich diet which provides for extensive bacterial fermentation leading to caries; as a result of under use it also causes atrophy of the periodontium and this may lead to periodontal disease. These dietary associations are reinforced by epidemiological studies in developing countries which show that an increase in the sugar content and degree of refinement of the diet is associated with a marked increase in the incidence of plaque-induced diseases (Table 36.1). Thus in Westernized societies only a few individuals

Table 36.1 The rapid increase in caries in developing countries.
Average number of decayed, missing and filled teeth (DMFT) per child age 12

	1950–1960	*1970–79*
Kenya	0·1	1·7
Uganda	0·4	1·5
Ethiopia	0·2	1·6
Iraq	0·7	3·5
Thailand	0·7	4·5
Vietnam	2·0	6·3
Polynesia	Approx. 0	8·0
Industrialized countries (for comparison), children aged 13–14:		
Sydney, Australia		6·7
Canterbury, New Zealand		10·7
Trondelag, Norway		12·6
Hanover, Germany		8·8
Yamakashi, Japan		7·5
Bristol, England		9·5

After Barmes (1977) *Journal of Clinical Periodontology*, **4**, 80, and Andlaw *et al.* (1982) *Caries Research*, **16**, 257

retain a complete and healthy dentition throughout their life and methods of preventing dental disease become increasingly important. These can be divided into a number of different categories and include dietary control, plaque removal, treatment of the enamel surface and various antibacterial measures. Effective prophylaxis is usually only obtained by a combination of several of these methods.

Dietary control

The fact that the enamel dissolution which occurs in caries is caused by organic acids produced by plaque bacteria from dietary carbohydrate is supported by the following evidence.

1. Dietary carbohydrates cause the pH at the tooth surface to fall below the critical pH for enamel dissolution.
2. Artificial carious lesions in enamel produced by acid–gels *in vitro* are indistinguishable from natural lesions.
3 Germ-free rats do not develop caries unless they are infected with bacteria from an animal with caries and are also fed a carbohydrate-rich diet.
4. Animals fed a cariogenic carbohydrate diet by mouth develop caries; those fed the same diet by stomach intubation do not.
5. The proportion of acid-forming bacteria in plaque samples from caries-active individuals is greater than in samples from caries-inactive individuals (Table 36.2). This ratio of acidogenic to total plaque organisms is significantly increased by supplementing the diet with sucrose.

Since dietary carbohydrate is now accepted as an essential element in the carious process it should, in theory, be possible to prevent or at least reduce the incidence of caries by reverting to a diet in which more fibre and less refined carbohydrate is consumed. Evidence as to the feasibility of preventing caries by controlling the diet of human populations is not easy to come by for practical and ethical reasons but, when in many European countries the sugar intake was severely restricted during the two World Wars, caries incidence decreased. This was due to a local effect on the teeth rather than a general nutritional effect since already erupted teeth benefited as much as developing teeth during the period of sugar rationing.

Observations at Hopewood House (1952–1956), a children's home in Australia which maintained a nutritionally adequate but mainly vegetarian diet in which refined carbohydrates

Table 36.2 The ratio of acidogenic to total organisms in plaque samples from individuals with different caries histories

Group	*Mean ± standard deviation*
Children	
Caries-free	0·35 ± 0·01
Caries-prone	0·63 ± 0·01
Students	
Caries-free	0·42 ± 0·04
Caries-prone:	
no recent lesions	0·39 ± 0·07
recent lesions	0·59 ± 0·05

and sucrose were excluded, showed that the children had a low DMFT index which was not related to fluoride nor to good oral hygiene. When the children left the home at age 12–13 and were no longer under dietary control, their caries experience rapidly increased to match that of other children from state schools. A 2-year study at Turku Dental School, Finland, in 1976, in which caries-prone subjects totally replaced the sucrose in their diets with xylitol showed that this eliminated further caries progression when compared to a control group given sucrose- or fructose-containing diets (Figure 36.1). These studies show that increasing or decreasing the amount of fermentable carbohydrate in the diet has a profound effect on caries experience.

Other studies have shown that, in fact, it is not so much the amount of sugar that is eaten that is important but rather the frequency with which it is eaten and the length of time over which appreciable amounts of fermentable carbohydrate are present in the mouth. The Vipeholm experiment (page 133) clearly demonstrated that the consumption of sugar, especially in a sticky form between meals, promoted caries development.

Experiments in rodents, which do not normally develop caries, have shown that sucrose is the most cariogenic carbohydrate while other common mono- and di-saccharides and cooked starch are generally less cariogenic. Monkeys fed a typical child's diet developed caries, and attempts are being made to assess the cariogenicity of foods so that snacks may be chosen for eating between meals which do not increase the risk of caries. Stephan curves prepared for each food show the ranking of a number of snacks according to their acidogenicity (Table 36.3). Sucrose-containing sweets, fruit drinks and sugared tea and coffee are among the most acidogenic snacks

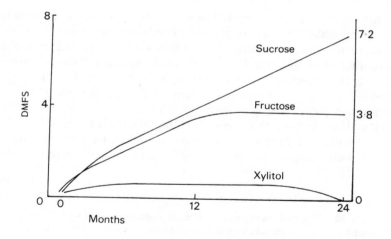

Figure 36.1 Turku sugar study. The cumulative development of decayed, missing and filled tooth surfaces (DMFS) over a 2-year period

and a comparison of rat caries scores produced by different foods also showed that those containing sucrose were the most cariogenic. Perhaps surprisingly, many 'natural' foods were also highly cariogenic, particularly if they are acidic in nature. Honey, dates, raisins, grapes, apples and figs produced high caries scores; apples, grapes, iced lollies and cola drinks also produced acid erosion of the enamel surface. In general, starchy foods produced the least caries (bread alone) while a sugar supplement (bread and jam; sweet biscuits) increased the caries

Table 36.3 Ranking of different snack foods according to their minimum pH values achieved in the Stephan curve

Snack	Minimum pH
Boiled sweet	5·33
Sugared coffee	5·41
Toffee	5·43
Orange drink	5·51
Plain biscuit	5·56
Sugared chewing gum	5·59
Chocolate-coated biscuit	5·62
Chocolate	5·63
Ice cream	5·66
Apple	5·81
Mars bar	5·82
Unsugared coffee	6·10
Ice-lolly (frozen)	6·11
Potato crisps	6·19
Bread and butter	6·28
Salted peanut	6·50
Strong cheese	7·50

Adapted from Rugg-Gunn *et al.* (1978) *British Dental Journal*, **145**, 95

score in proportion to the sucrose content. Analyses have also shown that many unexpected foods contain sucrose, e.g. some tomato soups contain 10% sucrose.

One of the main factors influencing the degree and duration of the fall in pH is the rate of salivary flow (page 481); if flow is stimulated during or immediately after sugar exposure the associated rise in salivary bicarbonate helps to buffer plaque acid and promotes a more rapid return of the pH to neutrality. Figure 36.2 shows the effects of saliva-stimulating foods such as an apple (a), and salted, roasted peanuts (b) on Stephan curves produced by a sugar lump and by strong cheese (c) given after tinned pears. Cheese eaten after sugar reduced caries in animals and it is possible that apart from reducing the acid the cheese also acts as a source of calcium and phosphate and other protective factors.

Sucrose is included in a wide variety of processed foods for reasons other than its sweet taste (page 134), and this often makes it difficult for the manufacturers to use an alternative sweetener. Sorbitol, mannitol and xylitol (page 136) have, however, been successfully incorporated into 'sugar-free' chewing gums and, since plaque bacteria metabolize them only very slowly, if at all, acid production is negligible. They have the additional advantage of stimulating salivary flow which causes a rise in pH and this may help in the remineralization of early lesions. Unfortunately, the consumption of large quantities of sugar alcohols leads to osmotic diarrhoea which has prevented their use in a wider range of confectionery. However, a whole range of alternative sweeteners is becoming available (page 135) and it is possible that some of them will be found to be suitable sucrose substitutes.

Maintenance of salivary flow and access

The importance of saliva in oral clearance, pH control, increased mineral ion availability and the provision of acid-neutralizing substrates such as urea and arginine peptides was considered in

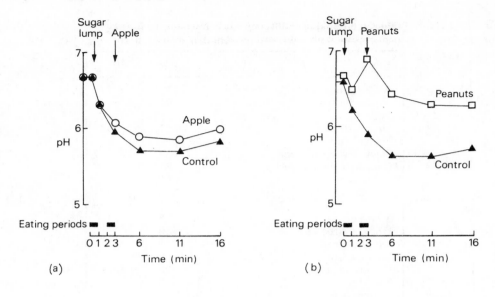

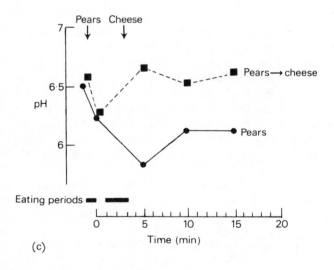

Figure 36.2 The effects of saliva-stimulating foods on the pH of plaque. (a) The effect of an apple after eating a lump of sugar; (b) the effect of peanuts after a sugar lump; (c) the effect of eating cheese after tinned pears. (After Geddes *et al.* (1977) *British Dental Journal,* **140**, 317 and Rugg-Gunn *et al.* (1975) *British Dental Journal,* **139**, 361)

Chapter 35. In addition, saliva has specific microbial defence mechanisms which make the mouth a hostile place for bacteria. These, in the absence of fermentable carbohydrate, ensure that there is limited bacterial growth in the saliva.

(i) Saliva contains *dissolved oxygen* and this is the main factor limiting the growth of potentially pathogenic anaerobic organisms. These require a reduced oxygen content for growth and the redox potential has been shown to fall from +200 mV to −140 mV as plaque develops on a clean tooth surface. This is associated with a gradual increase in the plaque anaerobic community and is especially noticeable at the gingival margins and in periodontal pockets. Values which may be as low as $-300\,\text{mV}$ have been reported, and are to be expected, since spirochaetes which require a redox potential of $-185\,\text{mV}$ for growth can be isolated in this area.

Plaque possesses a range of oxygen tensions depending on the site and on salivary access. A good oxygen supply is important since hydrogen peroxide produced by bacterial oxidase reactions limits the growth of catalase-negative bacteria. These include many Gram-positive cocci and rods such as *Actinomyces* and lactobacilli. Hydrogen peroxide is also produced by neutrophils (derived mainly from the gingival crevice area) under aerobic conditions as a result of superoxide generation (page 159):

$$O_2 + e^- \rightarrow O_2^{-\cdot}$$
$$2O_2^{-\cdot} + 2H^+ \rightarrow H_2O_2 + O_2$$

The hydrogen peroxide can then react with ferrous ions to produce the hydroxyl radical which is highly toxic to bacteria:

$$H_2O_2 + Fe^{2+} \rightarrow Fe^{3+} + OH^{\cdot} + OH^-$$

Alternatively, a reaction catalysed by neutrophil-derived *myeloperoxidase* produces hypochlorite a chemical which kills all known germs:

$$H_2O_2 + Cl^- \rightarrow OCl^- + H_2O$$

In saliva, in the presence of hydrogen peroxide, *salivary peroxidase* oxidizes salivary thiocyanate to hypothiocyanate:

$$H_2O_2 + SCN^- \rightarrow OSCN^- + H_2O$$

This and other short-lived oxidation products also inhibit bacteria.

(ii) Saliva contains various proteins that inhibit bacterial growth; these include *immunoglobulins* synthesized locally and derived from the serum via the gingival fluid (page 477), the enzyme *lysozyme* (page 409) and *transferrin*, a Fe^{3+}-binding protein which is capable of depriving organisms of this essential metal. The Gram-negative bacteria are particularly susceptible to iron deficiency but recent work has shown that the bactericidal effect is not a simple one since the inhibition of *S. mutans* is independent of iron deprivation. It has also been suggested that saliva contains specific *agglutinins* which cause clumping of bacteria, reducing their ability to colonize surfaces and favouring their removal by salivary wash-out. It also seems likely that all salivary organisms are coated with a variety of salivary glycoproteins in a non-specific manner.

Apart from its microbial defence mechanisms saliva may help to reduce calculus formation since the tendency for the spontaneous precipitation of calcium phosphates *in vitro* is reduced by peptides such as *statherin*. Statherin contains 47 amino acids and the highly charged *N*-terminal third of the molecule has the amino acid sequence:

$$\text{Asp-SerPO}_3^- \text{-SerPO}_3^- \text{-Glu-Glu-Lys-Leu-Phe-Arg-Arg-Ile-Gly-Arg}$$

The remaining two-thirds is mainly hydrophobic and it is this polar region, and particularly the two phosphoserine residues, which seem to provide a unique configuration for binding to nucleation and growth sites. Experiments have shown that a concentration of $1\,\mu\text{M}$, which is less than the concentration in saliva (2–$6\,\mu\text{M}$), is sufficient to inhibit crystal growth completely. Salivary pyrophosphate has also been shown to be an effective inhibitor at low concentrations ($7\cdot5\,\mu\text{M}$) and it has been proposed that this and the peptide inhibitors act by binding to calcium phosphate nuclei and to growth sites on seed crystal surfaces thus preventing crystal growth (page 456). A number of other molecules also inhibit and it is not easy to define the characteristics which make an effective inhibitor; the minimum requirement seems to be a phosphate group and an adjacent acidic group which can either be another phosphate or a carboxylate group. An interesting example of a naturally produced inhibitor is *phosphocitrate* which is found in the urine and is synthesized within the mitochondrion:

$$\begin{array}{ccc} O & & CH_2COO^- \\ \parallel & & | \\ ^-O-P-O-C-COO^- \\ | & & | \\ O^- & & CH_2COO^- \end{array}$$

For the reasons given above it will be apparent that the design and placement of fillings, crowns, bridges, partial dentures, orthodontic appliances etc. should be such as to ensure a good salivary access to all surfaces at all times. Reduced salivary flow in *xerostomia* is associated with an increase in plaque accumulation, caries, periodontal disease and infections of the oral mucosa, and various formulations are available for an 'artificial' saliva. These are usually slightly viscous aqueous liquids containing a mixture of salts, flavouring agents and an antimicrobial preservative. The viscosity is adjusted by adding macromolecules such as methyl cellulose. Buffers to control the pH and salivary stimulants to encourage the flow of the patient's own saliva are often included. The latter are usually organic acids such as citric, malic or lactic acid which have a low pH, and one preparation contains additional calcium in the form of calcium lactate to reduce the risk of enamel demineralization. Antimicrobial agents may be added to prevent the growth of potential pathogenic bacteria and yeasts but no real attempt has yet been made to match natural saliva, and 'dry mouth' remains a chronic problem for patient and dentist.

Plaque removal and the use of toothpaste

The ideal antiplaque agent has been described as one that would not stain the teeth but would work on all species of plaque-forming organisms, be non-toxic, have no adverse systemic effects, be effective in a short time, be cheap and have the approval of the drug-licensing authority. A well-designed toothbrush meets all these requirements and when used properly with a dentifrice is very effective in eliminating plaque. Considerable effort has gone into the formulation and marketing of dentifrices; aqueous suspensions of alginate, tragacanth, propylene glycol, glycerol and hydroxyethylcellulose have been used to form the body of the paste and to act as a vehicle for a variety of abrasives such as calcium carbonate, various calcium phosphates and aluminium and zinc oxides. These represent about 40–50% by weight and detergents are added at 1–2% to aid dispersion. The latter are surface active agents which are amphiphilic and, when dissolved in water, form an oriented monolayer at the air–water interface which allows the liquid to spread over the surface to be cleaned. Certain soaps which are anionic detergents are used in dentifrices, e.g. *sodium ricinoleate*, a hydroxy unsaturated 18-carbon fatty acid salt derived from castor oil:

$$CH_3[CH_2]_5CHOHCH_2CH{=}CH[CH_2]_7COO^- \cdot Na^+$$

and *sodium dodecyl(lauryl) sulphate* derived from lauric acid by sulphonation:

$$CH_3[CH_2]_{10}CH_2OSO_3^- \cdot Na^+$$

In addition, toothpastes contain a variety of flavouring agents such as menthol, a preservative to extend shelf-life and a therapeutic agent, usually sodium fluoride at a concentration of about 2·2% by weight (1000 ppm fluoride ion).

Toothpastes containing fluoride are considered on page 528 and those containing antibiotics on page 531.

Attempts have been made to incorporate into toothpastes enzymes such as *dextranase* and *mutanase* (α-1 : 6- and α-1 : 3-glucosidase respectively) which degrade plaque polysaccharides. These enzymes work well in laboratory tests, but seem to be unable to penetrate plaque *in situ* due to the molecular-exclusion properties of the plaque matrix (page 497).

An enzyme-containing toothpaste is however available which is claimed to promote the salivary peroxidase reaction (page 525). The paste contains *amyloglucosidase* which hydrolyses retained starch to free glucose, which is then acted upon by added glucose oxidase (page 94) to produce hydrogen peroxide under aerobic conditions. This in turn reacts with a potassium thiocyanate supplement to generate the hypothiocyanate anion:

$$\text{Soluble starch} \rightarrow \text{glucose}$$
$$\text{Glucose} + O_2 + H_2O \rightarrow \text{gluconate} + H_2O_2$$
$$H_2O_2 + SCN^- \rightarrow OSCN^- + H_2O$$

The manufacturers claim that 'this enzyme system helps to restore the natural protection of the saliva against bacteria' and, while it is true that hypothiocyanate inhibits bacterial growth and acid production and destroys DNA and membrane phospholipids, the system is not bactericidal under the anaerobic conditions existing in acid-producing plaques and in the periodontal pocket owing to the lack of oxygen.

An attempt has been made to reduce calculus formation by incorporating *diphosphonate* into a toothpaste. Diphosphonate is an analogue of pyrophosphate. It acts as a non-physiological inhibitor of calcification and is resistant to enzymic hydrolysis.

$$
\begin{array}{ccccc}
 & O & R & O & \\
 & \parallel & | & \parallel & \\
{}^-O- & P & -C- & P & -OH \\
 & | & | & | & \\
 & O^- & R' & O^- &
\end{array}
$$

It has proved to be moderately successful in clinical trials but its stability may lead to toxicity problems as, if inadvertently swallowed, it will be absorbed and could inhibit bone formation. An alternative approach has been to use fluoride as a *pyrophosphatase inhibitor* in the presence of pyrophosphate supplements in order to prolong the effects of pyrophosphate. It should be noted that these techniques will not remove preformed calculus, but should serve as useful aids in reducing further accumulation once calculus has been removed by scaling.

Modification of the enamel surface

Surface films

The possibility of changing the physicochemical nature of the enamel surface and thus of reducing bacterial colonization is a promising area of research which has been encouraged by the success of *fissure-sealants* in reducing pit and fissure caries in children. In this technique a plastic film is used to coat sound, but caries-susceptible, surfaces, in effect redesigning the tooth to remove stagnation areas and encourage self-cleansing. The surface has to be thoroughly cleaned, isolated from the saliva and etched with phosphoric acid to give a partially demineralized surface which provides for adhesion. A plastic methacrylate monomer is then allowed to flow into the fissures and polymerized *in situ* using chemical or u.v.-stimulated catalysis. Unfortunately, the plastic film tends to wear away quickly, particularly at the edges and has to be replaced at frequent intervals to avoid the accumulation of plaque at broken margins. New materials are being developed which can chemically bond to the surface and have a high fluoride content; these should allow the dentist to seal in early carious lesions as an alternative to conventional fillings.

The idea of a hydrophobic film covering the exposed enamel is attractive. In theory a charged 'head' group would bind to the apatite and a hydrophobic 'tail', such as the hydrocarbon chains found in fatty acids and in phospholipids, would be presented to the saliva. In this way bacterial adhesion and plaque formation could be reduced. The precipitation of specific salivary proteins to produce the acquired pellicle has much the same effect and it is interesting to note that treatment of an apatite surface with hydrophobic salivas reduced the attachment of *S. mutans* and other hydrophilic streptococci.

Fluoride

The normal maturation process of a newly erupted tooth surface can be speeded up by the application of fluoride ions. Ideally, fluoride should be incorporated during enamel formation by the provison of fluoridated drinking water (page 149). Alternatively, dietary supplements can be provided in areas where the water contains less than $700\mu g$ of fluoride ion per litre (0·7 ppm). Sodium fluoride tablets (2·2 mg) each provide 1 mg of fluoride ion and the following are the daily fluoride ion doses for children in areas where the water contains less than 0·3 ppm: for children 0–2 years $250\mu g$ (quarter tablet); 2–4 years $500\mu g$ (half tablet); 4 years and over 1 mg (one tablet).

Fluoride-containing toothpastes became generally available in the early 1970s and have proved to be an effective means of caries prevention. For example, between 1973 and 1983 the mean decayed, missing and filled teeth (DMFT) index of 12-year-old children in England and Wales fell from 4·8 to 2·9. Reductions occurred in communities supplied both with and without fluoridated water and it is believed that the use of fluoride-containing toothpastes was largely responsible. High fluoride concentrations of up to 1200 ppm are provided, usually as sodium or stannous fluoride, although sodium monofluorophosphate (Na_3PO_3F) has also been used. Fluoride in this form is compatible with the calcium-containing abrasives usually used, such as calcium carbonate or calcium phosphates. Fluorophosphate is soluble, readily retained by plaque by ionic interactions as PO_3F^{3-} and is subsequently hydrolysed into phosphate and fluoride ions by plaque phosphatase activity.

It is likely that most small children swallow some of the paste and this possibility should be considered when fluoride tablets are prescribed due to the dangers of an excessive dose (page 147). Topical application may also be carried out by dentists and dental auxillaries using acidic phosphate–fluoride gels applied to the tooth surface for several minutes. A low pH value is needed to drive the reaction

$$Ca_{10}(PO_4)_6(OH)_2 + 2F^- \rightarrow Ca_{10}(PO_4)_6F_2 + 2OH^-$$

by removal of the OH^- ions.

There is also the possibility of a double decomposition reaction leading to the precipitation of insoluble calcium fluoride:

$$CaHPO_4 + 2\,NaF \rightarrow CaF_2 + Na_2HPO_4$$

Excess phosphate in the gel helps to suppress this reaction in favour of fluoroapatite formation.

Fluoride also has effects on remineralization (page 519) and on bacterial growth (page 500). Although the success of fluoride treatment in giving large average reductions in total caries experience is not in doubt, this does not necessarily mean that all teeth benefit equally. A public health report in 1978 on caries reduction in individual teeth by water fluoridation showed an

80–100% protection of the anterior teeth and 56–75% protection of the premolars, but only 34–54% protection of the molar teeth, the lower molars being the least protected. Other studies indicate about 80% protection of approximal and smooth surfaces but only 43% in pits and fissures. Consequently, there is a need to provide additional protection against primary caries of intact surfaces and particularly against secondary caries occurring around existing fillings and on exposed root surfaces in older subjects.

Remineralizing solutions

A comparison of teeth shed by Bristol children before 1960 and after 1975 showed a 1·3-fold increase in enamel surface fluoride levels. This was presumably due to the increased use of fluoride-containing toothpastes since the water supply has remained non-fluoridated. However, no differences were observed in the rates of penetration of acid–gel-induced caries-like lesions of the enamel and it appears that the raised fluoride concentrations do not reduce enamel solubility sufficiently to account, by themselves, for the recently reported reductions in caries. For example, the DMFT index for 11 year olds in Bristol was 4·6 in 1970 and 2·9 in 1979, a reduction of 37%. It seems more likely that an increase in plaque fluoride ion concentrations is a more important factor as this is known to catalyse the reprecipitation of calcium phosphates capable of repairing the enamel (page 511) as well as inhibiting bacterial acid production. It has long been known that enamel, if softened with dilute acid solutions *in vitro*, will reharden to some extent after subsequent immersion in saliva. Similarly, early enamel lesions will revert in the mouth when salivary access is improved. These observations suggest that the enhancement of remineralization is as important in preventing caries as is a reduction in enamel solubility. Experiments have shown that if real or artificial carious lesions are exposed to saliva or a calcifying fluid, there is a reduction in the porosity and an increase in the radio-opacity of the lesions. Remineralization due to saliva was restricted to the surface layers but extended throughout the lesion with an inorganic calcifying fluid. A 1 mM calcium concentration was more effective than a 3 mM solution suggesting that the degree of supersaturation is important. If the solution is saturated or supersaturated with respect to all the calcium phosphate phases (Table 35.1) rapid surface precipitation occurs which reduces surface porosity and restricts further penetration into the body of the lesion. If, however, the solution is only supersaturated with respect to hydroxyapatite, a slower but more extensive mineralization occurs throughout the lesion. This favours growth of existing hydroxyapatite crystals rather than nucleation.

Table 36.4 shows that the presence of fluoride ions enhances the rate and extent of remineralization. Increasing the fluoride concentration had no further effect. This supports the idea that fluoride helps to reduce caries by enhancing the remineralization of microscopic enamel lesions so that they never become clinically detectable. If fluoride is not available the lesions increase in size until they can be seen on X-ray examination. Similarly small enamel lesions can be made to 'disappear' from radiographs following the use of recalcifying mouthwashes. At present these are based on calcium phosphate–fluoride solutions adjusted to

Table 36.4 Effect of the presence of fluoride ions on remineralization

Calcifying fluid	Reduction in area of lesion
3 mM Ca^{2+}	11%
3 mM Ca^{2+} + 53 μM F^-	20%
1 mM Ca^{2+}	28%
1 mM Ca^{2+} + 53 μM F^-	69%

neutral pH values, and active research is being undertaken to assess the effect of including ions, such as magnesium and bicarbonate, and organic compounds, such as proteins and phospholipids.

Colonization of an early lesion by acidogenic organisms such as *S. mutans* can prevent effective remineralization by lowering the local pH to such an extent that calcium phosphate precipitation will no longer occur. As well as catalysing remineralization fluoride ions act as inhibitors of bacterial metabolism and the effect of fluoride on acid production by *S. mutans* has been studied in some detail (see below).

General inhibition of plaque organisms

Antiseptics

Various antiseptics and chemical agents are used in dentistry in mouthwashes, sprays, lozenges and dentifrices but for them to be effective in preventing bacterial growth they must be retained in the mouth for long periods. Charged molecules are able to bind to plaque proteins and to bacterial surfaces by ionic interactions, and anionic detergents such as fatty acid salts and sodium lauryl sulphate have proved to be useful against Gram-positive bacteria but less so against Gram-negative bacteria. For example, sodium ricinoleate solutions have been reported to decrease the accumulation of plaque and the formation of calculus but their taste is so unpleasant that it requires great self-discipline to maintain regular use.

Cationic detergents generally have a more potent antiseptic action than anionic agents since they bind directly to negatively charged bacterial surfaces causing increased permeability and membrane disintegration. Many of them are quaternary ammonium salts which incorporate hydrophobic groups such as fatty acid chains and aromatic rings in their structures, e.g. *cetylpyridinium chloride* which is used in an aqueous 0·05% solution as a mouthwash or gargle:

$$\text{N}^+-[CH_2]_{15}CH_3 \cdot Cl^-$$

and *cetrimide* which is useful for skin disinfection in a 1% solution as it has excellent detergent properties:

$$CH_3[CH_2]_{14}-\overset{\overset{\displaystyle CH_3}{|}}{\underset{\underset{\displaystyle CH_3}{|}}{N}}{}^{\pm}CH_3$$

Chlorhexidine is another cationic agent which is used extensively in periodontal therapy to suppress Gram-negative plaque organisms since it is non-toxic, readily retained and is very effective at low concentrations even though it has a poor detergent capability. Structurally it is a substituted 1,6-bisguanidohexane which contains both hydrophilic and hydrophobic components.

$$\begin{pmatrix} & H & NH_2^+ & NH & \\ R-N-C-N-C-NH \\ & | & & & \\ & H & & \end{pmatrix}$$
$$\begin{pmatrix} & H & NH_2^+ & NH & \\ R-N-C-N-C-NH \\ & | & & & \\ & H & & \end{pmatrix}$$
$$[CH_2]_6 \qquad \text{where } R = \text{Cl}$$

Each bisguanido group has an associated proton which confers two strong positive charges on the molecule. At physiological pH values each of these groups exists in a monocationic form and the compound has pK values of 2·2 and 10·3 in which the bound proton is actually extensively delocalized over the five nitrogen atoms. Consequently, the molecule interacts strongly with negatively charged groups on the surface of bacterial cells and, on addition to a bacterial suspension, is immediately adsorbed, causing membrane damage, an irreversible loss of cytoplasmic constituents and enzyme inhibition.

At present chlorhexidine is the agent of choice in the short-term control of supragingival plaque although it is not without its disadvantages. It adsorbs to a pellicle-covered enamel and to the surface of calculus and subsequently reacts with dietary components to produce a persistent brown stain. In addition, some patients report a burning sensation and loss of taste after prolonged use.

Antibiotics

These are naturally occurring toxic chemicals that are produced and secreted by micro-organisms. Many of them are highly specific inhibitors of biological processes and some are clinically useful since they can inhibit infecting bacteria without damaging the host cells. Penicillin is a broad-acting antibiotic which was developed for clinical use in the early 1940s, and in 1946 it was shown that rats that were fed a caries-producing diet containing penicillin in either the food or water supply failed to develop caries whereas animals on a similar but penicillin-free regime developed decay as usual. This experiment showed clearly for the first time that bacterial, rather than inadequate nutrition, were the cause of caries.

Further studies confirmed that a number of antibiotics were potent inhibitors of caries in animals and their effectiveness seemed to be related to their ability to interfere with the growth of Gram-positive bacteria. This led to their use in Man and in 1950 the results were reported of a clinical trial which had produced a 58% reduction in caries in 6–14-year-old children after 2 years supervised toothbrushing with a powder containing 500 units of penicillin per gram. Subsequent observations on children receiving long-term penicillin therapy for the control of rheumatic fever or chronic pulmonary disease revealed that these patients had up to 40% less caries than healthy children of comparable ages; they also had less plaque and gingivitis.

As a result of these and other laboratory and animal studies penicillin-containing dentifrices were produced commercially. However, it was found that they could lead to the development of resistant organisms and allergic states; consequently they were withdrawn from the market.

Nevertheless, penicillin or other antibiotic-based preparations may still have a use in the short-term treatment of selected patients with otherwise uncontrollable decay, e.g. physically handicapped or mentally retarded patients, where ordinary methods of caries control cannot be used.

In spite of its clinical shortcomings, antibiotic therapy established beyond doubt that caries is a bacterial disease and the experimental use of selective antibiotics has shown that Gram-negative bacteria, yeasts and fungi have no significance in the initiation of rat caries.

Antibiotics, particularly broad-spectrum antibiotics, can prevent plaque accumulation and gingivitis in Man. The use of mouthwashes containing selective antibiotics showed that plaque could form with either a predominantly Gram-positive or Gram-negative flora. For example, *vancomycin rinses*, which specifically inhibit the caries-producing Gram-positive bacteria, allowed the development of as much Gram-negative plaque and gingival inflammation as did control water rinses after 22 days without oral hygiene, indicating the importance of Gram-negative types in periodontal disease. Currently, short-term *metronidazole* therapy, which has good activity against anaerobic bacteria, is used to treat acute, ulcerative gingivitis but the use of antibiotics should be limited to short-term therapy in carefully selected cases. The medically important antibiotics should be reserved for more serious infections. It must also be remembered that many of the antibiotics are bacteriostatic rather than bactericidal, i.e. they prevent growth but do not kill the bacteria. Therefore, they help to subdue the organisms but leave the host defences ultimately to overcome the infection. The danger is that if antibiotics and antiseptics are used indiscriminately the elimination of most of the normal commensal bacteria will allow other organisms such as the fungi to become dominant, often with pathological effects.

Selective inhibition of bacteria

Immunological protection

A dental vaccine?

Current evidence supports the idea that the initiation of caries is associated with specific acidogenic streptococci, and periodontal disease with the toxic products of anaerobic proteolytic organisms such as *Bacteroides* species and spirochaetes. In theory therefore it should be possible to control these diseases by long-term selective inhibition of the pathogenic bacteria rather than by the elimination of all plaque organisms.

The strain of streptococcus identified as *S. mutans*, so-called because of its varying morphology, has been shown to be more cariogenic than any other plaque isolate. In pure culture *S. mutans* is strongly acidogenic at pH values which are sufficiently low to inhibit other organisms and it is also capable of producing considerable amounts of insoluble extracellular glucan from sucrose.

The role of S. mutans *in the aetiology of dental caries*

Epidemiological studies in which comparisons were made of plaque samples from two human populations, one with a high and the other with a low caries incidence, often showed a relationship between the presence of *S. mutans* and the incidence of carious lesions.

In one study, 71% of carious fissures had *S. mutans* counts greater than 10% of total organisms whereas 70% of caries-free fissures had no detectable counts. Results were less convincing on smooth surfaces and a consistent feature of these studies was that a number of sites remained caries-free and yet had a high *S. mutans* count; in addition, a few caries-active sites were always found in which the organism was not detected. It was not clear which came first, the carious lesion which was subsequently invaded by the bacterium or the bacterium which then caused the lesion. The results of longitudinal studies on individuals in which the microbiological composition of caries-free sites was assessed at regular intervals until a lesion appeared failed to show a clear relationship between the presence of *S. mutans*, or any other organism, and lesion initiation. Although domination of a site with *S. mutans* sometimes occurred before initiation, more often a rise in *S. mutans* took place after radiographic detection of caries. As in the other studies, in some cases high numbers of *S. mutans* were present without subsequent lesion development and in other cases lesions occurred in the absence of the organism. Progression of the lesion through the enamel was associated with an increase in both *S. mutans* and lactobacilli and it was concluded that 'no single species appears to be uniquely associated with the onset of caries'.

It is probable that caries initiation is the result of a combined attack by all the acid-forming plaque organisms but there is no doubt that *S. mutans* is one of the more virulent bacteria in this respect. A simple microbiological technique which relies on changes in a pH indicator to measure plaque bacterial acidogenicity showed that individuals with active or recent lesions had a high ratio of acid-forming to total organisms, whereas individuals who were either caries-free or had no recent fillings had a lower ratio although the total organism count was similar (Table 36.2). The ratio remained constant from day to day in any individual but was increased by frequent exposure to sugar. As well as contributing to the overall acidogenicity the colonization of an early lesion by *S. mutans* may interfere with subsequent remineralization by helping to maintain an unfavourably low pH. Consequently, the specific elimination of *S. mutans* by vaccination might help to prevent the development rather than the initiation of the disease.

Natural immunity to S. mutans

Evidence for a degree of natural immunity to caries has been observed in some patients. A group of subjects with low caries experience maintained a persistently higher serum antibody titre to *S. mutans* than a high caries experience group which had no active lesions. The development of open carious lesions in a third group of patients seemed to be associated with a transient increase in *S. mutans* serum antibodies, but this failed to be maintained once the lesions had been filled. This suggests that immunity can be acquired but does not normally persist unless the organism is present in high numbers in open lesions. Consequently, while there is no doubt that the presence of *S. mutans* can induce a systemic immune response with the production of *S. mutans*-specific IgG molecules, this seems to be ineffective in the majority of individuals since the antibodies do not prevent the development of new lesions nor do they persist after the lesions have been filled. However, this may not be true for the small number of fortunate individuals who are relatively caries resistant due to their natural immunity.

Normally the systemic immune system is activated by the entry of antigen into the capillaries or lymphoid tissue, and its transport to the lymph nodes where activation of the humoral (B-lymphocytes, IgA, IgM, IgG) and cellular (T-lymphocytes, macrophages, polymorphonuclear leucocytes) components, takes place to produce the full immune response. In the mouth, bacteria or bacterial cell wall components can cross the mucous membranes, particularly in the gingival crevice region, and so enter the lymphatics or be transported there by phagocytes to induce an immune response. B-lymphocytes will proliferate and become plasma cells and secrete antibodies, while the T-lymphocytes become transformed into lymphoblasts and secrete *lymphokines*. These are soluble chemotactic factors which act largely through the macrophages to establish cell-mediated immunity.

Anti-(*S. mutans*) serum antibodies (IgG, IgM) and sensitized lymphocytes have been found in the peripheral blood of humans and it is now known from radioactive-labelling experiments that these molecules can pass via the gingival crevice into the oral fluids. To date, IgG, IgA and IgM, phagocytic monocytes, polymorphonuclear leucocytes, macrophages, complement (C3), blast cells and T- and B-lymphocytes have all been detected in crevicular fluid so that the immunoprotective components necessary for bacterial opsonization and phagocytosis are concentrated into this area.

Estimates from measured rates of crevicular fluid flow suggest that the total available volume from all crevices is between 0·5 and 2·0 ml per day, the flow rate increasing with the degree of gingivitis. The immunoprotective components present in such small volumes will be diluted rapidly by saliva to ineffective concentrations, but a local 'gingival domain' has been proposed in which a degree of naturally acquired protection can be expected. This almost certainly plays a role in protection against periodontal pathogens and, if sufficiently high antibody concentrations to *S. mutans* could be achieved in this area, a degree of caries protection might be possible at the gingival margins and interproximal areas, but it seems unlikely that this process would affect occlusal fissure caries. An alternative mechanism of protection by salivary-secreted IgA has largely been discounted.

Vaccination experiments

Attempts to boost this uncertain degree of natural immunity by vaccination against *S. mutans* were unsuccessful when carried out in rats. However, later experiments on monkeys injected subcutaneously with formalin- or heat-killed *S. mutans* cells showed a marked degree of protection against smooth surface caries which was associated with the appearance of anti-(*S. mutans*) IgG molecules in their crevicular fluid. These are thought to promote the phago-cytosis of *S. mutans* by polymorphonuclear leucocytes which emigrate from the gingival crevice. Perhaps surprisingly, however, the total number of *S. mutans* was not reduced to any significant extent. This may have been because *S. mutans* and other oral streptococci can mutate to give antigenic variations which are able to survive antibody attack and may also be less cariogenic than the original wild-type strains, so that the proportion rather than the total number of cariogenic organisms is reduced. These early experiments were unsatisfactory since the crude *S. mutans* preparations also contained antigen that cross-reacted with heart tissue, with the consequent risk of infective endocarditis. Moreover, they required simultaneous adjuvant injections to stimulate general antibody production and organisms other than *S. mutans* may have been affected. More recently, however, specific antigens have been isolated from the cell walls of *S. mutans* which are claimed not to cross-react with human tissue and should be safe for human trials. Results of these experiments are awaited with interest but it must be emphasized that there is considerable disagreement as to how the protective effect operates and many people doubt whether, even if it is possible to eliminate *S. mutans* completely, this will have any useful effect on human caries. Other antigenically dissimilar acidogenic organisms might well take over the ecological niche vacated by *S. mutans* so that, in the long term, there would be little or no overall change in the total acidogenic community of the plaque. Only a human clinical trial will resolve this problem and it has been pointed out that 'a vaccine against caries is a vaccine against a life-style* rather than a disease'. Many researchers question the social and moral desirability of vaccination against an avoidable disease, arguing that vaccination should be reserved for diseases which have such serious consequences that acceptance of possible damage from the vaccine itself is entirely justified.

Selective inhibition by fluoride

The phosphotransferase (PTS) system for the active transport of sugars which is found in many bacterial membranes is the rate-limiting step in energy production by streptococci growing at low extracellular sugar concentrations. The system is highly specific, has a high affinity for sugars and catalyses the group translocation of phosphate from phosphoenolpyruvate (PEP) to the sugar as it is transported into the cell:

$$\text{Sugar}_{out} + \text{PEP} \rightarrow \text{sugar phosphate}_{in} + \text{pyruvate}$$

The phosphorylated sugar is used as a substrate for glycolysis to generate two moles of PEP, one of which is used to phosphorylate a further sugar molecule and the other to produce ATP (Figure 36.3).

* i.e. inadequate dental hygiene and inappropriate diet.

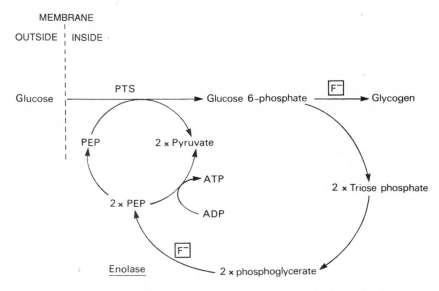

Figure 36.3 The active transport and metabolism of sugars by bacteria. PTS, membrane-associated phosphotransferase sugar-transport system; PEP, phosphoenolpyruvate; F⁻, sites of fluoride inhibition

The glycolytic enzyme *enolase* is inhibited by fluoride ions, which are rapidly taken into the cell in a lipid-soluble protonated form when the external pH is lower than the internal pH:

$$H^+ + F^- \;\rightleftharpoons\; HF \;\rightleftharpoons\; HF \;\rightleftharpoons\; F^- + H^+ \quad (pK \text{ of HF} = 3{\cdot}4)$$

Membrane

In entering, fluoride acts as a proton conductor, dissipating the transmembrane pH gradient and lowering the internal pH of the cell. Under these conditions the high intracellular fluoride ion concentration will inhibit sugar transport and ATP synthesis by a direct action on enolase and indirectly by internal acidification and inhibition of those glycolytic enzymes, particularly phosphofructokinase, which are inactivated by a reduction of the intracellular pH. The cell attempts to maintain the pH of the cytoplasm by extruding protons using a membrane-bound ATPase and this aggravates its already energy-depleted state and will eventually lead to the death of the cell.

Fluoride ions also inhibit a number of other magnesium-dependent enzymes including phosphoglucomutase, kinases and most phosphatases. Inhibition is rapid but reversible if the ion is removed and it is thought to result from the formation of an insoluble magnesium–phosphate–fluoride complex.

Plaque fluoride concentrations are very high when compared with salivary concentrations (page 499) and the ability of plaque to concentrate fluoride seems to be related to the formation of insoluble complexes so that not all of the fluoride is in ionic form. Even so, the ionic concentrations are still sufficient to modify the plaque bacterial composition and it is interesting to note that many of the less acidogenic plaque bacteria, for example *Actinomyces*, *Veillonella* and some streptococci, are able to tolerate higher fluoride ion concentrations than *S. mutans*. This property may help them to compete with the more acidogenic types since the high fluoride concentration will prevent excessive acid production and allow the less acid-tolerant and less cariogenic flora to become established.

Selective inhibition by fatty acids

The high-affinity phosphotransferase system (PTS) responsible for sugar uptake by many bacteria becomes saturated at relatively low external sugar concentrations (cf hexokinase, page 330) but there is an alternative sugar transport system which was first discovered in a mutant strain of *S. mutans* with a defective phosphotransferase system. Unlike the normal PTS this lower-affinity system operates at acidic pH values and is inhibited by uncoupling agents (page 220) and ATPase inhibitors. This suggests that the maintenance of a transmembrane pH gradient, and therefore a protonmotive force (pmf) across the membrane, is essential for activity (Figure 36.4).

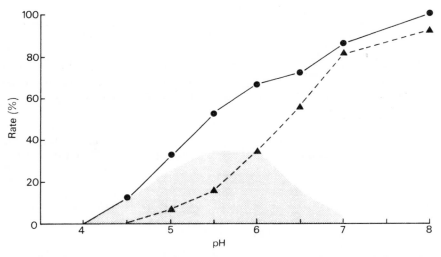

Figure 36.4 The effect of pH on the initial rates of acid production by *S. mutans*. Rates are expressed as a percentage of the maximum at pH 8·0. ●, measurements in the presence of 3·5 mM glucose; ▲, measurements with glucose plus the uncoupling agent CCCP (carbonyl cyanide *m*-chlorophenylhydrazone) (p*K* 6·0–6·5). The shaded area shows the difference between the two curves and represents the pH range over which the pmf is important

It is believed that the pmf helps to drive carrier-mediated sugar transport in symport (co-transport) with an inward flow of protons across the membrane. Consequently, a natural or imposed pH gradient, with the outside made acidic, leads to the internal accumulation of sugars (Figure 36.5). Protons are subsequently ejected in exchange for potassium ions by a mechanism that involves a membrane-bound ATPase. This sytem operates in the reverse direction to that found in mitochondria (page 221) since the energy of ATP hydrolysis is used to set up a pmf by ejecting protons. Since *S. mutans* appears to be slightly 'leaky' with respect to protons, glycolysis needs to be active at low extracellular pH values to provide for continuous proton ejection and the maintenance of the cytoplasm at a relatively alkaline pH.

Acidogenic plaque organisms are relatively resistant to the acid they produce and *S. mutans* has been found to retain 50% of its maximum acid-producing capacity at pH 5·0–5·5. The addition of an uncoupling agent (page 220) has a similar effect to fluoride in that it inhibits acid production below pH 6·0, suggesting that uncoupling agents might provide an effective means of inhibiting acid production by cariogenic organisms. While most uncoupling agents are toxic to

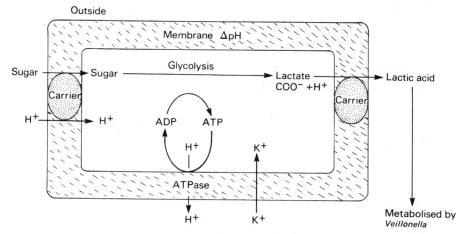

Figure 36.5 A proton gradient drives the active transport of sugars in some streptococci. The gradient is generated by the external accumulation of acids so that the external pH is lower than the cytoplasmic pH

mammalian cells, fatty acids, which are readily protonated ($pK \simeq 5\cdot0$) at the pH values seen in acidogenic plaques, are not. Protonation converts them into a neutral lipophilic form (HA) which dissociates on entering the cell thus shuttling protons across the membrane when the external pH is lower than the internal pH:

$$HA \xrightarrow{} HA$$

Outside H$^+$ $\quad$ $\quad$ H$^+$ inside

$$A^- \qquad\qquad A^-$$

Membrane

where A$^-$ = CH$_3$[CH$_2$]$_n$COO$^-$

The rate at which a fatty acid can recross the membrane depends on its concentration and mobility within the membrane. The latter is determined by the hydrophilic–hydrophobic properties of the molecule which depend on the chain length and pH. Fatty acids with a medium chain length of 9–12 carbons possess the best balance between water and lipid solubilities at pH 5·5, and produce maximum inhibition of plaque bacterial acid production.

The effect of mouth rinses containing potassium decanoate and glucose on the growth of acidogenic plaque bacteria is shown in Figure 36.6. The glucose acts as a bacterial substrate for the generation of a low plaque pH which facilitates fatty acid uptake. A negatively charged fatty acid such as decanoic is first retained within the plaque matrix by ionic interactions which probably involve Ca^{2+} and other divalent cations. If and when glucose is metabolized to acid, the fatty acid is converted into its lipid-soluble protonated form and is subsequently taken up by the cell to inhibit further acid production. Mouth rinses containing medium-chain fatty acids have the advantage that inhibition is directly related to acid production from the sugar and, unlike most antiseptic mouthwashes, produce preferential inhibition at potentially cariogenic sites. Areas of the plaque in which the pH does not fall remain unaffected. The use of a fatty acid–glucose rinse by caries-prone subjects for several days selectively reduced the proportions of *S. mutans* and other plaque acidogenic organisms to values associated with caries-inactive individuals without the unwanted suppression of the rest of the plaque flora.

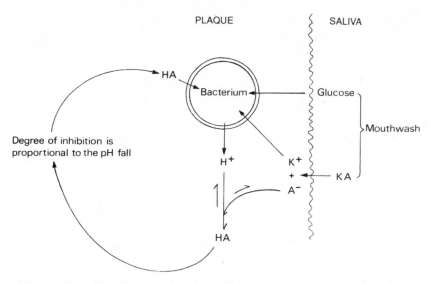

Figure 36.6 The inhibition of acidogenic plaque bacteria by a combination of glucose and the potassium salt of a medium chain fatty acid (KA)

These fatty acids have now been shown to inhibit caries in the rat. They are safe to use and compatible with fluoride and it is hoped that fatty acid–glucose mixtures, which also contain fluoride, applied in this way will become a useful aid in the long-term control of caries.

Concluding remarks

In conclusion it may be said that if all, or even some, of the suggestions given above were to be followed, the incidence of dental caries would almost certainly be significantly reduced if not entirely eradicated. Dental practitioners must, however, be resigned to the fact that, human nature being what it is, it is almost certain that a large number of people will continue to eat sugar-containing foods between meals, fail to maintain adequate oral hygiene and also fail to take fluoride tablets, use specially formulated mouthwashes or subject themselves to immunological protection for many years to come.

Suggestions for further reading

General

Rose, S. (1979) *The Chemistry of Life*, 2nd edn, Penguin Books, London.
Stryer, L. (1988) *Biochemistry*, 3rd edn, W. H. Freeman.
Lehninger, A. (1982) *Principles of Biochemistry*, Worth, New York.
Montgomery, R., Dryer, R.L., Conway, T.W. and Spector, A.A. (1983) *Biochemistry: A Case-Orientated Approach*, 4th edn, C.V. Mosby, St. Louis.
Morris, G. (1974) *A Biologist's Physical Chemistry*, 2nd edn, Edward Arnold, London.

Nutrition

Passmore, R. and Eastwood, M.A. (1986) *Human Nutrition and Dietetics*, 8th edn, Churchill-Livingstone, Edinburgh.
Waterlow, J.C. (ed.) (1981) *Nutrition of Man. British Medical Bulletin* **37**, No.1. Churchill-Livingstone, Edinburgh.
Manual of Nutrition, 8th edn (1985) Her Majesty's Stationery Office, London.
Paul, A.A and Southgate, D.A.T. (1978) McCance and Widdowson's *The Chemical Composition of Foods*, 4th edn, HMSO, London.

Molecular organization and interactions

Alberts, B., Bray, D., Lewis, J., Raff, M., Roberts, K. and Watson, J.D. (1983) *Molecular Biology of the Cell*, Garland, New York.
Chappell, J.B. (1977) *ATP*, Carolina Biology Readers, No. 52.
Chappell, J.B. (1979) *Energetics of Mitochondria*, Carolina Biology Readers.
Adams, R.L.P., Knowles, J.T. and Leader, D.P. (1986) *The Biochemistry of the Nucleic Acids*, 10th edn, Chapman and Hall, London.
Harris H. (1980) *Principles of Human Biochemical Genetics*, 3rd edn, Elsevier/North-Holland, Amsterdam.

Denton, R.M. and Pogson, C.I. (1976) *Metabolic Regulation. Outline Studies in Biology*, Chapman and Hall, London.

Oral biology

Jenkins, G.N. (1978) *The Physiology and Biochemistry of the Mouth*, 4th edn, Blackwell Scientific Publications, Oxford.

Williams, R.A.D. and Elliott, J.C. (1979) *Basic and Applied Dental Biochemistry*, Churchill-Livingstone, Edinburgh.

Glimcher, M.J. (1976) *Composition, Structure and Organization of Bone and Other Mineralized Tissues and the Mechanism of Calcification. Handbook of Physiology–Endocrinology*, VII, American Physiological Society.

Marsh P. and Martin, M. (1984) *Oral Microbiology*, Van Nostrand Reinhold, London.

Newbrun, E. (1983) *Cariology*, 2nd edn, Williams and Wilkins, Baltimore.

Silverstone, L.M. (1981) *Dental Caries: Aetiology, Pathology and Prevention*, Macmillan, New York.

Elliott, J.C. (1973) The problems of the composition and structure of the mineral components of the hard tissues. *Clinical Orthopaedics and Related Research*, **93**, 313.

Simpson, D.R. (1972) Problems of the composition and structure of bone minerals. *Clinical Orthopaedics and Related Research*, **86**, 260.

Index